EMERGING AND RE-EMERGING INFECTIOUS DISEASES

Professor Azza Fahmy

ALLIED
HEALTH
PRESS

Emerging and Re-emerging Infectious Diseases

Author: **Professor Azza Fahmy**

Allied Health Press
4164 Lakeshore Road
Burlington ON L7L 1A4
Canada
www.alliedhealthpress.com
Email: orders@arclereducation.com

ISBN: 978-1-77956-795-6

ABOUT THE AUTHOR

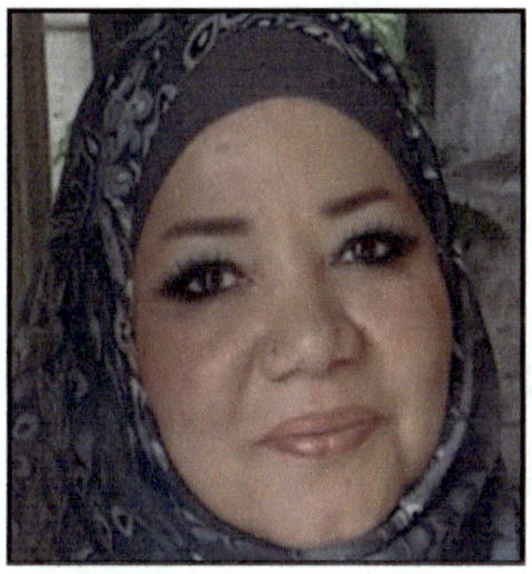

Professor Azza Fahmy is a distinguished Egyptian parasitologist and senior academic at the Theodore Bilharz Research Institute, with a PhD in Comparative Physiology and a distinguished record of contributions to parasitic disease research, diagnostics, and experimental therapy. Her work has significantly advanced both laboratory and clinical approaches to parasitic infections, with a focus on novel therapeutics, smart diagnostics, and host-pathogen interactions.

Professor Fahmy has authored numerous peer-reviewed publications covering a wide range of research themes, including:

- Experimental therapies for schistosomiasis, trichinellosis, cryptosporidiosis, toxoplasmosis, and giardiasis using agents such as GABA, Lepidium sativum, Albendazole, Mefloquine, and Commiphora molmol.
- Nanotechnology-based drug delivery systems in cancer therapy.
- The role of the microbiome in human health, and the immunomodulatory effects of parasitic antigens.
- Stem cell-based interventions for hepatic granuloma reversal in schistosomiasis models.
- Evaluations of plant-derived antiparasitic compounds (e.g., Cyperus rotundus, Syzygium aromaticum).
- Public health and policy-focused studies on antihypertensive medication adherence and its economic burden.
- Pioneering reviews on AI applications in healthcare, including the early diagnosis of diabetic foot ulcers and chronic disease prediction.

Her diagnostic innovations, such as antigen-based ELISAs, have improved the detection of various parasitic infections. She also engages in molecular diagnostics, immunopathology, and host-parasite interaction studies, enriching the field with both basic and translational insights.

An active reviewer for several leading parasitology and biomedical journals, Professor Fahmy contributes to maintaining rigorous academic standards across disciplines. She is committed to professional development and global collaboration, frequently presenting at international symposia and fostering research partnerships.

Brief Table of Contents

Detailed Table of Contents

CHAPTER 5

Global Health and Infectious Disease Surveillance 139

CHAPTER 6

Zoonotic and Vector-borne Diseases 173

CHAPTER 7

Antimicrobial Resistance (AMR) 207

CHAPTER 8

HIV/AIDS 243

CHAPTER 9

SARS, MERS, and COVID-19 281

CHAPTER 10

Ebola and Marburg Viruses 317

CHAPTER 11

Zika and Chikungunya 351

LIST OF FIGURES

PREFACE

Infectious diseases have had a profound impact on the course of human history, modulating demographic trends, economic development, and the progress of public health interventions. During the past century, advances in sanitation, immunization, and antimicrobial treatment have greatly diminished the prevalence of many infectious diseases. However, pathogens continue to evolve, and completely new infectious agents still arise. The term "emerging infectious diseases" refers to diseases that newly appear in a human population or those that, having occurred before, are undergoing a sudden increase in incidence or geographic spread. In contrast, "re-emerging infectious diseases" refer to diseases that previously were well controlled but have reappeared, often with enhanced resistance to presently available treatments or changed epidemiologic patterns. Causative factors for emergence and re-emergence are urbanization, deforestation, international travel, changes in agriculture, and climatic fluctuations. Microbial genetics and selective pressures—especially from antibiotic overuse—have accelerated the development of drug-resistant organisms, making it more challenging to implement measures to maintain global health security. Understanding these processes requires an integrative program incorporating microbiology, immunology, ecology, epidemiology, and health system administration. This book attempts to bridge the gap by presenting a complete review of the biological, environmental, and social determinants of emergence, persistence, and control of infectious threats worldwide.

In "Emerging and Re-emerging Infectious Diseases", a wide-ranging review of both fundamental principles and cutting-edge challenges in the science of communicable diseases is provided. The book begins with foundational material on definitions, historical progress, and fundamental concepts, further proceeds to discuss pathogen dynamics, host immunological responses, and measurement and monitoring of disease trends. Subsequent chapters assess global monitoring systems, the role of animal reservoirs and insect vectors, and the mounting threat of antimicrobial resistance (AMR). The latter part of the book comprises in-depth case studies of individual diseases—covering HIV/AIDS, re-emerging coronaviruses, hemorrhagic fevers, arboviral events, tuberculosis (TB), vaccine-preventable infections, and waterborne infections. Each chapter distills the latest research findings, recognizes the gaps in our knowledge, and suggests areas for policy development, research agendas, and practical application. Throughout the book, there is a clear focus on translating scientific outcomes into effective measures that can strengthen detection, prevention, and response efforts at the local, national, and international levels.

Chapter 1 provides a context for the magnitude and importance of infectious diseases, including prominent milestones from initial bacterium discoveries to the creation of modern surveillance systems. It defines essential terms, like incidence, prevalence, and patterns of transmission—and recounts hallmark outbreaks that rewrote public health practice.

Chapter 2 explains microbial pathogenesis and host interactions, which explain how bacteria, viruses, fungi, and parasites infect, evade immune defenses, and lead to clinical disease. Adherence mechanisms, invasion, toxin production, immune evasion, and tissue damage are discussed as well as an overview of innate and adaptive host responses.

Chapter 3 covers epidemiology, including study designs (case–control, cohort, cross-sectional) for epidemiologic investigations, measures of association (odds ratios, risk ratios), and statistical methods used in outbreak investigations. Surveillance, data collection, and principles of interpretation are highlighted as the backbone to disease control.

Chapter 4 explains the difference between newly emerging pathogens and re-emerging pathogens after a dip. It examines the drivers behind both trends—genetic mutation, ecological perturbation, human behavior, and health system vulnerabilities—and addresses criteria for classification and priority-setting in public health.

Chapter 5 addresses the environment of global health and infectious disease surveillance. It explains the architecture of global reporting systems, the coordination of laboratory and field data, applications of digital technology in real-time monitoring, and approaches aimed at early detection and rapid response. The chapter also points out obstacles like underreporting, data integrity, and unequal access to diagnostic centers.

Chapter 6 explores the domain of vector-borne and zoonotic diseases and explains how and why the pathogens are making the transition from animal reservoirs to humans. The life cycles of significant zoonotic diseases, the biological properties of vectors such as mosquitoes and ticks, and the environmental conditions that favor spillover events are discussed. Furthermore, control measures—wildlife management and integrated vector management—on sustainability and community participation are discussed.

Chapter 7 centers on AMR, following the molecular foundation of resistance mechanisms—enzyme manufacture, target alteration, efflux pumps—and surveying surveillance mechanisms that monitor resistant strains. The chapter assesses stewardship strategies, antibacterial development incentives, and alternative strategies like phage treatment and immunomodulation.

Chapter 8 tracks HIV/AIDS as a model for an emerging pandemic. It overviews the history of HIV discovery, viral and genetic character, transmission modes, pathophysiological mechanisms to immunodepletion, and evolution of antiretroviral therapy. In addition, it covers global trends in incidence, prevention measures (including pre-exposure prophylaxis), and continuing efforts toward a vaccine.

Chapter 9 shifts to severe acute respiratory syndrome (SARS), Middle East respiratory syndrome (MERS), and COVID-19. Each of their origins, zoonotic drivers, transmission patterns, clinical presentation, and public health responses are compared to emphasize lessons learned and gaps revealed by recent outbreaks.

Chapter 10 discusses Ebola and Marburg viruses, their filoviral morphology, high-mortality hemorrhagic presentations, and outbreak control logistics in the resource-poor environment. Therapy and vaccine advances are also discussed.

Chapter 11 discusses Zika and Chikungunya viruses, which are vector-borne by Aedes mosquitoes. In this chapter, vectors' ecology, congenital and neurological presentation of Zika, the Chikungunya chronic arthralgia, and vector control strategies in communities are discussed.

Chapter 12 discusses TB, including the distinctive cell wall of *Mycobacterium tuberculosis*, granuloma formation, diagnostic tests (e.g., GeneXpert), and the problem of drug-resistant TB. Public health approaches of case finding and directly observed therapy are outlined.

Chapter 13 discusses malaria and dengue fever, comparing Plasmodium life cycles and malaria vector control strategies with the serotype-dependent issues of dengue and the promise of vaccines.

Chapter 14 discusses measles and polio, two diseases targeted for eradication by vaccination. It connects the success stories of worldwide immunization campaigns, the issue of vaccine refusal and controversy, and the maintenance of herd immunity.

Chapter 15 also looks at cholera and typhoid fever, waterborne diseases that remain prevalent in much of the low-resource world. Chapter 15 discusses the transmission of pathogens by fecal-contaminated water and food, clinical management options, and the role of sanitation infrastructure and vaccination in long-term prevention.

This book is designed for a broad audience of professionals and students whose work intersects with infectious disease control. Graduate and advanced undergraduate students in public health, medicine, veterinary science, and microbiology will find foundational material alongside current case studies. Epidemiologists and field investigators can use the practical guidance on outbreak investigation and surveillance. Clinicians will benefit from concise reviews of pathogenesis, clinical features, and therapeutic advances. Policy-makers and program managers can draw on analyses of global health strategies and governance mechanisms. Laboratory scientists and researchers will appreciate the in-depth discussion of microbial mechanisms and resistance trends. Finally, educators may adopt individual chapters as teaching modules or reference points for curriculum development. Whether the reader seeks a comprehensive introduction or a targeted update, this book offers a resource that bridges theory and practice in a rapidly evolving field. It aims to support informed decision-making, encourage interdisciplinary collaboration, and strengthen capacity at every level—from local clinics to international agencies—to meet the continuing challenges posed by infectious diseases.

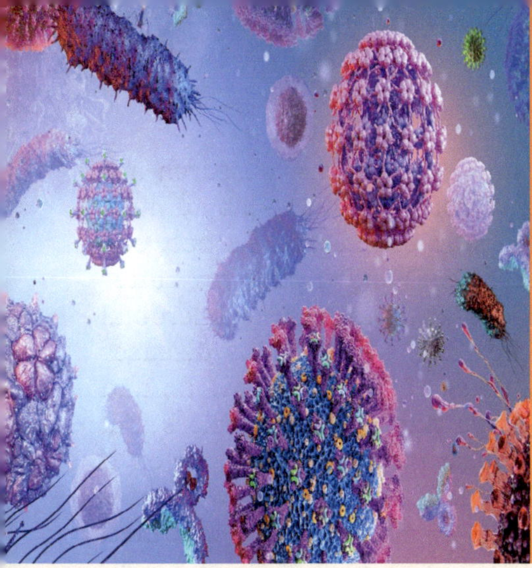

Chapter 1

INTRODUCTION TO INFECTIOUS DISEASES

Contents

Introduction

Microscopic life and our own health have always had a curious, tangled connection—one that's caught the eye of science for ages. There's several friendly and harmful microbes living with us, and sometimes, some of these bacteria, viruses, fungi, or parasites get the upper hand. They invade, multiply, and throw our bodies off balance, usually by moving from one person to another in direct or roundabout ways. In most cases, when these tiny bugs evolve and even get resistant to our immune defenses, they present a real headache for both doctors and public health teams (Murray et al., 2022). So, getting a grip on these infections means not only identifying the germ but also piecing together how it spreads and affects people worldwide. Infectious diseases aren't just about the microbes themselves—they cover a vast area of public health that touches on how microbes and people interact in often unpredictable ways. One nagging problem is antimicrobial resistance (AMR), which generally makes existing treatments less effective, leading to more disease and even deaths. Research has pointed out that resistant bacteria—think *Escherichia coli* or *Staphylococcus aureus*—play a huge role in infection-related fatalities (Murray et al., 2022). This tangled web of interactions between microbes, human bodies, and the environment calls for continuous monitoring, a push for better healthcare systems, and interventions that are tailored to local needs, combinationing microbial behavior with clinical and global impacts. In clinical pathology, the story of infectious diseases dives deep into the cellular and molecular realm that drives how these conditions show up and progress. Advances in molecular biology have opened the door to spotting genetic markers and specific traits in pathogens—details that now help shape more precise treatment plans, even if the good old histopathological exam still holds strong; sometimes the mix of old and new creates a bit of confusion. It's also clear that infections aren't always just a quick, acute issue; sometimes, the same microbes or the resulting inflammation stick around, blurring the lines between short-term sickness and chronic conditions. Recent studies, generally speaking, highlight a push-and-pull where genetic alterchanges in either the host or the microbe change the game entirely. Over time, combinationincorporating these molecular insights into routine pathology is proving critical for better diagnosis, treatment decisions, and prevention strategies in everyday clinical practice (Figure 1.1).

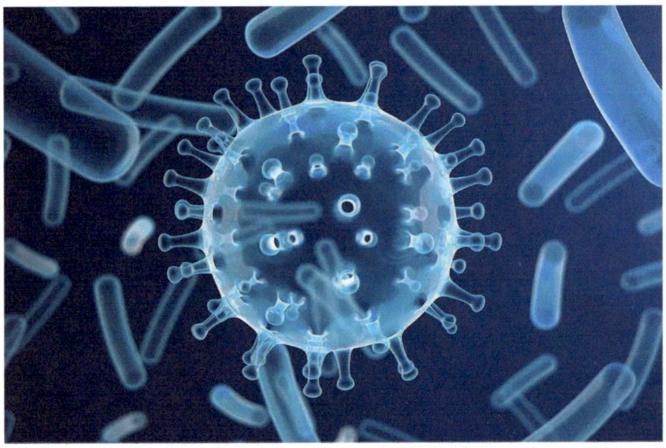

Figure 1.1. Infectious diseases.

Source: Sysmex Europe. (n.d.). *Infectious Disease Illustration.*

Explanation of Infectious Diseases

Disease spread over the ages shows how our everyday social ties mix with the movement of bacteria. People were on the move—trading, migrating, simply living—long before the term "globalization" even popped up, and in doing so, they carried little invaders with them. In many cases, infections weren't just random biological hiccups; they were part of the everyday hum of human life, a sort of constant background noise woven into history. Early outbreaks, in a way, hinted at the borderless nature of our modern world, where sickness can ignore maps and cultures alike. You really have to see that figuring out infections means looking at the complex web of human activity that still drives disease spread today (Dellana et al., 2014). Not everyone gets hit the same by these diseases. Wealth, where you live, access to good health care and education—all these social bits turn out to be big factors in how badly infections can affect someone. Life expectancy and sickness rates differ, sometimes striking starkly across countries and even within communities. Generally speaking, this shows that bacteria don't knock on every door with the same force; they take advantage of social inequalities. Fighting infections, then, isn't just about medicine—it's about mending the social cracks that leave some groups more exposed. In short, smart strategies to curb diseases always have to consider these deeper, often complex social roots (Marmot et al., 2005). Several tiny pathogens—bacteria, viruses, fungi, and parasites—are behind most infections by slipping into our bodies and manipulating with how everything works. The tricky part isn't only their biological characterestics but also how they team up with their hosts and the environments around us. Some of these microbes hit fast, sweeping through communities, while others stick around quietly in one spot or even hide out in people for long stretches. In most cases, new strains emerge while old ones make surprising comebacks, keeping public health workers on constant alert. To really get what infections are all about, you've got to reckon with the wild variety of these microscopic troublemakers and all the different ways they weave through both our bodies and our world.

Types of Infectious Agents

Infectious diseases hit you with several different troublemakers, and the first step is really getting to know what these agents are all about. It isn't just about memorizing names—viruses, bacteria, fungi, parasites, and even prions each come with their own characterestics. Viruses, for instance, are these almost ghost-like particles that need a host to do anything at all; they can trigger anything from that annoying cold to more severe, brain-related issues, where inflammasome activation is said to play a notable role in disease progression (Voet et al., 2019). Meanwhile, bacteria, being self-sufficient single-celled organisms, prompt our immune systems by revealing patterns our bodies have learned over time (commonly known as pathogen-associated molecular patterns, or PAMPs). All this variation means that figuring out which pathogen is at work isn't straightforward, and it keeps the challenge of diagnosis, treatment, and prevention on its toes. Detecting these infectious pathogens is, in most cases, crucial for managing outbreaks and keeping epidemiologists on their toes. Traditional methods that look at how cells behave can work, but they tend to be slow, laborious, and require a lot of specialized know-how—a situation that can sometimes be a real pain. Then came modern molecular diagnostics, especially techniques that amplify nucleic acids, which generally bump up both the speed and accuracy of finding pathogens. DNA microarray technology, for example, lets labs check for many different infectious agents at once—be they bacteria, viruses, or fungi. There are different platforms too, like those based on oligonucleotides or PCR products, that allow for a high-throughput romp through genetic material, making it easier to sort out infections, spot drug resistance, and even track how an epidemic spreads. Ultimately, these advances have shortened lab time while boosting the specificity and sensitivity of identifying the troublemakers, leading to more targeted treatments. Then you have prions, which really stand out because they're just misbehaving proteins with no nucleic acids at all. Rather than carrying instructions like other bacteria, prions spread by coaxing normal proteins into folding the wrong way, which can result in harmful clumps and lead to diseases such as Creutzfeldt–Jakob disease. Lately, researchers have been noticing how these abnormal protein folds correlate with neurodegenerative problems, especially since inflammasomes—those tiny intracellular complexes—seem to sense these misfolded proteins and trigger inflammatory responses (Voet et al., 2019). When inflammasomes go off, they release pro-inflammatory cytokines that add insult to injury, causing more neuroinflammation and damage. This mix-up between infectious agents and neurodegenerative processes shows just how complex the world of pathogens can be, influencing not only our approach to direct infections but also opening up questions in immunology and neurobiology.

Importance of Understanding Infectious Diseases

Humans, animals, and nature mix in ways that make it really important to get what's happening with infections – sometimes the way they interact just makes it easier for bacteria to move around. Wild organisms like boars naturally keep viruses, bacteria, and parasites around; these bacteria can sometimes jump to people, stirring up problems for both animal care and public health. We still don't have the full scoop in many areas – details like how pathogens spread, where they show up, and which animal movements matter aren't completely clear, so researchers from different fields need to team up to fill in those gaps. New diagnostic gadgets and broad monitoring efforts are starting to help catch problems early, which is generally speaking a big plus. Figuring out these details is crucial for building strong biosecurity steps that protect both animals and us, and can stop outbreaks before they spin out of control (Nissanova et al., 2025). Take schools, for example – these places show just how quickly bacteria can move in crowded settings. When people are crammed together in classrooms and hallways, even a little lapse in keeping things clean can let infections take off. Learning how tiny agents work and why a clean environment matters builds a solid base for stopping diseases early on. Community programs that teach these ideas often manage to boost understanding and encourage actions like regular handwashing and mask-wearing; these small changes add up to lower infection rates. Such efforts help individuals feel better while also easing the overall strain on public health, especially in spots where risks are higher (Fahdi & Sari, 2024). Grasping how infectious diseases work lets public health teams target their efforts better to cut down on outbreak impacts and improve overall wellbeing. Knowing how bacteria evolve, jump from one host to another, and sometimes build up resistance, helps steer vaccine creation, shape treatment plans, and inform policy moves. At the same time, taking into account things like economic pressures and environmental characterestics nudges us toward control strategies that fit the situation at hand. Without these insights though, our fight against infections might miss the mark entirely, leading to longer bouts of disease and extra economic headaches. It ends up being a group effort – microbiologists, epidemiologists, doctors, and policymakers all need to hash out ideas together, even if sometimes the interaction isn't perfectly clear, to turn theory into real-world fixes. In the end, keeping awareness of these diseases both deep and practical is a must if we want to ease their toll on society and beef up global health security (Figure 1.2).

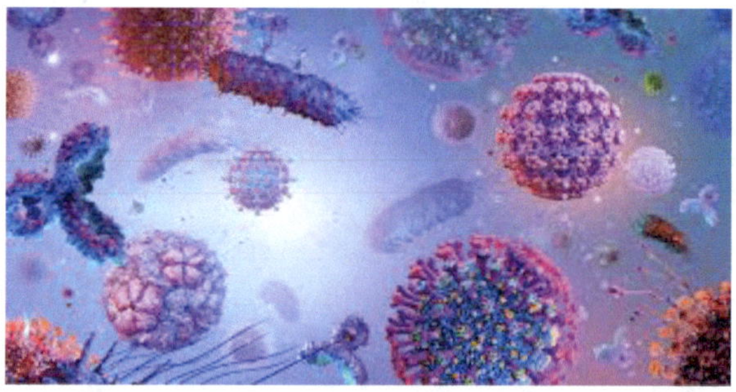

Figure 1.2. The importance of understanding infectious diseases.

Source: Genomics Education Programme. (2023). *Illustration of DNA Double Helix Structure.*

1.1. History of Infectious Diseases

In human history, diseases have played a wild hand in reshaping societies—alteraltering population shifts, economic paths, and even how medicine gets better over time. Ancient groups fought off brutal epidemics while hardly knowing what sparked them or how diseases spread; it was all very mysterious. Then, around the 19th century, germ theory emerged, letting scientists finally point to the microbes behind the sickness and figure out their roles. That newfound insight was the spark for life-saving tools like vaccines and antibiotics, which, in most cases, helped cut down disease and death rates dramatically. Still, things aren't ever straightforward; bacteria learn to dodge our drugs, and this emerging resistance keeps global health in a tough spot. Recent deep studies even show that resistant bacteria are behind millions of deaths ,a sobering reminder that continuous research and solid healthcare systems are key (Murray et al., 2022).

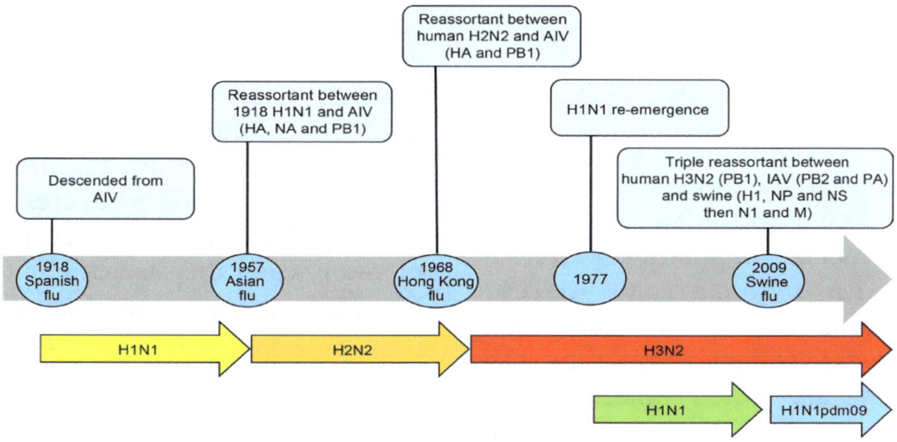

Figure 1.3. Pandemics and their impact.

Source: Frontiers in Microbiology. (2020). *The Evolutionary Origins of Influenza Viruses: A Historical Perspective.* Frontiers in Microbiology, 11, 631736.

Technology and robust public health moves have danced closely with breakthroughs in science when fighting infectious threats. Vaccines, for instance, have become a top defense—blunting the impact and spread of diseases. The worldwide reaction to SARS-CoV-2 shows how studying vaccine performance and its ripple effects across communities can help steer efforts during outbreaks. One set of models suggests that if a vaccine works at about 70% against infection, it might just cut off COVID-19's spread, though less effective shots need backup measures like lower contact rates or a bit of natural immunity in the crowd (Makhoul et al., 2020). This way of tackling threats fits a longer history in which knowing what makes a germ tick or how it passes along guides us in fine-tuning responses as both pathogens and our defenses evolve. Even with these gains, history reminds us—often quite bluntly—that infectious diseases remain stubborn foes, especially in places where resources for surveillance and treatment are limited. Regions with less robust healthcare often end up with a heavier load of drug-resistant infections, which only deepens the struggle (Murray et al., 2022). And, truth be told, pathogens are always alteraltering through mutations and picking up resistance, which can catch our current treatments off guard. This flip side of medical progress means we need to boost lab abilities, gather better global data, and keep the wheel turning on new vaccines and antibiotics. Each breakthrough seems to open the door to fresh challenges, and that ever-present tug-of-war calls for constant vigilance and sometimes a bit of creative alteraltering in public health strategies. Ultimately, the ongoing saga of infections is a complex combination of human ingenuity and microbial change, continuously shaping how we understand and respond to health threats over time (Figure 1.3).

1.1.1. Major Pandemics and Their Impact

Pandemics have, throughout history, left indelible marks on our world. Such outbreaks have tended to remake population patterns, overwhelm health systems, and disrupt economies and communities. At other times, the spilling of disease is connected to the way we live around animals—when climate change, urban development, or intensive agriculture bring people closer to animals, new diseases come into human populations. In a chaotic mix of factors, such spillovers—where animal infections enter into our daily lives—give public health a head-scratching headache. Wrapping our heads around the complicated relationship is essential; a combination of public health mobilization and community mobilization can be rather crucial in preventing subsequent outbreaks (Djoko et al., 2010). And if you examine carefully, pandemics appear to have their beginnings rooted deep in our ecology as well as social structure. Examples such as HIV/AIDS, SARS, and several influenza pandemics remind us that animal pathogens have the power to unleash global health emergencies. Behavioral changes, habitat destruction, and our increasingly linked world appear to accelerate the spread of such diseases. Despite modern smart science and cutting-edge technology, these outbreaks continue to emerge suddenly, too often evading early detection. This type of unpredictability arises from the complex interplay between hosts, pathogens, and pressures in the environment—factors that, quite frankly, are only imperfectly known. In general, addressing these challenges requires many strategies: mathematical modeling, enhanced diagnostic methods, and careful monitoring of where humans and animals come into close contact with one another (Carroll et al., 2012). The tentacles of these pandemics reach far beyond short-term health impacts. They contort economic systems, redefine social mores, and compel policymakers across the globe to re-evaluate priorities. In the past, the enormous burden of pandemics has prompted governments to restore public health infrastructure and strengthen response measures. However, there is not yet a firm, integrated global system to monitor when the diseases shift from animals to humans, and often this causes delays in essential interventions. In most instances, promoting small behavioral changes and more open communication can assist communities in handling emerging infections better. In the future, it appears essential that ongoing initiatives combine integrated surveillance with educational programs to identify early warning signals and reduce the broader economic and social impacts of pandemics (Djoko et al., 2010).

1.1.2. Historical Advancements in Medicine

Throughout history, many struggles have oddly helped shape our approach to fighting infectious diseases. Wars, for instance, weren't just brutal conflicts—they often made things worse by creating crowded conditions, malnutrition, and poor healthcare, which in turn sped up infections. Yet, in many cases, these tough times also nudged scientists toward new, sometimes unexpected ways to handle disease. Think about how tuberculosis (TB) wreaked havoc during

World War I and II; that crisis underscored a desperate need for better tests and treatments. This push led the research community to try out more effective methods for controlling infections. In a way, those chaotic moments and the responses that followed highlight just how adaptable our strategies for managing disease have become over time (Egli et al., 2024). Back in the late 1800s and early 1900s, shifts in clinical methods began to reshape medical research and treatment in pretty significant ways. Clinicians like Achille de Giovanni were busy trying to connect how our bodies work with how diseases develop, relying on careful measurements and a close eye on observations.

His work—often called clinical anthropometry—was all about understanding why people differ, using detailed looks at body shapes to tease apart normal functions from things going wrong. Even though his ideas eventually lost some of that appeal, they still mark one of the first real attempts at personalizing medicine. Generally speaking, this period set the stage for moving from one-size-fits-all approaches to strategies that take individual differences into account when battling infections (Zampieri et al., 2018). A major turning point came when scientists finally pinpointed bacteria as the real pathogens behind many diseases. Recognizing specific microbes, like *Mycobacterium tuberculosis*, gave a fresh, clear direction to how we tackled these health issues. Then came vaccines and antibiotics, which changed public health dramatically—they provided practical tools for preventing and treating diseases that once seemed untreatable. These breakthroughs didn't come out of nowhere but were built up over many years of trial, error, and observation. Still, it's worth noting that the battle continues, as drug-resistant strains now require ongoing international cooperation and inventive public health strategies to keep up the momentum (Egli et al., 2024).

1.1.3. Evolution of Public Health Responses

Public health has always been on some sort of ongoing path—constantly changing as diseases and our knowledge about them change. In the old days, people primarily relied on simple sanitation and straightforward quarantine strategies because, simply put, they saw how diseases spread within communities. As time went by, and in most instances, as our understanding of bacteria and transmission grew, these general steps were replaced by more specific strategies. Vaccination campaigns and the judicious application of antibiotics began to appear rather than the deployment of one-size-fits-all treatments. This slow-burn transformation comes from mixing traditional epidemiology with dives into molecular biology and a hefty dose of data analysis; essentially, we're now able to pinpoint disease carriers and patterns much more precisely—even though new challenges with managing data in real-time have cropped up, pushing public health to innovate new systems (Lewnard & Reingold, 2019). Today, infectious disease control is almost a collaborative sport that cuts across disciplines. Digital monitoring, genetic sequencing, and, yes, predictive modeling have flipped the game on its head and enabled us to predict outbreaks before they get out of hand. terms, this implies that epidemiological techniques, which previously concentrated on chronic disease, are now compelled to retool for the quick dynamics of infections—considering how diseases are transmitted and how individuals vary. Public health interventions have become more anticipatory than merely reactive, using vaccines and treatments in manners intended not only to contain outbreaks but to prevent them altogether. This is a nuanced but actual change towards precision public health, wherein ongoing innovation becomes central to deterring emerging as well as recidivous threats (Lewnard & Reingold, 2019). But shadowing these new innovations are obstacles that stubbornly persist. Despite having molecular diagnostics that rapidly detect pathogens, the infrastructure necessary to deliver aid to multiethnic populations typically remains behind. It is still challenging, for instance, to pinpoint a unique cause when clinical syndromes may arise from several microbes—a scenario further obscured by the intricate interplay of the human microbiome. The balance between the promise of scientific advances and ground-level realities requires not just good technology but also firm socio-political resolve and authentic community participation. For the most part, the public health future will hinge on integrating these new scientific findings into comprehensive, inclusive policies that address both biological and social drivers of infectious disease (Lewnard & Reingold, 2019) (Figure 1.4).

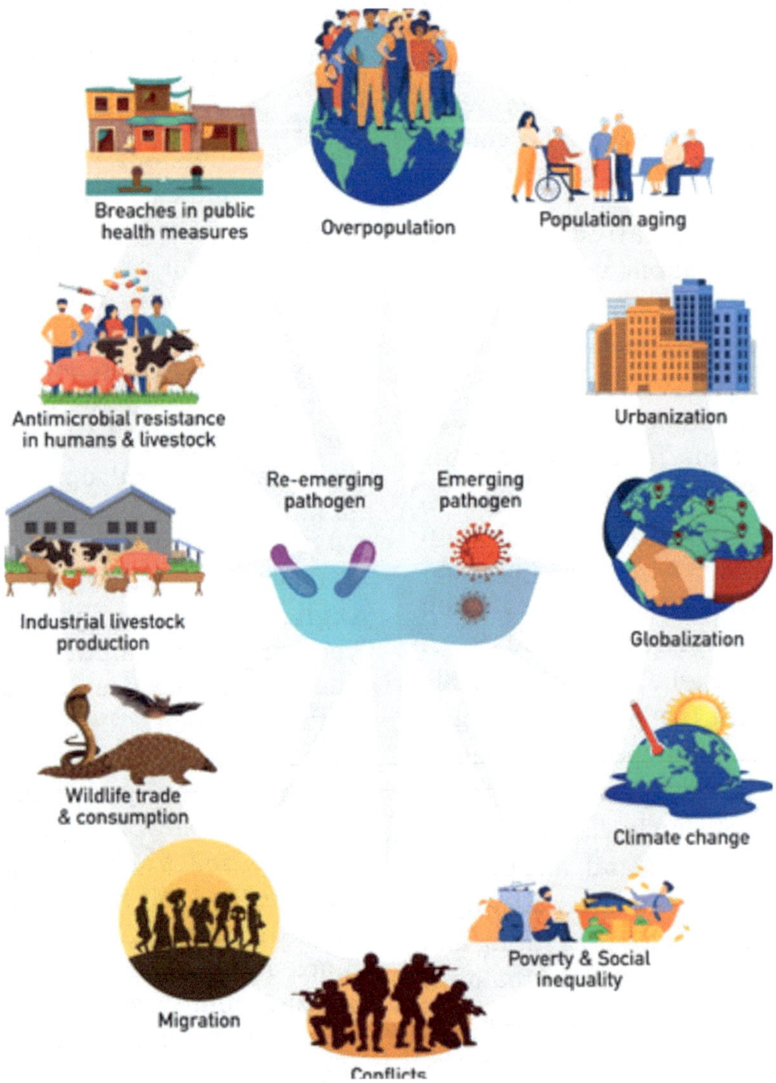

Figure 1.4. Public health responses in infectious diseases.

Source: Spernovasilis N, Tsiodras S, Poulakou G. Emerging and Re-Emerging Infectious Diseases: Humankind's Companions and Competitors. *Microorganisms*. 2022; 10(1):98. https://doi.org/10.3390/microorganisms10010098

1.2. Transmission of Infectious Diseases

Understanding how diseases spread isn't a straightforward matter. There's several factors at play—everyday human actions, shifts in our surroundings, and even our global travel habits all influence the journey of pathogens among us. The COVID-19 outbreak, for example, showed that measures like lockdowns, keeping our distance, and mask requirements not only slowed the virus itself but also altered the transmission of other infections. In the early days of the pandemic, reports of diseases fell dramatically—by as much as 86.73% across several transmission routes. Respiratory droplets, insect vectors, and even infections linked to food were especially affected. These facts generally underscore how our day-to-day actions are woven into disease dynamics, hinting that tackling one threat might unintentionally change the behavior of others (Spaziante et al., 2025). Recognizing these intricacies is crucial for creating public health strategies that are both flexible and effective. People's reactions to the threat of infection play a major role in stopping diseases from spreading. How well individuals stick to practices like handwashing, proper cough etiquette, and keeping physical distance can influence transmission rates. Research has shown, in most cases, that having solid ways to measure these behaviors is key to encouraging healthy practices. One tool that fits the bill is the Emerging Infectious Diseases Preventive Health Behavior (EID-PHB) Scale. Developed through careful analysis and expert feedback, it sorts preventive actions into six areas—covering droplet, contact, airborne, bloodborne, environmental safety, and even how people cope psychologically. This all-around approach captures prevention in its many forms, helping to guide targeted measures and behavioral studies. Its impressive statistics—a Cronbach's alpha of 0.92 and strong criterion validity—support its use in clinical settings, educational environments, and public policy work aimed at reducing disease spread (Lee et al., 2024). The ways bacteria make their way from one host to another are varied and depend a lot on the situation, so digging into these details is essential for effective control. Pathogens can travel through direct contact, by riding droplets, via airborne particles, be ferried by vectors, or even hitch a ride in contaminated food and water—each path posing its own challenges. Notably, the COVID-19 crisis didn't just affect the spread of its own virus; it also scrambled the usual routes for other diseases. In the recovery phase, infection rates didn't bounce back uniformly.

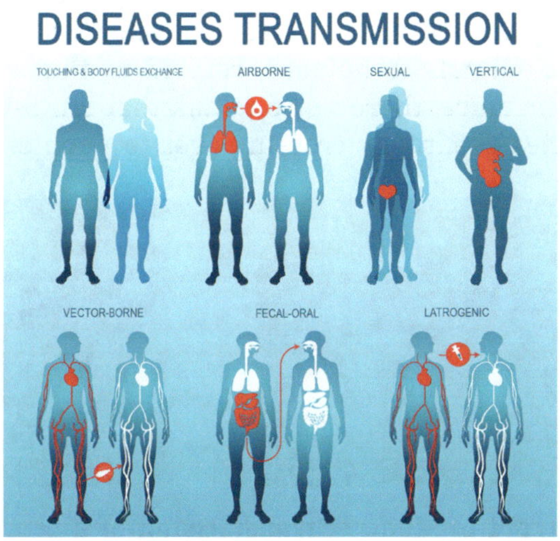

Figure 1.5. Transmission of infectious diseases.

Source: Dreamstime. (n.d.). *Disease Transmission: Infectious Disease Transmission Landscape Poster – Virus Pandemic Transfer via Different Types.*

For example, sexually transmitted and bloodborne diseases even went up, perhaps reflecting shifts in behavior and some hiccups in healthcare access. These shifting patterns signal that bouncing back from a pandemic isn't simply a matter of returning to old norms—it involves a complex transition between different disease scenarios (Spaziante et al., 2025). All things considered, keeping a constant watch and staying agile in our public health responses is essential to managing the ever-evolving ways diseases travel (Figure 1.5).

1.2.1. Modes of Transmission

Pathogens move between hosts in ways that really shape how outbreaks play out and how our control measures work—even if it isn't always obvious. Direct contact, meaning a simple touch or the exchange of bodily fluids, can start the chain, but microbes also manage to hitch a ride on everyday objects (fomites, as some call them) that end up as unintentional messengers. A cough or sneeze sends out respiratory droplets that, in crowded spots, push infections along at a surprising clip. Then there's airborne spread with those ultra-tiny particles that drift further and stir up extra challenges, as seen in diseases like TB. In most cases, grasping these different transfer methods lets health officials design counter steps such as social distancing, frequent handwashing, and surface cleaning—a lesson brought home by COVID-19. SARS-CoV-2, after all, sped its spread through droplets (and perhaps aerosols too) so rapidly that urgent global measures became necessary (Shereen et al., 2020). Sometimes, though, the process is even more layered than it first seems. Infection pathways can include an intermediary host or a vector, which makes the spread trickier and control efforts more muddled. Zoonotic diseases, where pathogens jump from animals to humans, remind us that environmental and ecological factors are also at work. For instance, there's strong talk that SARS-CoV-2 began in bats, with an unidentified intermediary species eventually crossing over to people.

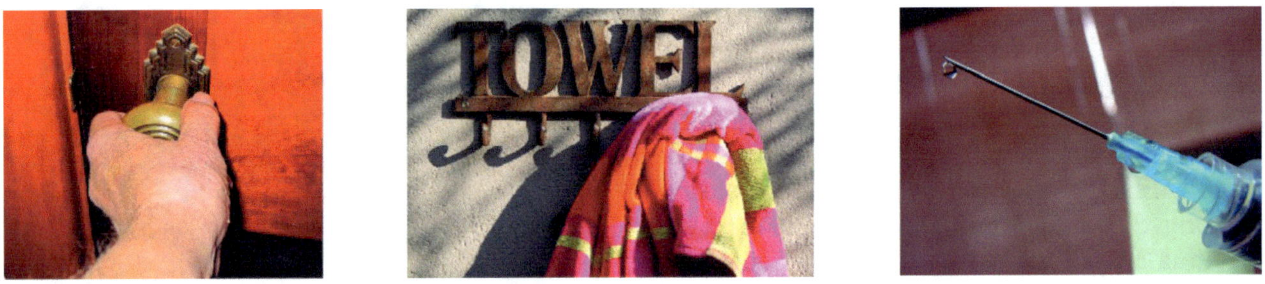

Figure 1.6. Mode of transmission of diseases.

Source: https://courses.lumenlearning.com/suny-microbiology/chapter/modes-of-disease-transmission/

These spillover events emphasize the need to monitor wildlife and even reconsider our interactions with animals that might harbor infectious agents. Further there are vector-borne diseases—mosquitoes or ticks, for example, that ferry bacteria along a different route. All this variety shows why our containment strategies must be as diverse and adaptable as the ways infections move; past experiences with SARS and MERS have generally pushed researchers and policymakers to better predict risks and prepare for future hazards (Shereen et al., 2020). Human behavior and society's layout also have a huge say in how infections spread. Think about the close settings we live in—households, healthcare centers, public transport—where bacteria can move more easily if prevention isn't taken seriously. It doesn't help that some people show few or no symptoms at first, making them unwitting spreaders and complicating efforts to track down cases. The recent COVID-19 pandemic was a clear reminder of just how fast a new pathogen can circle the globe when movement and contact aren't properly managed. That's why responses so often lean on quick case detection, diligent contact tracing, isolating cases, and ramping up vaccinations to break the transmission chain. Overall, assessing risks and rolling out evidence-based measures have been critical steps, with lessons drawn directly from earlier coronavirus outbreaks guiding today's public health strategies (Figure 1.6).

1.2.2. Factors Influencing Transmission

Infectious diseases don't just jump around randomly—they tend to spread through several biological characterestics and everyday environmental factors. Pathogens, for instance, use specific tricks to move from one host to another, and in most cases, getting a handle on these tricks is key to nipping outbreaks in the bud. You might see this in physical transmission, which happens through direct contact, airborne particles drifting in the air, or even microbes that act as little carriers; each of these paths shifts when factors like how long the germ can last outside a body or the surrounding conditions come into play. Human actions add another layer—overcrowded spaces or frequent travel can boost exposure risk. And sometimes, muddled ideas about disease spread only make things worse, because if people believe wrong things, they might not take the proper precautions.

A look at seafarers on cruise ships shows that even though overall knowledge may be decent, risky behaviors and biased attitudes still creep in and push the disease along (Siame et al., 2025). All of this points to the need for tackling not just the science but also the social habits behind disease spread. Socioeconomic factors also have a big say in how infections move among communities. Generally speaking, having solid access to healthcare, education, and sanitation doesn't just lower an individual's risk—it also helps keep outbreaks from growing out of control in neighborhoods. It turns out that lower education levels often mean folks are less aware of how diseases spread or what they can do to prevent them, which may leave them more vulnerable. Other aspects such as age, gender, and marital status join the mix, subtly shaping who might be exposed and how. For example, research at a major hospital in Kabul revealed that younger adults—especially males and those who are married—seem to have higher rates of hepatitis C infections, hinting at how social roles and personal behaviors intersect with the spread of diseases (Danish et al., 2025). In many cases, this suggests that public health strategies can't adopt a one-size-fits-all approach; rather, they must be tailored to meet the unique needs and risks of different groups by keeping social factors in mind. How people understand health, feel about disease, and act on that understanding all mingle together to shape the ways infections spread. When folks have solid health literacy, they tend to notice symptoms early and take precautions that can help stop the contagion. Still, persisting misunderstandings and stigma often get in the way of effective outbreak control. Educational campaigns—especially those that actively involve at-risk groups—can help bridge these gaps. For instance, participatory health literacy projects among seafarers have shown promise in sharpening understanding of transmission routes and encouraging safer practices (Siame et al., 2025). Such community-based initiatives often help steer people away from risky habits while chipping away at discriminatory views that might otherwise let infections run free. In the end, combining these educational efforts with practical improvements, like better screening and cleaner sanitary conditions—offers a well-rounded approach to curbing disease spread (Figure 1.7).

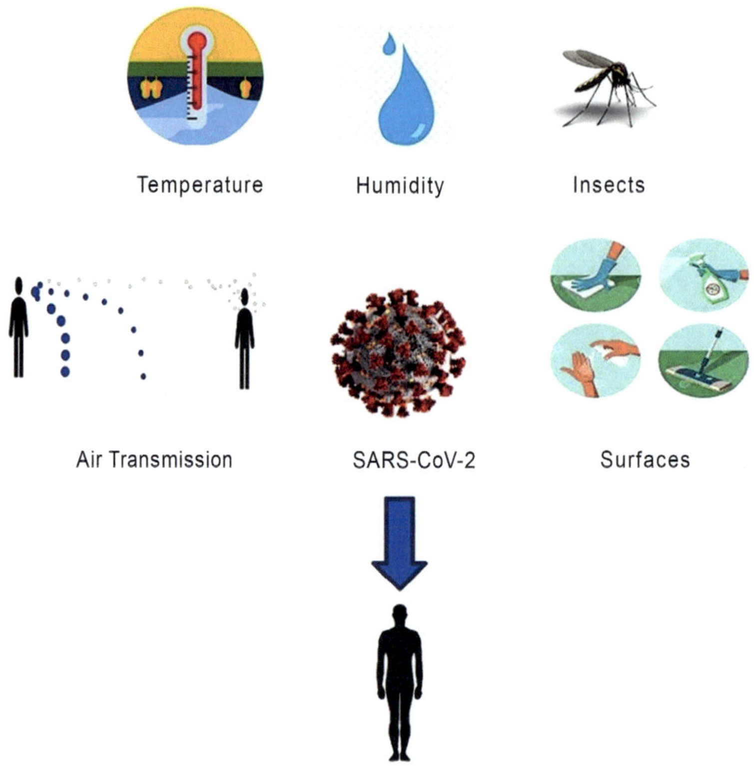

Figure 1.7. Factors influencing transmission for diseases.

Source: Valsamatzi-Panagiotou, A., & Penchovsky, R. (2022). Environmental factors influencing the transmission of the coronavirus 2019: a review. *Environmental Chemistry Letters,* 20(3), 1603–1610. https://doi.org/10.1007/s10311-022-01418-9.

1.2.3. Role of Vectors in Disease Spread

Infectious diseases don't just spread from person to person in a neat, orderly way. Sometimes, the process is a bit complex—various routes come into play, and those pesky carriers, like mosquitoes, ticks, and fleas, jump the gun by ferrying bacteria past natural limits that would otherwise hold them back. These tiny microbes, acting like biological shuttles, open doorways in unexpected spots, letting pathogens roam across diverse regions. It isn't only a matter of treating those who fall ill; you've got to worry about these vectors too, since their indirect role in transmission makes controlling outbreaks a tougher, more layered challenge. Generally speaking, grasping this indirect mode is key, as the mix of ecological and biological forces tends to complicate disease dynamics in real, unpredictable ways. Those same vectors really do star in the spread of heavy-hitting diseases like malaria, dengue fever, Lyme disease, and even plague. Their lifecycles—when they breed, where they feed—play a huge part in how efficiently these pathogens travel and where infections flare up. For instance, think about the Anopheles mosquitoes, which carry the Plasmodium parasites that cause malaria; their breeding spots and feeding routines drive regional and seasonal shifts in disease incidence. Most experts agree that an effective strategy has to be several environmental alterchanges, chemical treatments, and biological fixes—a patchwork approach often dubbed integrated vector management (Murray et al., 2022). In many cases, this all serves as a reminder that the way these microbes behave can really mess with our public health plans, creating unexpected hurdles along the way. Recent global health scares like COVID-19 remind us that while microbes are big players in some diseases, human-to-human transmission can dominate when a respiratory virus takes the stage. Still, it's important to note that animal reservoirs and vectors might still tip the balance in those initial spillover events and even in ongoing transmission cycles for different pathogens (Shereen et al., 2020). When you look at the bigger picture, you're dealing with a combination of ecology and evolution that demands a broader, more flexible view. Keeping a watchful eye on where these vectors hang around—and pairing that with steady vaccine improvements and new treatments—remains a core part of stopping future outbreaks. In the end, accepting and addressing the role vectors play is just a crucial piece of the giant jigsaw puzzle that is global health security.

1.3. Symptoms and Diagnosis

When doctors first try to figure out what's causing an infection, they usually start by checking how the patient feels—looking at the symptoms. It's not always a neat process because many microbes trigger signs that overlap one another. Think about upper respiratory issues: a blocked or runny nose plus a fever often show up, but the details can change depending on the germ and the person's unique traits. In many cases, extra clues come from inflammation markers, which offer a kind of backup to the initial assessment by showing just how hard the immune system is fighting back. For example, sometimes a spike in the neutrophil-to-lymphocyte ratio along with higher C-reactive protein levels lines up with zinc shortages in kids with COVID-19 , hinting that something as basic as nutrient status might alter how the disease unfolds (Perestiuk et al., 2025). These lab numbers add depth to what the doctor sees and help steer treatment in a more personalized way. Then there's the lab testing that really fine-tunes the diagnosis. Targeted tests have become even more critical nowadays, especially when different pathogens might be responsible for similar symptoms. Rapid antigen tests, PCR, and serological assays—each one plays a key role when trying to tell apart viruses like SARS-CoV-2, influenza, or respiratory syncytial virus. During the ups and downs of symptom trends over an infection season, these tests help clear up some of the confusion. For instance, in a surveillance study from the 2023/2024 season, COVID-19 patients generally showed fewer nasal complaints than those with influenza or colds, and immunized folks even exhibited more nasal mucosal responses, suggesting that prior immunity can nudge symptom expression in unexpected ways (Straburzyński & Romaszko-Wojtowicz, 2024).

To summarize, matching lab findings with what's observed clinically makes the diagnosis a lot more precise. CombinationIncorporating what you see in the patient with lab results really rounds out the approach to handling infections. Catching even the smallest variations in symptoms alongside inflammatory markers gives doctors extra hints about disease severity and its potential twists. In pediatric cases, noting the link between zinc levels and inflammation serves as a reminder—sometimes nutritional and immune factors go hand in hand (Perestiuk et al., 2025). Looking at how previous vaccinations might alter the way an infection shows itself provides helpful context for predicting what might come next (Straburzyński & Romaszko-Wojtowicz, 2024). Ultimately, pairing symptom observation with lab diagnostics is the bedrock of effective infectious disease management—it cuts down on uncertainty and aims for better outcomes for everyone (Figure 1.8).

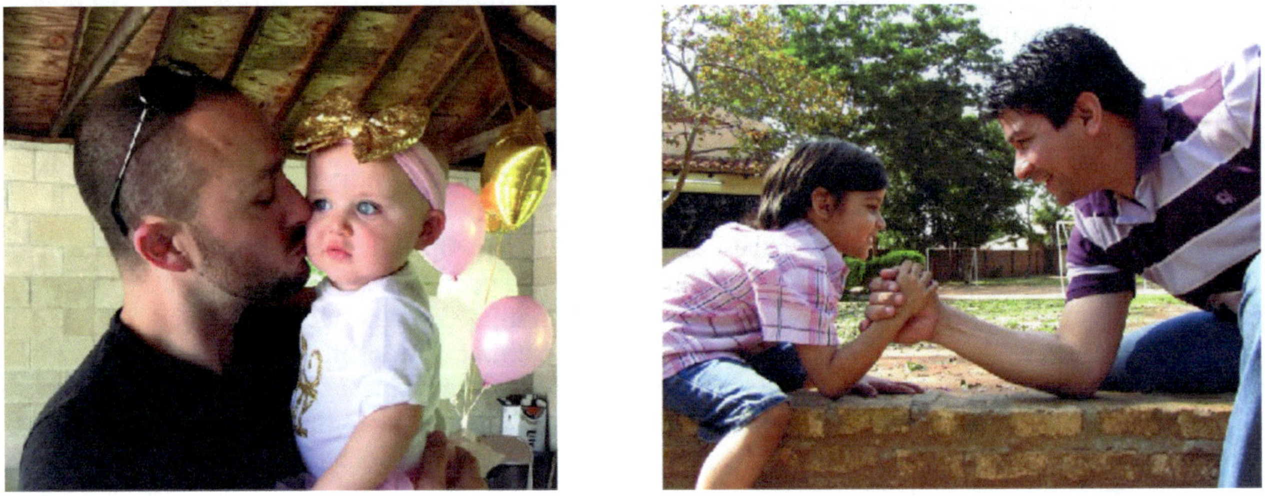

Figure 1.8. Symptoms and diagnosis of infectious diseases.

Source: **https://courses.lumenlearning.com/suny-microbiology/chapter/modes-of-disease-transmission/**

1.3.1. Common Symptoms of Infectious Diseases

When bacteria attack, the body communicates the invasion in a random assortment of ways instead of adhering to some clear checklist. Fever, for instance, is one of the earliest telltale signs—it's as though the body turns up the heat to make things more difficult for the microbes. Chills, tiredness, and that nagging feeling of being "off" usually accompany it, suggesting a full-blown immune boost and inflammation. You may also see red, swollen, or painful areas where the infection is persisting. In children, for example, oral infections tend to accompany clear lesions and pain (Kułaga et al., 2025), which informs us that symptoms can combination and combine depending on the pathogen and the affected tissue. Identifying these diverse cues allows physicians to move quickly with diagnostics and treatments, which is essential to maintaining the disease under control. Occasionally, the scenario becomes even more complex with neurological or metabolic symptoms. Consider polyphagia—that abnormally persisting hunger, which can be a sign of metabolic imbalances associated with a systemic infection or even hormonal reactions (Kułaga et al., 2025). In general, although these symptoms don't necessarily take center stage, they emphasize the complexity of infections; in most instances, the overt symptoms combination with underlying changes in behavior and physiological functions. They might, in time, erode a patient's quality of life and complicate management, emphasizing the importance of examining beyond the expected symptoms when formulating a treatment plan. Once infection establishes residence within a given tissue, it typically leaves a footprint of its own. Pedodontic oral infections, for instance, will leave painful ulcers, erythema which can be quite palpable, and—on very bad cases—necrotizing activity interfering with everyday oral functions (Aljohani et al., 2024). Such messages not only provide pain, but if unchecked, can facilitate system spread; truly, then, the importance of early discovery comes into its own. In addition, fungal infections such as candidiasis introduce their own set of symptoms—white plaques and even angular cheilitis—that can indicate problems with the immune system or even cleanliness. By interlacing symptom observations with laboratory testing, clinicians can more accurately determine whether they're working with a virus, bacteria, or fungus, further direct treatment accordingly, ultimately cutting down on further complications.

1.3.2. Diagnostic Methods and Technologies

Diagnosing infectious diseases hasn't seen huge leaps in recent decades; most places still lean on old-school methods like microscopy and culture. PCR did shake things up a bit once upon a time, but most of the new tools have only nudged the field forward. There's a growing clamor for tests that are rapid, sensitive and don't depend on big, resource-heavy labs. Immunoassays and molecular approaches are now added to the mix, offering faster results with better specificity. Some folks are even exploring proteomic techniques using mass spectrometry to tease out pathogen signatures with even more precision. Generally speaking, these innovations aren't just about boosting sensitivity—they also aim to make point-of-care testing workable in both high- and low-resource settings, trying to plug long-standing holes in our diagnostic routines (Ndao et al., 2009). In the end, getting these tests right is vital for acting rapidly and keeping disease spread in check. TB, for example, really puts the spotlight on these challenges.

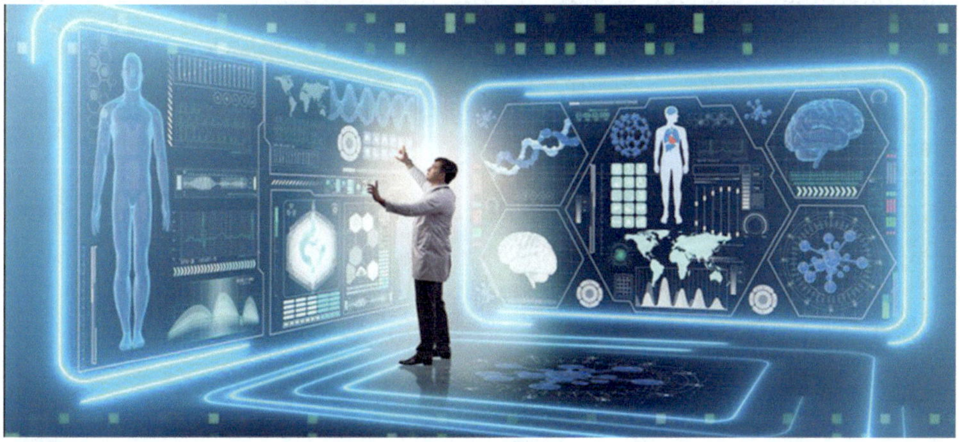

Figure 1.9. Diagnostic methods and technologies.

Source: ARTiBA. (n.d.). *Diagnosis and Predicting.*

It's a disease where catching it quickly is critical, yet doing so remains profoundly difficult. Traditional methods for TB still rely on lab-based tests that tend to be slow and often need repeated runs, which can delay starting treatment attemptively. Without a trustworthy rapid test that works at the point of care, TB transmission can sneak along undetected in communities. Recently, however, there's been some progress with new assays better at spotting active disease, screening for latent infections, and even picking up drug-resistant strains. Still, the complex nature of TB diagnostics calls not only for further technical upgrades but also for coordinated political and financial backing to make these tests broadly accessible in affected areas. Beating these hurdles is essential for catching cases sooner and lightening the global TB load. When trying to weave new diagnostic tools into everyday clinical practice, there's another layer of complexity. The price tag, complicated procedures, and need for specialized personnel all emerge as hurdles. Even though modern molecular and immunological methods do offer improvements in speed and accuracy, they demand infrastructure and training that aren't available everywhere. Ideally, a diagnostic test should be fast, easy to use, and affordable—letting doctors run tests on the spot without skimping on sensitivity or specificity. Researchers are still chasing down new biomarkers and working on multiplex tests that can spot several pathogens or diseases at once. In most cases, striking the right balance between cutting-edge technology and practical accessibility remains a major sticking point in infectious disease diagnostics. Addressing these operational and technical snags is critical for rolling out fair, effective diagnostic solutions worldwide (Ndao et al., 2009) (Figure 1.9).

1.3.3. Challenges in Diagnosing Infectious Diseases

Infectious disease diagnosis often gets muddled by the tangled interplay between microbes and the environments they call home. Take, for example, multi-drug resistant Tuberculosis (MDR-TB)—traditional testing methods generally miss or delay spotting the resistant strains, especially when resources are tight. In many parts of the world, like India, long-established TB control programs sometimes prove too rigid, making it hard for new, smarter tests to take hold (Engel et al., 2025). This clash between sticking with standard, familiar biomedical routines and the need to adjust to ever-changing microbial behavior usually means that diagnoses end up delayed or simply off, creating serious roadblocks in managing diseases.

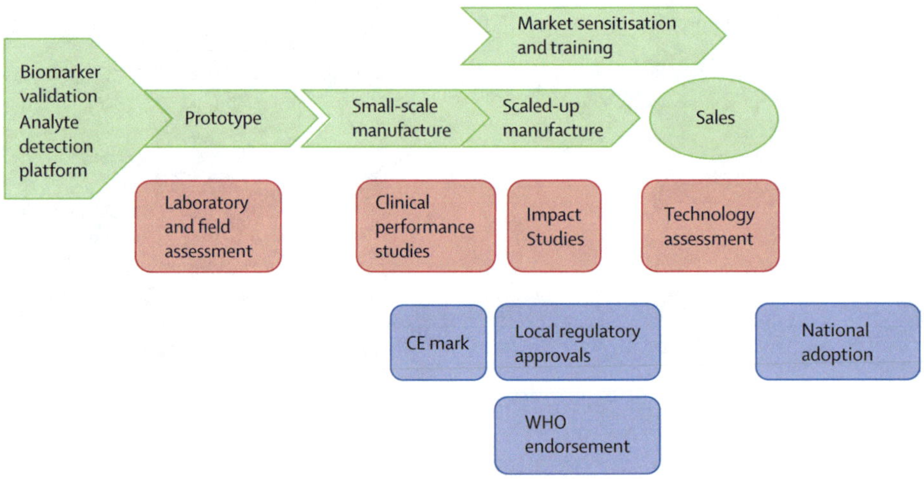

Figure 1.10. Challenges in diagnosing infectious diseases.

Source: Elsevier Health. (n.d.). *Gr1 Image*. Elsevier Health.

Overall, addressing these issues needs not just technical upgrades but also health systems that can flex and learn locally, in most cases adapting to unexpected challenges. The hurdles in diagnosing infectious diseases aren't only about fancy tech falling short—they also come from social and operational snags that shape how healthcare gets delivered. Patients might show up with symptoms that are either totally absent or all over the place, sometimes misleading clinicians who then struggle to pinpoint the exact cause. Plus, geographic differences mean that folks in remote or impoverished areas rarely get the quick, accurate tests they need. Such disparities, it seems, make a strong case for professionals working together—often in informal chats or even international meetings among infectious disease experts, where sharing case studies and ideas happens in a pretty natural, sometimes unpolished way (Myrvang & Newport, 2009). In many instances, bridging these gaps means incorporating top-notch lab techniques with improved communication and ongoing learning among healthcare providers. On top of clinical and logistical bottlenecks, diagnosing infections has to grapple with bacteria that just won't stay the same. New infectious agents and strains resistant to drugs routinely upend diagnostic tests designed with older profiles in mind, forcing constant innovation and revalidation of methods. There's always that balancing act between a test's specificity and sensitivity—too many false results can really steer treatment and containment efforts off course. Generally speaking, this dynamic situation calls for a steady stream of research investment and a willingness on the part of health systems to switch things up in real-time. Recognizing these layered challenges—from the unpredictable evolution of microbes to somewhat inflexible public health infrastructures—can pave the way for approaches that sharpen detection accuracy and, ultimately, help ease the global burden of infectious diseases (Engel et al., 2025) (Figure 1.10).

1.4. Treatment and Management

Recent leaps in fighting infections have boosted patient outcomes, even though we still wrestle with stubborn challenges like evolving resistance and shifting environmental factors. It all often kicks off when an disease is caught early, letting doctors step in quickly to ease things up. A simple rehydration method, for example, is still a go-to fix for diarrheal issues—especially for kids prone to dangerous dehydration. That said, the rise in antibiotic-resistant strains keeps shaking up treatment plans, which means new guidelines and careful use of antibiotics are a must. In some areas where typhoid and diarrhea hit hard, mixing quick clinical fixes with broader public health moves, like ramping up sanitation and sharing health tips with locals—proves vital. In most cases, keeping an eye on treatment strategies and alteraltering them as resistance patterns shift is key to holding onto all the progress made (Arnold, 2024). Tech breakthroughs have changed the game in infection control, and artificial intelligence (AI) is at the heart of that shift. AI diagnostic tools can zero in on pathogens faster and more precisely, setting the stage for prompt treatment moves. Oddly enough, machine learning systems even dig into massive data troves to predict outbreaks, fine-tune treatment plans, and sometimes even shape therapies to suit individual patient characterestics—all of which boosts overall effectiveness and drops unwanted side effects. AI is also speeding up the drug-discovery process, opening up fresh ways to counter antibiotic resistance and tackle emerging microbes. Still, weaving AI into healthcare isn't all smooth sailing; there are ethical, privacy, and accessibility wrinkles that need ironing out along with rigorous clinical testing. Generally speaking, using AI to its fullest might just transform how ready and responsive our healthcare systems are against infections (Srivastava et al., 2024). Winning the fight against infectious diseases isn't just about clinical interventions—it also means doubling down on prevention to cut down the spread and recurrence of these diseases. Vaccination programs have long been the unsung heroes, slimming down infection rates worldwide. Meanwhile, basic public health moves like better hygiene, easier access to clean water, and stronger sanitation systems are crucial for shielding at-risk communities. When folks learn more about preventing disease, they tend to seek help sooner if symptoms flare up. It's clear that teaming up with doctors, researchers, and policymakers is essential to keep these comprehensive plans rolling. And, of course, steady funding for monitoring and research is needed to quickly spot new threats and adjust treatments sponteneously, ensuring our strategies stay effective as challenges evolve (Arnold, 2024).

1.4.1. Antimicrobial Therapies

Antimicrobial therapies have really reshaped how we handle infections, directly targeting the bacteria and, in most cases, cutting down the rates of disease and death worldwide. At first, treatments leaned mostly on antibiotics, antivirals, antifungals, and antiparasitics – each of these designed to disrupt key processes inside microbes. Yet, with their heavy use—and sometimes even misuse—there's been a notable rise in resistant strains, which, frankly, limits how well these drugs work. As microbes evolve clever ways to sidestep our current treatments, a need for fresh strategies becomes crystal clear. Research is now turning to alternatives like bacteriophage therapy, which harnesses viruses to attack specific bacteria. Still, even though the promise is there, moving these ideas from the lab into real-world care gets tangled in regulatory, financial, and patent hurdles, prompting a rethinking of innovation incentives within pharmaceutical development (Todd et al., 2014, 2019).

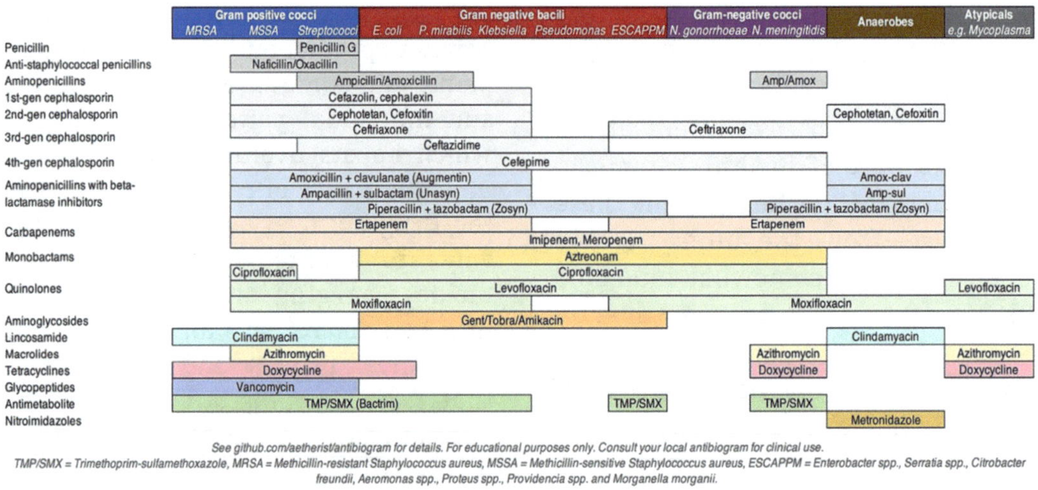

Figure 1.11. Antimicrobial therapies.

Source: By EricAtSHH - Own work, CC0, https://commons.wikimedia.org/w/index.php?curid=142081284

Digging into the details of antimicrobial treatments shows a surprisingly tangled mix of microbial biology, how drugs interact in the body (pharmacodynamics), and the strict regulatory settings. Traditional antibiotics typically hit bacterial cell walls, interrupt protein-making machinery, or block DNA replication. But over time, bacteria have wedded clever tactics—think efflux pumps or enzymes that break down drugs—that set them up for this ongoing evolutionary arms race. Generally speaking, this reality highlights the limits of our old antimicrobial approaches and makes phage therapy, which selectively infects and kills bacteria, even more attractive as a precision tool. Still, getting solid patent protection for phage-based products under today's intellectual property laws is a real challenge; that forces investors and developers to consider other routes like regulatory exclusivities and trade secrets to keep research moving forward (Todd et al., 2014, 2019). Given the mounting global threat of antimicrobial resistance (AMR), our future in infectious disease management likely rests on mixing traditional drugs with newer tactics to outmaneuver resistance and extend the life of treatments. Innovative therapies - including those using bacteriophages - have emerged as exciting options that could work alongside or even replace conventional drugs. In most cases, though, seizing this opportunity means big shifts in funding, regulation, and patent policies are on the table. Policymakers and scientists must, albeit sometimes in a slightly complex collaboration, lay down comprehensive frameworks that embrace alternative protections and inventive payment models. Without these systemic changes, the goal of keeping effective antimicrobial therapies available to protect global health against resistant infections remains in serious jeopardy (Todd et al., 2014, 2019) (Figure 1.11).

1.4.2. Vaccination and Preventive Measures

Controlling diseases in farm animals isn't just about throwing a vaccine at the problem. Vaccines play a critical role, sure, but their impact depends a lot on day-to-day management, the environment animals live in, and even their genetics. Look at organic farms—there, issues like parasite invasions and animal social stress emerge, challenging farmers in unexpected ways. In many cases, fixing these issues means rethinking housing, nutrition, and even breed choices along with adding immunizations into the mix. The tangled system of organic systems generally calls for studies that really nail down how these prevention tactics shape immune responses and boost disease resistance. Without incorporating management with preventive protocols, even the best vaccine might just cover part of the risk (Eijck et al., 2003). Even though everyone agrees that vaccines are important, putting them to work isn't always straightforward. Research on Bovine Viral Diarrhea Virus (BVDV) in cattle, for instance, shows that a lot of farms aren't even sure if their herds are infected, and many jump into vaccination without a first look at diagnostics. These lapses in checking are wedded to the overall impact of vaccines, if testing isn't synced up with immunization, their benefits get watered down. So, understanding local disease trends and linking them neatly to vaccine use is pretty crucial; without that, disease control programs can easily risk falling short of expectations, leaning too much on guesswork rather than solid, data-driven decisions (Booth et al., 2013). At the same time, as vaccine technology marches forward, it ends up bumping into ethical and regulatory hurdles—especially on operations like organic farms.

In these cases, GMO-based vaccines, despite all their scientific promise, are largely off-limits, cutting down the options for disease prevention. There are also alternative approaches, like phytotherapy, which sometimes get praise based on anecdotal evidence, even though they don't have a rock-solid track record yet. This broader scenario shows that vaccines run in a complicated arena where they need to jive with established farming values and be backed by other evidence-based practices, like robust biosecurity and sound animal welfare measures. To summarize, a well-rounded strategy combining immunization, attention to biosecurity, proper animal care, and environmental control really seems to be the best bet for keeping infectious diseases at bay in diverse livestock systems (Eijck et al., 2003) (Figure 1.12).

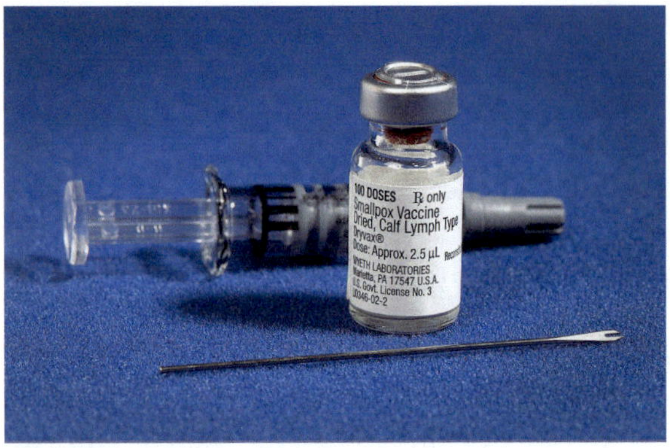

Figure 1.12. Most common vaccine preventable diseases.

Source: By Photo Credit: James GathanyContent Providers(s): CDC - This media comes from the Centers for Disease Control and Prevention's Public Health Image Library (PHIL), with identification number #2674.Note: Not all PHIL images are public domain; be sure to check copyright status and credit authors and content providers.العربية | Deutsch | English | македонски | slovenščina | +/−, Public Domain, https://commons.wikimedia.org/w/index.php?curid=367791

1.4.3. Role of Healthcare Systems in Management

Efficiently handling infectious diseases kicks off with a strong, well-linked healthcare system that stands as our first shield. These systems don't just treat patients—they also jump in with steps like mass immunizations and cleaning-up protocols. Hospitals, local clinics, public health groups, and even neighborhood networks mix in unexpected ways to keep diseases at bay. This kind of teamwork, by the way, lets us notice shifting infection trends and alter how we use antibiotics, reacting quickly when new threats emerge. In most cases, beating infections has less to do with piecemeal efforts and more with a big, all-encompassing plan that boosts open talk and resource sharing across every level of care (Ahmad et al., 2019). To summarize, such an approach can help patients get better and slow the spread of bacteria both inside medical settings and out in the community. Local healthcare is only one piece of the puzzle, though.

Across borders, our battle against infectious diseases calls for plans that stretch into global governance. Pathogens aren't known for respecting borders—they zip around populations faster than you'd expect. As a result, we need solid policies that spot, report, and respond to outbreaks in a hurry. Recent pandemics really highlighted how lacking investment and readiness can leave us hanging, which is why stepping up global health security—through infrastructure, better-trained workforces, and more research—is a must to lower disease, death, and economic setbacks (Ayala et al., 2017). Governments, international bodies, academic circles, and even everyday communities all play parts in crafting a resilient system for today's and tomorrow's challenges.

When it comes to curbing AMR, healthcare systems are front and center, rolling out programs that guide antibiotic use sensibly. These antimicrobial stewardship efforts—or AMS as some call them—need to spread across all healthcare sectors if we're to really embrace a "One Health" view that links human, animal, and even environmental factors. While many AMS projects still hone in on individual institutions, broader, more connected approaches are slowly gaining ground. There's emerging evidence (mostly from high-income areas) that these integrated moves can trim down unnecessary prescriptions and cut hospital infections (Ahmad et al., 2019). To truly hit the mark, though, barriers like coordination hiccups, patchy data sharing, and funding issues need to be ironed out by moving toward system-wide plans that invite multisector cooperation. In short, tightening up AMS integration is crucial if we're going to keep pace with ever-evolving microbial threats.

1.5. Global Impact of Infectious Diseases

Infectious diseases do more than just attack our health right away—they reshape societies and shake up economies all over the world. When these diseases spread uncontrollably, health systems can get overloaded, which means that resources meant for managing long-term diseases or running essential services get pulled away. The result is that the burden falls harder on those already at risk, as these communities typically suffer from higher exposure and fewer options for care. There's also a problematic side to this story: widespread misunderstandings and distorted facts about these diseases end up slowing down public health efforts by interfering with vital vaccination drives and other control measures. For example, health literacy, or the general understanding people have about medical issues, seems to play an important role in how vaccines are viewed—in many cases, a lack of clear information helps nasty myths stick around. All of this really underscores why educational programs—ones that take into account things like education background and professional training—are so important, as they can change how people receive health messages (Lubej et al., 2025). Ignoring these tangled issues could very well leave our efforts against infectious diseases falling short on a global scale. There's another twist here that we can't ignore. As societies age and the number of non-communicable diseases grows, especially among older adults, a whole new set of challenges shows up. In many regions, populations are growing older at a pretty fast clip, and chronic diseases are climbing too, making it tougher for those individuals to fend off infections. The mix of mental health issues, activity levels, and even body weight creates a sort of complicated puzzle. Think about long-term care environments, where it's not unusual to see depression and obesity side by side—this combo can ramp up a person's vulnerability to infections and muddle treatment efforts. On the brighter side, initiatives that encourage physical activity can hit two birds with one stone by easing depressive symptoms and boosting metabolic health, which might even help fend off infections better (Naidoo & Naidoo, 2025). Altogether, such a multifaceted situation suggests that we really need integrated strategies, ones that tackle both the infectious threats and the surge in chronic conditions in our aging communities, if we're aiming to lessen the overall disease burden worldwide. Look at the bigger picture: the fight against infectious diseases is a global issue that calls for policies and healthcare responses that aren't confined by national borders.

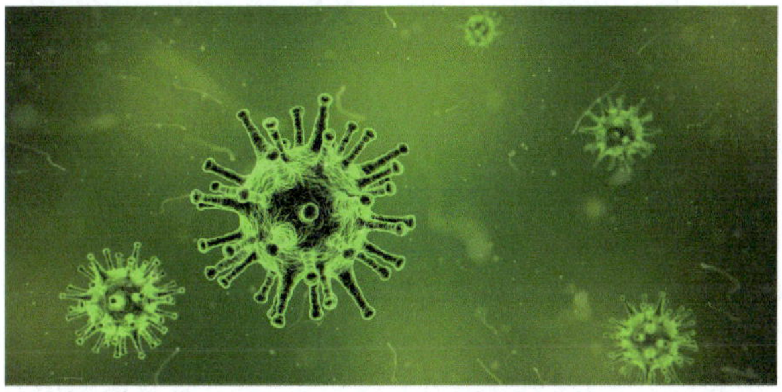

Figure 1.13. Global impact of infectious diseases.

Source: Journalists Resource. (2016). *Virus Close-up.*

These troublesome pathogens don't pay any regard to country lines, so it's clear that international cooperation is a must for effective monitoring, rapid action, and fair distribution of key resources like vaccines and treatment drugs. On top of that, socioeconomic differences only make it harder to implement proper preventive measures, since regions with fewer resources often struggle most. By boosting global health infrastructure and mixing in community-level education, we can help slow the spread of diseases—this happens partly by spreading sound, accurate health information and by getting more people on board with vaccination guidelines. Getting health professionals more involved and widening educational access seems to make a noticeable difference as well, given that better-informed individuals and trained caregivers tend to have higher vaccine acceptance rates (Lubej et al., 2025). In short, nurturing a globally aware and proactive public health scene is critical if we hope to lessen the deep-rooted impact these infections have on our world (Figure 1.13).

1.5.1. Economic Consequences

Economic struggles often mix up more than just bank accounts; they end up stirring the spread of diseases in ways that aren't obvious at first glance. When money runs tight, everyday living can get rougher and access to healthcare plummets, which in turn makes it easier for infections to take root. Migrants, the homeless, and people in prisons tend to suffer even more because cramped conditions and weak health services are common in these spots. During lean times the public health purse usually shrinks too, letting prevention programs and treatment fall by the wayside, which only adds fuel to the fire. Some research points in different directions, but generally speaking, tough economic times are often linked with more disease cases. This unique mix hints that governments should get ahead of the problem and keep pouring support into health systems (Abubakar et al., 2011). Farmers and those in the livestock business feel this pinch too. When diseases hit, it's not just about a drop in earnings on a single farm—it can ripple out and shake up entire trade networks. Take Johne's disease, for example, this incurable and easily spread disease drags down dairy farms by reducing output and hiking up costs for management. Economic models tend to show that putting money into disease control pays off better over time rather than simply turning a blind eye. In many cases, mixing different control methods that fit the disease's own characterestics turns out to be the most budget-friendly way to cut down infection rates while keeping farms in business. These ideas really drive home how important it is to combine a bit of biology with smart money moves in agriculture (Cho et al., 2009). Beyond the direct expenses of treatment and prevention, infections can throw labor productivity, markets, and public health systems into disarray, creating broad economic headaches. Outbreaks might even lead to trade limits or make consumers steer clear, which naturally squeezes market access and slashes revenues for the industries involved. On top of that, there are hidden costs like long-term disabilities, lost wages, and a greater need for social support that together put extra strain on government budgets and slow down economic progress. When you add up all these aspects, it's clear that planning ahead is key—and that means balancing health priorities with keeping the economy steady. Evidence-backed interventions and a well-kept eye on disease trends are crucial for keeping both health and financial disruptions in check.

1.5.2. Social Implications

Sometimes disease outbreaks reveal deep cracks in society rather than just causing disease. Take COVID-19 as an example: people's experiences split wide apart, with some groups hit harder early on by economic setbacks, fewer chances at medical care, and risky jobs. Lockdowns and travel bans reshaped daily lives and personal freedoms, sparking heated talks on whether these moves were fair. In Sweden, authorities leaned on voluntary measures, trying to juggle public well-being with personal responsibility—even though critics pointed out delays and gaps in care for vulnerable folks, especially elderly residents of nursing homes. That mix of obligatory rules and self-chosen actions shows just how tangled it is to handle public health crises, with community trust and cohesion playing a big role (Björkman, 2022). Handling infectious diseases often calls for a layered social response—one that can sometimes stray into broader issues of control and human rights.

Policies meant to slow the spread might end up singling out certain behaviors or whole groups as high-risk, which can push them to the edges of society. Meanwhile, systems originally set up for health monitoring can stretch into broader social oversight, quietly chipping away at personal freedoms under the banner of safety. We see this trend in policing and urban management, where health issues combine with strict disciplinary tactics, raising questions about just how far these measures should reach. In most cases, taking a closer look at this overlap reminds us that while keeping communities safe is key, it's equally important to protect basic rights through thoughtful, nuanced policies (Program on Human Rights and the Global Economy, 2010).

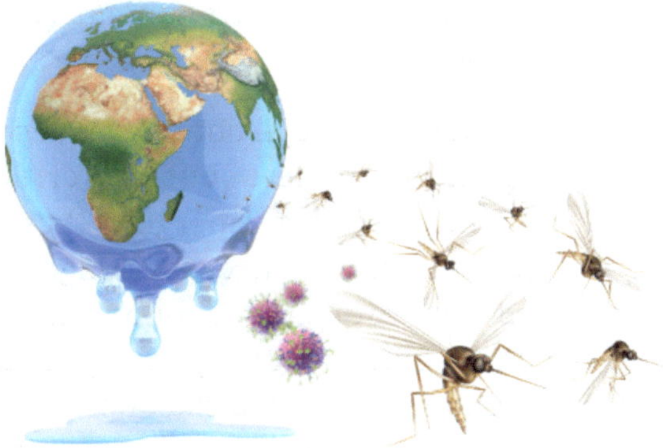

Figure 1.14. Social implications.

Source: Research Outreach. (2020). *Florence Fouque Figure 1.*

Outbreaks don't just spread bacteria—they shake up how communities live and interact every day. They shift routines, stir up economic changes, and sometimes even erode trust in our institutions. The fear of getting sick can spark discrimination and exclusion, particularly when certain groups, rightly or wrongly, are blamed for the spread. Whether steps taken are voluntary or enforced, the ripple effects often change the public's view of authority and their willingness to follow guidelines. Recognizing these layered social impacts is critical if we want solutions that not only curb infections but also hold society together. Lessons from past epidemics remind us, generally speaking, that weaving social insights into health strategies helps build a response that's resilient, informed, and more inclusive (Björkman, 2022; Program on Human Rights and the Global Economy, 2010) (Figure 1.14).

1.5.3. Global Health Initiatives and Collaborations

Infectious diseases don't stick to one country's borders, so managing them means getting everyone on board—local groups, national agencies, and global players all have a role. Health projects nowadays aren't built on neat systems; they mix resources, share outbreak data, and even alter how they keep eyes on diseases. Quick spotting of outbreaks and getting teams moving fast is key, especially where health services are a bit thin. Sometimes, an odd mix of different experts and sectors working together ends up boosting disease tracking in unexpected ways. Studies, for example, show that these informal partnerships and smart use of resources (Gamon et al., 2013) can really help keep infections under control, linking efforts worldwide in a less clear, but effective, manner. In regions where diseases hit hard, interventions usually evolve based on what local clinics can manage and how strong those global links are. Take MDR-TB as an example—its fight is a complex but necessary dance between local practitioners, national health bodies, and international organizations. Countries with solid public health programs, rapid diagnostics, and ready access to decent meds tend to see better treatment adherence and slower spread. New, resistant bacteria keep making things trickier, so fast drug susceptibility tests become pretty crucial. Global cooperation can nudge countries like India to polish up their health systems, raise public health know-how, and settle on treatment styles that just work in their cultural context.

Drawing on previous successes helps slow down these stubborn pathogens and spreads more balanced health outcomes (Gamon et al., 2013). Looking at big, cooperative networks in disease surveillance shows how charity and international teamwork can change the game. Foundations and global agencies are increasingly backing projects that mix cross-border chats, shared know-how, and a bit of capacity building – sometimes in ways that feel a little improvisational. Independent evaluations often note, generally speaking, that measuring both the inner workings of these projects and their real-life health effects really guides where future funding should go. These reviews inform more organic grant strategies and encourage approaches that combine different skills for tracking diseases. Bringing together such varied disciplines ends up forming a creative hub for tackling infections, one where quick outbreak responses eventually lead to more durable, if slightly complex, surveillance systems that help keep new diseases from gaining ground (Kimball et al., 2011).

1.6. Emerging Infectious Diseases

Global health these days has been wrestling with a growing problem: AMR, where bacteria seem to learn new tricks to dodge antibiotics. This twist muddles treatment plans and makes infections turn more severe—contributing to lots of disease and, sadly, many deaths worldwide. A broad study roughly estimated that almost five million deaths in 2019 were linked to bacteria that had gotten resistant (Murray et al., 2022). What's striking is how low-resource places suffer even more; when healthcare systems are stretched thin and infections run rampant, these resilient microbes have room to thrive. Common offenders like *Escherichia coli* and *Staphylococcus aureus* keep tripping up usual treatments, urging us to deploy focused actions backed by solid infection data to rethink control measures and antimicrobial practices. New pathogens that trigger serious respiratory issues underline just how impactful infectious diseases can be. The 2019 outbreak of what became known as 2019-nCoV in Wuhan, China, really drove home how quickly zoonotic viruses can spread, making early detection and fast responses absolutely key. Early reports hinted at thousands of cases and hundreds of deaths cropping up within weeks, with clear signs of person-to-person spread that alarmed people everywhere. In the U.S., both federal and local teams jumped in—using aggressive case tracking, contact follow-ups, and travel screening—to delay widespread community spread, ultimately giving hospitals some much-needed time to prepare and researchers a boost in rolling out better tests and treatments (Patel & Jernigan, 2020).

In many ways, that episode continues to serve as a cautionary tale about the critical need for readiness against emerging threats. Managing new infectious diseases hinges on rapid science and coordinated public health moves. When scientists quickly mapped the coronavirus genome, it opened the door to new molecular tests emerging within weeks; this leap was central for tracking and managing the outbreak. Still, many uncertainties about transmission, severity, and who's most at risk persist, which can make targeted responses feel like navigating in the dark. Interim guidelines generally favor isolation and supportive care since there aren't always specific treatments or vaccines around. At the same time, strict screening at entry points and quarantine measures work together to block the entry and spread of these pathogens. Such combined efforts—bolstered by international teamwork—highlight just how critical preparedness is as these threats evolve in complexity and reach (Patel & Jernigan, 2020). To summarize, this evolving challenge reminds us that ongoing research, smarter data sharing, and stronger response capabilities are essential for facing future infectious risks effectively (Murray et al., 2022) (Figure 1.15).

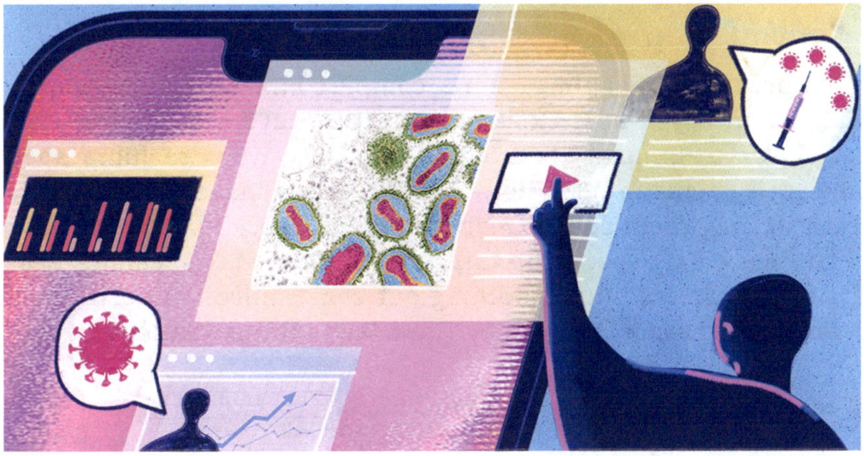

Figure 1.15. Emerging infectious diseases.

Source: University of Michigan School of Public Health. (n.d.). *Infectious Diseases.*

1.6.1. Definition and Examples

Infectious diseases hit us when pesky pathogens, like bacteria, viruses, fungi, or even parasites—find a way into our bodies. Once there, these unwelcome guests tend to throw our normal functions off balance and trigger a range of symptoms that, generally speaking, can go from just a bit of discomfort to something downright dangerous. Often, how we group these diseases depends on which germ is to blame and how it entered the body—maybe through a handshake, the air we breathe, microbes as vectors, or even a contaminated surface. For instance, TB shows one style of bacterial damage, while influenza, caused by viruses, paints a different picture. Add to this mix the growing challenge of AMR, which keeps muddying the treatment waters (Murray et al., 2022). Looking a bit closer at viral foes, one notices that some viruses, especially those that jump from animal hosts to people, pack extra punch. Consider SARS-CoV-2—this novel coronavirus, in most cases, sparked the global COVID-19 pandemic. It's been grouped with viruses like SARS-CoV, which was responsible for that severe outbreak back in the early 2000s. These scenarios reveal a kind of dynamic dance between humans and animal reservoirs; new bacteria can suddenly appear and spread with surprising speed.

Recognizing features such as their genetic makeup and how they tend to move through populations is crucial for catching outbreaks early and acting fast. On the bacterial side, things don't get any easier (Gorbalenya et al., 2020). AMR is a real headache, complicating treatment and pushing up disease and death rates all over the world. Take bacteria like *Escherichia coli*, *Klebsiella pneumoniae*, and *Staphylococcus aureus*—they've increasingly found ways to dodge multiple antibiotics, and, as a result, millions of lives are impacted every year. Lower respiratory infections caused by these stubborn microbes present serious challenges, particularly where healthcare resources are thin. Not to mention, MRSA and carbapenem-resistant *Klebsiella pneumoniae* stand out as especially worrisome because they often leave doctors with very few treatment choices.

Clearly, beefing up microbiological surveillance, practicing smarter antibiotic use, and digging into new treatment options isn't just a nice idea—it's absolutely essential (Murray et al., 2022).

1.6.2. Factors Contributing to Emergence

Infectious disease outbreaks come about from a complex mix of factors—social, environmental, and biological—that often defy a neat explanation. Cities have exploded in size over the years, and as people get closer to animals, pathogens find new ways to jump species. Meanwhile, crumbling public health systems in many low-resource areas make it tough to catch and contain these outbreaks early, letting them spread more or less unchecked. Modern travel, with its rapid and far-reaching movement, only speeds up this process. Generally speaking, experts now tend to agree that ramping up lab checks and smoothing out communication networks are critical steps in catching these emerging threats before they run away with us (Satcher et al., 1995).

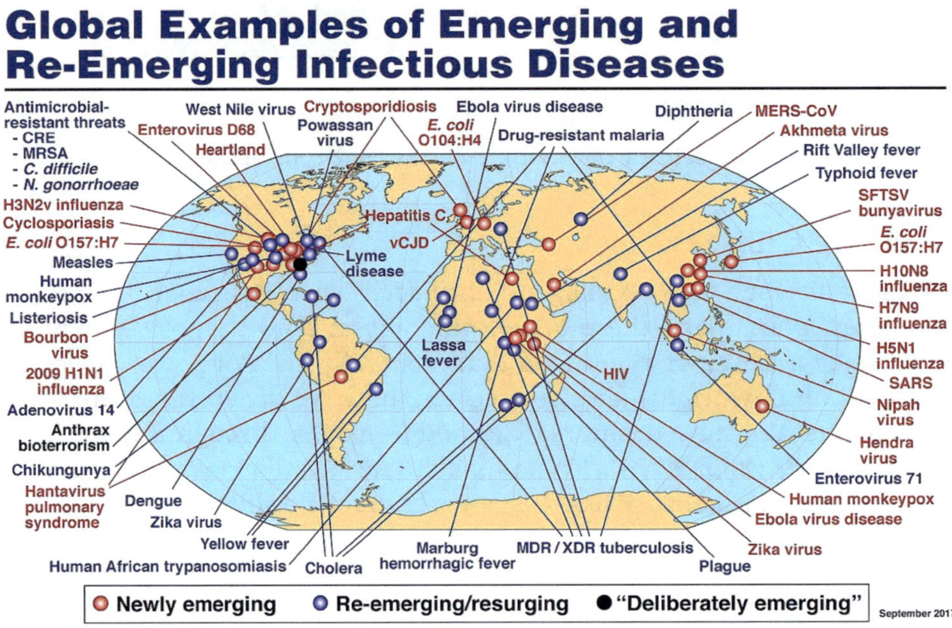

Figure 1.16. Factors contributing to the emergence of infectious disease.

Source: By Anthony Fauci (Q573246) - https://www.niaid.nih.gov/sites/default/files/main%20map.jpg, Public Domain, https://commons.wikimedia.org/w/index.php?curid=89608427

Migration adds its own complicated layer to the mix. In places like Malaysia, for instance, the steady flow of migrant laborers has been linked with rises in diseases such as TB, malaria, and a host of other infections. Even with mandatory health screenings in place, cramped living spaces, spotty sanitation, and limited access to healthcare mean that infections keep cropping up among these communities. On top of that, cultural and language differences can slow down the process of getting timely medical help, further deepening health disparities. In many cases, these intertwined issues show just how powerfully human movement can shake up disease patterns (Azman et al., 2023). Environmental changes play a major, if unpredictable, role too. Widespread deforestation, shifting climates, and new ways of using land throw natural systems off balance, often giving pathogens a leg up. When wildlife habitats shrink, people and animals end up rubbing shoulders more than ever, which can lead to zoonotic diseases making the jump between species. Weather and climate shifts also tend to re-map where disease-carrying insects and ticks can survive, complicating things even further. Mix these factors with globalization and everyday human habits, and you get a recipe that continually stokes the emergence of new infections. Generally speaking, addressing such a tangled set of issues means embracing integrated monitoring systems and joining forces across different sectors to stay one step ahead of potential outbreaks (Satcher et al., 1995) (Figure 1.16).

1.6.3. Strategies for Surveillance and Response

Timely, spot-on surveillance is key when fighting infectious diseases. Health officials depend on systems that quickly grab and break down all sorts of information so they can catch new threats before they really spread. Sometimes local communities step in by noticing odd clusters or trends that might otherwise slip past. Modern tools like real-time data sharing, mapping via geosystems, and even checking things at the molecular level all help the system get sharper—this boosts both its sensitivity and capacity to focus on real problems. Being able to follow disease movement across several layers, from animal carriers to humans, gives us a full picture that's crucial for easing outbreaks and lowering the number of cases and fatalities. Generally speaking, these broad-ranging plans need regular rechecks and alterchanges to keep up with shifting challenges (International Conference on Emerging Infectious Diseases. 2008). Preparing for health issues means more than just having plans on paper; it's about being ready to jump into action whenever something goes wrong. There are pre-set rules for looking into outbreaks, rapid moves for sending out medical help, and even special tactics to keep those at risk informed—often, these plans get better when government groups, hospitals, and community organizations work together seamlessly. Using the One Health idea, which weds human, animal, and environmental well-being, naturally spins the wheel on sharing information and sparking joint responses. All these measures, when mixed, build our understanding of what's happening on the ground and set up a system that can quickly block an epidemic's path (Chaula et al., 2016). In regions more exposed to new infectious threats, ramping up both surveillance and the backup response isn't just useful—it's essential for global health security. In many cases, countries with tight budgets must focus on showing healthcare pros and local members how to detect and report mishaps early on. Building a solid lab network goes a long way by expanding our ability to confirm outbreaks and even keep an eye on trends in antibiotic resistance. Moreover, linking up with international data systems speeds up the sharing of critical information and paves the way for a coordinated worldwide effort. With investments in decent public health systems and supportive political policies, an environment is created where sustainable control efforts can really take root. This sort of all-around prep not only cuts down the risk of full-blown crises but also helps ensure that when infections emerge, the response is both fast and effective (Chaula et al., 2016; International Conference on Emerging Infectious Diseases, 2008).

CLOSER LOOK

EMERGING INFECTIOUS DISEASES

Emerging infectious diseases (EIDs) are infections that have newly appeared in a population or are rapidly increasing in incidence or geographic range. They represent one of the most critical challenges to global health in the 21st century.

Many EIDs arise due to zoonotic spillover, where pathogens jump from animals to humans, often facilitated by deforestation, wildlife trade, or intensive farming. Viruses such as Ebola, SARS, MERS, and most recently COVID-19, demonstrate how disruptions in ecosystems can create opportunities for cross-species transmission. Additionally, antimicrobial resistance (AMR) contributes to the emergence of diseases once thought controllable, as bacteria and parasites evolve to withstand existing drugs.

Globalization has accelerated the spread of infectious agents. Increased international travel and trade enable pathogens to cross borders within hours, while climate change alters the habitats of vectors such as mosquitoes, expanding diseases like dengue, chikungunya, and Zika into new regions. Urbanization, poor sanitation, and overcrowding further amplify the risk of outbreaks, particularly in low- and middle-income countries.

The consequences of emerging infectious diseases go beyond health. They impose enormous social, economic, and political burdens, as witnessed during the COVID-19 pandemic, which disrupted economies, overwhelmed healthcare systems, and reshaped societies. Addressing these threats requires robust surveillance systems, rapid diagnostics, coordinated public health responses, and investment in vaccine and therapeutic research.

EIDs is not solely a medical task but a multidisciplinary effort involving public health, ecology, policy, and community engagement. Strengthening global preparedness and fostering cooperation among nations is vital to detect threats early, contain outbreaks swiftly, and build resilience against future pandemics.

Summary

Infectious diseases aren't exactly straightforward; they need real scientific digging mixed with hands-on teamwork at both local and global levels. Recent checks in the Asia-Pacific hint at a pretty wild spread of funding and priorities—investments are high, yet most of the cash flows into social science areas, leaving animal and environmental health (key to zoonotic spread) a bit neglected. This uneven split, in most cases, suggests we really ought to mix ethical and ecological angles into our research plans. Bringing together different funding groups and stakeholders seems pretty necessary if we want to up our overall impact and get ready for future outbreaks (Antonio et al., 2023). The complex link between diseases and our environment reminds us that weather data shouldn't be left on the sidelines. Research from tropical, developing countries shows that everyday climate measures like temperature and humidity really shape how diseases such as dengue fever roll out. It turns out that folding in climate details with standard disease data can help set up more flexible, context-specific systems that keep an eye on outbreaks based on local weather characterestics. Generally speaking, this kind of combined approach offers us a smarter way to predict and manage disease spikes in vulnerable areas. When you really think about it, fending off infectious diseases means pulling together coordinated funding, multi-disciplinary research, and a solid grasp of environmental influences. Efforts like those led by GloPID-R paint an encouraging picture of how research can be rallied and preparedness boosted—especially in high-risk spots like the Asia-Pacific region. Adding climate insights into our usual monitoring not only fine-tunes predictions but also sharpens our response tactics. Overall, dealing with both long-standing and emerging disease threats comes down to steady, cross-sector collaboration and welcoming diverse scientific views. These steps, taken together, pave the way for stronger public health systems and a more secure global health future (Antonio et al., 2023).

Modern progress in modeling infections keeps changing how we see disease spread, but you still have to read the outputs with a grain of salt. A lot of older models stick to simple exponential assumptions for latent and infectious periods—or sometimes skip the latent phase entirely, which, generally speaking, puts the basic reproductive number on the low end. These oversimplifications can lead to predictions that are a bit too upbeat about control measures, potentially putting public health responses at risk. It turns out that taking a closer look at these foundational assumptions is pretty important if we're going to predict outbreak trends accurately. In many cases, alteraltering the models so they mirror more realistic disease progressions lets epidemiologists offer guidance that's far more reliable, helping to improve outbreak management strategies and resource allocation during epidemics. Lately, mixing in ecological along with socio-environmental factors has really broadened our approach to studying infectious diseases. Frameworks like Ecohealth—, methods for looking at how human, animal, and environmental health jostle with each other—remind us that things like urban sprawl, intensified agriculture, and environmental shifts push disease emergence and shape transmission patterns. In Southeast Asia, where emerging diseases are a common challenge, Ecohealth initiatives have sparked some pretty broad multidisciplinary collaborations to tackle these issues. Researchers in the region have even upped their game in capacity-building, which shows that embracing a more inclusive framework can, in most cases, deepen our understanding of disease drivers while paving the way for steadier, more sustainable prevention and control efforts (Doria et al., 2015). Even with these advances, there are still many hurdles when it comes to fully incorporating these integrated methods into infectious disease control. Challenges emerge in harmonizing project designs, boosting interdisciplinary teamwork, and translating research insights into policies that can scale. It's an ongoing struggle to make sure every research team not only grasps the basics of Ecohealth but can also navigate the contextual differences from one country to the next. Plus, keeping the momentum of these initiatives demands solid regional cooperation and a strategic nod to frameworks like One Health, which also champion a broad view of health management. In most cases, future efforts will need to laser-focus on turning scientific findings into practical public health strategies that can really address the complex realities of disease emergence and spread (Doria et al., 2015).

References

1. Abubakar, I., Basu, S., Desai, M., Hunter, B., Orcutt, M., et al. (2011). The impact of economic crises on communicable disease transmission and control: A systematic review of the evidence. *PLOS ONE, 6*(6), e20724. https://core.ac.uk/download/13093583.pdf (accessed on 7 May 2025).

2. Ahmad, R., Holmes, A., McLeod, M., Micallef, S., et al. (2019). A whole-health-economy approach to antimicrobial stewardship: Analysis of current models and future direction. *PLOS Medicine, 16*(3), e1002774. https://core.ac.uk/download/323306206.pdf (accessed on 7 May 2025).

3. Aljohani, H. R., Almansour, S. H., Mobarki, A. S., Jaafari, W. A., Al-mohaya, D. A., Ali, M. W., Aldaini, B. O., Nogali, N. A., Almimony, H. A., Hafez, M. H., & Almazariqah, S. A. (2024). An overview of oral pediatric infectious diseases. *International Journal Of Community Medicine And Public Health, 12*(1), 477–481. https://doi.org/10.18203/2394-6040.ijcmph20243796 (accessed on 7 May 2025).

4. Antonio, E., Hagen, H. E., Lee, J., Norton, R., et al. (2023). Mapping regional funding for COVID-19 research in the Asia-Pacific region. *BMJ Global Health, 8*, e013551. https://core.ac.uk/download/591800975.pdf (accessed on 7 May 2025).

5. Arnold, N. (2024). Evaluating treatment and management strategies for diarrhea and typhoid fever in Uganda. *IDOSR Journal of Science and Technology*. https://www.semanticscholar.org/paper/77f331e665c9a640a32fbfe8faa837fce0e4ecca (accessed on 7 May 2025).

6. Ayala, A., & Gostin, L. O. (2017). *Global Health Security in an Era of Explosive Pandemic Potential* (Georgetown Law Faculty Publications and Other Works, No. 1943). https://core.ac.uk/download/74539397.pdf (accessed on 7 May 2025).

7. Azman, A. S., Lewis, J. W., Mohd Putera, N. W. S., Mohd Zain, S. N., et al. (2023). Current status of infectious diseases among migrants and non-citizens in Malaysia. *Tropical Biomedicine, 40*(2), 138–151. https://core.ac.uk/download/599576003.pdf (accessed on 7 May 2025).

8. Björkman, A. (2022). The Swedish COVID-19 control measures and the national commission report. *Acta Pediatric, 112*, 8–10. https://www.semanticscholar.org/paper/2f133c4699cf2b46f80edcae35a73c09472c761e (accessed on 7 May 2025).

9. Booth, R., De Vliegher, S., Deprez, P., Dewulf, J., et al. (2013). *Assessment of Two Essential Elements of Bvdv Control on Selected Flemish Dairy and Beef Farms*. https://core.ac.uk/download/55761867.pdf (accessed on 7 May 2025).

10. Carroll, D., Daszak, P., Karesh, W. B., Lipkin, W. I., et al. (2012). Prediction and prevention of the next pandemic zoonosis. *The Lancet, 380*(9857), 1956–1965. https://doi.org/10.1016/S0140-6736(12)61684-5.

11. Chaula, G., Maboko, L., Mangu, C. D., Manyama, M., et al. (2016). Emerging viral infectious disease threat: Why Tanzania is not in a safe zone. *Tanzania Journal of Health Research, 18*(3), 1–14. https://core.ac.uk/download/478317395.pdf (accessed on 7 May 2025).

12. Cho, J., Grohn, Y. T., Lu, Z., Schukken, Y. H., et al. (2009). Economic analysis of Johne's disease control strategies in dairy herds. *Preventive Veterinary Medicine, 90*(3, 4), 223–232. https://doi.org/10.1016/j.prevetmed.2009.04.009.

13. Danish, S. M., Asghari, S. J., Hashimi, S. A., Furmoli, M. E., Zamani, M. U., & Amiri, S. H. (2025).

The prevalence and associated demographic factors of hepatitis C infections among patients referred to the hospital of infectious diseases in Kabul, Afghanistan: A cross-sectional study. *Afghanistan Journal of Basic Medical Science, 2(1), 37–43*. https://www.semanticscholar.org/paper/afcdc5fa1c4ba4fb740dbd885c9d81629d9c453f (accessed on 7 May 2025).

14. Davison, N., Millett, P., & Nixdorff, K. (2004). *Technology and biological weapons: Future threats* (BTWC Science and Technology Report, No. 2). Bradford Disarmament Research Centre, Department of Peace Studies, University of Bradford. http://hdl.handle.net/10454/713 (accessed on 7 May 2025).
15. Dellana, C. J. (2014). Human disease–Unintended globalization. *Celebration, 26*. https://cupola.gettysburg.edu/cgi/viewcontent.cgi?article=1085&context=celebration (accessed on 7 May 2025).
16. Djoko, C. F., Fair, J. N., Lebreton, M., Pike, B. L., et al. (2010). The origin and prevention of pandemics. *Clinical Infectious Diseases, 50*(12), 1636–1640. https://doi.org/10.1086/652860.
17. Doria, S., Grace, D., Mallee, H., Nguyen-Viet, H., et al. (2015). Eco health research in Southeast Asia: Past, present and the way forward. *Infectious Diseases of Poverty, 4*, 5. https://core.ac.uk/download/33300685.pdf (accessed on 7 May 2025).
18. Egli, A., & Schulthess, B. (2024). Tuberculosis in times of war and peace. *Conexus, 7*(1), 186–212. https://core.ac.uk/download/636781636.pdf (accessed on 7 May 2025).
19. Egorova, M., Egorov, V., & Zabrodskaya, Y. (2024). Maternal influenza and offspring neurodevelopment. *Current Issues in Molecular Biology, 46*, 355–366. https://www.semanticscholar.org/paper/103e7c4058ded35abe716f03cf4807447c951a80 (accessed on 7 May 2025).
20. Eijck, I., Groot, M., Kasteel, D., Kijlstra, et al. (2003). Analysis of black holes in our knowledge concerning animal health in the organic food production chain. https://core.ac.uk/download/10919416.pdf (accessed on 7 May 2025).
21. Engel, N. (2025). Flexibility and innovation in response to emerging infectious diseases: Reactions to multi-drug-resistant Tuberculosis in India. https://core.ac.uk/download/pdf/6941410.pdf (accessed on 7 May 2025).
22. Fahdi, F., & Sari, H. (2024). Introduction to basic microbiology concepts in the prevention of infectious diseases at Yapim Biru-Biru private high school. *Jurnal Pengabdian Masyarakat Putri Hijau*. https://www.semanticscholar.org/paper/3c0ba05bf2960cbab82f682380da240b701632c1 (accessed on 7 May 2025).
23. Gamon, M. (2013). *Maribel Gamon–Multidrug-Resistant Tuberculosis in India: Solving A Problem by Reconstructing the Public Health Infrastructure*. Ronald E. McNair Scholars Program 2013, Book 12. https://core.ac.uk/download/67755957.pdf (accessed on 7 May 2025).
24. Gorbalenya, A. E., Baker, S. C., Baric, R. S., de Groot, R. J., Drosten, C., Gulyaeva, A., Haagmans, B. L., et al. (2020). The species severe acute respiratory syndrome-related coronavirus: Classifying 2019-nCoV and naming it SARS-CoV-2. *Nature Microbiology, 5*, 536–544. https://doi.org/10.1038/s41564-020-0695-z.
25. International Conference on Emerging Infectious Diseases. (2008). *Emerging Infectious Diseases*. https://core.ac.uk/download/144197853.pdf (accessed on 7 May 2025).
26. Kimball, A. M., Gugerty, M. K., Abernethy, N., & Curran, S. (2011). *Disease Surveillance Networks*

Initiative Global: Final Evaluation. https://core.ac.uk/download/86445037.pdf (accessed on 7 May 2025).

27. Kułaga, M., Kasprzak, A., Grzybek, M., Mazur-Lesińska, D., Szostak, B., Wielgosz-Biała, S., Tyszkiewicz, K., et al. (2025). Polyphagia as an accompanying symptom of various diseases: Overview and treatment options. *Journal of Education, Health and Sport*. https://www.semanticscholar.org/paper/8b8e9bd35e19ce18b4c7e906698c27c3f1fceab5 (accessed on 7 May 2025).
28. Lee, W. K., & Shin, S. R. (2024). Development of Emerging Infectious Diseases Preventive Health Behavior (EID-PHB) Scale and validation of the complex models. *Journal of Multidisciplinary Healthcare, 17*, 445–460. https://www.semanticscholar.org/paper/1c4f255219132e39fc6cce07ae2db07e22b2bac8 (accessed on 7 May 2025).
29. Lewnard, J. A., & Reingold, A. L. (2019). Emerging challenges and opportunities in infectious disease epidemiology. *American Journal of Epidemiology, 188*(5), 873–882. https://doi.org/10.1093/aje/kwy264.
30. Lubej, M., & Kirbiš, A. (2025). Why does health literacy matter, and for whom? Explaining the differentiating impact of health literacy on vaccine attitudes. *Frontiers in Psychology, 16*. https://www.semanticscholar.org/paper/b8b77803c3515eb41d04d5442d13b439e33a6baa (accessed on 7 May 2025).
31. Makhoul, M., Ayoub, H. H., Chemaitelly, H., Seedat, S., Mumtaz, G. R., Omari, S. A., & Abu-Raddad, L. J. (2020). Epidemiological impact of SARS-CoV-2 vaccination: Mathematical modeling analyses. *Vaccines, 8*(4), 668–668. https://doi.org/10.3390/vaccines8040668.
32. Marmot, M. (2005). Social determinants of health inequalities. https://core.ac.uk/download/1669331.pdf (accessed on 7 May 2025).
33. Murray, C. J. L., Ikuta, K. S., Sharara, F., Swetschinski, L. R., Robles Aguilar, G., Gray, A. P., Han, C., et al. (2022). Global burden of bacterial antimicrobial resistance in 2019: A systematic analysis. *The Lancet, 399*, 629–655. https://doi.org/10.1016/S0140-6736(21)02724-0.
34. Myrvang, B., & Newport, M. J. (2009). Proceedings of a joint meeting held between the Norwegian Society of Infectious Diseases and the Royal Society of Tropical Medicine and Hygiene, Oslo, 20th June 2008. *Transactions of the Royal Society of Tropical Medicine and Hygiene, 103*(4), 321–324. https://doi.org/10.1016/j.trstmh.2008.11.010.
35. Nagtegaal, I. D., Odze, R. D., Klimstra, D. S., Paradis, V., Rugge, M., Schirmacher, P., Washington, K., et al. (2019). The 2019 WHO classification of tumors of the digestive system. *Histopathology, 76*(2), 182–188. https://doi.org/10.1111/his.13975.
36. Naidoo, S., & Naidoo, N. (2025). Depression's double-edged impact on body mass index: A hidden catalyst for non-communicable diseases in South Africa's aging population in long-term care facilities. *PLOS ONE, 20*. https://www.semanticscholar.org/paper/3258f3d4c85f330cfc42481bde8987c956fa7bac (accessed on 7 May 2025).
37. Ndao, M. (2009). Diagnosis of parasitic diseases: Old and new approaches. *Interdisciplinary Perspectives on Infectious Diseases, 2009*, 278246. https://doi.org/10.1155/2009/278246.
38. Nissanova, R., Orynbaev, M., Bashenova, E., Nakhanov, A., Mamanova, S., Akshalova, P., Baidavletov, E., et al. (2025). Wild boar infections and parasites, risks for veterinary medicine and public health. *Микробиология және вирусология*. https://www.semanticscholar.org/pa

per/38aec936497f05ec712b318258810ba09383c5cf (accessed on 7 May 2025).

39. Patel, A., & Jernigan, D. B. (2020). Initial public health response and interim clinical guidance for the 2019 novel coronavirus outbreak—United States. *American Journal of Transplantation, 20*, 889–895. https://doi.org/10.1111/ajt.15805.

40. Peeri, N. C., Shrestha, N., Rahman, M. S., Zaki, R. A., Tan, Z., Bibi, S., Baghbanzadeh, M., et al. (2020). The SARS, MERS, and novel coronavirus (COVID-19) epidemics, the newest and biggest global health threats: What lessons have we learned? *International Journal of Epidemiology, 49*(3), 717–726. https://doi.org/10.1093/ije/dyaa033.

41. Perestiuk, V. O., Kosovska, T., Volianska, L., & Boyarchuk, O. (2025). Association of zinc deficiency and clinical symptoms, inflammatory markers, severity of COVID-19 in hospitalized children. *Frontiers in Nutrition, 12*. https://www.semanticscholar.org/paper/2001864437a63d537d52e575d79ad5c33f22f2cb (accessed on 7 May 2025).

42. Program on Human Rights and the Global Economy. (2010). Modes and patterns of social control: Implications for human rights policy. *Human Rights & the Global Economy eJournal*. https://www.semanticscholar.org/paper/757ca43d6914cf9732a9b9a8e5f29047af6b8ebd (accessed on 7 May 2025).

43. Rocha, I. V., Bezerra, M. F., Sobreira, M., & de Almeida, A. M. D. (2025). 125 years of the plague in Brazil: Lessons learnt, historical insights, and contemporary challenges. *Memórias do Instituto Oswaldo Cruz, 120*. https://www.semanticscholar.org/paper/6ffa80a2745f156903e40b6312faa3ce01018c40 (accessed on 7 May 2025).

44. Satcher, D. (1995). Emerging infections: Getting ahead of the curve. *Emerging Infectious Diseases, 1*(1), 1–6. https://doi.org/10.3201/eid0101.950101.

45. Shereen, M. A., Khan, S., Kazmi, A., Bashir, N., & Siddique, R. (2020). COVID-19 infection: Emergence, transmission, and characteristics of human coronaviruses. *Journal of Advanced Research, 24*, 91–98. https://doi.org/10.1016/j.jare.2020.03.005.

46. Siame, S., Bygvraa, D. A., Hulse, L. M., Mouchtouri, V., & Hadjichristodoulou, C. (2025). Factors influencing the occurrence of infectious diseases among crew members on board cruise ships: A systematic review. *International Maritime Health, 76*(1), 63–70. https://www.semanticscholar.org/paper/17d5931745210a4526be2a7415a464087e9f5d66 (accessed on 7 May 2025).

47. Spaziante, M., Leone, S., D'Amato, M., De Carli, G., Tonziello, G., Malatesta, G. N., Agresta, A., et al. (2025). Interrupted time series analysis to evaluate the impact of COVID-19 pandemic on the incidence of notifiable infectious diseases in the Lazio region, Italy. *BMC Public Health, 25*. https://www.semanticscholar.org/paper/dbf9b11317873073d2548d9bdcf3eccfd442664a (accessed on 7 May 2025).

48. Srivastava, V., Kumar, R., Wani, M. Y., Robinson, K., & Ahmad, A. (2024). Role of artificial intelligence in early diagnosis and treatment of infectious diseases. *Infectious Diseases*. https://www.semanticscholar.org/paper/778e1cc1cce627e48a9d9c5aa1b6cf844be68b94 (accessed on 7 May 2025).

49. Straburzyński, M., & Romaszko-Wojtowicz, A. (2024). Comparison of sinonasal symptoms in upper respiratory tract infections during the infectious diseases season of November 2023 to March 2024—A cross-sectional study. *Frontiers in Medicine, 11*. https://www.semanticscholar.org/paper/e526cfb0a2bc442b72c65a7eb8ad65d83bc39486 (accessed on 7 May 2025).

50. Todd, K. (2014). The promising viral threat to bacterial resistance: The uncertain patentability of phage therapeutics and the necessity of alternative incentives. *Duke Law Journal, 68*, 767–805. https://core.ac.uk/download/213020895.pdf (accessed on 7 May 2025).

51. Voet, S., Srinivasan, S., Lamkanfi, M., & Loo, G. (2019). Inflammasomes in neuroinflammatory and neurodegenerative diseases. *EMBO Molecular Medicine, 11, e10248*. https://doi.org/10.15252/emmm.201810248.

52. Wearing, H. J., Keeling, M. J., Rohani, P., & Ellner, S. P. (2005). Appropriate models for the management of infectious diseases. *PLOS Medicine, 2*(7), e174. https://core.ac.uk/download/44114.pdf (accessed on 7 May 2025).

53. Zampieri, F. (2018). Rise and fall of Achille de Giovanni's clinical anthropometry. *Society and Politics, 12*(1), 66–80. https://core.ac.uk/download/157767229.pdf (accessed on 7 May 2025).

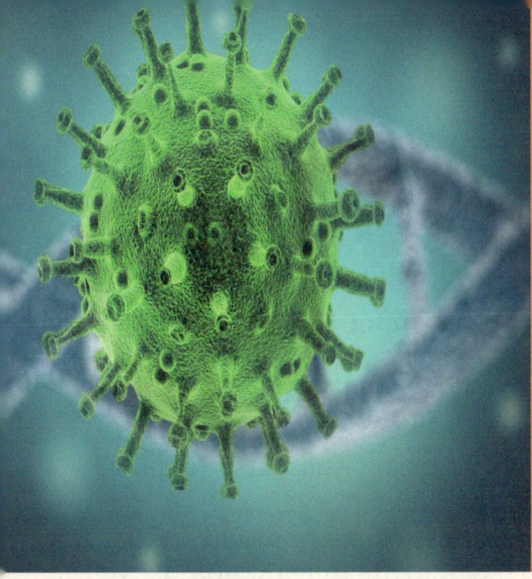

Chapter 2

MICROBIAL PATHOGENESIS AND HOST INTERACTIONS

Contents

Introduction

If we consider the mechanism by which microbes induce disease, it's a two-way mess of interactions between the tiny invaders and the hosts they infect. It's not simply a matter of finding the microbes; rather, you need to go back and investigate how there is a day-to-day give-and-take that ultimately results in health or sickness. In general, both the microbe's deadly equipment and the host's immune defenses define this balance, so it's not so hard to see that knowing about this interaction is central to understanding how diseases progress. New pathogens continue to emerge while resistant strains make a surprising resurgence, which usually indicates why combining host and microbe dynamics into contemporary studies can sharpen our concepts for treatment and prevention. At the core of it all is the notion that disease never really comes down to cause-and-effect—it's more a tug-of-war between the offensive tactics of a microbe and the counterattacks of the body. The damage-response paradigm, for example, has become a kind of standard by considering disease in the unorganized context of host–pathogen interactions, where the extent of damage itself provides a quantifiable indication of what is transpiring. terms, this model pushes researchers to consider more than merely concentrating on the bug; rather, it encourages them to take into consideration such factors as the immune status of the host and even the number of microbes. By doing so, this viewpoint facilitates the opening up of new research strategies and therapeutic concepts toward the goal of reestablishing a rough balance in host–microbe interactions (Nosanchuk, 2025). Aside from the glaring infections, the daily interaction between hosts and microbes overflows into quieter parts of our body's ecosystem—particularly in congested areas like the gut. Dysbiosis, or an out-of-balance microbiota, has been associated with chronic inflammatory issues like inflammatory bowel disease, where the frequently complex communicating between cells and microbes appears to induce and forge the sickness. In general, advances in multi-omics approaches have taken our understanding beyond, providing fine-grained views of microbial communities, active genetic processes, and even their metabolic outputs. When you put all this information together, you get a more complete picture of host–pathogen cross-talk that eventually broadens the scope of microbial pathogenesis research from single microbes to the whole microbial community and their constant interaction with the host (Su et al., 2025) (Figure 2.1).

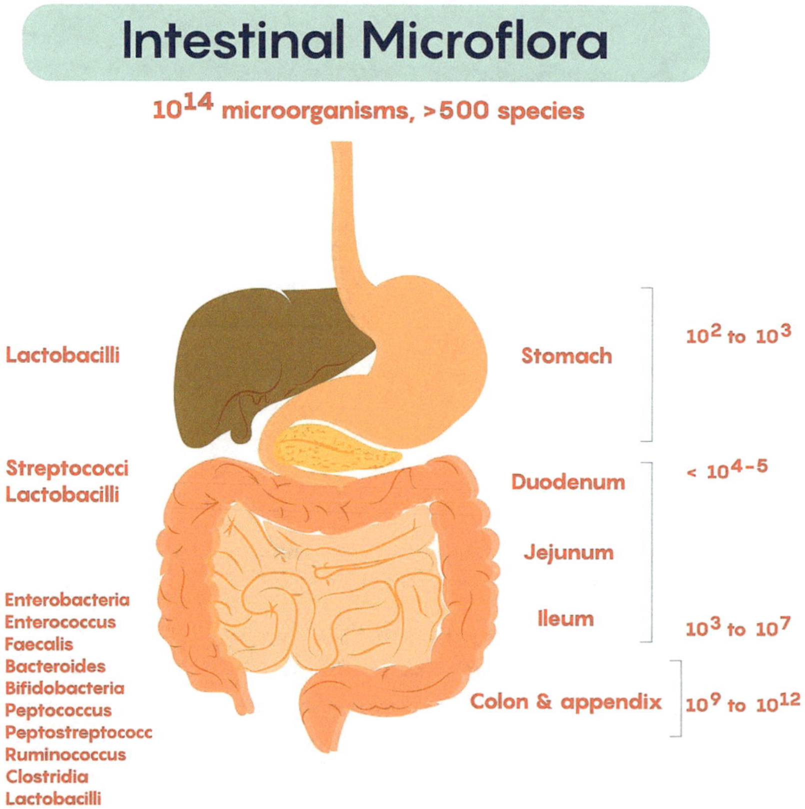

Figure 2.1. The microbial pathogenesis and host interactions.

Source: By Dr William Ju, University of Toronto - http://neuroscience.openetext.utoronto.ca/chapter/chapter-1-the-gut-microbiome-and-its-impact-on-the-brain/, CC BY 4.0, https://commons.wikimedia.org/w/index.php?curid=139935345

Definition of Microbial Pathogenesis

Microbes and their hosts share a tangled relationship that isn't easy to pin down. To really get what's going on, you've got to dive into microbial pathogenesis—a term that wraps up everything from harmless colonization to serious tissue damage, elves; it's also about how what they do meshes up with our body's defenses. Some pathogens sneak in, dodge immune attacks, and even siphon off our resources, eventually sparking the full cascade of disease. When you look closer, you see these microbial groups can also alter reproductive functions and overall fitness in both sexes—a continuous, complex web of interactions rather than a simple on/off switch (Rowe et al., 2020). To summarize, molecular and ecological scales, microbes pull off a variety of clever moves. In many cases, some of them directly mess with cell processes by pumping out enzymes and metabolites that throw off normal function—think of it as a kind of hyperparasitism or antibiosis. Then there are those that, without physically bumping into the target pathogens, nudge the host's resistance by inducing or priming immune responses. You might notice these actions unfold as a string of loosely regulated metabolic events right in specific micro-environments of the host. Essentially, it isn't just about unleashing toxins; it's a coordinated, if sometimes unique, combination of biological interactions and environmental factors that we need to grasp if we're going to tackle diseases effectively. Traditional ideas pinned microbial pathogenesis solely on harmful pathogen-host clashes, yet these days it's clear microbes play a far richer role. Many of these tiny organisms coexist with us in supportive, even symbiotic, ways—contributing to our development, overall physiology, and yes, even our reproduction. This broader view challenges the old notion of microbes as just troublemakers, highlighting the importance of context in shaping their effects. Take the reproductive microbiome, for instance—microbial communities in reproductive tissues can influence sexual selection, host fitness, and maybe even nudge evolutionary paths. To summarize, it turns out that understanding microbial pathogenesis means looking at a whole tapestry of interactions between host, microbe, and ever-changing environmental conditions (Rowe et al., 2020) (Figure 2.2).

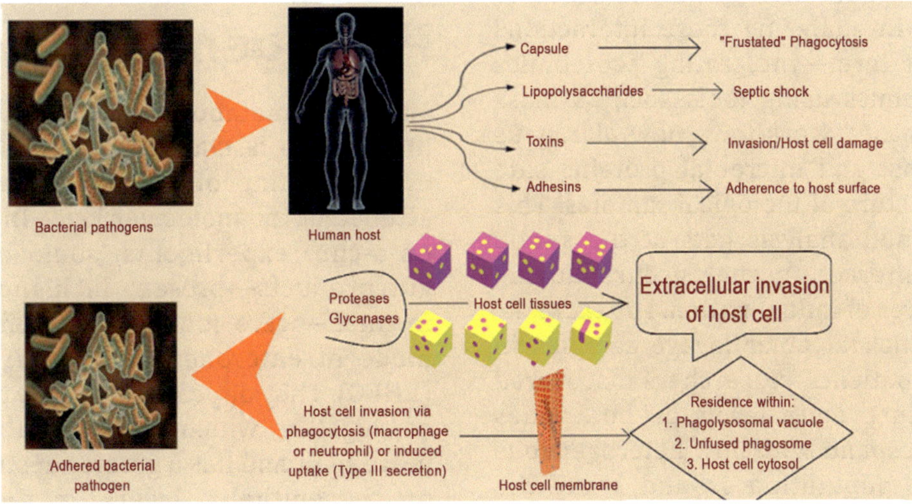

Figure 2.2. Stages of microbial pathogenesis: The bacterial components.

Source: Devi, S. (2023). *Stages of Microbial Pathogenesis: The Bacterial Components.*

Importance of Studying Host Interactions

The relationship between microbes and their hosts is rather interesting—It's not only that pathogens invade alone but also that they are part of this complex, dynamic interaction with our immune systems. Rather than believing in microbial pathogenesis as something isolated, think about how these tiny microbes and our defenses are constantly adapting to each other. In general, observing how microbes and hosts interact provides us with hints as to how invaders evade our natural defenses, establish themselves, and initiate disease. Consider the gut microbiota, for example; our small intestinal friends have been more and more recognized for their ability to fine-tune both metabolism and immune responses, particularly in cases such as acute myeloid leukemia (AML) (Nowicka & Gil, 2024). Studies even suggest that the chemicals synthesized by microbes could sometimes accelerate or even retard disease advancement at times. All of this implies that exploring these host-microbe interactions could unlock therapies that act by subtly tipping that balance. New technology has taken us to the next level in analyzing these interactions at a molecular level—integrating proteomics with metagenomics using tools such as mass spectrometry-based workflows now allows us to visualize host and microbial proteins side by side in a mixture of biological samples. This type of combined analysis gets at the subtle biochemical interaction that occurs during infection or flares of inflammation. For example, examining bronchoalveolar lavage samples in cystic fibrosis patients, researchers discovered that changes in protein levels on both sides appear to correspond with how heterogeneous the microbial population is and what the status of the disease appears to be (Kruk et al., 2024). These approaches not only facilitate easier identification of the nefarious players responsible for an infection but also shine a light on when the host's own reactions get a little out of hand, revealing a richer and sometimes surprising picture of how the disease functions. In terms of successful treatment, getting a handle on the dynamic between hosts and their microbial inhabitants is an important piece of the puzzle. An individual's immune status and the composition of microbes they carry can powerfully influence how effective treatments are, particularly in situations where immune issues or microbial imbalances are involved. Dysbiosis, an upset in the typical microbial community, has, for instance, been associated with increased infections and poorer prognosis in AML patients (Nowicka & Gil, 2024). Equally, entering the space of host and microbial protein mixture in airway disease presents new opportunities for treatments that are response and pathogen-specific (Kruk et al., 2024). Overall, understanding these interactions not only enhances our foundational comprehension of microbial pathogenesis but also pushes us toward precision medicine that addresses the gritty messiness of host biology.

2.1. Mechanisms of Pathogenicity

Microbial metabolites added to host tissues introduce a fascinating new dimension to our understanding of how bacterial behavior is attuned at the molecular level. In recent organ-on-a-chip experiments, some of the human gut products—present in higher levels than in mice—were found to influence the attack mode of enterohemorrhagic *Escherichia coli* (EHEC). They appear to increase the production of flagellin, which is essential for bacterial movement and has a greater destructive impact on the epithelial layers. In the majority of instances, this species distinction illustrates how such compounds render the pathogens more virulent and are directly responsible for more severe infections in individuals. It also nudges us to consider new treatment approaches; by alteraltering these microbe-derived chemicals, we might lower the risk of infection (Tovaglieri et al., 2019). Overall, this chemical interplay in our microbiome plays a big part in steering bacterial virulence. Beyond the gut, microbes also hang around on our skin, where they help keep the barrier strong and stop invaders from settling in. The balance between commensal (or friendly, for that matter) insects and pathological ones such as *Staphylococcus aureus* is not a specific one, it shifts and occasionally veers in directions that influence disease outcomes. Commensal bacteria quietly modulate our fundamental and specialized immune responses, slowing down the development of pathogens and even stymying conditions such as atopic dermatitis (AD). When the microbial diversity of the skin declines, these conditions worsen. A few initial clinical trials employing topical doses of friendly bacteria even suggest a promising means of strengthening our own defense system against colonization (Paller et al., 2018). In brief, the actions of these microbes rely on a combination of competitive and cooperative relationships between the societies that reside within our body. When infections begin, the process is an complex one involving both bacterial components and our immune response, all of which are shaped by early microbial experiences. In infants, the initial wave of skin-colonizing microbes plays a dominant role in how the immune system learns its equilibrium. For instance, regulatory T cells activated within those initial days assist the body in accepting its resident microbes while suppressing excessive inflammation. If this first encounter is delayed or goes wrong, it could trigger an immune reaction that sets the stage for greater inflammation and easier bacterial invasion. Further, some molecules produced by skin bacteria appear to engage innate immune receptors, dialing up or down inflammation, and directly determining how nasty a pathogen can be. In essence, pathogenicity is not simply a matter of the bacteria's own weaponry—the timing and character of our early immune dialogues with these microbes are also very important, and propose new possibilities for perhaps preventing or minimizing bad infections (Paller et al., 2018) (Figure 2.3).

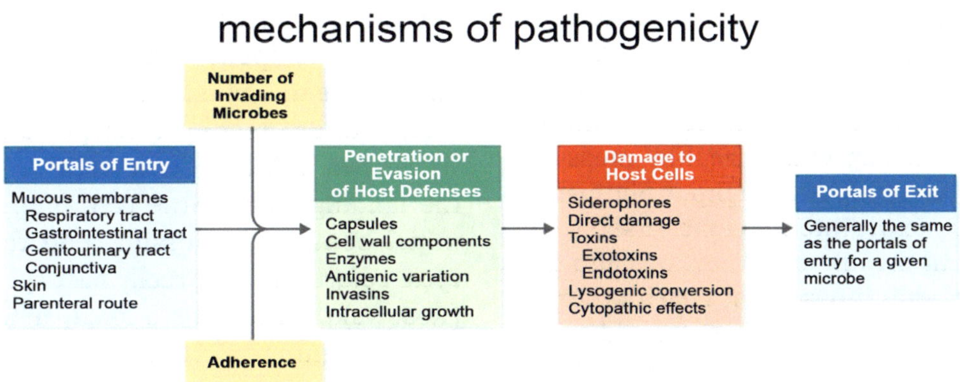

Figure 2.3. Mechanisms of pathogenicity.

Source: SlideServe. (n.d.). *Mechanisms of Pathogenicity.*

2.1.1. Adherence to Host Cells

Pathogens start an infection by attaching themselves to host cells – a kind of initial greeting that typically paves the way for colonization and subsequent disease. They do this with peculiar, specialized structures such as pili, fimbriae, and adhesins that locate and bind to specific receptors that are distributed on the cell membrane. This type of specific binding usually results in the microbes getting into tissues that are somehow just right for them so they can survive a hostile world. It isn't just a physical anchor, either; occasionally that initial contact initiates a cascade of signals within the cell that can, most of the time, adjust immune defenses in favor of these intruders. When you factor in that a host's genetic profile may tip the balance of how likely these microbes are to persist (Rosowski, 2023), it comes back to really just how interconnected microbial strategies and host defense may be. Essentially, these findings point toward novel mechanisms for getting in ahead of the infection – disrupting that attachment could well prevent the infection from gaining purchase. Unraveling the complex specifics of bacterial sticking requires new, sometimes unorthodox approaches. Instead of adhering to aged, time-consuming tests that are as unreliable as they are time-consuming, scientists now employ automated systems to test bacterial sticking with a healthy measure of precision. These high-throughput platforms, which move experiments fast, assist in identifying both the microbial portions and the host receptors that interact with each other in adhesion. There are times when the old ways of doing assays just can't keep up with it all, so these new instruments allow researchers to see anything from the smallest molecular link to large cell-to-cell interactions. In a sense, these strategies untangle that subtle symphony between the microbes' sticky components and host cell surfaces – an important step toward devising brighter antimicrobial tactics against initial infection. .

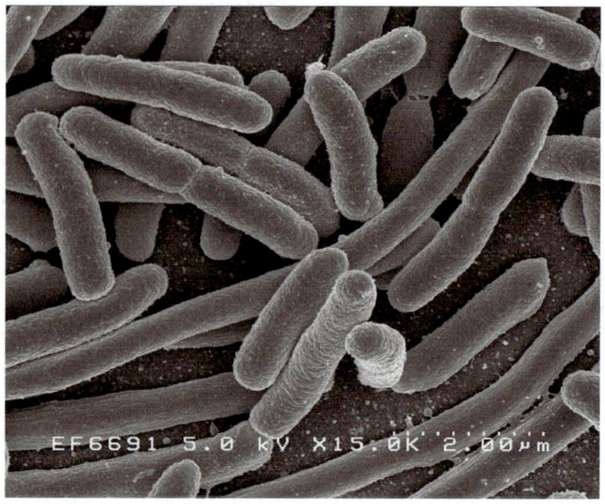

Figure 2.4. Host cell.

Source: By NIAID - E. coli Bacteria, Public Domain, https://commons.wikimedia.org/w/index.php?curid=39933215.

Adhering to a host isn't merely the first move; it tends to initiate subsequent actions such as biofilm accumulation, immune avoidance, or even deeper invasion. Once microbes adhere, they may create protective groups or turn the host's own signaling pathways upside down to shield themselves from immune attacks, thereby making their visit longer. That initial adhesion not only provides the pathogen with a physical hold but also opens a strategic window for it to manipulate the cellular terrain. All of this is why scientists are testing concepts on interfering with these sticking structures or on blocking the landing pads of the cell. Interrupting that initial bond could possibly end the infectious cycle before anything really nasty gets underway (Rosowski, 2023). It's a small detail, perhaps, but preventing microbes from sticking might be a watershed moment in our battle against infectious disease (Figure 2.4)

2.1.2. Invasion Strategies Employed by Pathogens

Pathogens tend to move in and establish residence within a host, primarily by outwitting the defenses of the body. They get things started by sticking to tissues—hanging onto stuff like pili, fimbriae, and adhesins with which to attach to receptors—simply for evading mechanical clearance. Once they're stuck, they proceed to bypass the epithelial barrier. For instance, certain bacteria sort of deceive the host into ingesting them by manipulating its cell skeleton, whereas others resort to an enzyme assault—releasing, for instance, hyaluronidases to degrade the extracellular matrix so they can slide through. In most instances, these tactics allow pathogens to slip into safer niches where they can proliferate, all the while avoiding early immune alarms. It's a strange dance at the host-pathogen interface that truly flaunts just how complex microbial pathogenesis is (Pandey, 2024). Once they breach the first line of defense, these microbes then encounter the unforgiving terrain of body tissues and immune reactions. Most of them secrete virulence factors that interfere with phagocytosis or allow them to survive within phagocytic cells, effectively avoiding immune clearance. Intracellular pathogens tend to become sneaky, hijacking the host cell's functions to evade lysosomal breakdown and even utilizing the host cell's own resources for propagation. Additionally, certain bacteria secrete toxins that disrupt cellular junctions, enabling them to penetrate further into tissues and even throughout the body systemically. This phase of spreading is quite pivotal—it's typically associated with an increase in pathogenicity and disease exacerbation. In a bit of back-and-forth, the interaction between these invasion stunts and the host's immune retaliation determines the end game of the infection, highlighting how crucial it is to truly understand these molecular interactions (Pandey, 2024). Our immune system, shaped over decades of socializing with millions of microbes, becomes both a barrier and an opportunity for invaders. The microbiota, of course, has its role to play in shaping our defenses against infection—and pathogens sometimes must navigate around or even warp these reactions. In typically speaking genetically predisposed individuals, when microbial balance goes haywire, the body's defense may get slightly slack, leading the way for opportunistic infections to fill in. In a few instances, microbes even take advantage of an overactive or uncontrolled immune response to establish long-term infections. As research continues, understanding precisely how pathogens hijack these sophisticated host-microbe interactions should serve to galvanize novel therapies that rebuild healthy immunity and repel invasions.

2.1.3. Evasion of Host Immune Responses

Microbial pathogens have developed some clever means of evading our immune system and persisting long enough to produce chronic problems. One big trick they employ is to interfere with the local community of microbes, which then upsets the way our defenses would otherwise function.

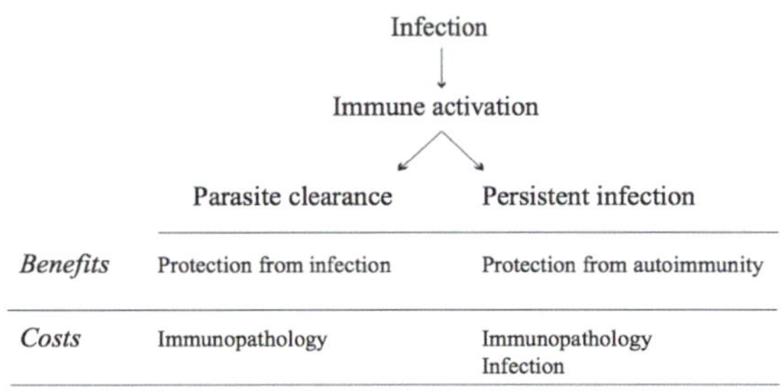

Figure 2.5. Evasion of host immune responses.

Source: Sorci G, Cornet S, Faivre B. Immune Evasion, Immunopathology and the Regulation of the Immune System. *Pathogens*. 2013; 2(1):71-91. https://doi.org/10.3390/pathogens2010071

Consider the chaos in our oral biofilms, say: when the normal balance is disrupted, pathogens such as *Porphyromonas gingivalis* and *Tannerella forsythia* can proliferate out of control and cast a monkey wrench into both our immediate and acquired immune responses. These bacteria produce chemicals that degrade the signal molecules our body relies on and even destabilize neutrophil function—so defeating invaders becomes much more difficult. In a turn of events that could sound quite strange, this chronic inflammation not only causes damage to tissues but somehow produces an area where these microbes may live.

2.2. Types of Pathogens

Microscopic pathogens responsible for disease exist in a wide range of shapes, and you have to examine how various pathogens play havoc with a host's internal mechanisms. Viruses, bacteria, fungi, protozoa, and helminths all have their own uniqueness to bring to the party—each with distinctive characteristics that determine how much damage they can do and how they are transmitted. Consider viruses: they depend virtually solely on the cells of the host to replicate themselves, frequently provoking immune responses that contribute to the overall condition. Bacteria, inherently prokaryotic and sometimes a wanderer or even in a type of cooperation, contain strains that invade tissue or produce toxins disrupting normal body function. These diverse behaviors don't just impact clinical outcomes but also fashion the day-to-day, dynamic interactions between our bodies and those nasty microbes.

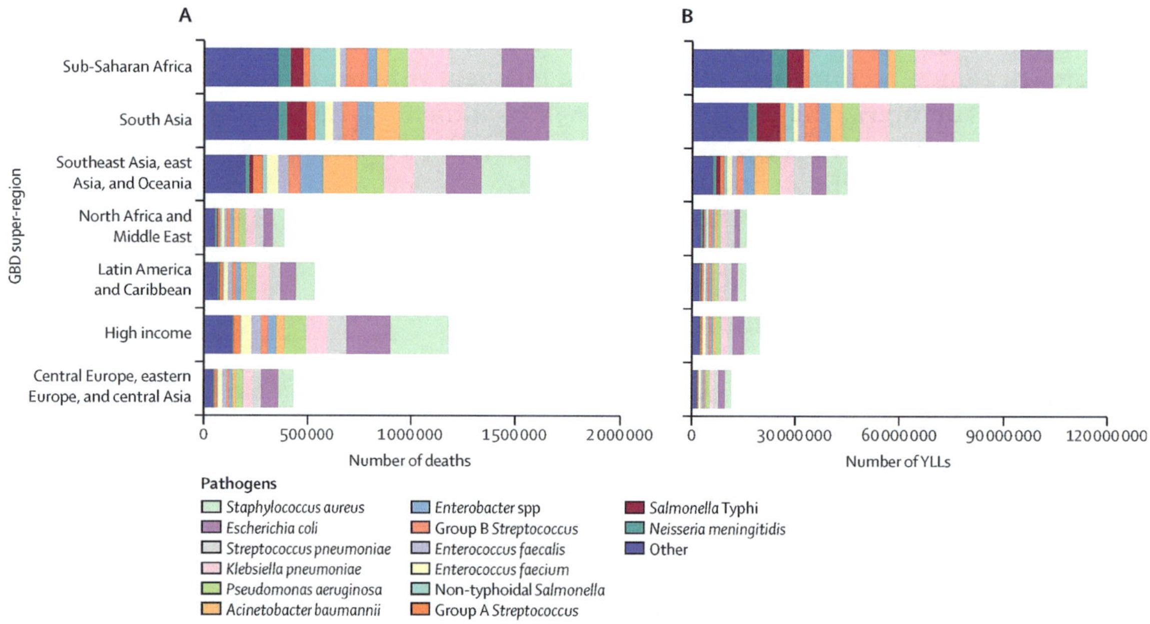

Figure 2.6. Types of pathogens.

Source: By Authors of the study: GBD 2019 Antimicrobial Resistance Collaborators - https://www.thelancet.com/journals/lancet/article/PIIS0140-6736(22)02185-7/fulltext, CC BY 4.0, https://commons.wikimedia.org/w/index.php?curid=127577217 SlideServe. (n.d.). *Types of Pathogens.*

Fungi and protozoa add even more complexity to the big picture. For the most part, fungi—being eukaryotic and often opportunistic—can penetrate epithelial barriers, particularly when a person's defenses are compromised, and they produce infections that may very well remain superficial or become systemic. Protozoa, variable single-celled organisms, tend to employ ruses such as switching surface proteins to evade immune detection and persist longer. Both kinds can affect and, conversely, be influenced by the host's own microbiota and immune systems. In most instances, the chemicals released by our gut residents tend to regulate the intestinal barrier and immune activity, something researchers have noted in several studies (Ghosh et al., 2021). Helminths, the bigger parasitic worms, provide yet another spin by frequently modulating the immune system in the long term. Not only do they function to destabilize our immune defenses to survive but sometimes even provide small regulatory advantages, forming conditions of tolerance and imbalance. This tug-of-war between our immune system and the microbes, including those quietly dwelling in us, highlights the role of variables such as genetics and our surroundings in determining the trajectory of an infection. With scientists ongoingly unscrambling these complex dynamics—and, let's be honest, sometimes muddling through in the process—there's hope that future treatments will also address the host's immune configuration (Zheng et al., 2020). Ultimately, classification of pathogens based on how they respond to us continues to be an important step in furthering our knowledge about disease and designing new treatment strategies (Figure 2.6).

2.2.1. Bacterial Pathogens and Their Characteristics

Bacterial interactions with their hosts demonstrate a complexcomplex association—guided by an extensive history of evolution in which both parties continue to push back. Bacteria have acquired some quite specific tools that allow them to colonize tissues, evade immune defenses, and just hang around. They may construct slimy biofilms, splash out toxins, or even manipulate the host's immune signals to their own advantage. In most instances, opportunistic perpetrators such as those within the *Burkholderia cepacia* complex yield a variety of outcomes, and cells such as macrophages become busy little centers for bacterial growth and inflammatory triggers. Experiments with zebrafish models have, in most cases, allowed us to see these processes in real-time, visualizing bacteria and innate immunity within an active, living environment (Gomes et al., 2019). Obviously, these bacterial characteristics aren't static—they shift with the host's own environment. Looking at the host's internal ecosystem, the composition and balance of gut microbes truly emerge in the role of how pathogenic bacteria can be. A person's gut community behaves like an ecological armor, managing nutrient processing, maintaining the integrity of the gut lining, and even modulating immune responses.

And when this balance gets a little out of whack—what we tend to refer to as dysbiosis—it sometimes opens the door to infections, as the usual microbial crowd loses its ability to keep invaders at bay. Early life and daily routines both cast a long shadow on how this microbial combination ends up, putting a personal spin on the host-microbe relationship (Rinninella et al., 2019). In this dirty microbial universe, bacteria need to adapt or overwhelm the local defenses, something important to grasp to make therapies that rebalance these essential communities and strengthen host defenses. Bacterial adroit truly comes into view when you look at how they deal with the body's first responders such as phagocytes and the mechanisms that activate the inflammasome. Some bacteria even hijack cells such as macrophages and neutrophils—either by compromising their capacity to kill or by entering and exploiting them as sheltering sites to avoid clearance and spread further. Mycobacterium species, for example, have been seen distorting the granuloma formation process to survive longer, whereas *Staphylococcus aureus* can efficiently hijack phagocytes to evade immune assault. Minutepositive alterations in the bacterial cell envelope or modifications of second messenger machinery further demonstrate ways these microorganisms avoid immune surveillance, exhibiting biochemical acumen difficult to disregard (Gomes et al., 2019). Throw in the concepts of trained innate immunity and host epigenetic changes, and you have a battleground that is constantly in flux where both bacterial strategy and host response continue to change, ultimately dictating how infections establish themselves and progress.

2.2.2. Viral Pathogens and Their Modes of Action

Viruses in the body don't simply drift around—they engage in a complexcomplex association with our cells. You can see that when you consider how viral portions and host cell processes combine in unexpected combinations. Consider influenza, for instance; its infectivity largely depends on the uniqueness of its hemagglutinin protein. Different strains need different pH levels to get going, and those that activate at higher pH tend to break into a wider variety of cells—this is one reason why strains like H5 and H7 can be extra aggressive.

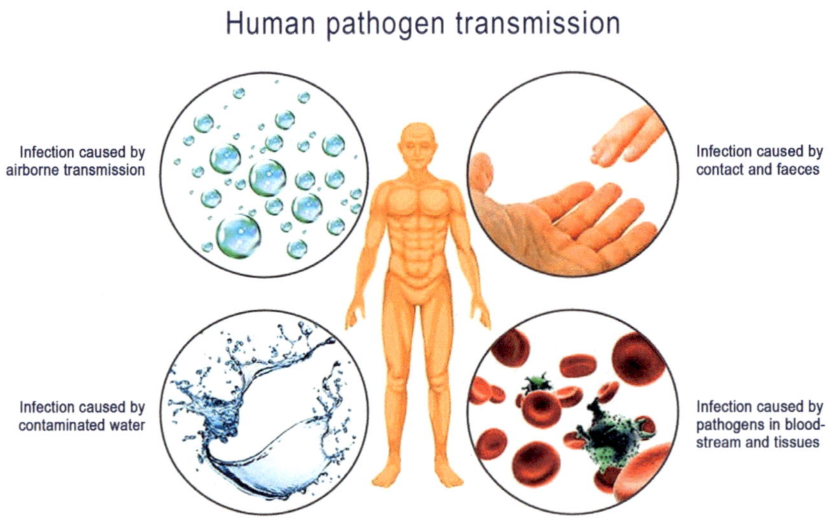

Figure 2.7. Mode of transmission and main portal of pathogens.

Source: Blogger. (n.d.). *Mode of Transmission and Main Portal of Pathogens.*

Hepatitis C, of course, sticks around somehow by attacking the lymph system, keeping the immune system revved up all the time and, in the long run, producing tissue damage well beyond where it first entered (Takamura, 2017). The body's immune reaction isn't one-size-fits-all protection—it can be a two-edged sword. Epithelial cells, macrophages, dendritic cells and other such players are constantly on the lookout, employing receptors to pick up even the slightest hint of a virus. When they pick up any viral signal, a chain reaction begins, releasing cytokines and initiating inflammation. To summarize, this reaction requires a delicate balance: too many cytokines tend to intensify tissue damage, while too few may allow the virus to wreak havoc. Also, the adaptive component—with the CD4 helper T cells and the tissue-resident memory T cells—is called upon to organize a more targeted cleanup, particularly in areas such as the bronchus-associated regions where localized immune centers produce high-affinity B cells and sustain antibody production (Takamura, 2017). Current drug strategies are beginning to flip the script, calling for an emphasis not only on the virus but on host factors that it depends upon. Older antimicrobial therapies addressed just viral enzymes or structures, but emerging resistance has made that an increasingly harder fight. Currently, reassigning attention to the host—by aiming for the central interactions that allow viruses to penetrate cells—has caught on. Scientists are using genome-wide scans and proteomic analysis to identify host targets that could be targeted with new drugs, a step that could reduce the threat of resistance over time. Combining classic antiviral meds with host-targeted therapies may just increase efficacy and knock down chronic infections. In all, this new approach to therapy is a more sophisticated understanding of the host–virus relationship, boundary-pushing in therapy design, albeit with some natural, human-like errors (Figure 2.7).

2.2.3. Fungal and Parasitic Pathogens

Fungal and parasitic infections truly highlight the give-and-take struggle that occurs between our immune defenses and microbial evasion strategies. You see, these microbes have, over the years, developed sneaky tricks to evade detection, and one of the major players here is interleukin-17 (IL-17). For the most part, IL-17 comes in to mobilize proinflammatory molecules that keep these nasty invaders in check, but—ironically—it can also cause excessive inflammation. This overreaction, in most instances, could result in tissue damage and persistent inflammation, making a protective response one that hinders healing. In short, IL-17 emphasizes that delicate balance where protection by the immune system can sometimes tip over into damage (Das et al., 2017). As for the genetic aspect of things, new research has shed light on the evolutionary pathways that shape fungal pathogenicity, particularly within Onygenales. Consider fungi such as *Histoplasma capsulatum* and Coccidioides species, not just do they live, they evolve to fit their mammalian host host-like.

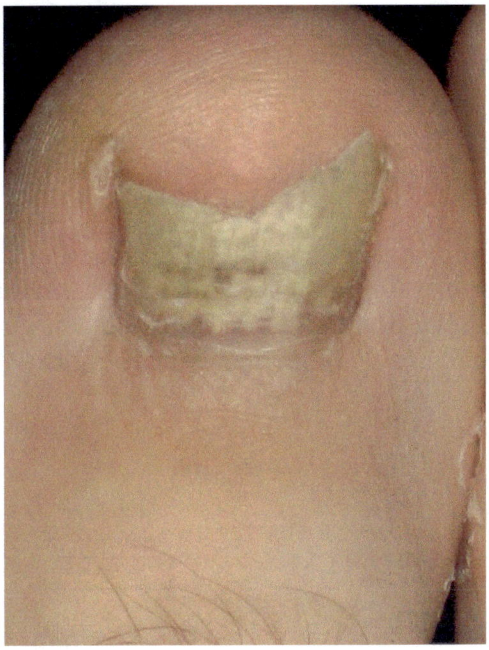

Figure 2.8. Fungal infections.

Source: By Medguy at English Wikipedia - Transferred from en.wikipedia to Commons., Public Domain, https://commons.wikimedia.org/w/index.php?curid=7678638.

Comparative genome sequencing, which examines both pathogenic and nonpathogenic relatives, has revealed unexpected trends of gene family reduction and expansion. Mostly, such patterns contain specialized clusters in pathogenic Coccidioides spp., which are associated with certain phases like the formation of endospores that enhance their virulence. On the whole, this genomic plasticity allows fungi to decipher methods of exploiting their host's vulnerability and evade immune attacks, providing greater insights into the molecular underpinnings of fungal pathogenesis (Taylor & Whiston, 2015). Parasites, too, add to the mix by subtly turning the tables in their favor. Unlike many bacteria and viruses, they often settle in for the long haul by alteraltering the host's immune system just enough to avoid clearance without causing too much collateral damage—after all, they don't want to wreck their own habitat. This is a devious strategy that entails a variety of adaptations, from changing surface proteins (antigenic variation) to interfering with cytokine signals such as those from IL-17. The host reacts by increasing proinflammatory mediators, trying to clear the intruders while maintaining inflammation under control. All of this creates a picture of a constantly developing evolutionary arms race that ends up determining how bad an infection could get and how it propagates between people (Das et al., 2017) (Figure 2.8).

2.3. Host Immune Response

The tango between the living host and invading microbes depends on the efficiency with which the immune system balances taking out intruders without harming its own tissues. When the balance is lost, the body either will not be able to knock out the pathogen or will overdo it and harm its own cells as well, further worsening the disease.

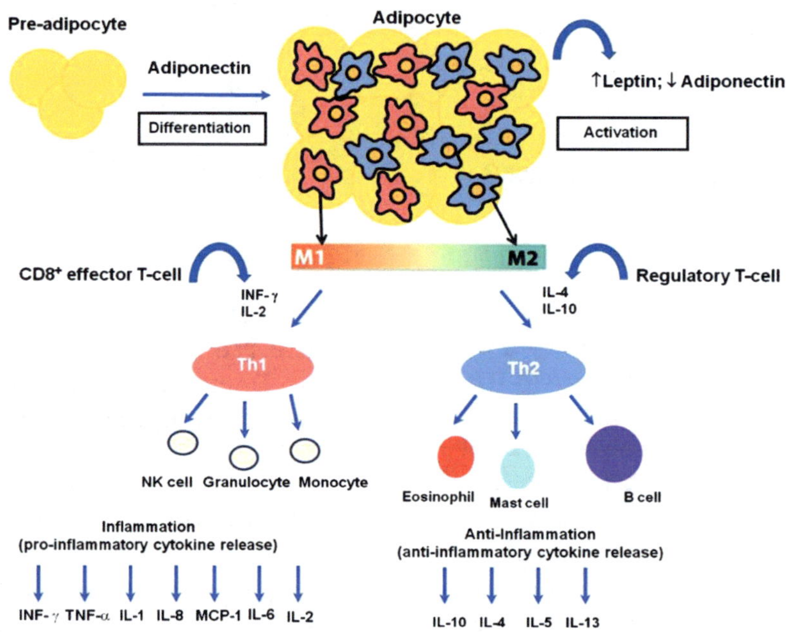

Figure 2.9. The human host immune response to a variety of inflammatory states.

Source: Kim, S. K. (2015). *The Human Host Immune Response to a Variety of Inflammatory States.*

You can observe this two-edged problem in fungal infections – individuals with a compromised immune system can't mount an adequate defense, allowing the fungus to run rampant. But when the immune response gets out of hand, it induces inflammation that damages the host, illustrating just how delicate balancing this act is. Examining these interactions with the use of tools such as the damage response framework (DRF) provides us a glimpse of how our defenses guard us but, at times, harm us by accident (Pruksaphon et al., 2024).

The immune work of the body doesn't end with just killing harmful invaders; it also plays an enormous role in maintaining a cordial relationship with the microbes that naturally reside on us, particularly in areas such as the gut. Innate immunity is not just about destroying bad microbes, it assists in maintaining tolerance towards our resident microbiota, allowing the intestine to function properly.

When dysbiosis occurs and microbial diversity is reduced, this equilibrium is disrupted and can open the door for inflammatory conditions like inflammatory bowel disease (IBD). In these cases, abnormal immune function against microbes in the gut results in ongoing inflammation and tissue damage, demonstrating once more how changes in the microbial community can wildly impact our body's responses and the disease process as a whole (Fu et al., 2024).

When treating microbial diseases with treatments designed to target the host immune response, the need is to tread an extremely fine line. Overall, clinicians attempt to soothe the destructive inflammation without losing the ability to expel the intruders—a delicate balancing act. In a majority of situations, the definition of discrete virulence factors and critical immune messages has led to immunomodulatory therapies (yes, even the occasional typo) that will reset the immune system. By combining our knowledge of microbial mayhem with host defense mechanisms, these approaches are designed not only to suppress the infection but also to reconstitute a normal, healthy immune state, which in turn can result in improved patient outcomes for diseases driven by intricate host-pathogen interactions (Fu et al., 2024; Pruksaphon et al., 2024) (Figure 2.9).

2.3.1. Innate Immune Response Mechanisms

Our gut health relies upon a fragile tug-of-war between our body's defenses and encroaching microbes. Sudden innate responses are the initial line of defense against unwanted colonization, launching rapid, unspecific attacks when pathogens arrive on the scene. Everything depends upon crucial immune players—macrophages, dendritic cells, and neutrophils—that not only detect danger but also control the traffic of inflammatory signals, which go on to guide more specialized defenses. Maintaining the gut lining intact is at the center of all these; when that barrier breaks or the signals become out of order, chronic inflammation ensues—commonly observed in inflammatory bowel disease (Mousa et al., 2024). When you consider gut immunity, another critical piece is how our innate defenses communicate with the resident microbiota—organisms that are both beneficial and pathogenic. In most instances, the immune system must choose between the friendly, helpful microbes and those that could cause us harm. This choice occurs with pattern recognition receptors (PRRs) that recognize familiar microbe components, initiating a defensive yet cautious response that, in a sense, spares the good ones. Of course, if there is a dramatic change in microbial diversity, dysbiosis, as it is referred to, the balance could be disrupted, creating an overactive immune response and damaging tissues. Studies commonly indicate such imbalances escalate inflammation, a contributor to diseases such as ulcerative colitis (Fu et al., 2024). Undoubtedly, the ongoing give-and-take among microbes and our immune systems is central to maintaining gut health. Innate immunity in the gut is not simply a matter of detecting invaders but also listening to cues from the environment and from surrounding microbes to fine-tune its behavior. Immune cells not only respond passively but also secrete a cocktail of cytokines and chemokines that summon reinforcements and assist in the establishment of an organized defense system. Recent research, in many instances, points out that our internal system even dictates which microbes get to stay, promoting a kind of necessary, albeit imperfect, symbiosis. New therapies are currently looking at these very channels and microbial interactions as promising means of turning down chronic inflammation. A closer examination of how all these components interact is important in finding new ways to regain balance and repel dangerous microbes (Fu et al., 2024; Mousa et al., 2024).

2.3.2. Adaptive Immune Response and Its Components

Microbial pathogens and our immune system tango in a manner that quite determines the direction of an infection. When a germ gets past our first line of defense, the body quickly triggers a specialized response that homes in on the intruder. B cells and T cells—our own immune system's team—leap into action in unpredictable capacities; sometimes B cells produce antibodies to catch the danger, while T cells may attack the infected cells directly. This specialized defense finds a way to keep collateral damage at a minimum, even as it struggles to destroy the intruder. It's a form of the biological balancing act in which fighting the infection doesn't necessarily have to involve destroying our own tissues. At its core, the adaptive immune system weaves together a disorganized web of cells and molecules that recall previous experiences to attack more quickly next time. Occasionally, cells such as dendritic cells pick up bits of the infection and parade them around in front of naïve T cells, who then change shape into experienced fighters capable of dealing with the task. Helper T cells release a combination of chemical signals, but the cytotoxic type enter and destroy infected cells; B cells, on the other hand, work on making themselves better and more efficient with fine tunes such as affinity maturation and class switching. In most instances, this memory of the immune system operates like a much-traveled shortcut—useful if the same pathogen attempts to enter again.

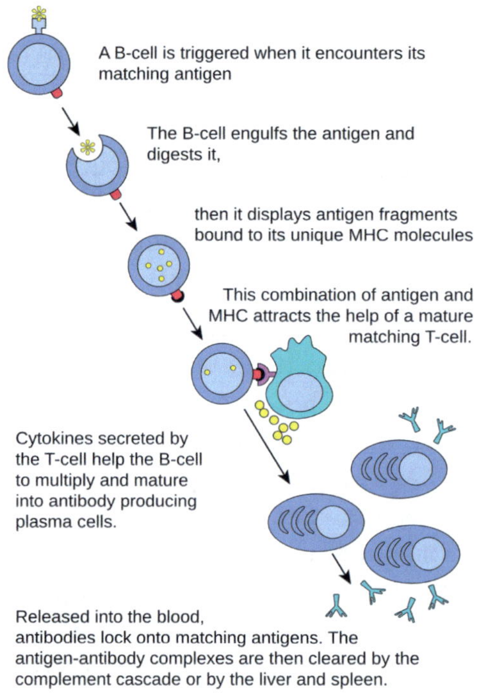

Figure 2.10. Adaptive immune responses.

Source: By Fred the Oyster - The Immune System (pdf), Public Domain, https://commons.wikimedia.org/w/index.php?curid=36367201

Not all components of our immune system act out in a neat script, however. A few sensors within our cells, for example, detect small bits of bacteria and trigger inflammatory responses that are essential for protection. Intracellular receptors—such as those NOD proteins—may sound complicated, but they serve as early warning systems; if their signals go haywire or mutations set in, it can cause issues such as inflammatory diseases (Cucchiara et al., 2018). Even everyday aspects, like applying ozone to sterilize surfaces, adjust the combination by lowering the amount of microbes and subtly altering the antigen levels the adaptive arm must work with (Goudie et al., 2003). In general, understanding how these cues interact with our immune response aids in determining cleverer, more natural strategies for fighting infection without causing undesired damage (Figure 2.10).

2.3.3. Role of Cytokines in Host Defense

Pathogens and our immune responses are in a constant, unpredictable dance, with cytokines really taking center stage. These little secreted proteins jump into action when microbes show up, acting like messengers that sometimes shout for more inflammation, call in reinforcements, or fine-tune the activation of our defense cells—all depending on the situation. When a germ is found, molecules such as interleukins, interferons, and tumor necrosis factors are rapidly produced, each transmitting messages that may turn the immune system up or down depending on the threat. It's sort of important that this dialogue remains focused, since if it gets damaged, not only can infected cells go untreated, but there's also potential to harm healthy tissue. In the majority of instances, grasping these pathways also allows us to comprehend how things may go out of control to form chronic infection or immune-mediated damage, thus informing new therapies for combating microbial disease (Hudson & Egan, 2024). Our body depends significantly on the timely, context-specific release of cytokines to control bacteria. In a sense, such molecules are the unheralded messengers that summon cells such as neutrophils and macrophages directly to the battle zones, preparing them for germ-cleansing duty. They do not rest there—cytokines also assist in constructing a bridge to the subsequent, more specific adaptive immune system by prodding T cells into specialized jobs against the causative microbes. This type of loosely coordinated collaboration tends to close the window on bacteria persisting and spreading. Even in environments such as marine or environmental ecosystems, where microbial intruders can disrupt natural equilibria and jeopardize food sources, venturing into cytokine roles is more than merely about our well-being—it's about learning life on a grander level (Hudson & Egan, 2024). It truly indicates that cytokines play a role in protecting a broad spectrum of host systems against microbial threats. While it's no secret that cytokines are instrumental in protecting the body from infections, determining precisely how their timing changes during an infection is still somewhat of an enigma. Research tends to concentrate on the most dramatic instances—those survival mechanisms in test subjects that are impossible to ignore—so the less conspicuous, yet perhaps equally significant, cytokine signals can fall through the cracks. This methodology sometimes muddies the distinction between the early "red alert" messages that initiate our immune system and the subsequent cues that sustain it or fine-tune it over time. A few researchers indicate that if we were able to strike cytokines at these various stages, we could better tailor treatments to eliminate pathogens more efficiently without too much immune overdrive that may harm tissues. Acknowledging that cytokine action isn't fixed but varies with the infection stage truly highlights their complex role in the host and pathogen battle, and it directs us toward new research directions (Cramer & Kowalski, 2021).

2.4. Microbial Virulence Factors

Microbes and hosts have a surprisingly complex symphonysystem that is not always clear and well-organized. They employ a mixed arsenal of devices—adhesins, toxins, enzymes, plus a few methods for evading immune attacks—to stick to tissues, sneak inside, and grab simple nutrients. Essentially, these are not euphemisms;

they're the mechanisms through which bacteria manipulate the host's own biochemistry to get the better of it, even outnumbering the indigenous microbial throng. In most instances, this evolution by counter-evolution, in which host defense and microbial strategy continually adjust to each other, implies that what we refer to as "virulence factors" represent a complex adaptive conflict. Studies, as most would concur, have progressively illuminated how these virulence factors increase disease intensity and facilitate the spread of infection.

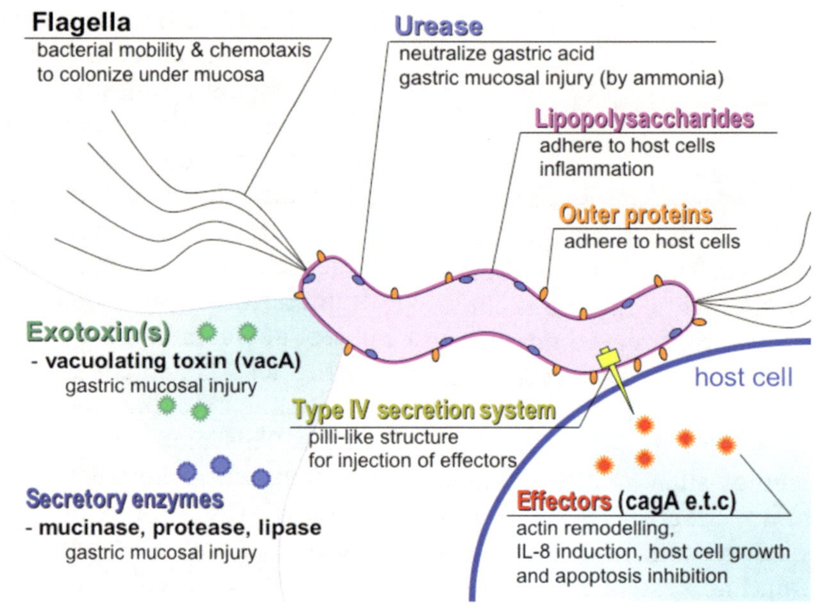

Figure 2.11. Microbial virulence factors.

Source: https://commons.wikimedia.org/wiki/File:H_pylori_virulence_factors_en.png

There's also increasing evidence that the functions of these microbial weapons extend way beyond one scene of infection. Consider chronic respiratory diseases such as cystic fibrosis, for instance—bacterial populations there tend to use overlapping sets of virulence genes so that even if the bacteria themselves rearrange taxonomically, the overall infectability remains relatively stable. Most often, this type of redundancy suggests that targeting a single pathway may, in practice, destabilize the entire system, potentially opening up new avenues for treatment. Concurrently, when various microbial populations interact—sometimes conflicting, sometimes collaborating—the resultant community effects become increasingly capricious and rich in subtlety. Elucidating these complex, molecule-to-molecule interactions within complex microbial consortia is a central frontier in our understanding of infection dynamics (Bevivino et al., 2019). At a larger scale, the evolution of such virulence strategies is deeply shaped by how microbes evolve to fit into the host environment. It's obvious that changes in levels of oxygen, nutrient availability, and even the fluctuating moods of the immune system force microbes to modify and diversify their virulent properties. In most instances, the dissemination of these factors is accelerated by horizontal gene transfer—a type of microbial give-and-take whereby these properties are transferred from one population to the next. Consider the reproductive microbiome, for example; it's a fairly specialized niche where host-microbe and microbe–microbe interactions, sometimes rather haphazardly, determine community structure and even influence reproductive fitness. In this context, virulence factors may assist microbes in maintaining their grip and being passed on, although their expression is guided by both deterministic pressures and stochastic, near chance-like events in the host–microbial metacommunity (Rowe et al., 2020). Finally, perceiving the entire ecological landscape in this way requires a research mindset that is not linear but instead accepts complexity and a little bit of serendipitous wisdom (Figure 2.11).

2.4.1. Toxins and Their Effects on Host Cells

Microbial toxins readily disturb the fragile balance between bacteria and host cells. They're notorious microbes that can, in most instances, harm cells directly—ripping apart membranes, inhibiting protein synthesis, or even scrambling the ways cells communicate with one another. When bacteria find their way into the mix, their toxins at times destroy the cell's outer wall or disrupt essential functions, which can eventually kill the cell or simply result in plain dysfunction. For instance, some bacteria secrete enterotoxins that manipulate the cell's internal messaging systems, triggering episodes of inflammation and diarrhea that allow the microbes to disseminate. Overall, these activities not only enhance microbial survival but also exacerbate tissue damage, making the diseases more serious. It is still a fundamental step in finding treatments that minimize the resulting damage to learn how these toxins affect cells. Host cells also come into contact with toxins that disrupt bodily defenses, particularly the epithelial layers of the gut. These layers are like natural gatekeepers—they allow nutrients to pass through while keeping unwanted visitors out. Toxins interfere with proteins like occludin and claudins that would otherwise keep these cells tightly attached, which in turn results in a leaky barrier. This leak allows microbes and their by-products to get through and awaken the innate immune system into action, usually leading to inflammation in the process. Toxins even change the makeup of the mucus layer at times, lessening its protective effect. Such interruptions not only compromise the body's defense but also lay the ground for chronic inflammatory conditions. All of this truly illustrates how significant microbial factors are in maintaining barrier integrity, and how toxins can deceptively subvert those protections (Ghosh et al., 2021; Hou et al., 2022). The consequences of toxin-induced cell death extend far beyond the immediate environment—it affects local tissues and sends shockwaves throughout the entire immune response system. When a cell dies, it sends out distress signals that amplify inflammation and summon immune cells to the site. Surprisingly enough, certain toxins adjust immune signaling just enough to enable microbes to evade detection, which can lead to chronic infections. In most instances, the overreactive immune response of the body winds up inflicting additional tissue damage far from the toxin's initial point of attack. This cycle of breaking down the barrier, microbial imbalance, and persistent inflammation seems to be at the core of most infection-related diseases. Existing research is currently exploring how to mend these damaged barriers and modulate the immune reactions, all in a bid to restore balance to the interaction between microbial invaders and our innate defenses (Ghosh et al., 2021; Hou et al., 2022).

2.4.2. Enzymes That Facilitate Invasion

Microbes have learned some really interesting ways to bypass our defenses. They will frequently hide a release of enzymes that enable them to slip through barriers, both physical and immunological. Consider hyaluronidases, for instance; they disintegrate the hyaluronic acid in the extracellular environment, effectively weakening the adhesive that holds our cells in place. Further collagenases that destroy the collagen fibers, which are responsible for our tissues' strength. In most instances, such enzymatic activity not only makes it easier for these invaders to pass through but also triggers an immune response—a kind of unintended tug-of-war between the invader and the host (Rinninella et al., 2019). The ability to dispense such invasion-friendly chemicals is inextricably linked with just how virulent an individual microbe can become. In general, pathogens regulate the secretion of proteases, lipases, and nucleases according to signals derived from the host environment. These enzymes not only degrade physical barriers but also wreak havoc on immune processes. For instance, certain bacterial proteases may attack immunoglobulins or even components of the complement system, thus rendering the host more vulnerable. Additionally, phospholipases begin to shred cell membranes by hydrolyzing phospholipids—leading cells to burst and tissues to get damaged; this, in turn, facilitates the microbes dispersing even further. Overall, the extensive range of these enzymes and their target specificity truly showcase the versatility of pathogens in bypassing host barriers (Rinninella et al., 2019). In addition to punching holes in tissues, these enzymes also mess around with cell survival and immune signaling. By disrupting cell membranes and the surrounding matrix, they can induce a variety of cell death types, such as necrosis and pyroptosis, which typically accompany a good amount of inflammation and a cascade of immune responses. The injury and consequent release of alarm substances not only activate the immune system but may even make the infection worse by allowing the spread of pathogens further. In general, gaining an understanding of how these enzymes induce cell death provides insight into the precarious balance between microbial invasion and host defense, suggesting possible therapies that could interfere with these enzymatic processes to reduce both the invasion and its toxic consequences (Figure 2.12).

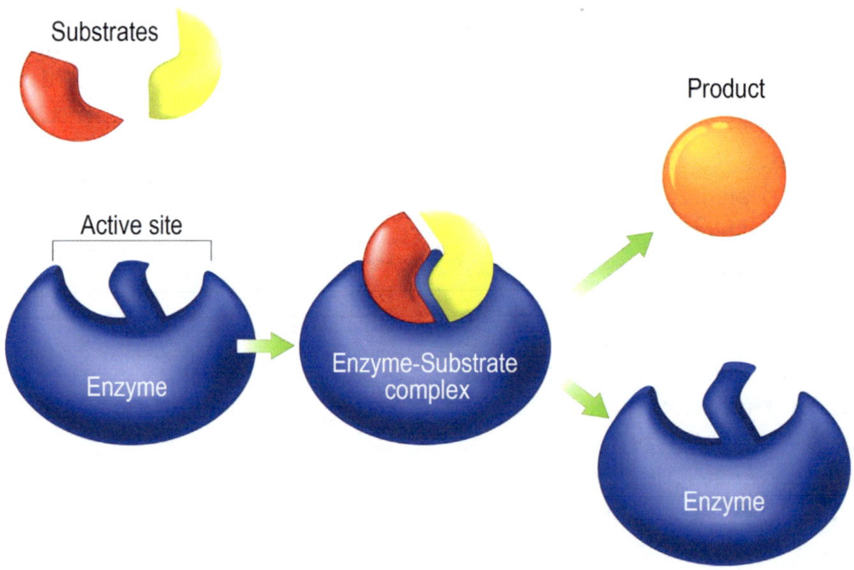

Figure 2.12. Enzymes that facilitate invasion.

Source: iBiologia. (2018, November). *Enzymes that Facilitate Invasion.*

2.4.3. Surface Structures That Enhance Pathogenicity

Microbes usually cause problems by employing a variety of special surface portions that allow them to enter and slide around our defenses. Consider all the tiny strands such as pili and fimbriae, slippery capsules, and outer membrane proteins—they essentially assist bacteria in sticking to our tissues instead of being carried away. They don't just enable them to adhere but also build warm little pockets where they can cling on no matter our built-in cleaning mechanisms. In certain instances, they even conceal the actual signals that would otherwise alert our immune system, either by masking the significant markers or by playing tricks with immune receptors. This mutual game between the tricks of the bug and the wary nature of our body makes all the difference in whether or not an infection spirals out of control (Zheng et al., 2020). Some microbes take it a step further by cosplaying themselves up in surface polysaccharide capsules. These carbohydrate-laden capsules tend to resemble the host's own molecules—kind of like wearing an intelligent disguise—to avoid the detection of phagocytic cells and complement proteins. For the most part, this molecular mimicry provides pathogens with additional time to establish themselves and makes them more virulent overall. How a capsule is produced can even influence the amount of inflammation or tissue destruction that occurs, providing another complexity to disease development. Studies have demonstrated at the microscopic level that these surface characteristics not only enhance the survival of the bug but also dictate how the host is able to remain balanced or develops immune problems (Zheng et al., 2020). In brief, these sugary, sticky shields are a clever tactic for bacteria to not be swept away. Beyond the more direct shields such as capsules and pili, surface proteins play their own naughty tricks. They may play the role of adhesins to allow bacteria to attach themselves to host cells, or be invasins, entering into cells in order to secure sanctuaries—sometimes even throwing in an additional role as immune modulators. For instance, certain of these proteins bind to certain receptors, holding the bacteria in position, while others assist them in breaking into cells where they can go underground. Sometimes, they even mess up the host's signaling mechanisms or cause a little inflammation that, ironically, makes the microbe more mobile. In the majority of instances, the battle between bacterial colonization and immune activation is reduced to whether and to what extent these proteins the microbe expresses. Knowing these specifics, as much as it is a problem sometimes, is key to developing new drugs that can break these critical steps in the infection process.

2.5. Host-Microbe Interactions

Inside our bodies, countless tiny organisms live side by side with us—and they do way more than just hang around. They churn out various byproducts from our meals that seem to alter how our guts work and even play with our immune system, sometimes subtly, sometimes in a rather noticeable manner. These chemicals, suspended very close to the lining of the gut, are able to directly affect our epithelial cells and move immune responses, usually keeping everything in balance. When this sensitive communication goes off-script, however, the barrier can get weaker and allow unwanted bacteria or particles that fuel inflammation to come in. New omics techniques have begun illuminating these host-microbe interactions, revealing to us common signaling pathways that appear to support the defenses of the gut. In the majority of instances, taking advantage of this information may ultimately provide new avenues for restoring our systems and alleviating gastrointestinal issues (Ghosh et al., 2021). Platelets were for years viewed primarily as the body's backup clot makers, but it appears they have a split personality when it comes to infection. In addition to their established function of halting bleeding, these platelet fragments also bear a combination of inflammatory and anti-inflammatory messages—essentially a little of both worlds. Once pathogens intrude, platelets move quickly: sometimes immobilizing the enemies in place, other times summoning reinforcements by attracting immune cells to the area. This mutual activity is able to limit the spread of bacteria while also establishing the groundwork for a general immune response. Conversely, there are some wily microbes with tricks to foul up platelet counts and behavior, which themselves may influence how a disease proceeds. As a whole, appreciation of this exchange provides interesting opportunities for novel therapy designed to tailor our immune defense in the setting of infection (Li et al., 2020).

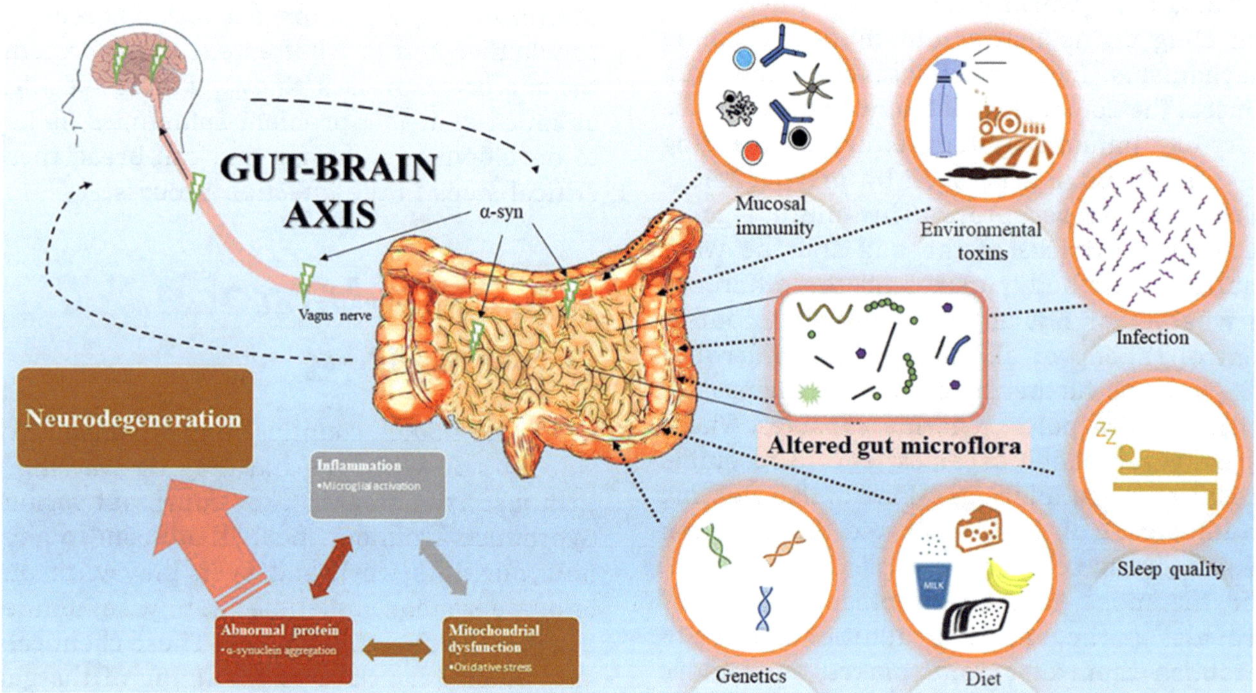

Figure 2.13. Host-microbe interactions.

Source: By Chao Yin-Xia, Gulam Muhammad Yaaseen, Chia Nicholas Shyh Jenn, Feng Lei, Rotzschke Olaf, Tan Eng-King - https://www.frontiersin.org/articles/10.3389/fneur.2020.00849/full, CC BY 4.0, https://commons.wikimedia.org/w/index.php?curid=112558306

Our gut lining isn't just an inactive barrier; it's an active checkpoint through which good stuff such as nutrients pass while spurning harmful intruders. This barrier is not one singular wall but several layers: a slippery mucus shield that discourages microbes from getting too close, a solitary layer of differentiated, specialized epithelial cells, and below them, an immune system silently patrolling the premises. Proteins such as occludin, claudins, and zonula occludens function as malleable glue between cells, managing what can pass through these minute holes. If something is amiss with these proteins—a change in their expression or a mess in their configuration—the barrier becomes compromised, permitting microbes to seep through and cause inflammatory surges. The tangled relationship between these microbial chemicals and the signals from our gut cells is complex, to say the least. Figuring out this intricate dance is essential if we're going to come up with ways to mend the barrier, especially in conditions like inflammatory bowel disease, where a damaged host-microbe interaction keeps inflammation nagging on (Ghosh et al., 2021) (Figure 2.13).

2.5.1. Symbiotic Relationships and Their Benefits

Microbes and their hosts have a sort of natural tug-of-war that maintains our inner equilibrium. In most instances, populations of small organisms—hanging around in the gut, on the skin, or even in our airways—do more than quietly coexist. They intervene to safeguard us by dominating space and resources, so that unwanted invaders struggle to get settled. Quite frequently, this comfortable arrangement ends up resetting our immune reactions and aiding in healing tissues. When this equilibrium falters, a condition referred to as dysbiosis can initiate a host of health problems, illustrating precisely how vital these interactions are. Some researchers even pursue treatments such as adjusting our microbe composition or carrying out fecal transplants to rectify matters (Hou et al., 2022). Beneficial microbial communities can also enhance host defenses in more concrete ways. Consider the zebrafish, for instance—its transparent nature and amenable genetics allow scientists to observe how particular bacteria influence immune responses to infection. In a few experiments, important bacteria in the cocktail were observed to fine-tune the function of phagocytes and modulate inflammation levels, sometimes cranking up defense and at others dampening it, depending on circumstance. These results remind us that the dance between our cells and these microbes is not a cut-and-dry relationship; there's usually a nuance back-and-forth that affects overall health. The zebrafish model, with its special transparency at single-cell resolution, has initiated a whole new window into these *in-vivo* interactions (Gomes et al., 2019). In addition to warding off infections, our microbial friends are also crucial for digesting food and regulating our metabolism. They assist in breaking down resistant food components, contribute to the synthesis of crucial vitamins, and even regulate how we store fat, all directly impacting our nutritional status and energy equilibrium. In many cases, these microbes also produce compounds that resonate throughout our bodies, associating microbe function with metabolic disorders when something goes wrong. It appears that such functions are conserved among a wide range of species, emphasizing just how embedded microbial symbiosis is in our existence. Exploring these cellular and molecular interactions not only enhances our knowledge of host-microbe dynamics but also suggests promising new methods for the prevention and treatment of disease (Gomes et al., 2019; Hou et al., 2022).

2.5.2. Commensal Organisms and Their Role in Health

Humans and their small microbial housemates have a remarkably balanced relationship—a true win-win that serves to keep our bodies in balance. A group of these microbes, particularly the commensals, are at the heart of many important functions, primarily in our gut. They contribute to the shaping of the immune system (you might say they have a hand in constructing lymph tissues and in establishing immune tolerance) and even digest our food to extract energy, which in turn adjusts nutrient absorption and overall metabolism. Their behavior appears to change with what we consume, our daily routines, and even the frequency at which we take antibiotics—so much that any disruption in this balance could pave the way for all sorts of health ailments (Gonçalves et al., 2014). Look beyond the gut, and you'll discover these same commensals hanging around on other mucosal surfaces as well. Take the mouth, for instance: here, fungi such as *Candida albicans* get along with bacteria such as *Streptococcus mutans*. There is evidence from dual-species biofilm studies which indicates that Candida seems to mellow out the acid-producing activity of *S. mutans* by changing the pH - an adjustment which turns out to be more protective of tooth enamel than when *S. mutans* occurs alone. It's like they, in concert, assist in making the mouth's ecosystem more stable and resistant to rot (Eidt et al., 2017).

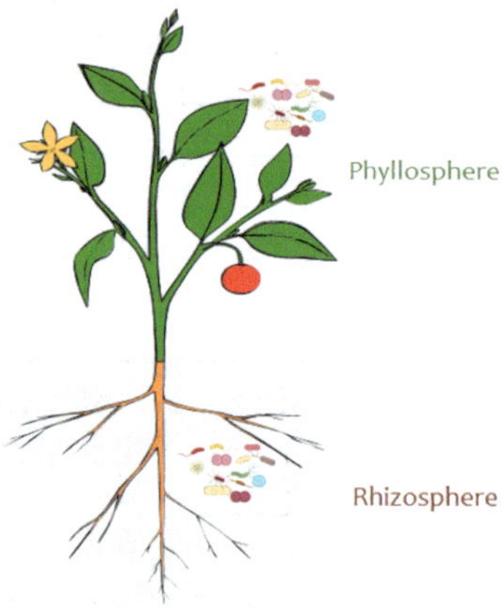

Figure 2.14. Commensalism interaction.

Source: By Sheng-Yang He - [1], CC BY-SA 4.0, https://commons.wikimedia.org/w/index.php?curid=93793003

Our microbial friends don't just help digest and clean our mouths—sensing unwanted intruders, they keep those nasty microbes at bay. By colonizing choice locations on our body, they prevent opportunistic pathogens from settling in and disrupting the mucosal barriers. This competitive atmosphere keeps the overall system stable, and therefore when something does disrupt it, the immune system is prepared to kick in. In general, these harmonious arrangements also de-escalate excessive inflammatory responses, which play a role in autoimmune conditions. New technologies in metagenomics and metaproteomics keep unraveling how much these small microorganisms play a role, not just in balancing metabolism but in showing our immune system its tricks. As such, treatments which involve bringing back a healthy balance of microbes—such as probiotics, prebiotics, or even fecal microbiota transplants—are receiving increasing scrutiny in contemporary medicine (Gonçalves et al., 2014) (Figure 2.4).

2.5.3. Dysbiosis and Its Implications for Disease

Our bodies harbor a complex community of microorganisms that keep everything in check—even though when that equilibrium is upset, a condition called dysbiosis appears to be connected to a multitude of health issues. When things get wobbly out of kilter, it can upset our immune system's ability to manage inflammation, which in turn provides opportunity for nasty microbes to make more damage. The intestine, for instance, produces a range of chemicals that not only direct our metabolism but also have an effect on immune reaction and stability of tissue. These small microbial by-products have been linked to problems with blood cell formation and life-threatening diseases like acute myeloid leukemia (AML). In general, there is growing evidence to suggest that even slight changes in the composition of microbes could alter disease progression and patient responses to treatment, highlighting the noted connection between a perturbed microbiome and increased infection risk in AML patients (Nowicka & Gil, 2024). Shifting gears from blood disease, scientists are now exploring how a faulty microbial community may influence how drugs function—particularly with autoimmune diseases such as rheumatoid arthritis. The gut bacteria are preloaded with a kind of enzymatic toolbox that can alter how drugs get absorbed and how potent they become, sometimes enhancing a drug's effect and sometimes dampening it. This variability translates to the fact that because each individual's microbial composition is slightly unique, reactions to disease-modifying anti-rheumatic drugs (DMARDs) can be extremely varied. And it doesn't go one way; the drugs themselves can push the microbial combination in various directions, opening up a give-and-take relationship with far-reaching implications for treatment regimens. In all but the most special situations, knowing this type of interplay is crucial to creating tailored therapies that consider microbial markers to predict if not positively influence, the success of treatments (Fan et al., 2023). Together, our increasing understanding of dysbiosis reveals its complicated role in how our bodies engage with pathogens and regulate disease. Pairing microbiome studies with analyses of metabolic products promises exciting new directions for identifying the biochemical and immune-based mechanisms underlying these outcomes. Such far-reaching strategies may even enable us to detect new microbial signatures that predict how diseases will unfold or how well a patient will respond to a particular treatment. As understanding develops, it's increasingly critical to account for the function of these microbial communities not just in the development and progression of disease, but also in determining how our bodies respond to treatment. This change of thinking, although a bit disorganized sometimes, has genuine potential for more customizing treatment and enhancing overall patient outcomes (Fan et al., 2023; Nowicka & Gil, 2024).

2.6. Emerging Infectious Diseases

Pathogen–host interactions are responsible for playing a gigantic part in revealing to us how infections arise and evolve with time. The old-fashioned approach to viewing bacteria has been discarded for a more complex perspective where both the bug's deceptions and our own mechanisms combination together to bring harm. Consider the DRF, for instance; it views disease as a consequence of the conflict between microbial virulence and the body's response. In most instances, it then implies that what we previously would have thought was the work of the enemy sometimes ends up being our own reaction fueling the fire. With new or even recurrent bacteria challenging our present diagnostics and treatments, an emphasis on damage – simple as it gets – provides us with new leads on how infections follow their course (Nosanchuk, 2025). In a further turn of events, new diseases also appear with every kind of symptom under the sun, sometimes affecting one particular area such as the eye. Ebola, Zika, and Nipah viruses have been associated with eye issues like uveitis and conjunctivitis. These annoying inflammations don't merely threaten vision; they also point to the ways pathogens travel in local tissues and how our immune system mobilizes to defend itself. *Toxoplasma gondii* and Plasmodium diseases that appear to return, time and again, only further emphasize that these problems aren't disappearing anytime soon. Integrating observations of the eyes with broader host–pathogen dynamics really emphasizes why we require a comprehensive, multidisciplinary perspective – the sort of thinking across the One Health framework that considers ecological and zoonotic factors (Blyden et al., 2024). Confronting new infections truly requires viewing the whole picture—where biological uniqueness combine with environmental uniqueness. Human hosts, animal reservoirs, and local environments all combine and influence how bacteria travel and make damage. In general, knowing not just the lifecycles of these insects but also how they evade our defenses allows us to chart targeted prevention and treatment plans. With globalization, global warming, and changing environments making waves, structures such as the DRF, and cross-disciplinary approaches, become essential weapons in the fight against both emerging and recurring microbial infections (Blyden et al., 2024; Nosanchuk, 2025) (Figure 2.15).

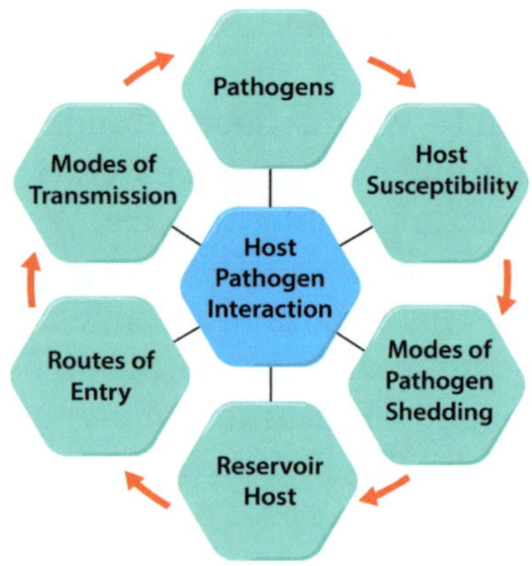

Figure 2.15. Bacterial pathogenicity.

Source: Oregon State University. (2019, August). *Bacterial Pathogenicity.*

2.6.1. Factors Contributing to the Emergence of New Pathogens

Hosts and microbes engage in a sort of wild dance that spurs the emergence of new diseases—nature's own brand of shaking things up. New studies employing living models such as zebrafish larvae reveal, in most instances, that the body's immune reactions and a pathogen's ability to do damage really evolve side by side (Gomes et al., 2019). Here, you notice that although our natural defenses may stave off these intruders at times, they also inadvertently provide them with a toehold, which in turn encourages the microbes to become even more ingenious. Environmental changes and the relentless pressure of antibiotics select for the microbes that resist the attack, and the immune status of the host itself fine-tunes how nasty these pathogens end up being. Tricks such as evading defenses, seeking refuge in safe intracellular havens, and manipulating with inflammation are all involved—emphasizing that both the host's condition and the genetic alterations of the microbes are equally important when fresh infections begin to appear. Plants are also included, but things happen slightly differently. They never truly exist alone; rather, an entire community of microbes inhabit them, both influencing their health and susceptibility to infection (Hacquard, 2015). Research on agave plants in different environments shows that the composition of microbes varies significantly depending on which part of the plant you examine and where it's cultivated. Interestingly, the effects of farming practices can disrupt these indigenous microbial communities, decreasing diversity and changing the competitive balance. Such disruption could lead to the emergence of cryptic pathogens, which is to say that both environmental pressures in the natural world and human activities can re-engineer how these micro-ecosystems function—not only in plants but in more general life forms. Further there is the internal life of the microbes themselves. Within these intricate communities, competition, cooperation, and even the sharing of genetic material (quite commonly through horizontal gene transfer (Hacquard, 2015)) assist them in adapting in times of stress. In such communities, microbes share portions of DNA and modulate their group behavior, which can increase virulence particularly when a host's defenses are slightly askew. In most instances, the combined power of an alert immune system and an evolving environment induces pathogens to experiment with new tricks for invading hosts or evading immune defenses. All these interwoven interactions form an endless cycle of emerging infections, rendering it a true challenge to keep up with and contain the spread of diseases efficiently.

2.6.2. Impact of Globalization on Disease Spread

The past decades have witnessed travel and communication alter the dynamics of how diseases are transported. Pathogens no longer confine themselves to their traditional areas—they find themselves in strange locations, interacting with new hosts and environments that can initiate larger epidemics. It's not just that individuals are more mobile; it's also the imperfect interaction of germ evolution and the ease with which hosts get infected. Genomic technology now assists in identifying new microbes in hospitals, providing us with a better picture of how infections leap across continents. These technologies even allow us to monitor outbreaks in real time, assisting public health efforts attempting to stem pandemics. Naturally, the mess of bioinformatics required to sort out all this genetic information demonstrates just how difficult contemporary epidemiology has it in the face of infectious hazards stoked by global changes (Chiu et al., 2013). Beyond the minute interactions of cells, a combination of social, cultural, and environmental determinants also influences the behavior of diseases in our interconnected world. Diseases aren't merely isolated cases—they propagate across populations driven by urban sprawl, patterns of migration, and socioeconomic disparities. These factors modify exposure risks, shifting clinical outcomes, and occasionally allowing diseases to persist in communities longer than anticipated. Ecological change and back-and-forth host adaptation complicate epidemic patterns. Researchers tend to use mathematical models in order to sift through that complexity, modeling various scenarios that help determine interventions and inform public health policies in our globalized reality (da Costa et al., 2019). Piling on top of all of this, international trade and travel mix with microbial adaptation to fuel a feedback loop that accelerates the development of diseases with actual pandemic potential. Rapid identification of new microbes by next-generation sequencing is imperative for prompt reactions, but demonstration that these microbes are pathogenic usually requires considerable epidemiological effort and laboratory confirmation. This combination of circumstances reminds us that globalization not only extends the geographical spread of pathogens but also increases the difficulties for scientists in investigating them. Finally, confronting these risks involves using a combination of disciplines—clinical microbiology, genomics, epidemiology, and even the social sciences—to mitigate the ill effects of globalization on disease transmission and create an adaptive balance between hosts and pathogens in today's closely linked world (Chiu et al., 2013) (Figure 2.16).

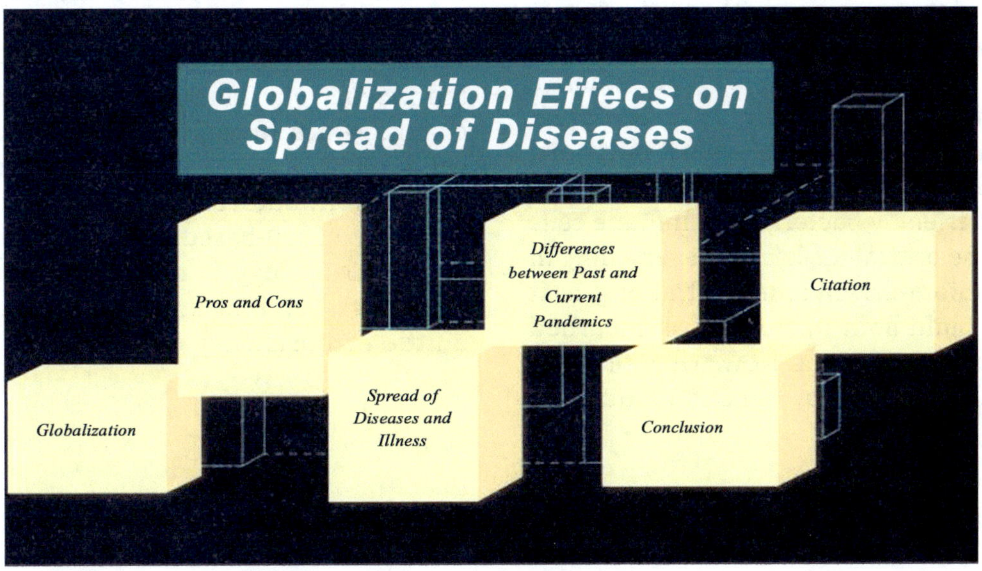

Figure 2.16. Impact of globalization on disease spread.

Source: Prezi. (n.d.). *Impact of Globalization on Disease Spread.*

2.6.3. Strategies for Prevention And Control

Preventing infection from microbes essentially comes down to recognizing how our body's immune system gets around with pathogens. One concept is to modify the gut bacteria since the combination of those microbes appears to determine how susceptible you are to disease. When the microbial community becomes disrupted, it can even put you at higher risk for Clostridioides difficile infection (CDI)—a big hospital issue. Adding in tests that screen for both problems with your microbiome and immune markers appears to catch CDI earlier and distinguish it from other gastrointestinal problems. Certain diagnostic tests that combine microbe information and immune indicators perform quite well better, which may mean pursuing both directions initially would be a good idea. These findings, in general, reveal the potential for tailored measures that not only attempt to restore the microbial balance but also stimulate the immune system, hence reducing infections and enhancing outcomes (Ke et al., 2021). Obviously, you can't create good prevention strategies without looking at both the microbes and our body's response. Besides the improvements in diagnosis, there's also growing enthusiasm for ways to adjust and train our immune system against microbial invaders. The back-and-forth communication between our friendly bacteria and immune cells turns out to be critical for keeping everything in check. Microbiota-driven immune training, as it were, helps build both immediate and learned defenses against pathogens. Now, when that fine balance is thrown off—by genetic uniqueness or the day-to-day stress of our environment—it can cause immune hiccups and make us more vulnerable to infection. For the most part, it has fueled interest in treatments that attempt to rebalance it using something like probiotics, prebiotics, or even fecal microbiota transplantation. These strategies, which focus on the modulation of host-microbe interactions to control disease progression, demonstrate how crucial a supported immune system is (Zheng et al., 2020). Speaking of which, implementing infection control measures on the basis of findings from molecular biology and immunology is essential in responding to microbial challenges head-on. Vaccination, judicious use of antibiotics, and even improved sanitation measures all must be shaped by what we now know about how bacteria and the body interact. Vaccines that induce the appropriate immune response against the most important microbial targets can prevent colonization and fend off disease. Concurrently, judicious use of antibiotics reduces the likelihood of developing resistant strains while maintaining the beneficial microbial diversity. And enhanced cleaning protocols reduced the ways in which bacteria spread within hospitals and community settings. When all these strategies—along with monitoring our immune status and microbial changes—are brought together, they create a solid, multi-pronged plan to manage infections and prevent outbreaks. In practice, this hybrid approach of cell-based immunity combined with microbial ecology is crucial to maintaining us healthier, even if at times it requires tolerating a little inconsistency of approach.

CLOSER LOOK

BACTERIAL PATHOGENICITY

Bacterial pathogenicity refers to the ability of bacteria to cause disease in a host. Not all bacteria are harmful; many are harmless or even beneficial. However, pathogenic bacteria possess specific traits, known as virulence factors, that allow them to invade host tissues, evade immune defenses, and produce toxins leading to illness.

The process of pathogenicity usually begins with adherence, where bacteria attach to host cells using pili, fimbriae, or adhesins. This step is crucial for colonization, as seen in Escherichia coli binding to the urinary tract or Streptococcus mutans adhering to teeth surfaces. Once attached, some bacteria can form biofilms, which provide protection against antibiotics and immune responses.

Following attachment, bacteria may employ invasion mechanisms, penetrating host cells or spreading through tissues. For example, Salmonella and Shigella invade intestinal epithelial cells to establish infection. To survive within the host, pathogens often produce molecules that inhibit or escape immune defenses. Mycobacterium tuberculosis can survive inside macrophages by preventing phagosome-lysosome fusion, while Neisseria meningitidis uses a polysaccharide capsule to resist phagocytosis.

Another critical aspect of pathogenicity is toxin production. Exotoxins, secreted by bacteria like Clostridium botulinum or Vibrio cholerae, can cause severe tissue damage or disrupt normal physiological processes. Endotoxins, mainly lipopolysaccharides (LPS) from Gram-negative bacteria, trigger strong immune responses that may result in fever, inflammation, or septic shock.

Ultimately, bacterial pathogenicity is a complex interplay between microbial strategies and host defenses. The outcome of infection depends on the strength of the bacterial virulence factors and the effectiveness of the host's immune response. Understanding these mechanisms is essential for developing targeted treatments, vaccines, and preventive strategies against bacterial diseases.

Summary

Understanding infectious diseases means looking closely at how microbes and hosts interact – it's a tangled and lively process. You can see that a host's unique genetic makeup and its immune response really matter when microbes make their move. Plus, the mix of bacteria inside us, like in the gut, not only bumps up disease risk in many cases but also alterchanges our immunity. All this hints that perhaps we could do better by incorporating different sources of information—genomic, metagenomic, and even metabolomic information—to get what is going on between host and pathogen, and which might potentially lead to more intelligent methods of diagnosis and disease treatment. More recent research has suggested a two-way interaction between our genes and the microbes we carry. For instance, in diseases such as systemic lupus erythematosus (SLE) the gut microbiota manifests changes—particular groups of bacteria and their metabolic pathways become significantly damaged (Tomofuji et al., 2021). Just the same, scientific studies of IBD reveal that genetic variants with effects on immune regulation appear to go hand-in-hand with changes in what the microbiome performs, and therefore our genetic script assists in choosing which bacteria thrive, and along the way these microbes can turn the disease outcome (Hu et al., 2020). This sort of interdependence, in general, is a good candidate for therapy in terms of alteraltering one aspect maybe having a beneficial impact on the other. Overall, advancing our understanding of how microbes are disease-causing through interactions with hosts is a major biomedical frontier. A balanced perspective is to consider genetic predispositions, microbial diversity, and their metabolic status. Current research suggests that such complex networks may hold the key to new, individualized medicine approaches aimed at blocking detrimental processes while enhancing the body's defenses. Future research should, in general, emphasize longer-term and multi-omics approaches to provide better predictive and adaptive regulation of disease outcomes, ideally towards better infection care as well as management of immune-related disorders by specifically targeting host parameters and the microbes with which they coexist (Hu et al., 2020; Tomofuji et al., 2021).

Microbes and their hosts maintain a surprisingly complex dialogue – one that goes far beyond merely falling ill. Small chemical signals, immune adjustments, and even nerve-associated signals are all part of the mix. You wouldn't think so, but the gut-brain link is no joke; microbial byproducts gently nudge our nervous system with immune messages, local nerve circuits, and the vagus nerve that can mold our body and mood in the long term. Birth processes, antibiotic exposure, and daily stress just put more spice into all this microbial action, altering the microbial combination now further and, for most of us, boosting our likelihood of developing disorders from early brain development problems through later neurodegenerative afflictions. In general, this increasing understanding indicates that controlling these microbial communities may reveal new avenues to address diseases associated with mis-communications between hosts and microbes (Cryan et al., 2019). Taking another aspect into consideration, some beneficial microbes appear to hold the uglier ones at bay – a delicate balancing act that is particularly significant in agriculture. Here, beneficial microbes use several tricks: they outcompete harmful ones for nutrients, prime the host to better resist invaders, or even directly attack pathogens through antibiosis or hyperparasitism. These actions usually hinge on delicate metabolic signals acting right at the infection site, often at very low levels. What's fascinating is that outcomes observed in the lab aren't always mirrored in the wild, reminding us that observing microbes in their native environment is key. This discrepancy not only refines biological control plans but also indicates directions through which we can avoid issues such as resistance and unforeseen environmental side effects—domains where old-school fungicide doctrines simply don't measure up. Everything considered, microbes function within a maze of interactions, ranging from overt battles with pathogens to long-term effects on immunity, metabolism, and even neurobiology. Confronting these interconnected processes requires a combination of intensive laboratory work and *in vivo* observation. In a majority of instances, future investigations must focus on particular molecular blueprints, enhance how we detect microbial antagonists, and create bespoke microbe-based remedies. Integrating firm microbiological evidence with clinical and environmental perspectives could well lead to creative solutions in controlling health and disease (Cryan et al., 2019).

References

1. Goudie, A.C. and Olateju, F. and Anderson, J.G. and Rowan, N. and MacGregor, S.J. (2003) Inactivation of pathogens on food and contact surfaces using ozone as a biocidal agent. In: Society for General Microbiology – 152nd Meeting – –, 2003-04-07 - 2003-04-11. (accessed on 7 May 2025).
2. Bevivino, A., Bacci, G., Dřevínek, P., Nelson, M. T., Hoffman, L. R., & Mengoni, A. (2019). Deciphering the ecology of cystic fibrosis bacterial communities: Towards systems-level integration. *Trends in Molecular Medicine, 25,* 1110–1122. https://doi.org/10.1016/j.molmed.2019.07.008.
3. Blyden, K. K., Thomas, J., Emami-Naeini, P., Fashina, T., Conrady, C. D., Albini, T., Carag, J., et al. (2024). Emerging infectious diseases and the eye: Ophthalmic manifestations, pathogenesis, and one health perspectives. *International Ophthalmology Clinics, 64,* 39–54. https://www.semanticscholar.org/paper/d5fa7d390dc3942f3f374406d2b46af41b6e87f1 (accessed on 7 May 2025).
4. Chiu, C. Y. (2013). Viral pathogen discovery. *Current Opinion in Microbiology, 16*(4), 468–478. https://doi.org/10.1016/j.mib.2013.05.001.
5. Cramer, R., & Kowalski, C. H. (2021). Is it time to kill the survival curve? A case for disease progression factors in microbial pathogenesis and host defense research. *mBio, 12.* https://www.semanticscholar.org/paper/598f8499bf3da08d51fb7ccb2a63816a2becea1f (accessed on 7 May 2025).
6. Cryan, J. F., O'Riordan, K. J., Cowan, C. S. M., Sandhu, K. V., Bastiaanssen, T. F. S., Boehme, M., Codagnone, M. G., et al. (2019). The microbiota-gut-brain axis. *Physiological Reviews, 99,* 1877–2013. https://doi.org/10.1152/physrev.00018.2018.
7. Cucchiara, S., Negroni, A., Pierdomenico, M., & Stronati, L. (2018). NOD2 and inflammation: Current insights. *Journal of Inflammation Research, 11,* 49–60. https://core.ac.uk/download/153371188.pdf (accessed on 7 May 2025).
8. Cui, Z., Wang, P., & Gao, W. (2025). Microbial dysbiosis in periodontitis and peri-implantitis: pathogenesis, immune responses, and therapeutic. *Frontiers in cellular and infection microbiology, 15,* 1517154. https://doi.org/10.3389/fcimb.2025.1517154da Costa, A. L. P., Neto, O. A. R., & Silva-Júnior, A. C. S. (2019). Conditioners of the infectious disease's dynamics. *Macapá, 8*(3), 9–23. https://core.ac.uk/download/233924077.pdf (accessed on 7 May 2025).
9. Das, S., & Khader, S. (2017). Yin and yang of interleukin-17 in host immunity to infection [version 1; referees: 2 approved]. *F1000Research, 6,* 741. https://core.ac.uk/download/84911322.pdf (accessed on 7 May 2025).
10. Eidt, G. (2017). Papel da Candida albicans na desmineralização do esmalte dental e no potencial acidogênico de biofilmes de Streptococcus mutans: Estudo *in vitro.* https://core.ac.uk/download/293611733.pdf (accessed on 7 May 2025).
11. Fan, J., Jiang, T., & He, D. (2023). Advances in the implications of the gut microbiota on the treatment efficacy of disease-modifying anti-rheumatic drugs in rheumatoid arthritis. *Frontiers in immunology, 14,* 1189036. https://doi.org/10.3389/fimmu.2023.1189036 (accessed on 7 May 2025).

12. Fu, Q., Ma, X., Li, S., Shi, M., Song, T., & Cui, J. (2024). New insights into the interactions between the gut microbiota and the inflammatory response to ulcerative colitis in a mouse model of dextran sodium sulfate and possible mechanisms of action for treatment with PE&AFWE. *Animal Models and Experimental Medicine, 7*, 83–97. https://www.semanticscholar.org/paper/0b223fe201959e728797d2ebaac24fdcb3801d98 (accessed on 7 May 2025).

13. Galluzzi, L., Vitale, I., Aaronson, S. A., Abrams, J., Adam, D., Agostinis, P., Alnemri, E. S., et al. (2018). Molecular mechanisms of cell death: Recommendations of the Nomenclature Committee on Cell Death 2018. *Cell Death and Differentiation, 25*, 486–541. https://doi.org/10.1038/s41418-017-0012-4.

14. Ghosh, S., Whitley, C. S., Haribabu, B., & Jala, V. R. (2021). Regulation of intestinal barrier function by microbial metabolites. *Cellular and Molecular Gastroenterology and Hepatology, 11*, 1463–1482. https://doi.org/10.1016/j.jcmgh.2021.02.007.

15. Gomes, M. C., & Mostowy, S. (2019). The case for modeling human infection in zebrafish. *Trends in Microbiology, 28*, 10–18. https://doi.org/10.1016/j.tim.2019.08.005.

16. Gonçalves, M. A. P. (2014). Microbiota: Implicações na imunidade e no metabolismo. https://core.ac.uk/download/61017571.pdf (accessed on 7 May 2025).

17. Hacquard, S. (2015). Disentangling the factors shaping microbiota composition across the plant holobiont. *New Phytologist, 209*, 454–457. https://doi.org/10.1111/nph.13760.

18. Hou, K., Wu, Z. X., Chen, X. Y., Wang, J. Q., Zhang, D., Xiao, C., Zhu, D., et al. (2022). Microbiota in health and diseases. *Signal Transduction and Targeted Therapy, 7*. https://doi.org/10.1038/s41392-022-00974-4.

19. Hu, S., Vila, A. V., Gaćeša, R., Collij, V., Stevens, C., Fu, J., Wong, I., et al. (2020). Whole exome sequencing analyses reveal gene–microbiota interactions in the context of IBD. *Gut*. https://doi.org/10.1136/gutjnl-2019-319706.

20. Hudson, J., & Egan, S. (2024). Marine diseases and the Anthropocene: Understanding microbial pathogenesis in a rapidly changing world. *Microbial Biotechnology, 17*(1), e14397. https://www.semanticscholar.org/paper/2524565b3f2263016e780a47770d8bab95e9e3c3 (accessed on 7 May 2025).

21. Ke, S., Pollock, N. R., Wang, X. W., Chen, X., Daugherty, K., Lin, Q., Xu, H., et al. (2021). Integrating gut microbiome and host immune markers to understand the pathogenesis of *Clostridioides difficile* infection. *Gut Microbes, 13(1), 1935186*. https://doi.org/10.1080/19490976.2021.1935186.

22. Kruk, M., Mehta, S. P., Murray, K., Higgins, L., Do, K., Johnson, J. E., Wagner, R., et al. (2024). An integrated metaproteomic workflow for studying host-microbe dynamics in bronchoalveolar lavage samples applied to cystic fibrosis disease. *mSystems, 9*. https://www.semanticscholar.org/paper/e7f7fa0ae19710d9d945b389e3917d83511122b9

23. Li, C., Li, J., & Ni, H. (2020). Crosstalk between platelets and microbial pathogens. *Frontiers in Immunology, 11*. https://doi.org/10.3389/fimmu.2020.01962.

24. Mousa, R. S., Invernizzi, P., & Mousa, H. (2024). Innate immune cells in the pathogenesis of inflammatory bowel disease–From microbial metabolites to immune modulation. *Frontiers in Gastroenterology, 3*. https://www.semanticscholar.org/paper/350e5954b88bde968640376deef384158ca6d126 (accessed on 7 May 2025).

25. Nosanchuk, J. (2025). mGem: A quarter century with the Pirofski–Casadevall damage response framework—A dynamic construct for understanding microbial pathogenesis. *mBio, 16*(3), 1–7. https://www.semanticscholar.org/paper/46cd3736d326cf259e7ac757f780bbd27e626c5f (accessed on 7 May 2025).

26. Nowicka, A., & Gil, L. (2024). Microbial metabolomics in acute myeloid leukemia: From pathogenesis to treatment. *Advances in Clinical and Experimental Medicine, 33*(10). https://doi.org/10.17219/acem/191559.

27. Paller, A. S., Kong, H. H., Seed, P. C., Naik, S., Scharschmidt, T. C., Gallo, R. L., Luger, T. A., et al. (2018). The microbiome in patients with atopic dermatitis. *Journal of Allergy and Clinical Immunology, 143*, 26–35. https://doi.org/10.1016/j.jaci.2018.11.015.

28. Pandey, N. (2024). Bacterial pathogenesis. https://doi.org/10.58532/nbennurmmch1.

29. Pruksaphon, K., Amsri, A., Jeenkeawpieam, J., Thammasit, P., Nosanchuk, J., & Youngchim, S. (2024). The microbial damage and host response framework: Lesson learned from pathogenic survival trajectories and immunoinflammatory responses of *Talaromyces marneffei* infection. *Frontiers in Immunology, 15, 1448729*. https://www.semanticscholar.org/paper/6d1198e999b8ddb7abbbcc0c6e79451b814dd228 (accessed on 7 May 2025).

30. Rinninella, E., Raoul, P., Cintoni, M., Franceschi, F., Miggiano, G. A. D., Gasbarrini, A., & Mele, M. C. (2019). What is the healthy gut microbiota composition? A changing ecosystem across age, environment, diet, and diseases. *Microorganisms, 7*, 14. https://doi.org/10.3390/microorganisms7010014.

31. Rosowski, E. E. (2023). mSphere of influence: How host genetics impact microbial pathogenesis and treatment of infectious disease. *mSphere, 9*. https://www.semanticscholar.org/paper/40e92301569b368ffef44ac1095b2571622a71ba (accessed on 7 May 2025).

32. Rowe, M., Veerus, L., Trosvik, P., Buckling, A., & Pizzari, T. (2020). The reproductive microbiome: An emerging driver of sexual selection, sexual conflict, mating systems, and reproductive isolation. *Trends in Ecology & Evolution, 35*, 220–234. https://doi.org/10.1016/j.tree.2019.11.004.

33. Schwegmann, A., & Brombacher, F. (2008). Host-directed drug targeting of factors hijacked by pathogens. *Science Signaling, 1*, re8. https://www.semanticscholar.org/paper/3fc9df87905a781172c8ca0025bd9da8283937ad (accessed on 7 May 2025).

34. Su, F., Su, M., Wei, W., Wu, J., Chen, L., Sun, X., Liu, M., et al. (2025). Integrating multi-omics data to reveal the host-microbiota interactome in inflammatory bowel disease. *Gut Microbes, 17*(1), 2476570. https://www.semanticscholar.org/paper/f1fc709e419a2af22e2e4bad5c7b0cd3fd1e6a2e (accessed on 7 May 2025).

35. Takamura, S. (2017). Regional immune responses in the lung after respiratory virus infections. *Viral Immunology, 30*(6), 397. https://www.semanticscholar.org/paper/13714efa126543aea5820a0f7ca74ce98af2a52d (accessed on 7 May 2025).

36. Taylor, J. W., & Whiston, E. (2015). Comparative phylogenomic of pathogenic and nonpathogenic species. *G3: Genes, Genomes, Genetics, 6*(2), 235–244. https://doi.org/10.1534/g3.115.022806.

37. Tomofuji, Y., Maeda, Y., Oguro-Igashira, E., Kishikawa, T., Yamamoto, K., Sonehara, K., Motooka, D., et al. (2021). Metagenome-wide association study revealed disease-specific landscape of the gut microbiome of systemic lupus erythematosus in Japanese. *Annals of the Rheumatic Diseases, 80*, 1575–1583. https://doi.org/10.1136/annrheumdis-2021-220687.

38. Tovaglieri, A., Sontheimer-Phelps, A., Geirnaert, A., Prantil-Baun, R., Camacho, D. M., Chou, D. B., Jalili-Firoozinezhad, S., et al. (2019). Species-specific enhancement of enterohemorrhagic E. coli pathogenesis mediated by microbiome metabolites. *Microbiome, 7*. https://doi.org/10.1186/s40168-019-0650-5.

39. Wang, X., Wang, J., Mao, L., & Yao, Y. (2024). *Helicobacter pylori* outer membrane vesicles and infected cell exosomes: New players in host immune modulation and pathogenesis. *Frontiers in Immunology, 15, 1512935*. https://www.semanticscholar.org/paper/ad7041ab35c03cfd75ad6d364fdc746c84d853d0 (accessed on 7 May 2025).

40. Zheng, D., Liwinski, T., & Elinav, E. (2020). Interaction between microbiota and immunity in health and disease. *Cell Research, 30*, 492–506. https://doi.org/10.1038/s41422-020-0332-7.

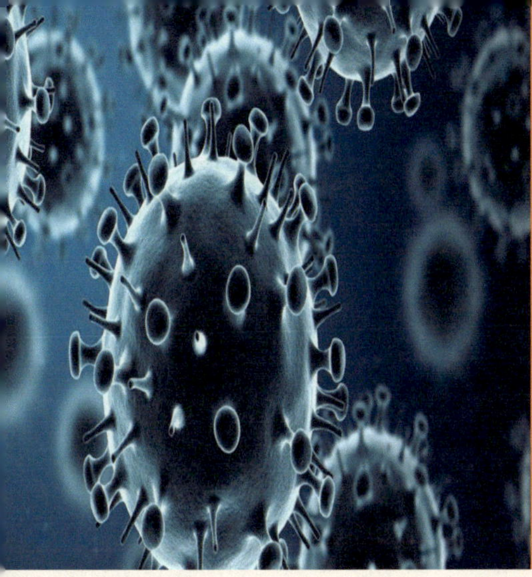

Chapter 3

EPIDEMIOLOGY OF INFECTIOUS DISEASES

Contents

Introduction

Humans have traditionally peered into how sickness and health appear and travel through certain populations—it's really the center of what public health is all about. You could say that exploring how diseases begin, spread, and impact communities has provided us with a tool called epidemiology. It's most often applied by researchers and policymakers to determine what risks promote infections to move from one individual to another. They acquire counts of disease cases and observe where they form clusters, usually detecting associations among bacteria and those they infect. This technique doesn't only uncover how a bug directly strikes us; it also suggests how larger social elements may be involved. All this comes into play when determining where to invest resources and what control measures to implement, to decrease the rates of disease and mortality worldwide. A major piece in all of this is weighing the disease—tabulating new cases, total incidence, deaths, and even disability effects. A major headache today, in general, is that bacteria are developing resistance to our treatment, and it is becoming increasingly harder to halt infections. Seriously, many large-scale studies have worked their way through mountains of data from across the world to estimate deaths attributed to these persistent pests. What they have discovered is that some areas are hit far harder than others, and a few bacteria are usually to blame (Murray et al., 2022).

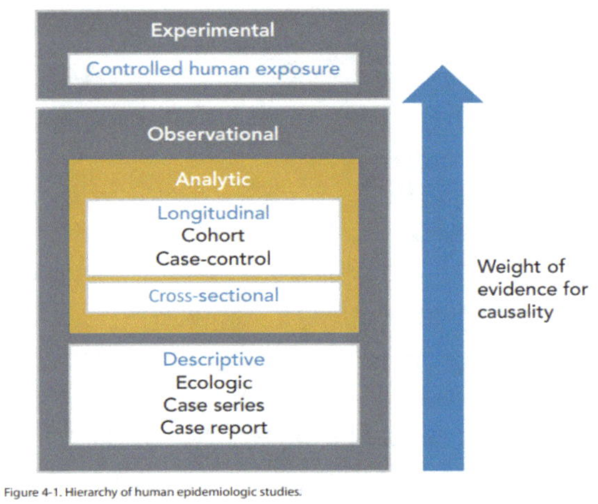

Figure 3.1. Epidemiology of infectious diseases.

Source: By National Institute for Occupational Safety and Health - https://www.cdc.gov/niosh/docs/2020-106/pdfs/2020-106revised032020.pdf, Public Domain, https://commons.wikimedia.org/w/index.php?curid=150471869

This highlights just how crucial reliable surveillance systems and properly equipped labs, particularly in areas with fewer resources, are for monitoring resistance trends. Having a sense of what to anticipate, however, health authorities can usually respond promptly and appropriately to ward off more contamination of these difficult-to-kill diseases. Considering infections is also trying to comprehend why some people get ill more frequently than others. Consider autoimmune diseases such as systemic lupus erythematosus, for instance; if the immune system isn't optimally functioning, individuals become increasingly susceptible to infections (Barber et al., 2020). It's kind of counterintuitive in a way since interventions intended to dial down over-activity within the immune response have the ability at times, ironically, to raise the threat of infection, and that confuses clinicians. In most situations, identifying who's at greater risk is crucial, and epidemiology work aids in mapping out preventive measures—whether it's through vaccination campaigns targeted at specific groups or refining treatments. By marrying knowledge from individual patient profiles with wider information on full populations, this discipline informs strategies that seek to reduce both serious diseases and fatalities within groups with unique health burdens (Figure 3.1).

Definition of Epidemiology

Deciphering why diseases arise in clusters can illuminate which public health action to take. Epidemiology examines where and why diseases emerge in certain groups, examining what triggers diseases, what exposes people, and how microbes travel from person to person. Most of the time, by aggregating and parsing data, scientists in this branch detect outbreaks and track disease trends, while simultaneously checking whether our health and medical endeavors are doing their part. This sort of work is not all about infections—environmental and chronic conditions also have a turn taken at the turntable, with the mix of host, agent, and environment receiving attention. Such situations as the COVID-19 pandemic, with its sudden changes, show us just how crucial epidemiology is when it comes to anticipating and managing international health emergencies (Cheema et al., 2020). Delving slightly further, epidemiology combines a variety of approaches to unravel cause-and-effect in the spread of infections. At times, plain case review and some contact tracing can yield why an outbreak starts, giving authorities a clue on how to craft interventions such as quarantines or immunization campaigns to delay the chain reaction. Clinical observations, laboratory analysis, and ground-level surveillance all contribute to the puzzle, explaining finer details such as incubation periods, modes of transmission, and characteristic symptom patterns. There have even been instances where unusual eye symptoms appeared before other infection signs, which typically highlights why medical professionals need to remain vigilant for unanticipated trends to prevent further transmission (Cheema et al., 2020). Beyond merely explaining what occurs, epidemiology now leans towards predicting and forestalling disease using sophisticated statistics and large-scale trials. In general, by monitoring numbers such as the primary reproductive number (R0), incidence, and prevalence, experts can estimate how an infection may develop and guide public health policy accordingly. The rapid transmission of new pathogens across the globe serves as a reminder that a small local epidemic can rapidly become a pandemic if not contained. Work in modeling has identified that highly infectious diseases require concerted international efforts and rapid, anticipatory actions to reduce cases of disease and death. Overall, the discipline combines the science of disease tracking with realistic action for safeguarding populations, and it is an essential tool in our globalized world (Wu et al., 2020).

Importance in Public Health

Knowing where diseases spread and what fuels their transmission is important to establishing effective public health strategies. Epidemiology provides us with a means of detecting outbreaks, tracking their unglamorous routes, and determining which populations may be at risk. In most instances, this type of information allows public health professionals to redirect resources rapidly and make decisions about interventions that may reduce transmission. It even acts as a check on existing measures, frequently proposing subtle changes for improved results. Occasionally, when surveillance systems combination in epidemiological information, the early warning signs come to life—essential for quick response. And when you combination in advanced molecular techniques with new diagnostic technologies, you arrive at a much clearer perspective of pathogens and resistance patterns. All of these innovations, by and large, illustrate why monitoring disease behavior is so key to safeguarding populations from infectious threats (International Conference on Emerging Infectious Diseases, 2008). The COVID-19 pandemic, for example, truly showcased the strength of modeling disease transmission in informing public action. Models that simulate the way infections rise and fall provide insight into what could occur under various circumstances, informing strategies such as containment or moderation. Recent advances in machine learning and simulation-based inference have made these predictions more accurate and easier for policymakers to understand, enabling models to update in real time as new information becomes available. This type of technology advance even enables policymakers to have input on steps—such as social distancing, vaccination campaigns, or border controls—before they're implemented. Additionally, user-friendly platforms like COVID-sim and OpenMalaria made these modeling tools accessible to a broader population, calling for effective, evidence-based solutions for different infectious diseases. Most of the time, this changing alliance between epidemiology and computational science is precisely what contemporary public health responses require (Baydin et al., 2020). Backing away from the urgency of current outbreaks, epidemiology also extends its reach to longer-term health concerns. Chronic diseases such as antimicrobial resistance (AMR), zoonotic spillovers, and infections that vaccines can prevent all require constant surveillance and continuous intervention. Research in the field unties the complicated intertwined trio of host, pathogen, and environment that drives the emergence and sustainment of diseases—albeit with the photograph sometimes not clearly focused. With that knowledge in hand, scientists can inform the equitable health policy measures taken to stem inequalities among exposed groups. Further, developing the health capacities and establishing sustainable systems for surveillance against disease danger. To summarize, the union of policy, laboratory support, and community engagement guarantee that epidemiology continues to contribute to public health security and the journey toward international health equity (International Conference on Emerging Infectious Diseases, 2008) (Figure 3.2).

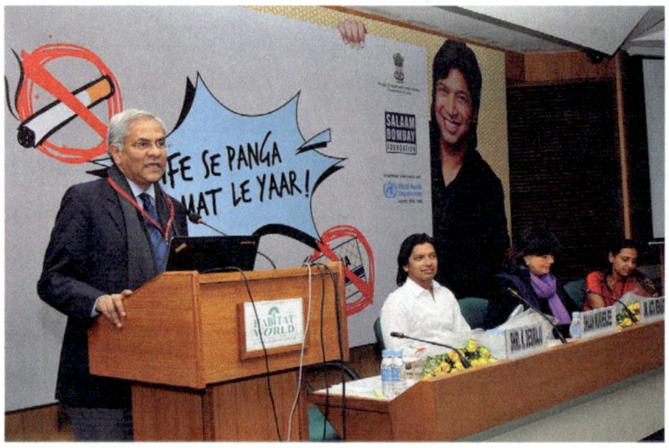

Figure 3.2. The importance in public health.

Source: By Ministry of Health and Family Welfare (GODL-India), GODL-India, https://commons.wikimedia.org/w/index.php?curid=71789278

3.1. Types of Infectious Diseases

To get a grip on infectious diseases, begin by considering what causes them. They generally arise from various kinds of bacteria—bacteria, viruses, fungi, or parasites—that each have their own uniqueness. Consider tuberculosis (TB), for instance; the bacteria that cause it disseminate on very small airborne droplets, whereas viruses such as the flu sneak around undetected on respiratory droplets. You can see that fungal infections tend to appear from exposure to the environment, and parasitic infections tend to be accompanied by a side of dirty food or water. At times, these microbes even trigger allergic reactions or even tamper with the nervous system, really proving just how diverse their effects can be (Sayfullayevna et al., 2024). Peering closer at the people who become ill, disease patterns among populations tend to be everywhere and nowhere. terms, the numbers of cases and where they are help draw out the broad disease burden and identify particular remedies. Geography, finances, and the local health infrastructure all have big effects. For example, vector-borne diseases—malaria being a case in point—are typically hard on tropical areas, while respiratory diseases, although more widespread, peak and trough seasonally. Recently, sophisticated tools such as machine learning and sophisticated predictive analytics have begun to chew through massive amounts of data to extract these trends and provide early warnings that could really hone our response plans (Santangelo et al., 2023).

It's obvious that dividing infections based on what they're caused by determines how we attack them head-on. Successful methods rely heavily on determining exactly how an disease is spread, how long it lays in wait before causing symptoms, and how the body may react. With viruses, vaccination attempts generally do a bang-up job, but bacterial issues tend to require antibiotics in addition to improved sanitation. Parasitic cases, on the other hand, often need things like vector control and cleaner water supplies. New tech—machine learning included—helps predict these threats a bit earlier, allowing us to tailor interventions more precisely. Overall, this layered strategy not only boosts our ability to manage diseases but also underpins research into fresh, emerging challenges (Santangelo et al., 2023; Sayfullayevna et al., 2024) (Figure 3.3).

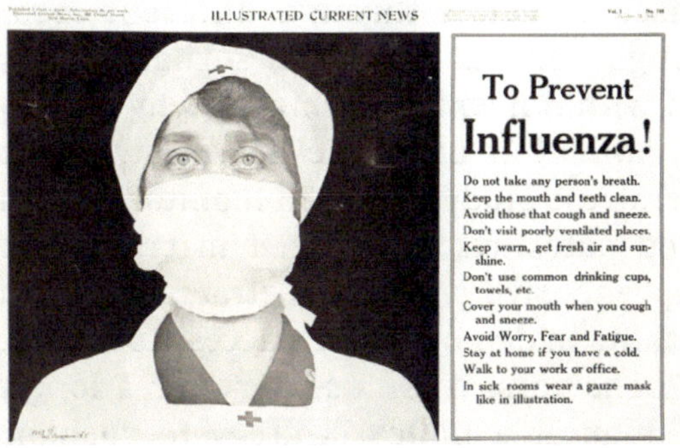

Figure 3.3. Types-of-infectious-disease.

Source: By Paul Thompson - https://collections.nlm.nih.gov/catalog/nlm:nlmuid-101580385-imgOriginally published in "Illustrated Current News", New Haven, CT. Volume 1, no. 785 (or 788), 1918., Public Domain, https://commons.wikimedia.org/w/index.php?curid=107373257

3.1.1. Bacterial Infections

Bacterial diseases have been a significant public health concern for years, and understanding their patterns involves examining a combination of influences that don't always fit easily into categories. Various areas, populations, and social circumstances all influence how frequently these diseases show up. For instance, statistics emerging from Saudi Arabia tend to identify brucellosis, TB, and salmonellosis as leading suspects, although each of them has some peculiar twists. You may observe that males are harder hit with brucellosis and TB, while salmonellosis appears more frequently among Saudi nationals. It's fascinating, : this irregular distribution suggests a complicated interaction between the host, the insect itself, and environmental factors. And, overall, the recent pandemic, with its blanket public health interventions, caused significant declines in a range of bacterial infections (Alhumaid et al., 2024), which is some indication that how we act and the policies we implement can have an impact. Ultimately, this type of variation appears to necessitate surveillance systems as malleable as the diseases they monitor. Beyond raw quantities, how our immune system responds to these bacterial pathogens is central to discerning who becomes ill and how severe the disease can become. As our bodies get older, our immune systems weaken, so elderly individuals are more vulnerable when these microbes attack. Inflammaging and immune senescence, two words that, in general, go together, both erase both the immediate and learned immunity of our body, essentially depriving our body's capacity for combating such infection. Not only does this impairing increase the chance of contracting an infection but also renders vaccines weaker in fighting them off. Knowing these changes, although it sounds somewhat technical, assists public health professionals in predicting infection trends to change and in developing strategies that are more appropriate for an older population, ironically which may have longer life expectancy but a growing infection burden. In brief, integrating our understanding of how the immune system evolves with age into epidemiology models truly enhances our overall strategy for preventing bacterial infections in various populations. In the future, controlling bacterial infections will probably rely on redesigning our surveillance systems and collecting data that is more than just a mere head count. Recent research advocates a new approach to disease reporting—one that considers the origin of an infection, travel history, hospitalization information, and even mortality status. In doing so, we not only hone the sensitivity and precision of our tracking mechanisms, but we also have a better sense of which pathogens pose the most dangerous risks. Paying close attention to mortality from these infections, governments can more effectively prioritize action and allocate, for example, resources more meaningfully. It's also worth observing that although certain infections such as diphtheria and syphilis have declined, others remain or even reappear, reaffirming the fluid, constantly evolving nature of bacterial epidemiology (Alhumaid et al., 2024). In melding detailed epidemiological data with insights from clinical and immunological fields, we're likely to see a stronger, more flexible approach to tackling bacterial diseases around the globe.

3.1.2. Viral Infections

Recent pandemics, particularly COVID-19, have reconfigured the way we manage viral threats globally. Practices like social distancing and other public health measures, implemented primarily to curb SARS-CoV-2, wound up reducing instances of other infections like influenza, respiratory syncytial virus, parainfluenza, and adenovirus. It's fascinating how fighting one virus has a ripple effect to spread benefits in unexpected ways, even though it also adjusts the general composition of viruses we observe. In most instances, these developments remind us that viruses are by nature interconnected, and understanding these intersections is fundamental to developing adaptable responses in the future (Achangwa et al., 2022). Liver-diseasing chronic viruses continue to add significantly to global health issues. Hepatitis B and C, for example, are still the chief causes of chronic liver disease, despite vaccines and newer medications moving the landscape slightly. The decline in hepatitis B cases, due to childhood vaccination, demonstrates how prevention can pay off—but many infections are overlooked because of missed diagnoses or treatment lapses. Meanwhile, hepatitis C is a very real challenge, especially in regions where healthcare is not strong and risk behaviors such as intravenous drug use are prevalent. These facts highlight why good screening, vaccination, and treatment efforts, which are adapted to local needs, are so crucial in decreasing liver-related disease (Cheemerla & Balakrishnan, 2021). In addition to hepatitis, other viral diseases also contribute to global health issues in a manner that blends with lifestyle and environmental factors. For instance, liver issues associated with alcohol or nonalcoholic fatty liver disease increasingly overlap with viral hepatitis, rendering treatment less predictable. Viruses transmit through different means—through vertical channels, sexual activity, or even within hospitals, which is why we require a combination of public health strategies. In general, the study and keen monitoring of these varied pathways may assist in creating more comprehensive prevention strategies. In light of the shifts in demographics, access to healthcare, and behaviors, it is necessary for a long-term and adaptable policy strategy to cushion the overall effect on public health (Cheemerla & Balakrishnan, 2021) (Figure 3.4).

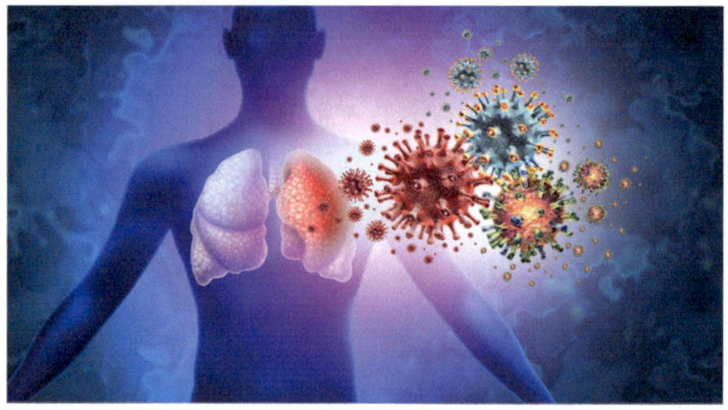

Figure 3.4. Viral infections.

Source: WW Medical Group. (n.d.). *Viral Infections.*

3.1.3. Parasitic Infections

Parasitic disease is a complicated affair – they're not just diverse in biology, but their life cycles curl around various hosts and even the environment in unforeseen manners. You know, in most of the tropical and subtropical regions, where there's poor sanitation and weather combined with economic distress, these insects are a giant pest for public health. Sometimes, the lines blur further when animal and insect routes overlap—making it hard to pin down where an outbreak started. Real monitoring? That means incorporating medical statistics with microbe and nature data to figure out both when and where things go wrong. And, in broad terms, world travel and changing migration routes continue to mix the pot, as infections leap into new regions and compel nations to collaborate on detection and control (International Conference on Emerging Infectious Diseases, 2008). In terms of prevention, the game plan essentially depends on reaching deep into what motivates such transmission cycles. Measures of health usually attempt to strike at the vectors, the in-between hosts, and even areas within the environment where the bacteria are found, but success invariably rests on local knowledge and active participation from the populace. Another complexity is added by drug resistance—a problem that's clouding treatment and driving researchers to continuously search for new therapies or vaccines. You also need to take into account that economic and social gaps tend to exacerbate the situation, adding additional risks to already at-risk communities. Therefore, increasing surveillance and adding in quick tests are important steps for preventing outbreaks from getting started, particularly where individuals are most vulnerable (International Conference on Emerging Infectious Diseases, 2008). Scientists nowadays are relying on molecular methods and geospatial resources to understand these infections more interactively. Most of the time, these technologies enable scientists to identify parasite strains accurately and track their paths across populations, thus making any specific response sharper. You may also hear of systems such as GIS or even remote sensing – these assist in mapping not only where vectors reside but also what environmental conditions lay the groundwork for outbreaks. All of these innovations assist in stretching public health budgets and preparing better for possible crises. That being said, gathering and mixing all the information together is still an actual challenge, particularly in low-resource areas. Closing these gaps requires additional investment in training, improved laboratory-to-field communication, and constructing networks that connect researchers, field workers, and public health officials (International Conference on Emerging Infectious Diseases, 2008).

3.2. Transmission of Infectious Diseases

Deciphering how bacteria spread between individuals is central to keeping outbreaks in check and preventing public health threats. There are a multitude of ways this occurs – bacteria can waft through the air, hit you in a cough or sneeze droplet, or even catch a ride on common objects. At times, the pathogens persist suspended in the air long enough to find their way to individuals even distant from the origin. Those heavier sneeze particles don't go very far but still have enough oomph to transfer an infection. Further there are contaminated objects (fomites, as they're sometimes referred to) that, when one touches them, transfer the microbe on indirectly. All these routes illustrate how complicated infection transmission can be, and why a combination of strategies is necessary to sever the chain (Fung et al., 2018). In the majority of instances, pinning down such pathways is what serves to sever the risk. An effective system for guarding things and being prepared for foul play is at the center of fighting epidemics. Surveillance is what health teams do to catch trends, identify outbreaks early, and verify whether their control actions are effective. This usually involves collecting data rapidly and passing it through computer simulations, mathematics, and statistics specifically programmed for monitoring disease. Such tools enable us to make estimates about where an outbreak will go next and choose control steps before things getting out of hand. Being proactive also involves taking measures such as isolating the ill, establishing quarantine, implementing vaccination drives, and even enhancing rudimentary hygiene. This combination of watchful waiting and rapid response—based on epidemiological knowledge—is essential to controlling outbreaks and protecting our communities (Fung et al., 2018). Bouncing a bit deeper, you see that there's a complex combination of biology, environment, and behavior that all influence how infections move and why it's so difficult to contain them. Parameters such as temperature, humidity, and whether or not a room receives enough fresh air can impact how long bacteria persist on surfaces or hang in the air. Social customs—crowding together, how we approach cleanliness, even the practice of healthcare—additional tune the chances of an infection taking hold. Finally, the manner pandemics come into being makes it certain that synchronized international effort is necessary, as pathogens can readily take advantage of travel and close social groups. Overall, combining all these aspects into our models assists in improved prediction and reduced disease transmission. It all reinforces the importance of continuous research and for health measures to continue adjusting as the landscape of transmission evolves (Fung et al., 2018) (Figure 3.5).

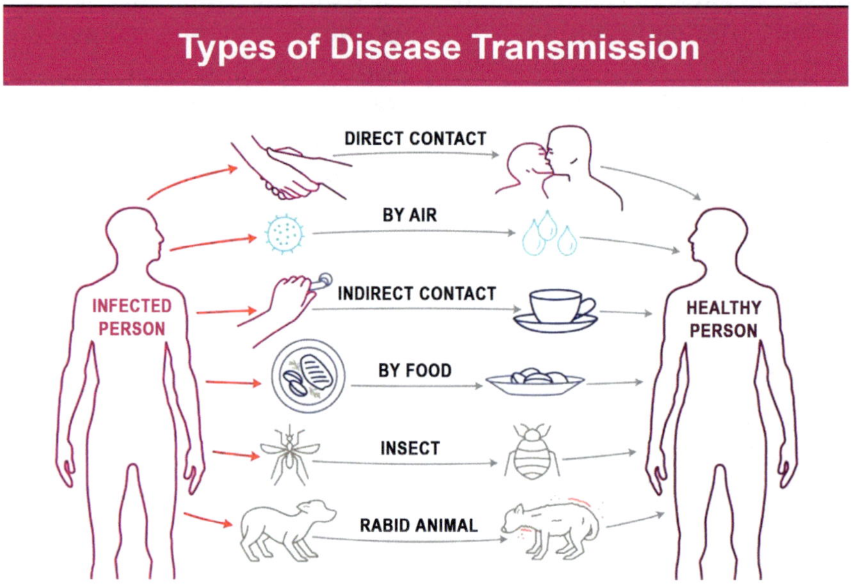

Figure 3.5. Transmission of infectious diseases.

Source: Shutterstock. (n.d.). *Transmission of Infectious Diseases.*

3.2.1. Modes of Transmission

Pathogens don't move in clear, linear paths; disease winds up spreading in patterns that combine nature and our daily environments. Viruses tend to ride on small droplets we emit when we speak, cough, or even breathe, and when individuals get too close, these droplets end up right on someone's face, typically on mucous membranes. Even if everyone does not appear to be sick—because carriers may be asymptomatic—the virus just keeps going, which makes it a great problem to contain outbreaks. Exposure to symptoms may have varying time windows, but it is an important detail in determining how quickly things progress and when to quarantine. Such simple behaviors as wearing a mask and standing a little apart significantly reduced transmission by reducing both the emission and intake of those infective particles. Public health planners in most instances apply this type of information to mitigate outbreaks, particularly in times of crisis such as COVID-19, when SARS-CoV-2 is transmitted globally so rapidly (Wiersinga et al., 2020). Moving the spotlight from mere breath droplets, there's a bigger picture in action. Other bodily fluids and secretions can also store those naughty viruses – occasionally in unexpected places. Recent studies have revealed infectious SARS-CoV-2 in eye fluids, identifying the eye as a relatively under-appreciated point of entry. The mucous surface of the eye could even permit the virus to grow, with viral RNA remaining in conjunctival swabs for longer than one would think. This has prompted numerous healthcare providers to employ additional protection such as eye shields and for all individuals to be even more careful, such as not rubbing their eyes and keeping hands exceptionally clean. These discoveries, for the most part, push us to reevaluate our concepts concerning transmission, expanding our horizon on how diseases are transmitted (Colavita et al., 2020). Further there is indirect transmission. Dirty surfaces, or fomites, become unwitting hand-offs as the virus persists on other objects until it reaches your mucosal surfaces. This form of transmission truly emphasizes why cleaning and handwashing are still essential. Also, anatomical connections such as the nasolacrimal duct—the tube connecting the eyes and the respiratory system, can enable the virus to transfer between areas in ways that make our general picture of patterns of infection more complex. Such unusual routes create levels of complexity and can go some way toward explaining why certain infections appear to recur even when we believe we've dealt with them. Comprehension of these myriad pathways is key to creating aimed interventions that address multiple fronts, ultimately bolstering public health efforts to stem the tide of disease.

3.2.2. Factors Influencing Transmission

Diseases seldom attack in a nice, neat fashion. They happen as a mess of causes—bacteria, individuals, and the environment around them all come into play. Age, gender, and even the amount of money one possesses can tip the balance in who becomes ill. For instance, among Kabul men, hepatitis C appears more commonly among young men aged 21 to 30. The trend suggests that work habits and daily routines may enhance exposure to infection. You also notice clues in the way marital status and education correlate with the population that becomes ill, implying that one's ability to access health information and services contributes to transmission. In most instances, we need to look at biology as well as the social environment if we are to develop prevention interventions that penetrate the true causes of disease and not merely the microbe (Danish et al., 2025). Tick-borne diseases show a rather fascinating picture of the confluence of nature and work environments. Crimean-Congo Hemorrhagic Fever (CCHF) is one such case, usually picked up from tick bites or from contact with animal blood—especially if you're working around livestock or in a slaughterhouse in the right conditions. The local climate, the mix of vegetation, and how many animals are around can all change where and when ticks show up. In addition, the reality that the CCHF virus exists in various genetic types only makes for an additional source of complication in keeping things in check. In general, this combination of viral adaptation and changing ecological circumstances makes for a complex and chaotic situation to be in charge of controlling outbreaks (Srivastava et al., 2024). And on top of that, human behavior and social organization contribute significantly to disease transmission. Where health systems are incomplete or resources are scarce, a lack of concise information regarding routes of infection can exacerbate the situation further—as with conflict areas beset by high levels of hepatitis C. Even diseases that rarely spread directly between people, such as CCHF, serve to remind us that even infrequent secondary transmission makes a measure of community watchfulness necessary. Designing interventions such as vaccines, antiviral medication, or educational programs relies on the availability of extensive, detailed data from a wide range of perspectives. In general, combining insights gathered from nature's uniqueness and ordinary human experience remains the only reliable means of slowing down outbreaks and improving overall public health outcomes (Danish et al., 2025; Srivastava et al., 2024).

3.2.3. Role of Vectors in Disease Spread

Vectors play a large role in how diseases spread. Small animals—mosquitoes, ticks, and flies, for instance—routinely transport bacteria from one host to another without getting sick themselves. What they do and where they live on a day-to-day basis determines when and where diseases erupt, so fighting against outbreaks is rather difficult. Consider malaria, dengue, or even leishmaniasis: how these insects operate isn't merely about transmitting bacteria but also about combining their innate ability to transmit with shifting environmental uniqueness. In all but the most straightforward instances, deciphering this tangled web—how vectors push pathogens to adapt and even increase infection rates—is the secret to fighting more effectively against disease. When you examine vector-borne disease more closely, matters become even more intricate. Such diseases as visceral leishmaniasis, transmitted by sandflies, rely on nailing down how infectious a host may be to its little carrier. Probes like xenodiagnoses, , which examine whether vectors acquire infections with a blood meal—illuminate the numerous turns of these cycle events. Yes, these methods provide important insights into the vector–host–pathogen interaction but at the cost of ethical and logistical challenges that may restrict their wider application, particularly with human samples. Overall, filling these gaps by establishing improved diagnostic facilities is essential for improving strategies to break transmission chains at their source (Singh et al., 2020). On top of that, vectors also play a surprising role in driving the spread of drug-resistant microbes. When these carriers sustain and move resistant strains around, it only adds to the public health headache by raising both death and sickness rates. Models that crunch the numbers on infections linked to resistance clearly point out that smart vector management is a must. Interestingly, certain bacterial species associated with vector-borne infections have a significant increase in resistance, and this only complicates treatment. Combining vector control with measures to use antibiotics more judiciously appears to be a balanced strategy to reduce the overall burden. Simply put, gaining a firm hold of the various functions vectors perform—whether they are carrying pathogens directly or disseminating resistance—is essential for designing evidence-based, locale-specific interventions (Murray et al., 2022) (Figure 3.6).

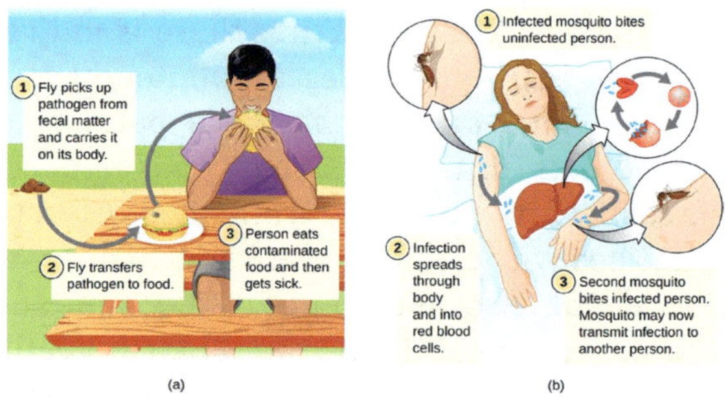

Figure 3.6. Modes of disease transmission.

Source: OpenStax. (n.d.). *Modes of Disease Transmission.*

3.3. Epidemiological Methods

Infectious disease is grasped best when professionals employ contextual, hands-on approaches that untangle both how pervasive a disease is and how it's transmitted from one individual to the next. Data arrives in lots of types, from lab results and surveillance feeds to studies of communities, and generally, these fragments combine incidence figures with death and morbidity statistics. Lots of times, when scientists combine disparate data points, they can identify risk factors and trends that otherwise wouldn't be apparent. Just consider the way modeling methods that draw information from lots of sources ultimately make estimates more reliable and inform public health decisions (Roth et al., 2020). With time, refining these methods means that frontline workers in public health can identify infections faster and use resources more efficiently. It isn't only a clinical acumen that pins down a diagnosis; there's also the help of modern molecular methods. Real-time quantitative polymerase chain reaction, RT-qPCR, for short, is a clear trick that identifies viral RNA in a variety of samples. In the COVID-19 crisis, this instrument pierced into the dirty cycles of viral shedding, even demonstrating that SARS-CoV-2 could persist in sputum and feces well after throat swabs test negative (Chen et al., 2020). This surprising turn of events reminds us that relying on only nasopharyngeal specimens sometimes creates a gap in the complete picture. A multi-site design strategy, in the majority of instances, refines the procedure for uncovering cases, provides hints on the duration of patients to remain in quarantine, and exposes transmission pathways that could have gone unnoticed. As our techniques change, scientists are now examining both risk factors and pathways of transmission with new, sometimes unexpected strategies. By combining analysis of clinical samples from different locations with the assessment of patient symptoms, scientists gain a more nuanced, if slightly unclear picture of disease behavior. For instance, the duration of viral RNA in gastrointestinal samples suggests an eventual fecal-oral route, which is a rather crucial fact for containing diseases such as COVID-19 (Chen et al., 2020). Assessing these routes of transmission typically involves continuous sampling and merging lab information with field-level modeling. In general, this type of experiential, cross-disciplinary research makes public health recommendations and isolation policies better attuned to the way pathogens act, so that our reactions remain as adaptive as the threats we encounter (Figure 3.7).

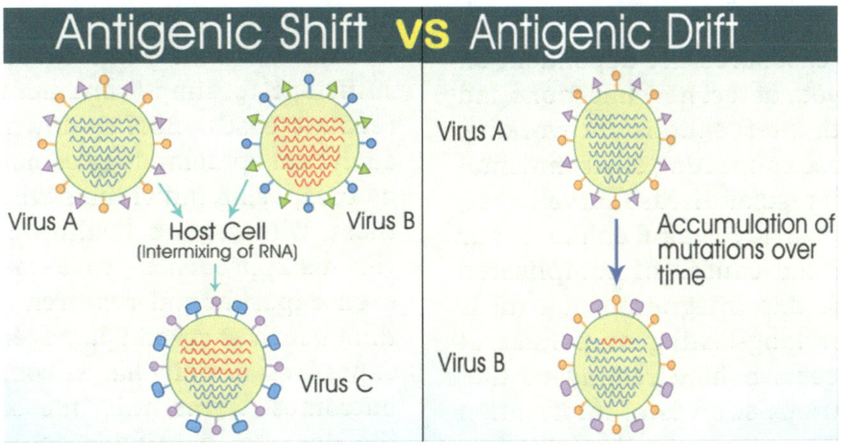

Figure 3.7. Epidemiology: Types of epidemiological studies.

Source: By Abuahmam - Own work, CC BY-SA 4.0, https://commons.wikimedia.org/w/index.php?curid=103320865.

3.3.1. Descriptive Epidemiology

Monitoring disease trends among communities is important when attempting to stop and prevent infection. Descriptive epidemiology comes to the rescue by providing the when, the where, and the who become infected—, it indicates what populations are infected, where the outbreaks originate, and when the cases peak. Through amassing and reviewing information in a structured but occasionally inexact manner, this method provides medical professionals with the foundation to speculate possible causes and create targeted remedies. In a majority of instances, combining molecular methods with this process further defines our perspective, enabling us to identify pathogen strains and track how infections circulate. One obvious instance is in aquaculture, where the combination of these methodologies with contemporary laboratory methodologies has made possible the revelation of viral trends in populations of commercial fish and enhancing disease control strategies (Snow et al., 2011). Overall, descriptive epidemiology remains a foundation for learning about infections as well as refining control measures within affected communities. Not only does descriptive epidemiology chart out who becomes ill, but it is also a large part of monitoring how disease patterns change over time. Systems of surveillance, they're designed to continuously gather and sort through information regarding disease cases and exposures, are dependent on these methods to both detect new infections and see if public health interventions are working. Others even propose connecting environmental exposure data with regular disease surveillance, since this additional layer can enhance our understanding of the causes of complicated diseases. Although this integration of data is more frequent for long-lasting or persistent diseases, the concepts behind remind us that the merging of various sources of information can fortify our battle against infectious diseases (Balmes et al., 2004). In general, descriptive epidemiology is not a once-and-done situation; it is constantly changing with new technology and new methods so that public health measures can keep up with new challenges. In addition to simply collecting and analyzing data, the efforts of descriptive epidemiology also inform public policy and determine where to allocate resources. By identifying specifically which groups are at greatest risk and when disease prevalence increases, these investigations inform interventions such as vaccination campaigns or public education campaigns to be implemented at the appropriate time. The level of specificity in mapping where and when disease takes place ensures the measures are equitable as well as effective, though the maintenance of these systems operating effectively requires continued investment and a willingness to evolve, particularly as pathogens evolve or entirely new threats rapidly emerge. The aquaculture scenario, in which the integration of traditional descriptive techniques with contemporary molecular information has truly honed outbreak investigations (Snow et al., 2011), is a clear example of this fact. Ultimately, descriptive epidemiology is still an indispensable tool in the epidemiologist's arsenal, necessary for making intelligent decisions regarding infectious diseases.

3.3.2. Analytical Epidemiology

In learning how infectious diseases are transmitted and what causes them, it's not sufficient to simply enumerate quantities or recount cases. Boring down a little deeper, analytical epidemiology comes in to tell us why by comparing individuals who become ill with those who remain healthy. Scientists employ various approaches , case–control, cohort, and even experimental research , to observe how things such as certain pathogens, environmental exposures, or daily habits connect with disease outcomes. terms, this line of thinking opens the door to identifying actual causal factors, a step that's fairly important for establishing interventions and informing public health policy. For instance, when confronting antimicrobial resistance (AMR), the discipline calculates additional deaths and lost healthy life years, explaining the effect of resistant insects and informing focused interventions (Murray et al., 2022). Research tends to blow up rapidly in epidemics – use the COVID-19 pandemic as one example – and this merely adds to the complexity of analytical epidemiology. A deluge of research comes out to inform clinical and public health choices, but many lack raw data or reflect limitations in their methodology that can invalidate their findings. A closer examination usually shows that opinion-based articles predominate while studies that do involve patient data are full of bias. There is a kind of tug-of-war between the pressing necessity to make rapid inferences to combat encroaching infections and the equally urgent necessity for robust, quality evidence. Analytical epidemiology in most situations must balance the speed of analysis with sufficient rigor to prevent misleading associations and maintain its conclusions valid and feasible (Raynaud et al., 2021).

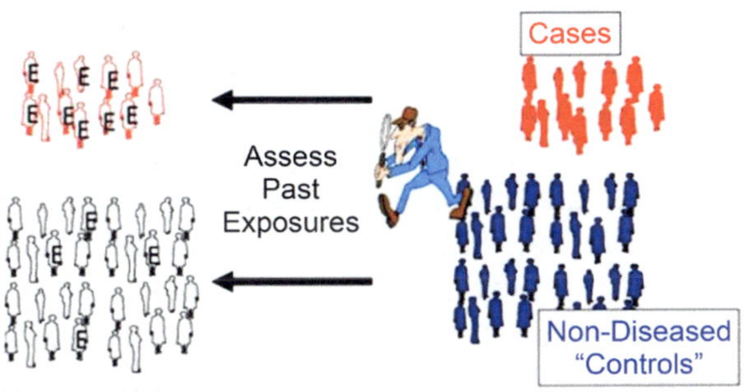

Figure 3.8. Basic strategies for analytical epidemiology studies.

Source: https://external-content.duckduckgo.com/iu/?u=https%3A%2F%2Ftse3.mm.bing.net%2Fth%3Fid%3DOIP.9YhIboFNuVmib33ynh5wYgHaD-%26pid%3DApi&f=1&ipt=a9a966912f44bdb787fbf04397a6377eb86970832acd415e586c9dc42db0856c.

Even when there is no large outbreak, analytical epidemiology remains at the forefront of addressing ever-present diseases. It deciphers how infections travel through various populations and identifies risk factors in the process. Its function even extends to monitoring the trends of antibiotic resistance, identifying high-risk groups, and testing prevention measures at the local and global levels. By applying cutting-edge statistical models and drawing data from different sources, this area offers important estimates for policy—such as demonstrating the enormous burden of AMR in low-resource settings. Initiatives such as these highlight the utmost need to enhance lab capabilities and strengthen surveillance systems so that choices are evidence-based. Finally, this area of research still motivates critical public health programs focused on managing infectious diseases and reducing their overall effects (Figure 3.8) (Murray et al., 2022).

3.3.3. Experimental Epidemiology

Experimental epidemiology is at the center of determining infectious diseases by allowing us to toy with concepts in a controlled environment. It's not like observational studies that just tell us about associations from what nature presents to us. In this case, scientists manipulate variables to pin down what precisely causes what. Take, for instance, pediatric unit studies where antimicrobial stewardship programs were pilot-tested under quasi-experimental designs—they reported significant reductions in antibiotic consumption and more informed prescribing without compromising patient outcomes (Fernández-Polo et al., 2024). This experiential approach allows public health practitioners to optimize resource distribution and calibrate clinical guidelines more accurately, thus decelerating disease transmission and reducing the rates of resistance among the higher-risk segments. Stringent experiments also have a significant role in investigating the effectiveness of vaccines for high-risk populations. Health workers, being exposed to infectious agents every time they work, are an ideal population for such studies. In the majority of instances, the combination of seroprevalence data with focused interventions demonstrates that disease immunity levels like those for rubella may differ significantly by age and profession—young healthcare providers, for example, are more susceptible (Borràs et al., 2014). The results tend to indicate generally that vaccination campaigns aimed at particular groups need to be employed, utilizing experimental designs to control hospital-acquired infections and more effectively shield staff and patients. The constant trial and error that goes into fine-tuning vaccine policies opens the door to public health action that is specific to local circumstances, which in turn contains outbreaks and increases overall immunity within healthcare settings. Experimental epidemiology is also crucial when it comes to determining how to maximize antibiotic use in our battle against increasing AMR—a concern that continues to mount worldwide. By subjecting stewardship programs to experiment in controlled trials, researchers have observed sustained changes in the prescribing of antibiotics and even cost benefits, demonstrating that resistance management need not be mutually exclusive with good patient care (Fernández-Polo et al., 2024). Such evidence typically supports the contention that hands-on, experimental methods balance treatment value against resistance issues. These findings set the stage for evidence-based policies, driving forward continuous monitoring and feedback in antimicrobial interventions. In brief, experimental epidemiology not only influences clinical interventions but also forms the basis of more general public health policies that are critical to keeping infectious diseases in check within various healthcare environments.

3.4. Surveillance and Data Collection

Control of infectious disease has evolved considerably over time. New methods of information gathering, such as contemporary surveillance and data collection, now enable us to detect outbreaks rapidly and distribute specific remedies nearly sponteneously. In the past, for so many years, we primarily worked off of standard clinical reports and laboratory findings; But now, with sources like social media and mobile phone apps (which weren't even initially created for health work), they're uncovering trends that older techniques may overlook. It's fascinating how these digital currents at times get ahead of us, particularly how we might observe with COVID-19 when rapid digestion of data provided input into public decisions as well as health responses. In short, combining old-school approaches with these online strategies increases our rapid response and early warning capabilities (Hamilton et al., 2021). Surveillance isn't only concerned with infectious diseases, either. More and more surveillance systems combine environmental exposure data with health outcomes to paint an even fuller picture of disease threat. By and large, although tracking environmental health has largely addressed chronic conditions, its strategy can provide insightful lessons for infectious disease work as well—particularly when it comes to combinationincorporating data and creating systems. National networks that connect disease surveillance with environmental variables are an important factor in identifying sources of exposure and vulnerabilities in populations. These linkages require systems that refresh frequently and disseminate new findings to the public. In fact, the task is not merely gathering information but even how to apply that data to guide strategies to minimize risk, as well as balancing costs and continuous improvements (Balmes et al., 2004). Staying adaptive to new threats means infectious disease surveillance must be adaptable. Digital tools must both scale and be fine-tipped enough to register even subtle changes in how disease spreads—in virtually real-time, as well. Meanwhile, such concerns as privacy concerns and data quality errors must be handled cautiously, because you can't count on trust and precision. Drawing together several sources of information—from clinical records and environmental signals to social interactions, can hone our capacity to identify who's most vulnerable and where interventions will be most effective. In the majority of instances, consistently monitoring and adjusting these strategies is central to staying up to speed on emergent threats. To summarize, this continuous process of testing novel ideas, assessing outcomes, and fine-tuning accordingly is the cornerstone of contemporary global strategy in the control of infectious diseases (Balmes et al., 2004; Hamilton et al., 2021) (Figure 3.9).

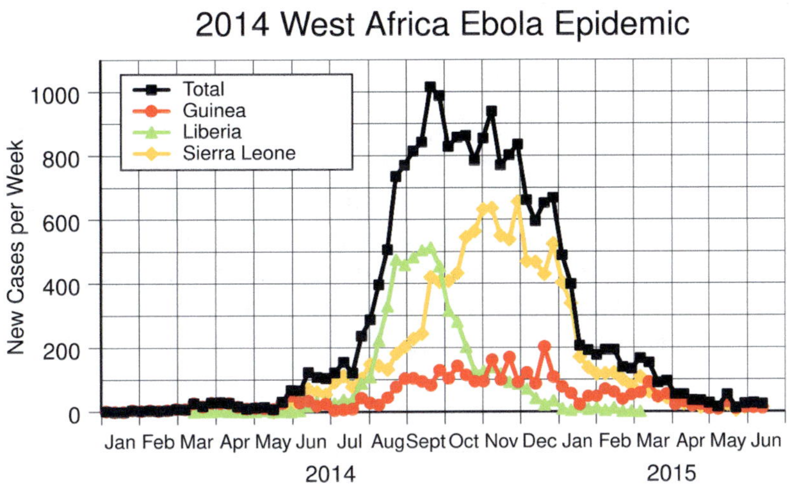

Figure 3.9. Alerting and surveillance for infectious disease.

Source: By Delphi234 - Own work, CC0, https://commons.wikimedia.org/w/index.php?curid=37007270

3.4.1. Importance of Disease Surveillance

Detecting infectious dangers early can be the difference between disaster and success. Disease surveillance, that vigilant monitoring of health statistics, has a lot to do with catching possible outbreaks before they take hold. Where medical care isn't always top-notch, such as in some parts of Sub-Saharan Africa, integrating findings from multiple disciplines has proven to be a good bet. One of these is training programs like FELTP (field epidemiology and laboratory training), which has been vital to developing epidemiologists working across the clinical, veterinary, and environmental domains in such a manner as to respond to the One Health concept. This sort of multidisciplinary cooperation, where emphasis is given on those diseases transmissible from animals to humans, is critical for ensuring quick responses and stronger health systems in threatened regions (Bingi et al., 2012). Digital technologies have also, over the past decade, entirely transformed the way we keep watch for these dangers. Information now streams in massive quantities from sources such as social media and mobile applications, providing us with new opportunities for monitoring problems as they develop. Digital epidemiology harnesses these flows of data and applies intelligent analytics to complement the traditional techniques, typically improving the pace and accuracy of alerts. For example, in the COVID-19 pandemic digital instruments were central in monitoring spread, supporting contact tracing, and even predicting potential hotspots. Often this combination of digital and classical methods has transformed public health monitoring into a quicker and more reactive system (Hamilton et al., 2021). Overall, monitoring disease is very much at the core of creating effective public health policy and wisely allocating resources. Ongoing checking for trends enables officials to identify patterns that can guide targeted measures such as vaccination campaigns, quarantine, or community talks. Rapid reporting with rapid investigation prevents outbreaks from getting out of control, lessening disease and death. By combining experts from various fields with digital innovation, we get a more complete picture of the behavior of disease. For that reason, we need to invest in solid, integrated tracking systems if we are to reduce the burden of infectious diseases worldwide and preserve public health security in our increasingly interconnected world (Bingi et al., 2012; Hamilton et al., 2021).

3.4.2. Types of Surveillance Systems

Monitoring infectious diseases isn't equal in all places; a combination of methods, each with its own uniqueness, is used. Frequently, cases are reported by medical professionals who report directly to central offices of health, a budget-friendly method but one that can lose information due to underreporting or delayed updates. At other times, officials take a more active approach by going directly to clinics and labs, an approach that consumes more resources but typically leaves one with a better overall view. There is also a type of monitoring that focuses on chosen sites or groups to detect trends and early warning signs of problems—a strategy that well complements the wider efforts.

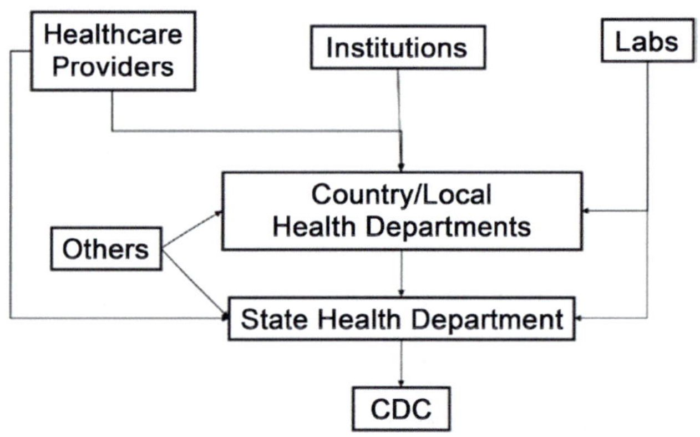

Figure 3.10. Surveillance for infectious disease.

Source: https://external-content.duckduckgo.com/iu/?u=https%3A%2F%2Ftse4.mm.bing.net%2Fth%3Fid%3DOIP.NWahegzsVMaxfp_CPepc8QHaF8%26pid%3DApi&f=1&ipt=4947e245f9c9cde5b92dd588c2d6569c152f08ed895e19c069c51c72a635f278.

For the most part, combining these various systems ultimately enhances early detection and simplifies containing an outbreak. New developments in molecular methods have truly changed the game when it comes to detecting and quantifying pathogenic bacteria. Conventional methods of tradition continue to have an elementary function, yet more recent technologies such as polymerase chain reaction (PCR) and genomic sequencing allow specialists to identify rapidly both the pathogens and genes driving drug resistance. For example, certain groups are now monitoring community sewage for evidence of infection; by examining biomarkers in the sewage, they can infer the prevalence of certain infectious agents. This type of approach—even when it sometimes grapples with the complexity of wastewater—can offer nearly real-time information on how infections are going, particularly for diseases that may otherwise go undetected. In most instances, continuous improvements are set to enhance accuracy, and this new tool is a reliable, scalable addition to disease surveillance (Zhang et al., 2021). With the emergence of drug-resistant insects, it has increasingly become apparent that surveillance of AMR has to accompany surveillance of infectious diseases. Information from hospitals, laboratories, and other surveillance programs—across different geographies—is used to develop public health regulations and clinical guidance. Frequently, such big data sets have identified a couple of resistant pathogens responsible for causing many deaths, making the necessity for focused, and occasionally geographically specific, intervention plans a pressing one. Increasing the capacity of microbiology laboratories and harmonizing data collection methods, especially where there is limited capacity, plays a long way in bridging the gaps. Overall, strong systems with AMR checks in place are not only essential for infection prevention, but they also direct more intelligent use of antibiotics and drive the creation of new therapies (Murray et al., 2022) (Figure 3.10).

3.4.3. Data Collection Methods

A good understanding of the ways that infection behaves begins with obtaining solid information. In general, the foundation for studying disease patterns is drawn from out-of-date procedures such as searching through literature, monitoring hospital and lab findings, and even conducting community surveys. These portions of information, gathered in ways that seem almost piecemeal, enable researchers to notice things such as how frequently a microbe occurs, its ability to withstand treatments, and how patients ultimately progress. When you combine data from multiple locations, you can even approximate the cost of resistant pathogens and identify geographical differences in effect, which reminds us that infectious risks are as varied as they come (Murray et al., 2022). As new technology emerges, such traditional approaches remain the foundation for predicting outbreaks and epidemiological trend mapping. Technological innovations have recently disrupted things by introducing an unforeseen element into disease monitoring. Today, digital epidemiology draws inspiration from social media interactions, mHealth apps, and even search engine trends to enhance earliness of warning signs and accelerate responses. This combination of unorthodox, big-data sources with old-fashioned surveillance—not to mention how it can track outbreaks in real time—creates a kind of dynamic picture of disease transmission. For most applications, combining these methodologies sharpens and sensitizes models, meaning public health responses can tend to be subtlesubtler. The COVID-19 experience, for instance, easily demonstrated that combining digital tools and methods can enhance control and preparation efforts (Kostkova et al., 2021). That being said, digital surveillance is not without its bumps. There remain concerns regarding data quality, standardization, privacy, and equitable access—particularly where lab capacities are already a little, well, constrained. It appears that strengthening lab infrastructure for consistent sample collection and testing remains vital if we're going to accurately assess the burden of resistance. Moreover, merging traditional and digital methods requires careful cross-checking to fend off biases that might sneak in from less conventional sources. By enhancing data systems and making sure that different platforms can "speak" to each other, researchers are more likely to draw out insights that are both specific and actionable. Overall, this balanced approach is central to adapting infection control measures to local contexts while addressing global issues such as AMR and emerging diseases (Kostkova et al., 2021; Murray et al., 2022).

3.5. Impact of Infectious Diseases

Infectious diseases have a tendency to distort our perception of health globally. They tend to strike hard—lots of individuals get very sick or even die, with the most vulnerable bearing the impact. Further, occasionally, our healthcare systems simply get bogged down when rising medical expenses, lost productivity, and disrupted social services all come together to hinder gains, particularly in low-resource settings. There's also the weight of stigma and residual stress that leaves communities out of whack and sometimes even resistant to seeking help. In the majority of instances, all these elements speak towards coordinated monitoring and rapid intervention that can stem the tide and leave communities healthier. Prevention, rapid diagnosis, and strong treatment continue to be the cornerstones in fighting these issues, both domestically and internationally. Really grasping how infections move means gathering solid data and keeping a watchful eye on shifting patterns. The Emerging Infections Programs (EIPs) in the U.S. show that when public health agencies, clinics, and research labs team up, it immediately boosts our outbreak-fighting know-how. These programs combine community-wide monitoring with hands-on lab work, offering important clues about how much disease is out there and how well vaccines perform. For the most part, findings from these initiatives assist in guiding policy—directing interventions to combat neonatal group B strep and crack down on foodborne pathogens, which in turn reduces disease and healthcare expenditures. In general, this holistic approach to surveillance reminds us why sustained investment in tracking mechanisms is necessary (Schuchat et al., 2003). In addition to tracking numbers, combating diseases relies on nations coordinating and exchanging information. The collaboration of the CDC with China, for instance, illustrates how combining forces—through developing effective workforces, implementing immunization programs, and applying effective risk communication—can address risks such as HIV/AIDS, influenza, and emerging infectious threats. Quite frequently, these international collaborations trigger both technological and scientific exchanges that enhance defenses at both local and global levels. By sharing information and preparing in advance for outbreaks, countries can suppress disease transmission and reduce mortality rates more efficiently. Evidently, such international collaboration highlights the necessity of vigilant monitoring and pooled resources in controlling infectious diseases (Figure 3.11).

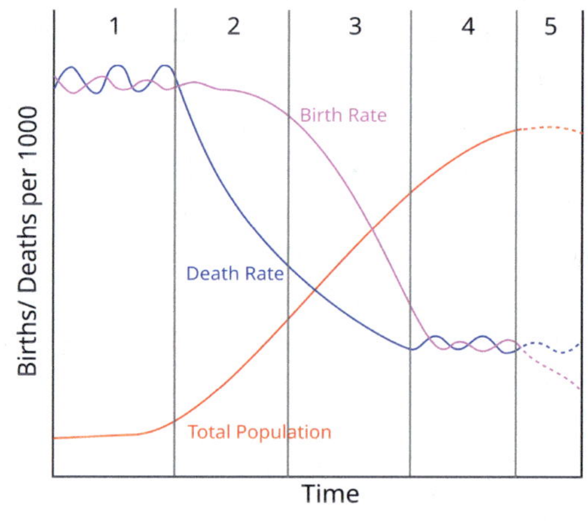

Figure 3.11. Emerging infections program (EIP).

Source: By Stage5.jpg: en:User:Charmed88derivative work: NikNaks93 (talk) - Stage5.jpg, Public Domain, https://commons.wikimedia.org/w/index.php?curid=5841448

3.5.1. Public Health Implications

Knowing how diseases get around isn't only science—figuring out useful public health strategies is important too. The study of bacteria and viruses informs us, informally, what path they travel, where they like to live, and how to deal with them. It influences decisions on uses of resources, vaccine campaigns, and public education efforts to keep outbreaks contained. In many cases, spotting where the risks are highest lets health officials zero in on measures that cut both disease and death. This idea becomes particularly important when new diseases emerge fast and quick info-sharing makes a real difference. Global meetings and reports—such as those summarized in recent infectious disease symposia (International Conference on Emerging Infectious Diseases, 2008)—remind us that the incorporating molecular leads, on-ground monitoring, and vaccine efforts is the very essence of preparing for health emergencies. Overall, combining these portions is fairly near the middle of reducing the overall burden of infectious diseases worldwide. Exploring how diseases spread, usually through dynamic modeling, is an essential tool when making public health decisions. These models kind of map out where an outbreak would head if various control measures are attempted, allowing decision-makers to look into the possible effectiveness of each action before leaping in. The mathematics of these models provides a good foundation for calculating things such as how long quarantine should last, what amount of vaccines may be required, and even how rigorous social distancing should become. And by inputting up-to-the-minute information, these models can change projections and recommendations as an epidemic evolves—keeping our responses agile. In general, particularly in times of crisis when disease increases rapidly and resources are limited, these analytical shortcuts facilitate streamlining where efforts are directed. Developing and refining models of transmission brushes against almost every aspect of preventing, controlling, and reducing the impact of outbreaks, highlighting just how critical they are in contemporary public health planning (Tam Tás). In a sense, the connection between theoretical calculation and actual health measures illustrates how our strategy in responding to epidemics is increasingly changing. Further there's the realization that looking at how diseases spread well exceeds the control of the outbreak at the time—it draws in broader concerns such as economic impacts and the burden on health systems. Systems that integrate rapid diagnosis with map information enable catching trouble early, which in a loose sense translates to fewer huge disruptions down the line. And when we gain an understanding of how microbes develop resistance to treatments, it informs programs designed to keep drugs effective against recalcitrant pathogens.

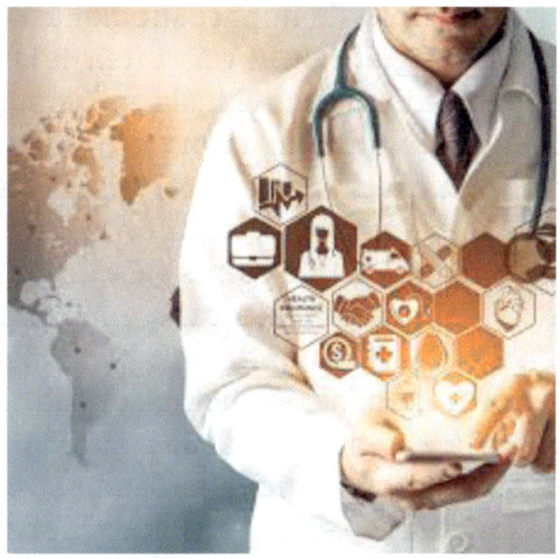

Figure 3.12. The public health implications.

Source: https://encrypted-tbn0.gstatic.com/images?q=tbn:ANd9GcRjmrqIRbEntnqxOs46c--z7A3Exhzqy9SaaA&s.

On top of that, difficulties such as disease spillover from animals, foodborne diseases, and even the volatile effects of climate change on insects transmitted through insects provide additional layers of complexity. In the majority of instances, strengthening our public health infrastructure and advocating for increased global equity—ensuring even the most marginalized receive the proper assistance and information—is totally essential. Global efforts aimed at vaccine-based prevention and new methods of disease tracking demonstrate a sincere commitment to a balanced health response, preparing us for threats in the future (International Conference on Emerging Infectious Diseases, 2008). Combined, this wide-ranging approach more or less charts the course for how we deal with infectious risks in an increasingly interconnected world (Figure 3.12).

3.5.2. Economic Consequences

Epidemics don't just strike our health—they end up affecting the overall economy in ways that may not be immediately clear. Consider SARS back in 2003; although it didn't kill massive numbers of people, its impact shook East Asia's markets quite significantly. Very often, it isn't the disease itself but how individuals and companies alter their habits in an effort to not get ill. Abruptly, panicked choices can disrupt trade, tourism, and general consumer confidence, and those economic hit points just accumulate on top of rampant healthcare expenditures. Occasionally, confused or downright misleading public information makes the risk appear larger than it is, and, in most instances, governments, fearful of an economic backlash, suppress vital information—ironically exacerbating the problem. Once transparency sets in, with several sources providing information, it tends to abate the panic and enable people to respond wisely (Brahmbhatt & Dutta, 2025). Evidently, incorporating economic measures alongside disease control isn't a choice anymore if we aim to secure health as well as financial well-being. When the economy falters due to outbreaks, it can trigger a bumpy cycle in which health problems and financial difficulties ultimately feed one another. During downturns, close living quarters, decreased availability of medical care, and individuals opting out of treatment regimens all can contribute to diseases spreading more quickly. Susceptible populations, , like migrants, homeless individuals, and even individuals in crowded detention facilities, tend to be at the center of such spirals. And with budget reductions taking a hard hit out of public health initiatives, the struggle to contain the spread just intensifies. For the most part, though, the connection between money woes and disease isn't destiny etched in stone; what governments do can significantly alter the outcome. With a good plan and adequate finances, a well-prepared state can stem disease resurgence amid economic crises, demonstrating just how important it is to marry economic policies with public health interventions (Abubakar et al., 2011). Taking the bigger picture, the dirty combination of economic forces and disease transmission informs us that epidemic control must be viewed from a socio-economic perspective. When a pandemic comes, it can drain productivity, overwhelm health systems, and disrupt social services—issues that disproportionately affect low-income and marginalized communities. Occasionally these epidemics even push consumer habits and market trends in unforeseen directions that persist. More often than not, it is important to get a grip on how people think about disease risk, and how that influences their behavior in the market, to craft responses that reduce both health and economic harm. That's why, in the end, relying on epidemiology, economics, and social sciences isn't just smart—it's necessary to develop policies that maintain disease at a distance while keeping economic performance and public trust in one piece (Abubakar et al., 2011; Brahmbhatt & Dutta, 2025).

3.5.3. Social and Psychological Effects

Infectious disease outbreaks are not merely a matter of physical health—epidemics also mess with individuals' feelings about themselves and others. When an epidemic occurs, individuals typically become more anxious, and that anxiety can warp into fear or even social ostracism. It is not just a personal ordeal; these emotions all too often permeate social life, disturbing the extent to which people trust health precautions or whether they are willing to comply with recommendations. Healthcare professionals, particularly those in the direct positions, can sense this more since the continuous influx of hazard tends to bring down both their individual well-being and the quality of their professional performance. Studies among nurses concerning infectious disease essentially indicate that although an acute perception of risk renders workaday activities more challenging, a shot of resilience coupled with good backup from colleagues can reduce the pressure. Overall, developing mental toughness and backing networks has become an essential part of maintaining such professionals healthy as well as effective (Zhang et al., 2024).

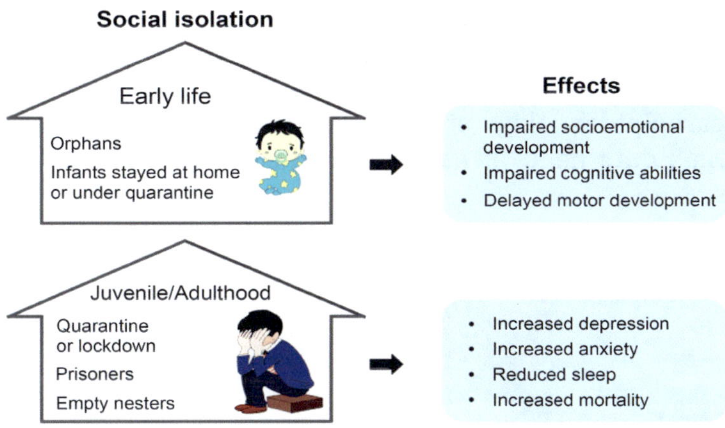

Figure 3.13. Social and psychological effects.

Source: Springer Nature. (2022). *Social and Psychological Effects.*

Working in healthcare has its own special dangers that aren't necessarily physical, there is a deep psychological aspect, as well. Various jobs have various problems; for instance, whether it's coping with biological agents, confronting chemical exposures, or dealing with ergonomic problems, the burnout and stress can accumulate quickly. Consider it: epidemiologists, nurses, pharmacists, and others all deal with layers of stress piling on in addition to physical danger. Consider epidemiologists who are tracing outbreaks—sometimes they have to make quick decisions in a stressful and uncertain environment, and that can absolutely erode their mental health unless things change. Most of the time, such complex social and psychological issues require solutions that extend beyond basic safety equipment, including mental health programs of support, transparent risk communication, and resilience training to make the work context slightly less of a strain on everyone (Al Sharif et al., 2024). Infectious disease fallout doesn't end with the individual, ranging far out into the broader community, disrupting relationships and the overall sense of community. Quarantine and the stigma that frequently accompanies disease tend to result in social isolation, causing individuals to feel lonely and emotionally exhausted. Such isolation will then interfere with public health interventions by discouraging individuals from seeking assistance or adhering to preventive measures. It's also important to note that stigmatized populations tend to bear a greater burden of these psychological disorders, one which only serves to further social inequalities and make control even more complicated. So public health interventions should incorporate psychosocial support and culturally attuned communication in an effort to resist stigma and foster a sense of solidarity. Identifying and intervening to assist with these mental and social issues is, simply, vital to mitigating the aggregate shocks of infectious disease and assisting communities in their recovery (Figure 3.13).

3.6. Prevention and Control Strategies

Efforts at prevention and control make a gigantic difference in the way we handle infectious diseases, particularly in hospitals since patients are especially vulnerable here. Hospitals shake things up by implementing multiple strategies to reduce infections such as surgical site issues. They make extensive use of thorough hand cleaning, distribute proper antibiotics before procedures, and invest in keeping things really clean during surgeries or other invasive procedures. Organizations like the Society for Healthcare Epidemiology of America in collaboration with the Infectious Diseases Society of America collaborate hand in hand, providing guidelines that are updated with new research as it emerges.

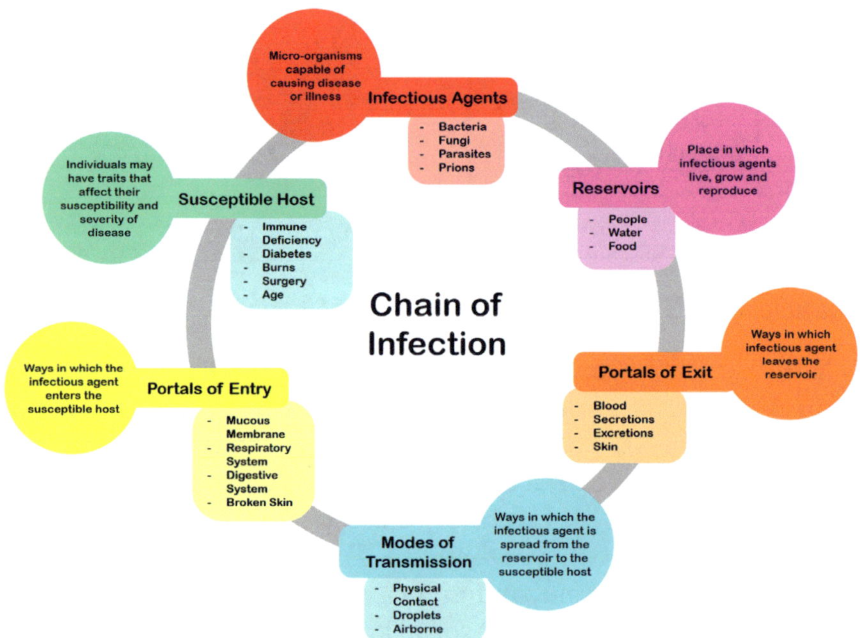

Figure 3.14. Infection prevention and control.

Source: Physio-Pedia. (n.d.). *Infection Prevention and Control.*

Overall, going through these steps results in hospitals focusing on infection control, keeping patients safe and reducing additional healthcare costs from complications (Calderwood et al., 2023). Beyond the hospital doors, halting outbreaks is largely up to synchronized public health actions and engaged community participation. Health authorities must remain vigilant, identifying emerging infectious threats rapidly and adjusting their strategies accordingly. Consider the initial COVID-19 days—isolating infected patients, tracing exposures, and even restricting travel were all components of the response. Though those strategies mimicked procedures during the 2003 SARS outbreak, COVID-19 introduced its own twists, such as numerous people remaining symptom-free. This compelled professionals to add in other precautions such as maintaining a physical gap, mass mask-wearing, and even remote working. In general, the World Health Organization continues to emphasize flexibility, on-the-spot evaluation, and a communication style that brings everyone along (Heymann & Shindo, 2020). Looking ahead even longer, the preparedness and resilience of our health systems are essential to sustaining these prevention efforts. Surveillance systems, which monitor disease trends and test how well interventions perform, assist in making sure additional resources can be mobilized quickly if demand surges. A part of this preparedness is ensuring that health workers have adequate protective equipment (even if sometimes the supplies aren't ideal) and proper training, that infection control measures are well maintained, and that life-saving devices such as ventilators and oxygen are available. In addition, public health campaigns that raise awareness on noticing symptoms, self-isolating as required, and receiving care early can empower individuals to slow down infections. At the same time, improved diagnostic equipment—such as serological tests—and continued research on animal-to-human transmission provide additional layers of protection. Overall, it's this combination of stringent hospital protocols and wider community measures that creates a strong, multi-layered response to containing infectious diseases (Heymann & Shindo, 2020; Calderwood et al., 2023) (Figure 3.14).

3.6.1. Vaccination Programs

Prevention of infectious diseases has always been a major concern in global public health. Vaccines, for instance, have proven to be a potent weapon—overall, they reduce the frequency of disease, save lives, and decrease the overall burden of disease that vaccines are designed to prevent. They're supposed to create incremental community protection (or herd immunity, if one prefers) which interrupts the regular chain of disease and assists those most vulnerable. In quite a few situations, immunization efforts have just about eradicated issues such as smallpox and even reduced some poliovirus strains to near nothingness. Nevertheless, the complete picture is not that easy; success doesn't just depend on how well a vaccine works—it relies on whether or not enough individuals get it. When health coverage is spotty or social and political concerns intervene, such programs falter, sometimes leaving behind reservoirs of disease and fomenting outbreaks that demonstrate how confused the mix is between health science, logistics, and public opinion. Consider polio as a case in point. Despite a precipitous decline in cases since the late 20th century, wild poliovirus continues to persist in some areas—largely due to immunization campaigns occasionally collapsing suddenly. In the case of Pakistan, for example, its vaccination schedules suffered at the time of the COVID-19 pandemic; mass immunization had to be suspended for a period of time, and millions of children missed their shots. This hiccup, in the majority of instances, ultimately reversed decades of effort and increased health threats in the region and further afield. Throw in people's reluctance to receive vaccines, stretched resources during a series of health emergencies, and poorly developed infrastructure, and you have an ingredient list for resumed outbreaks (Haqqi et al., 2020). These instances highlight the importance of having flexible, adequately funded vaccination programs. Vaccines also have a significant, but sometimes underappreciated, role to play in addressing AMR. By reducing the rates of bacterial infection—ones that would otherwise necessitate antibiotic therapy—vaccines reduce the pressure that fuels the development of resistant bacteria. Recent evidence highlights that many deaths globally are attributed to these resilient pathogens, with some low-resource settings particularly affected (Murray et al., 2022). Thus, concentrating vaccination on primary offenders can reduce the total burden of resistant infections. This two-pronged benefit—preventing the initial infections, as well as hindering the development of resistance—illustrates how critical vaccines are to our battle against infectious diseases. Scaling lab capacities for enhanced surveillance and streamlining vaccine distribution continue as highest-order priorities for international health systems fighting both AMR and more conventional infectious dangers.

3.6.2. Public Health Policies

Global public health policy has evolved quite dramatically over time with changing disease patterns. Chronic diseases dominated much of the 20th century, but infectious disease has made a bit of a resurgence. In the past, our epidemiological practices were designed primarily to examine long-term diseases, and therefore, when emerging outbreaks began to recur, researchers had to devise new study designs and statistical frameworks that more accurately describe how diseases transmit. This change in strategy has, in most instances, improved our capacity to track, suppress, and respond to outbreaks. With molecular and digital data now combinationed into such systems, outbreak detection (and indeed prediction) has become a lot more specific, allowing policymakers to implement targeted measures in almost immediate time. Overall, such advancements highlight how essential it is to have adaptive epidemiological tools when addressing infectious risks (Lewnard & Reingold, 2019). Contemporary public health interventions must also contend with the world where populations are closely interlinked, particularly owing to continuous migration and displacement. Migration trends, usually in geopolitically risky regions such as the Mediterranean, are their own source of problems when it comes to managing infectious diseases. Several nations now prioritize screening new migrants in an early stage as a preventive measure for disease detection and limitation. Data from other non-European Union countries bordering the Mediterranean and the Black Sea indicate that the majority of them have established screening programs, typically with a particularly keen interest in TB. Notably, the implementation of national guidelines appears to increase with higher numbers of refugees, suggesting a policy strategy that attempts to reconcile control of disease with humanitarian considerations. This combination of efforts emphasizes the necessity for concerted guidelines that preserve individual rights in the spirit of collective health security (Napoli et al., 2015). Looking in greater detail, infectious disease screening in migrant populations reflects larger epidemiological challenges. Although screening is generally regarded as beneficial, successful policy will need to combine cultural sensitivity, prudent resource allocation, and ethical concerns to provide equitable health outcomes for all. Add to that the fact that standardized protocols in varying geographic areas tend to make such interventions more efficient and effective. Aligning policy with sound epidemiology not only tends to bring the current scourge under control but also gains us an advance against novel pathogens as they surface. Ultimately, if public health policies are grounded in solid evidence and adaptive frameworks, they become critical tools for reducing the infectious disease burden in our increasingly connected, mobile world—emphasizing the critical role of policy in safeguarding community health (Lewnard & Reingold, 2019; Napoli et al., 2015).

3.6.3. Community Health Education

Seizing infections is not as straightforward as a clinic appointment; holding disease at bay typically requires a combination of strategies that have little to do with medicine. Education for health has a big impact—it's not just a footnote but provokes changes in how people perceive risk and modify behaviors. Informing individuals of the straight facts regarding how bacteria get around, what symptoms to look out for, and how to prevent contracting diseases creates an actual foundation for reducing disease at a community level. These programs tend to rely on local traditions and practices, which serves to debunk myths and combat the stigma that often attaches itself to disease. In most situations, allowing communities to get involved ends up being crucial—about as much of a secret recipe—as lasting health. At its core, this process takes hard, cold surveillance data and converts it into easy, mundane steps that may help stem an outbreak. In resource-constrained environments, incorporating participatory methods with what they had proved pretty effective. Some originate in such points as veterinary epidemiology, to remind us that local knowledge truly matters in picking up on patterns of disease (Alders et al., 2020). Health workers and community members find themselves discussing back and forth, exchanging findings in ways that honor daily habits and even some small uniqueness along the way. This type of interaction not only enhances the way we monitor diseases, but it also fosters trust—a crucial ingredient for individuals to adhere to public health guidance.

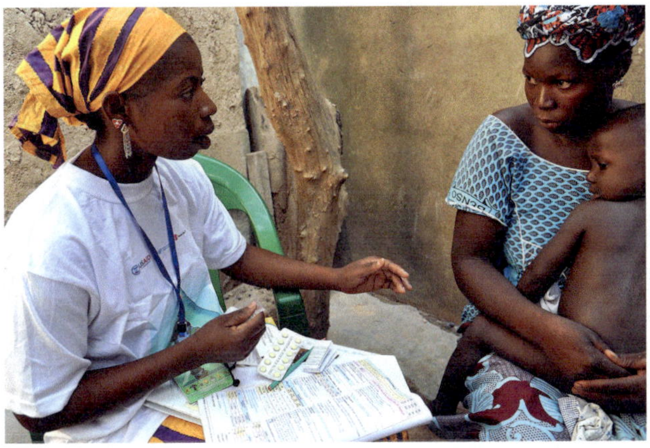

Figure 3.15. Community health education.

Source: By President's Malaria Initiative - Community Health Worker treats child, Public Domain, https://commons.wikimedia.org/w/index.php?curid=72085321

They also listen to gender dynamics and the interests of vulnerable populations so the message hits a diverse audience. Overall, whenever interventions are adapted to the specific feel of a community, things usually go much better. Diving into the nitty-gritty of disease transmission, community health education is not about flinging facts about; it is directly related to wider health objectives. Although noncommunicable diseases such as heart issues tend to make headlines (Roth et al., 2020), infectious diseases are an ongoing threat, particularly in most low- and middle-income areas. Typically, campaigns supported by sound evidence advocate for items such as immunization, improved sanitation, and safe food handling. Additionally, creating awareness on emerging disease risks will detect outbreaks early on, which saves big-picture problems from taking hold. It's also important to note, for the most part, that these activities are in line with wider sustainable development objectives, with preventing sickness being as important as curing it. Overall, community health education closes that difficult gap between the lab and reality, enabling individuals to act on real-life knowledge in a practical manner (Figure 3.15).

CLOSER LOOK

EPIDEMIOLOGY

Epidemiology is the branch of public health and medicine that studies the distribution, patterns, and determinants of health-related events in populations. It provides the scientific foundation for preventing and controlling diseases by examining how, when, and why illnesses occur. Unlike clinical medicine, which focuses on individual patients, epidemiology emphasizes groups of people, aiming to protect and improve community health.

At its core, epidemiology seeks to answer three key questions: Who is affected, where the cases occur, and when the disease arises. This helps identify risk factors and modes of transmission, enabling health professionals to design effective interventions. Epidemiologists use both descriptive epidemiology, which involves observing and describing disease trends over time, and analytical epidemiology, which investigates the causes and relationships behind health outcomes.

Several important concepts are central to epidemiology. Incidence measures the number of new cases within a specific period, while prevalence indicates the total number of cases in a population at a given time. Mortality and morbidity rates, along with other statistical tools, allow comparison across populations and regions. Epidemiologists also study epidemics, pandemics, and endemic patterns, which guide public health preparedness and response strategies.

Epidemiology has been crucial in uncovering the causes of major health problems. For example, John Snow's 19th-century study of a cholera outbreak in London laid the foundation for modern epidemiology by linking contaminated water to disease spread. Today, epidemiology plays a vital role in monitoring infectious diseases like HIV, COVID-19, and tuberculosis, as well as chronic conditions such as cancer, diabetes, and cardiovascular disease.

Epidemiology is an essential discipline that connects research, policy, and healthcare practice. By studying populations rather than individuals, it enables societies to prevent disease, promote health, and respond effectively to emerging global health threats.

Summary

Infectious diseases still come into play a great deal in the context of why health trends differ among populations. Given how our means of observing disease trends improve with each passing day, it's rather obvious now that microbes, particularly those that do not mind antibiotics, just keep switching their song. This implies that researchers and clinicians must continue changing the way they investigate and approach these topics. Spotting infections quickly, further handling them based on solid, up-to-date advice, is key. It also shows why folks from different fields need to team up, and why keeping an eye on what's happening worldwide is so important. New infection diagnosis and treatment methods appear to be promising, but meanwhile, the adroit aspect of how microbes develop warns us that our strategies must remain both flexible and resilient. In general, this method keeps us prepared for today's issues and those that may arise in the future. AMR – a true hard nut to crack – makes infection treatment even more challenging. The way patterns of resistance change means we really do need a closer examination of how these pathogens work, along with some knowledge of local trends. Clinical practice guidelines today encourage the judicious use of antibiotics and wiser, more targeted therapy, and specialists are saying that adhering to these standards, with assistance from susceptibility data, can really enhance outcomes by reducing disease and mortality associated with resistant microbes. But these regulations must be updated constantly, to remain current with new findings and the mechanisms by which resistance arises. This dynamic interplay between new science and how we treat antibiotics truly highlights the problem. To sum it all up, combating infectious diseases is always a moving target—pursued by both how microbes evolve and by what human behaviors, such as the habits we establish with antibiotic use and how far people move. Obviously, continuously funding research, monitoring closely through surveillance, and building up our healthcare infrastructure is essential to combating these threats. Incorporating methods from molecular research, real-time checks on data, and robust clinical guidance can genuinely hone the way we detect and treat infections. An anticipatory stance, one that attempts to anticipate resistance patterns and draws on concepts from many diverse experts—is vital if we are to reduce the worldwide burden of these infections. Ultimately, adhering to changing best practices (even when they're a little unorthodox at times) and basing them on sound research will assist us in protecting our communities more effectively from these continually changing threats.

Infectious diseases have been a substantial force on global well-being for centuries, warping death figures and dictating society's response over the centuries. Recently, studies in economic epidemiology tend to bifurcate disease behavior into short periods and long durations, and, more often than not, indicate that individuals' sensible decisions during outbreaks can turn the traditional patterns around in unexpected ways. This combination of human activity and disease transmission implies that health interventions must truly get under the skin of these uniqueness to strike the right note. Pursuing the fantasy of eradicating infections is still a priority, although it's full of obstacles attached to the disadvantages suffered by communities. Essentially, any strategy has to balance quick wins with the wider socio-economic waves in operation (Philipson, 2025). New methods in infectious disease research now rely on integrating ecological perspectives with a closer examination of microorganisms to get the whole story. Recurring problems such as time-honored infections, new outbreaks, and the development of antibiotic resistance heap up worldwide pressures that call for a new perspective. Novel tools let researchers dive deep into how tiny pathogens, our immune responses, and even the microbes that hang around with us interact, far beyond classic ideas. This gradual shift nudges us toward a patchwork of perspectives from biology, clinical insights, and social studies, aiming to boost both recognition and management measures. Despite all these technological strides, the pragmatic aspect of applying these advancements for routine public health work still trails behind, and there is a disconnect between lab breakthroughs and on-the-ground effects (Shahmaneshet al., 2020). Addressing these stacked problems entails transforming the way we train infectious disease control is rather critical. It begins by creating a curriculum that intertwines what's happening at the microscopic level, within populations, and even on a bigger environmental front. A spirit of team science, where various types of experts sit together—assists in combining various portions of data and viewpoints into actions that function. Along the way, one needs to develop the knack for scrutinizing new technologies and figuring out ethical dilemmas as diseases continue to morph. One of the most important turns in this training is ensuring that the most impacted have a voice, so research remains authentic to actual needs even when it becomes a little complex at times. Overall, this holistic training model seeks to prepare future epidemiologists to deal with the frequently unpredictable realm of infectious disease control (Shahmaneshet al., 2020).

References

1. Shahmanesh, M., Harling, G., Coltart, C. E. M., Bailey, H., King, C., Gibbs, J., Seeley, J., Phillips, A., Sabin, C. A., Aldridge, R. W., Sonnenberg, P., Hart, G., Rowson, M., Pillay, D., Johnson, A. M., Abubakar, I., & Field, N. (2020). From the micro to the macro to improve health: microorganism ecology and society in teaching infectious disease epidemiology. *The Lancet. Infectious diseases, 20*(6), e142–e147. https://doi.org/10.1016/S1473-3099(20)30136-5 (accessed on 7 May 2025).
2. Abubakar, I., Basu, S., Desai, M., & Hunter, P. R. (2011). The impact of economic crises on communicable disease transmission and control: A systematic review of the evidence. *PLoS ONE, 6*(6), e20724. https://core.ac.uk/download/13093583.pdf (accessed on 7 May 2025).
3. Achangwa, C., Park, H., Ryu, S., & Lee, M. S. (2022). Collateral impact of public health and social measures on respiratory virus activity during the COVID-19 pandemic 2020–2021. *Viruses, 14*, 1071. https://doi.org/10.3390/v14051071.
4. Al Sharif, N. A., Kabi, K. M. H., Alshayeb, H. A. A., Asiri, A. O. H., Asiri, J. A. H., Alzaid, E. D. I., Muqarbish, M. A. H., et al. (2024). Healthcare workplace hazards: A multilingual assessment of nursing, pharmacy, optics, social sciences, and epidemiology. *Journal of Ecohumanism, 3(8)*. https://www.semanticscholar.org/paper/a76366ae6740f2bdddb92dbc7852952230b46c36 (accessed on 7 May 2025).
5. Alders, R., Ali, S. N., Ameri, A. A., Bagnol, B., Cooper, T. L., Gozali, A., Hidayat, M. M., et al. (2020). Participatory epidemiology: Principles, practice, utility, and lessons learnt. *Frontiers in Veterinary Science, 7*. https://doi.org/10.3389/fvets.2020.532763.
6. Alhumaid, N. K., Alajmi, A. M., Alosaimi, N. F., Alotaibi, M., Almangour, T. A., Nassar, M., Memish, Z. A., et al. (2024). Epidemiology of reportable bacterial infectious diseases in Saudi Arabia. *Infectious Diseases and Therapy, 13*, 667–684. https://www.semanticscholar.org/paper/80889fccfb88b0b038f64bee778a60893cc8bd70 (accessed on 7 May 2025).
7. Balmes, J., Ritz, B., & Tager, I. (2005). Can lessons from public health disease surveillance be applied to environmental public health tracking? *Environmental Health Perspectives, 113*(3), 243–249. https://doi.org/10.1289/ehp.7450.
8. Barber, M. R. W., & Clarke, A. E. (2020). Systemic lupus erythematosus and risk of infection. *Expert Review of Clinical Immunology, 16*, 527–538. https://doi.org/10.1080/1744666x.2020.1763793.
9. Baydin, A. G., Darzi, A., de Witt, C. S., & Dokania, T. (2020). Simulation-based inference for global health decisions. https://core.ac.uk/download/396289157.pdf (accessed on 7 May 2025).
10. Bingi, A., Gitta, S. N., Mukanga, D., & Musenero, M. (2012). Paradigm shift: Contribution of field epidemiology training in advancing the "One Health" approach to strengthen disease surveillance and outbreak investigations in Africa. https://core.ac.uk/download/478428494.pdf (accessed on 7 May 2025).
11. Borràs, E., Campins, M., Esteve, M., Urbiztondo, L., Broner, S., Bayas, J., Costa, J., et al. (2014). Are healthcare workers immune to rubella? *Human Vaccines & Immunotherapeutics, 10*, 686–691. https://www.semanticscholar.org/paper/d612ad77058178bcc7b0f8aaa6b7b38ca7887b3f (accessed on 7 May 2025).

12. Brahmbhatt, M., & Dutta, A. (2025). On SARS type economic effects during infectious disease outbreaks. https://core.ac.uk/download/pdf/6372789.pdf (accessed on 7 May 2025).

13. Calderwood, M. S., Anderson, D. J., Bratzler, D. W., Delpersist, E. P., Garcia-Houchins, S., Maragakis, L. L., Nyquist, A. C., et al. (2023). Strategies to prevent surgical site infections in acute-care hospitals: 2022 update. *Infection Control and Hospital Epidemiology, 44*, 695–720. https://doi.org/10.1017/ice.2023.67.

14. Cheema, M., Aghazadeh, H., Nazarali, S., Ting, A., Hodges, J., McFarlane, A., Kanji, J. N., et al. (2020). Keratoconjunctivitis as the initial medical presentation of the novel coronavirus disease 2019 (COVID-19). *Canadian Journal of Ophthalmology, 55*, e125–e129. https://doi.org/10.1016/j.jcjo.2020.03.003.

15. Cheemerla, S., & Balakrishnan, M. (2021). Global epidemiology of chronic liver disease. *Clinical Liver Disease, 17*, 365–370. https://doi.org/10.1002/cld.1061.

16. Chen, C., Gao, G., Xu, Y., Pu, L., Wang, Q., Wang, L., Wang, W., et al. (2020). SARS-CoV-2–positive sputum and feces after conversion of pharyngeal samples in patients with COVID-19. *Annals of Internal Medicine, 172*, 832–834. https://doi.org/10.7326/m20-0991.

17. Colavita, F., Lapa, D., Carletti, F., Lalle, E., Bordi, L., Marsella, P., Nicastri, E., et al. (2020). SARS-CoV-2 isolation from ocular secretions of a patient with COVID-19 in Italy with prolonged viral RNA detection. *Annals of Internal Medicine, 173*, 242, 243. https://doi.org/10.7326/m20-1176.

18. Danish, S. M., Asghari, S. J., Hashimi, S. A., Furmoli, M. E., Zamani, M. U., & Amiri, S. H. (2025). The prevalence and associated demographic factors of hepatitis C infections among patients referred to the hospital of infectious diseases in Kabul, Afghanistan: A cross-sectional study. *Afghanistan Journal of Basic Medical Science*. https://www.semanticscholar.org/paper/afcdc5fa1c4ba4fb740dbd885c9d81629d9c453f (accessed on 7 May 2025).

19. Fernández-Polo, A., Melendo-Pérez, S., Larrosa Escartin, N., Mendoza-Palomar, N., Frick, M. A., & Soler-Palacín, P., on behalf of the PROA-NEN Working Group. (2024). Five-year evaluation of the PROA-NEN pediatric antimicrobial stewardship program in a Spanish tertiary hospital. *Antibiotics, 13*, 511. https://www.semanticscholar.org/paper/0b3ae6bf722a4ac2713ea6f14e00f38ee12df101 (accessed on 7 May 2025).

20. Fung, I. C. H. (2018). EPID 9131–Infectious diseases transmitted via inter-personal contact. *Public Health Syllabi, 275*. https://core.ac.uk/download/229147236.pdf (accessed on 7 May 2025).

21. Hamer, D. H., Rizwan, A., Freedman, D. O., Kozarsky, P. E., & Libman, M. (2020). GeoSentinel: Past, present and future. *Journal of Travel Medicine, 27*(8), taaa219. https://doi.org/10.1093/jtm/taaa219.

22. Hamilton, C., Borbolla, D., Novillo-Ortiz, D., Saigí-Rubió, F., Eguia, H., et al. (2021). Data and digital solutions to support surveillance strategies in the context of the COVID-19 pandemic. *Frontiers in Digital Health, 3*, 707902. https://core.ac.uk/download/480394162.pdf (accessed on 7 May 2025).

23. Haqqi, A., Zahoor, S., Aftab, M. N., Tipu, I., Rehman, Y., Ahmed, H., & Afzal, M. S. (2020). COVID-19 in Pakistan: Impact on global polio eradication initiative. *Journal of Medical Virology, 93*, 141–143. https://doi.org/10.1002/jmv.26240.

24. Heymann, D., & Shindo, N. (2020). COVID-19: What is next for public health? *The Lancet, 395*, 542–545. https://doi.org/10.1016/s0140-6736(20)30374-3.
25. International Conference on Emerging Infectious Diseases. (2008). *Emerging Infectious Diseases*. https://core.ac.uk/download/144197853.pdf (accessed on 7 May 2025).
26. Kostkova, P., Saigí-Rubió, F., Eguia, H., Borbolla, D., Verschuuren, M., Hamilton, C., Azzopardi-Muscat, N., et al. (2021). Data and digital solutions to support surveillance strategies in the context of the COVID-19 pandemic. *Frontiers in Digital Health, 3*. https://doi.org/10.3389/fdgth.2021.707902.
27. Lewnard, J. A., & Reingold, A. L. (2019). Emerging challenges and opportunities in infectious disease epidemiology. *American Journal of Epidemiology, 188*(5), 873–882. https://doi.org/10.1093/aje/kwy264.
28. Murray, C. J. L., Ikuta, K. S., Sharara, F., Swetschinski, L. R., Robles Aguilar, G., Gray, A. P., Han, C., et al. (2022). Global burden of bacterial antimicrobial resistance in 2019: A systematic analysis. *The Lancet, 399*, 629–655. https://doi.org/10.1016/s0140-6736(21)02724-0.
29. Napoli, C., Riccardo, F., Dente, M., Rossi, P., Declich, S., & Kärki, T. (2015). Screening for infectious diseases among newly arrived migrants: Experiences and practices in non-EU countries of the Mediterranean basin and Black Sea. *International Journal of Environmental Research and Public Health, 12*, 15550–15558. https://core.ac.uk/download/54525874.pdf (accessed on 7 May 2025).
30. Philipson, T. (2025). Economic epidemiology and infectious diseases. https://core.ac.uk/download/pdf/6822479.pdf (accessed on 7 May 2025).
31. Raynaud, M., Zhang, H., Louis, K., Goutaudier, V., Wang, J., Dubourg, Q., Wei, Y., et al. (2021). COVID-19-related medical research: A meta-research and critical appraisal. *BMC Medical Research Methodology, 21*. https://doi.org/10.1186/s12874-020-01190-w.
32. Rocklöv, J., & Tozan, Y. (2019). Climate change and the rising infectiousness of dengue. *Emerging Topics in Life Sciences, 3*, 133–142. https://doi.org/10.1042/etls20180123.
33. Roth, G. A., Mensah, G. A., Johnson, C. O., Addolorato, G., Ammirati, E., Baddour, L. M., Barengo, N. C., et al. (2020). Global burden of cardiovascular diseases and risk factors, 1990–2019. *Journal of the American College of Cardiology, 76*, 2982–3021. https://doi.org/10.1016/j.jacc.2020.11.010.
34. Santangelo, O. E., Gentile, V., Pizzo, S., Giordano, D., & Cedrone, F. (2023). Machine learning and prediction of infectious diseases: A systematic review. *Machine Learning and Knowledge Extraction, 5*, 175–198. https://www.semanticscholar.org/paper/3ff16e6b97f08229f0b58271c1c0ba752a1aa427 (accessed on 7 May 2025).
35. Sayfullayevna, X. G., Shahzodbek, K., & Usman. (2024). Analysis of the types of epidemiology diseases and incidence level in the population. *Texas Journal of Medical Science, 28, 18–20*. https://www.semanticscholar.org/paper/d747fa2899eea81edd0921b8fa99063fc84e0c2c (accessed on 7 May 2025).
36. Schuchat, A., Asnis, D. S., Baltimore, R. S., Rebmann, C. A., & Centers for Disease Control and Prevention. (2003). Disease surveillance and the academic, clinical, and public health communities. *Emerging Infectious Diseases, 9*(7), 781–787. https://doi.org/10.3201/eid0907.030083.
37. Singh, O. P., Hasker, E., Boelaert, M., Sacks, D. L., & Sundar, S. (2020). Xenodiagnosis to address

key questions in visceral leishmaniasis control and elimination. *PLOS Neglected Tropical Diseases, 14*, e0008363. https://doi.org/10.1371/journal.pntd.0008363.

38. Snow, M. (2011). The contribution of molecular epidemiology to the understanding and control of viral diseases of salmonid aquaculture. *Veterinary Research, 42*(1), 56. https://doi.org/10.1186/1297-9716-42-56.
39. Srivastava, S., Kumar, S., Sharma, P. K., Rustagi, S., Mohanty, A., Donovan, S., Henao-Martínez, A., et al. (2024). Control strategies for emerging infectious diseases: Crimean-Congo hemorrhagic fever management. *Health Science Reports, 7(9), e70053*. https://www.semanticscholar.org/paper/0070505be9f28cb5bfef53d331b24da065a5ce2c (accessed on 7 May 2025).
40. Tamma, P. D., Aitken, S. L., Bonomo, R. A., Mathers, A. J., van Duin, D., & Clancy, C. J. (2023). Infectious Diseases Society of America 2023 guidance on the treatment of antimicrobial resistant gram-negative infections. *Clinical Infectious Diseases, ciad428*. https://doi.org/10.1093/cid/ciad428.
41. Tekeli, T. (2025). Modelling and optimizing testing strategies for epidemic outbreaks. https://core.ac.uk/download/543227170.pdf (accessed on 7 May 2025).
42. Wiersinga, W. J., Rhodes, A., Cheng, A. C., Peacock, S. J., & Prescott, H. C. (2020). Pathophysiology, transmission, diagnosis, and treatment of coronavirus disease 2019 (COVID-19). *JAMA, 324*, 782. https://doi.org/10.1001/jama.2020.12839.
43. Wu, J. T., Leung, K., & Leung, G. M. (2020). Nowcasting and predicting the potential domestic and international spread of the 2019-nCoV outbreak originating in Wuhan, China: A modelling study. *The Lancet, 395*, 689–697. https://doi.org/10.1016/s0140-6736(20)30260-9.
44. Zhang, H. L., Wu, C., Hu, M., Ma, W. J., Xu, X. L., Shi, R. J., & Lang, H. J. (2024). Risk perception and quality of working life of nurses in infectious disease departments in China: The chain-mediating effects of psychological resilience and social support. *Nursing Open, 11(9), e70045*. https://www.semanticscholar.org/paper/87f7b66f61aa6d8f4158bf84533939951dd1b062 (accessed on 7 May 2025).
45. Zhang, S., Li, X., Wu, J., Coin, L., O'Brien, J., Hai, F. I., & Jiang, G. (2021). Molecular methods for pathogenic bacteria detection and recent advances in wastewater analysis. *Water, 13*(24), 3551. https://doi.org/10.3390/w13243551.

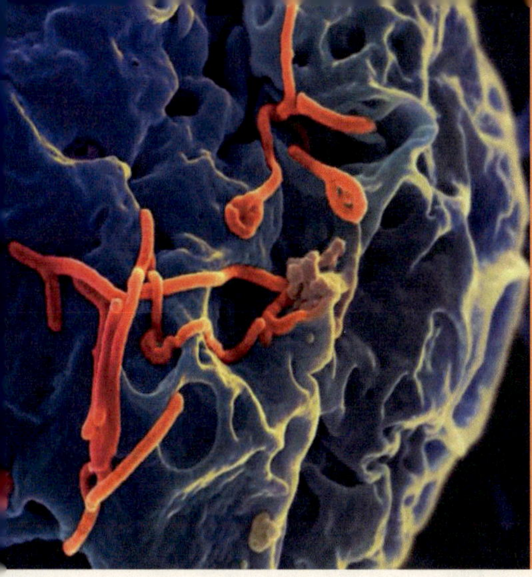

Chapter 4

EMERGING VERSUS RE-EMERGING DISEASES

Contents

Introduction

Infectious diseases are always a moving target, influenced by environmental changes, daily decisions, and microbes that continue to evolve in unexpected ways. You see, some infections emerge from nowhere—recently emerging and rapidly spreading—while others, previously believed to be under control, come back even more vigorous, often more resistant. This confusion is significant because it suggests various underlying causes and requires different measures to safeguard public health; it's all about the complex impact between biology and our social sphere. COVID-19 turned our assumptions upside down. The new coronavirus not only accelerated physical disease but also created a whirlwind of mental disease—social disruptions, economic anxiety, and restrictions on our liberty all came into play. Recent studies indicate an unmistakable surge in depression and anxiety directly attributed to the virus's spread and how we attempted to lock it down (Santomauro et al., 2021). Overall, this entire event demonstrates that pandemics affect us on more dimensions than disease and death. In contrast, comeback infections are another type of pain. When diseases we believed were brought under control recur—usually combinationed with issues such as aging population and shifts in healthcare—it turns out that even problems such as hospital-related delirium can exacerbate conditions such as dementia (Livingston et al., 2020). All of these considerations, stacked on top of one another, place genuine pressure on our health services and remind us that knowledge of both emerging and re-emerging diseases provides essential insights for constructing stronger defense systems in the future (Figure 4.1).

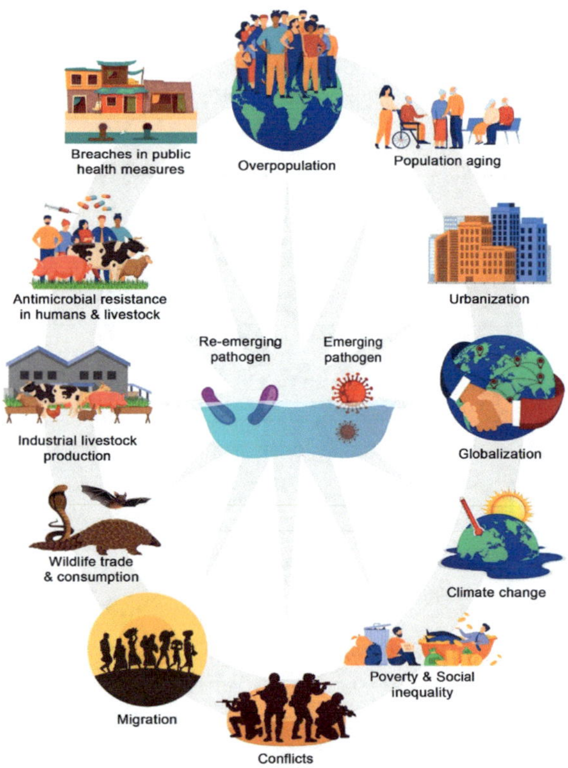

Figure 4.1. Emerging and re-emerging infectious diseases.

Source: MDPI (n.d.). *Emerging and re-Emerging Infectious Diseases Diagram.*

Definition of Emerging Diseases

Emerging diseases arise when new diseases start appearing in individuals or rapidly sweep through areas, typically taking us by surprise. They do not simply spring into existence; rather, they typically arise from a complex combination of alterations to our environment, changes in what humans do, and even small adjustments in microbes. Oftentimes, they are novel microbes to us – either because they acquired a mutation, trans-specied, or simply capitalized on new ecological niches. Consider SARS–CoV–2, for instance: this COVID-19 virus appears to have had an animal origin, but no one has been able to identify the specific animal reservoir. Such ambiguity, most of the time, compels us to redefine how we categorize diseases. The World Health Organization typically groups zoonoses (infections that naturally transfer from animals to humans) under the same banner, but SARS-CoV-2 sort of spoils that image, leading us to label COVID-19 an emergent infectious disease of probable animal origin instead of a paradigm zoonosis (Oran & Topol, 2021). Most emergent diseases will be a little different from classic infections. They often debut in communities with nearly zero natural immunity, which – quite frankly – lets them spread like wildfire and makes control efforts a real headache. Sometimes, these pathogens also develop new tricks, like enhanced virulence or clever ways to hop from person to person. When COVID-19 struck, its quick spread was not solely due to the virus itself; it was also facilitated by large numbers of individuals who felt perfectly healthy, unaware that they were passing it on. Studies have largely shown that those asymptomatic carriers contribute significantly to the spread, placing another layer on the difficulties of containment (Oran & Topol, 2021). It is all a reminder of just how essential it is to remain vigilant and respond fast. In other instances, new diseases appear when disease-causing agents suddenly find ways to infect people – usually following what can be termed a spill-over from animals or even the environment. Contrary to re-emerging diseases, which are sort of familiar faces returning after a hiatus, these new agents strike new populations or regions with unforeseen impacts. This disparity is quite important for determining public health policy, particularly in the realms of prevention and control. And when you can't identify an animal reservoir – as was the case with SARS-CoV-2 – tracing origins and disrupting transmission becomes even more difficult. At the same time, such diseases usually come from a combination of animal-to-human jumps, microbial alterchanges under the radar, and human interference like manipulating with their environment. Understanding all these factors, in most instances, enables us to better prepare for future epidemics and reinforces our general understanding of how these diseases arise (Haider et al., 2020) (Figure 4.2).

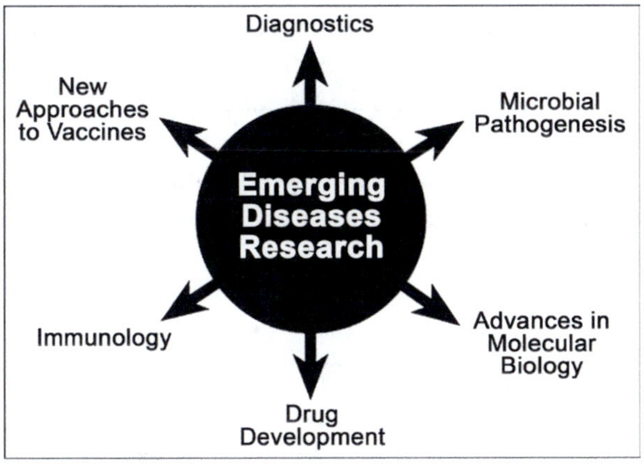

Figure 4.2. Emerging diseases.

Source: Centers for Disease Control and Prevention (n.d.). *Emerging Diseases Timeline.*

Definition of Re-emerging Diseases

Re-emerging infections feature surprisingly prominently in the way we conceptualize disease. They're not really new dangers; they just come back after a quiet spell. More often than not, microbes become a little resourceful—adapting just sufficiently—or gaps in vaccine regimens, changes in daily behavior, or even slight environmental changes all combine to usher these diseases back in. Health care systems occasionally find that what used to work no longer does. In general, getting your head around these diseases means looking at the ugly amalgam of hosts, adaptive microbes, and environmental uniqueness that collectively modify how disease appears over time. If you venture into the epidemiology, you observe an complex dance between pathogen evolution and human movement. Insects can grow resistant to medicines or become creative at finding a way to dodge our immune defenses, sometimes popping up in what we thought was a secure population. Combined with this, phenomena such as population movement shifts, urban sprawl, and even the times that health infrastructure lets us down stoke the fires. It's not a semantic distinction—whether an outbreak is a new issue or a re-emerging one makes a difference in how we respond. Further there's the added complexity of many of these diseases having animal origins, which allows disease spill-over to occur in unforeseen ways. Re-emerging diseases remind us that no control measure is ever permanent; ongoing vigilance and flexible public health strategies are a necessity. Consider the COVID-19 pandemic, for instance—it's typically dealt with as an emerging disease of probable animal origin, but it blurs borders and makes us question our definitions and approaches (Oran & Topol, 2021). Similarly, when diseases spread silently along asymptomatic carriers, our conventional models begin to falter; those silent spreaders can all too easily keep the chain rolling without warning, as in SARS-CoV-2 outbreaks (Oran & Topol, 2021). Overall, these nuances require a measured, multi-leveled strategy that combines knowledge of pathogen behavior, human activity, and environmental context to better inform prevention and control efforts.

Importance of Studying Both Categories

New diseases suggest new worldwide threats while recurring diseases recall old threats; both are worth our careful notice. New diseases tend to appear when animals transfer microbes to people, when our environment changes, or when microbes just choose to evolve—signs that something new is on the horizon. On the other side, returning diseases can partially be attributed to factors such as missed vaccinations, increasing resistance to medicines, or normal changes in society and the environment. Researchers who invest time to visit both types of sites usually observe patterns—such as how climate changes or fast urbanization drive the spread of disease. For the most part, monitoring both areas assists public health groups in developing stricter, more specific monitoring strategies. By monitoring only one side, we could overlook the delicate connections among infections and overlook preliminary indications of diseases that we believed were being contained or whole new dangers; in general, remaining vigilant on both sides is fairly important to be prepared. In most resource-constrained environments, it becomes even more imperative to monitor both new and recurrent infections. Consider dengue in most of Africa—it tends to go unnoticed because its symptoms can appear very similar to those of malaria, and therefore there are mix-ups and not-so-good responses. Current research, for the most part, highlights that climatic conditions and concerns such as urban waste disposal favor the breeding of mosquitoes, which only increases dengue striking harder; and genetic variability among populations may also adjust to what extent the disease becomes severe (Gainor et al., 2022). All this is a reminder of how neglecting the disheveled, complicated reality of these back-from-the-dead diseases can scramble our general picture of how infections get around, and how resources need to be allocated. Looking at both diseases in tandem just provides a more complete picture of recalcitrant diseases that might otherwise be overlooked, emphasizing the need for a wide and comprehensive approach to global health screenings. Also, leveraging wastewater-based epidemiology has become an innovative, early warning system that routine clinic-based surveillance could readily overlook. When researchers find viral RNA in wastewater, it provides a rapid glimpse of what's occurring in real-time within communities, all without invasive testing and at reduced expense (Mousazadeh et al., 2021). This approach proved its value during the COVID-19 pandemic, as it demonstrated that monitoring viruses in our wastewater can assist in real-time revising public health response nearly sponteneously. With testing backlogs and reporting delays sometimes a pest, observing both emerging and re-emerging pathogens through creative methods provides health systems with a more proactive advantage. Finally, combinationincorporating knowledge from both disease types not only makes us a better early detection game but also aids in establishing timely actions to minimize the health and economic bumps associated with outbreaks.

4.1. Historical Context

In the long past, infections have followed some surprising detours, changing with human ways. Take yellow fever in Brazil, for example, it once stuck primarily to some corners of South America and Africa but has rebounded in unexpected forms. Despite having a good vaccine in our back pocket, outbreaks have occasionally worsened, probably due to environmental changes and explosive urban growth. That 2016 outbreak in Brazil, which struck regions previously assumed to be secure, revealed some vulnerabilities in the public health system and emphasized how crucial it is to keep a continuous watch on diseases. These occurrences highlight that diseases thought to be relics are not only stuck in the past but can become new challenges, calling on scientists and authorities to maintain a continuous vigil (de Oliveira Figueiredo et al., 2020). Looking at recent coronavirus episodes really brings emerging and re-emerging diseases into sharp focus. The sudden rise of SARS-CoV-2—central to the COVID-19 crisis—marks only the third time in 20 years that a coronavirus has jumped from animals to us. This repeated animal-to-human leap hints at the persistent risk new microbes pose in our closely connected world. Attempts by organizations such as the Coronaviridae Study Group, which burrow into viral family relationships at the species level, serve to signal where the next spillover will occur. In general, these observations remind us that new diseases tend to emerge from a complex mix of changing natural processes and altering environments, and therefore addressing future threats requires sweeping, multidisciplinary collaboration (Gorbalenya et al., 2020).

In retrospect, the contrasts between emerging and re-emerging diseases provide important lessons in remaining ready. Frequently, completely new diseases emerge as conditions evolve, while old enemies return when vaccine campaigns falter or resistance accumulates. The return of yellow fever and the consistent presence of coronaviruses demonstrate that pathogens can take advantage of any weaknesses in our defenses, refuting the notion that control in the past ensures safety in the future. Most of the time, history has taught that continued investment in outbreak surveillance, vaccination campaigns, and international collaboration is essential when dealing with both new threats and recurring old ones. With these lessons remembered, maintaining our health systems on high alert and having the flexibility to respond is still the most important way to cope with the dynamic profile of biological threats (de Oliveira Figueiredo et al., 2020; Gorbalenya et al., 2020) (Figure 4.3).

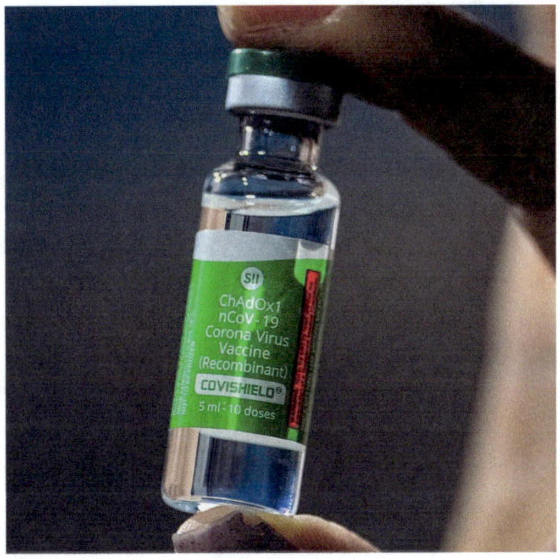

Figure 4.3. Solid vaccine in hand.

Source: By Agência Brasília - https://www.flickr.com/photos/64586261@N02/50870507747/, CC BY 2.0, https://commons.wikimedia.org/w/index.php?curid=99227214

4.1.1. Overview of Significant Emerging Diseases in History

In the long term, diseases have always arrived uninvited, making their presence felt in society. Surprise outbreaks tend to come in the wake of changes in our daily routines, local adjustments, and the rapidity of international travel. Remember the late 1900s—HIV/AIDS revolutionized public health overnight. Then there was that brief fright in 2003 when SARS taught us that an animal-to-human disease can become a global concern overnight. These emerging diseases tend to have mysterious perpetrators, so we scramble to learn how they are transmitted and what harm they can cause. In most cases, it's not just about treating a patient; it's also about steering social, economic, and governmental responses in uncharted waters. The way these diseases spread so unpredictably really drives home why our health systems need to keep one eye open 24/7. COVID-19 stands out as one of the most eye-opening examples of a disease emerging in our modern era, sparked by the novel SARS-CoV-2 virus. terms, it's an open-and-shut case of a virus that demonstrated how unpredictable infections can be—individuals who have no symptoms are still capable of spreading it, and its symptoms greatly differ from person to person.

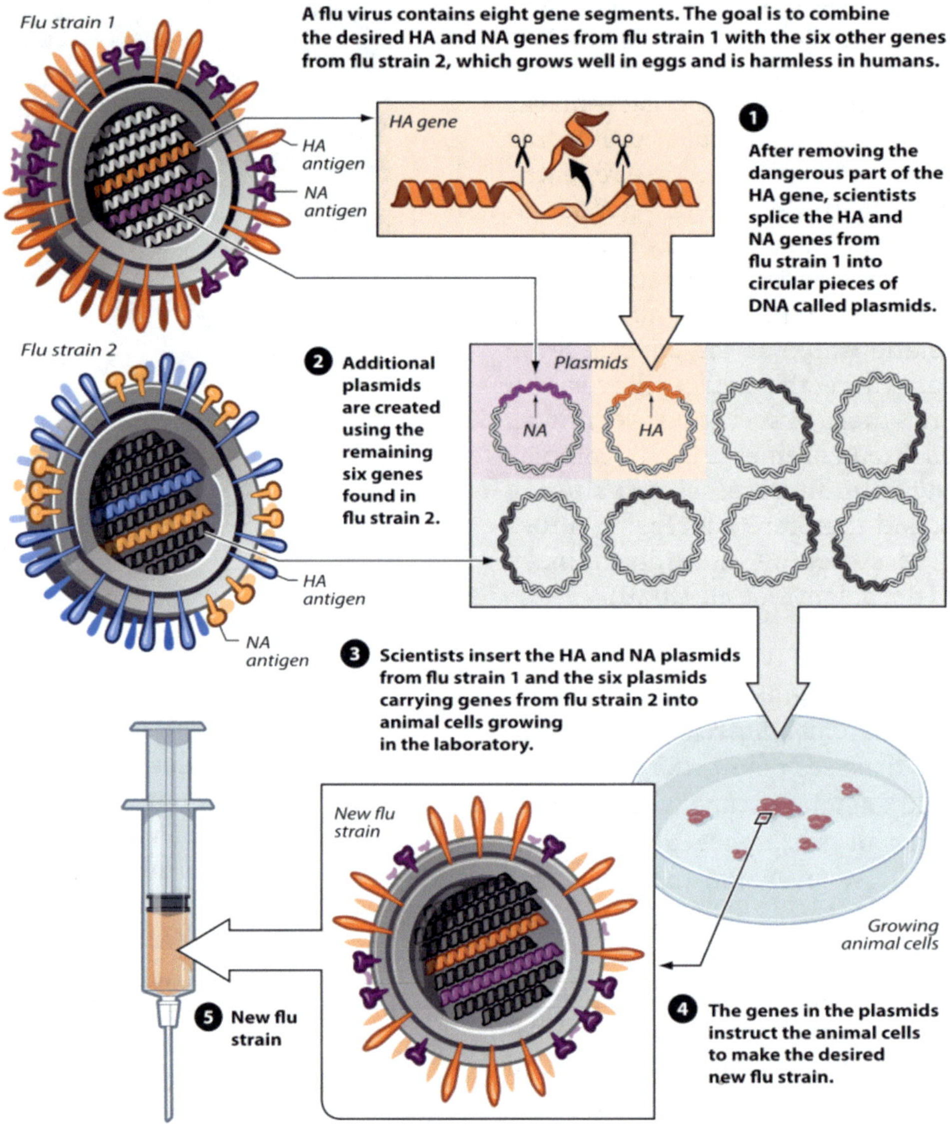

Figure 4.4. Immunotherapy targets emerging infectious diseases.

Source: By Mouagip - Own work(Link Studio for NIAID), Public Domain, https://commons.wikimedia.org/w/index.php?curid=13869477

Some recent instances even mention that even when one gets a clean bill of health in a respiratory test, remnants of the virus remain in cough samples or even stool (Chen et al., 2020). Such continuing viral shedding suggests other means the virus could be transported, confusing attempts to contain it. International air travel and densely populated cities only compounded things, reminding us that the more connected people become, the more easily a minor outbreak can balloon into a giant problem. This scenario drives home the reality that we require a combination of thoughts from various disciplines just to get our heads around such new enemies and determine how to prevent them. Sometimes, things that appear to be in hand come roaring back, this is what occurs with re-emerging diseases. And here we have ancient pathogens back again after a quiet period, often mutating or evading vaccines, and that blurs the distinction between what is so-called "new" and what is merely back in town. While new diseases that surprise us challenge us to face the unknown, these return diseases remind us that some dangers never leave so much as evolve their appearance or mode. It's noteworthy that even seemingly disparate problems, such as long-term conditions like dementia, can influence how susceptible a person is to infection (e.g., increased risk of delirium when in hospital (Livingston et al., 2020)). All these variables combination together, and it becomes apparent that any strategy to combat incipient diseases must have a wide perspective, encompassing everything from biology to daily life (Figure 4.4).

4.1.2. Overview of Significant Re-emerging Diseases in History

Diseases tend to return even when we believe we have them under wraps. Year after year, infections that we thought we had conquered resurface, sometimes leaving us unprepared. Sometimes the microbes mutate or our innate immunity declines with time; other times, our environment or social arrangements shift. Tuberculosis (TB), measles, and cholera—diseases we had repelled with vaccines and improved sanitation—now indicate renewed surges. Consider TB, for example; its resurgence is driven by drug-resistant forms and broader dissemination of HIV that undermines immune systems. All of this is a reminder that the struggle between small microbes and human vulnerability is more complex than perhaps it appears, and, by and large, there is much to be learned from these cycles to plan both today's and tomorrow's health initiatives (Livingston et al., 2020). Leaping forward to the end of the 20th and initial portions of the 21st century, our international connections appear to increase the threat of bygone diseases being revived. The SARS debacle in 2003 is one such case, an almost unknown coronavirus suddenly transformed itself into a re-emerging problem, with hospitals becoming hotbeds in many instances. In most developed regions, measles, too, is on the increase; lower coverage of vaccination, irregular economic climate, and a deluge of inaccurate news reports about vaccine safety are all in the mix. Further, of course, there's COVID-19, this pandemic necessitated healthcare staff embracing strict, and occasionally clumsy, safety measures to hold off the spread, a problem echoing from earlier instances of disease re-emergence (Ng et al., 2020). Those types of cases, in the majority of situations, illustrate how medical progress must be combined with strong public conduct and, quite honestly, with improved communication. Referring back even more years, epidemics such as cholera illustrate how events such as poor sanitation during wars or natural disasters can kindle a disease's resurgence, with results often very severe. It is our capacity to detect these infections early that depends so much on real-time monitoring of disease, rapid diagnostic tests, and availability of treatments and vaccines. However, as the recent past has demonstrated, gaps—such as in the safety of healthcare workers or the mismatched deployment of resources—can critically undercut our response in high-risk settings (Ng et al., 2020). In most cases, staying alert, investing wisely, and keeping the public well-informed are key to managing the ever-changing scene of reoccurring diseases (Livingston et al., 2020).

4.1.3. Impact of Historical Outbreaks on Public Health Policies

The diseases persist in resurfacing, incessantly compelling our public health institutions to reimagine their playbook. Prior outbreaks breaked most of our old control hypotheses so that, broadly speaking, policymakers had little other option than to amp up prevention and surveil closer to home. Consider, for example, those infamous influenza waves at the turn of the 1900s, and how they uncovered substantial weaknesses in international coordination as well as fundamentals in health architecture. That tough lesson prompted massive changes such as creating the World Health Organization and moving toward more thoughtful, systematic outbreak responses. In most instances, combining scientific advances with top-level policy served to address both new and old infectious threats, and governments ultimately began investing more in research and cross-sectoral collaboration, all to remain agile in our unpredictable health environment. Historical epidemics did more than force backstage change-of-the-century infrastructure improvements—they also reconfigured the way we perceive the role of our surroundings in medicine. As it happens, conditions like water quality, sanitation, and even mundane hygiene have enormous implications for disease transmission. You'd frequently see this during recurring rounds of diarrheal and parasitic disease. Low- and middle-income areas, which kept getting drummed into our faces. Consequently, interventions for increasing water, sanitation, and hygiene (WASH) found their way into mainstream prevention efforts, assisting in reducing the tide of diseases attributed to adverse environmental conditions, particularly among the most vulnerable. Public health concepts over time shifted from treating symptoms alone to excavating root causes, clearly indicating that our environment and infectious disease control are interconnected (Prüss-Üstün et al., 2019). Today, however, the trend of online communication has turned things around for epidemic response. Formerly, when there was a slow trickle of timely information, diseases used to spread faster; now, sources such as social media can carry awareness lightning-fast, even though at times, they transmit misinformation along. This is a challenge for policymakers today, that they have to balance leveraging those tools to energize people for good with pushback against fake content. They are generally forced to depend on measures that combine digital expertise, local coverage and rapid data tests to enhance disease monitoring and reaction. The outdated lessons remain well and alive, but contemporary policy revolves around harmonizing established conventions with new, often capricious tech innovations—acknowledging both the potential and the periodic setbacks of the new techniques in controlling outbreaks (Appel et al., 2019).

4.2. Factors Contributing to Emerging Diseases

Environmental changes and the way we live now have accelerated how new diseases emerge. Global warming and changing precipitation patterns disrupt our ecosystems and wildlife, creating conditions that allow many pathogens and their insect vectors to flourish. For instance, when the weather warms up, mosquitoes—these annoying disease carriers—can drift into new territories, threatening communities even if they previously only had to contend with tropical diseases. Deforestation for homes and urbanization also drive wildlife toward us, which in turn can induce those zoonotic jumps. In many cases, this mix of nature and human habits shows just how tightly our health is linked to the environment (Intergovernmental Panel on Climate Change, 2023). Understanding these connections is key if we're going to come up with public health moves that lessen environmental harm and keep a closer watch on disease spread. Global travel and trade add another twist to the emerging disease story. With so many people and products traveling so quickly and in such quantities, pathogens tend to hitch a ride into new areas, and old methods of preventing them simply don't work anymore. Urban environments, with their high concentrations of people, facilitate the spread of breathing-related and contact-transmitted diseases at a surprisingly quick rate. Cultural practices, accessible healthcare, and daily behavior all modify the way diseases establish themselves and spread through populations. For example, South Korea's early, aggressive move to mask-wearing amid the COVID-19 pandemic slowed transmission rates despite the virus initially racing through the nation (Lim et al., 2020). terms, this is proof that coordinated health responses—underpinned by public trust—are essential in our densely linked world. Further there is the deviousness of the bacteria themselves. Viruses and bacteria can shift sponteneously, mutating and even evading the defenses our bodies or medications create. This agile nature allows them to bypass our immune systems and often makes some treatments less effective, causing both the rise and resurgence of diseases. COVID-19, for instance, exposed the problem of a new virus that can easily spread from human to human. Lessons from past epidemics – such as MERS – have prompted some societies to embrace preventive actions like mask-wearing earlier, even if it was to feel slightly odd initially. All these variables—biological refinements, environmental shifts, and human behaviors—entwine in a complex manner to drive the direction of disease emergence, indicating the necessity for wide-ranging, adaptable public health interventions (Intergovernmental Panel on Climate Change, 2023; Lim et al., 2020) (Figure 4.5).

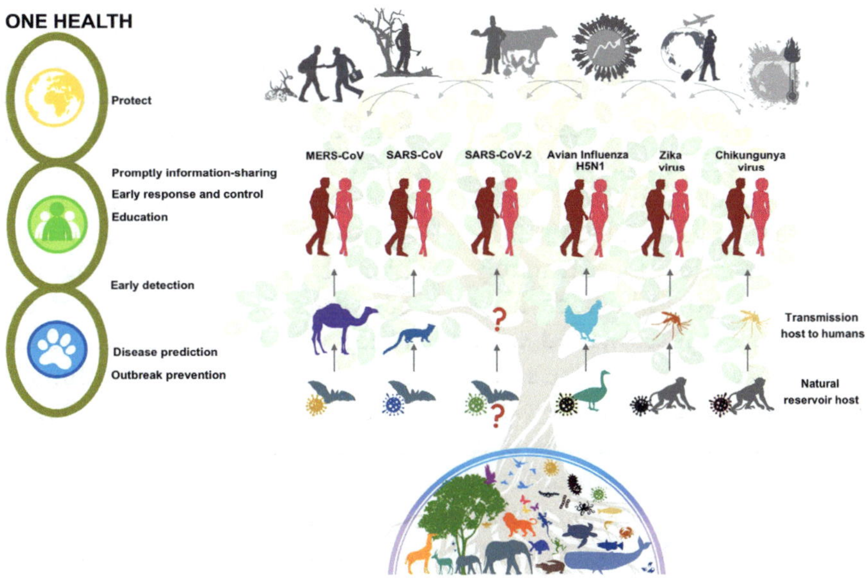

Figure 4.5. Emerging and re-emerging zoonotic viral diseases.

Source: Frontiers in Public Health (2023). *Zoonotic Viral Disease Emergence Map.*

4.2.1. Environmental Changes and Climate Impact

Climate change is mixing things up in ways that can't be ignored. Warmer days and goofy rain patterns are allowing microbes like mosquitoes and ticks to wander into new nooks, and these tiny hitchhikers tend to spread diseases like malaria and Lyme. Occasionally, these changes even drive diseases into areas where they hadn't been a significant issue previously. Severe weather—partially thanks to our warming climate—troubles both nature and our communities, causing congested areas and hygiene. Urban sprawl and environmental deterioration knock down aged, natural barriers that once protected from infection, allowing outbreaks to arise in new locations (Allam et al., 2022). Plant scientists have been feeling the same jitters as well. Changes in heat and moisture can mess with how plant insects and bacteria behave, sometimes bringing back diseases we'd hoped were over and threatening our crops and biodiversity. It's rarely a problem confined to one field; instead, it blurs the lines between ecology, weather science, and disease control, all needing a bit of teamwork. In most instances, warmer temperatures even create an opportunity for exotic insects that are very difficult to find and control. In most cases, responding to these interconnected challenges involves intertwining concern for the environment with intelligent medical and agricultural solutions (Jeger et al., 2021). There's a scramble globally to reduce harmful emissions and create more resilient cities, but strangely enough, these solutions tend to bypass how intensely our environment is intertwined with the spread of disease. Most of the emissions are produced by urban areas, and they get grittier air and strange little climate niches that can aggravate breathing and heart conditions, making people more susceptible to infections. Concepts such as the 15-minute city emerge as innovative solutions, seeking to reshuffle our environments so that the necessities are never far away and lengthy commutes are a relic of the past. By retaining resources locally and reducing frenzied transit, these proposals seek to alleviate the environmental pressures that fuel disease transmission. To summarize, mixing smarter policies with on-the-ground planning seems vital if we're going to keep both new and recurring diseases in check in this fast-shifting climate landscape (Allam et al., 2022).

4.2.2. Globalization and Increased Travel

Global linkages are exploding today, and humans are flying across borders like never before. This explosion of travel and trade isn't only opening up new markets and cultural contacts—it's also giving bacteria a speedy pass. New epidemic outbreaks can now hop between continents nearly as if borders didn't exist, keeping our public health systems on heightened alert. Even infections we'd thought were under control creep into new territories, reminding us that global travel and disease are two sides of the same coin. Diseases slip past geographic limits so easily that coordinated international efforts become essential, especially in jam-packed urban areas where risks seem to multiply (Allam et al., 2022). In most instances, gaining a better understanding of the role that international travel plays in determining these patterns is central to increasing our preparedness and reducing new and repeat infections. The effects of increased travel extend far beyond mere germ spread. Urban areas, now a primary mode of transit, are experiencing a combination of concerns not solely based on biology. Cities today are faced with additional stresses from such factors as air pollution and unpredictable weather, factors that undermine our natural barriers and render citizens more susceptible to infections. New diseases and old diseases both thrive in such an environment. Further there's the psychological toll: pandemic travel bans and isolation have seen a clear spike in instances of depression, anxiety, and other mental health concerns (Santomauro et al., 2021). Overall, international travel not only alters how disease travels but also its impact on our overall health. Mixing public health initiatives with intelligent city planning and better mental health care may just be the solution to addressing these interconnected issues. Reimagining disease management in today's era of constant global travel is becoming imperative. Old-fashioned public health paradigms just don't apply when individuals are in transit 24/7. Rapid solutions such as boosting airport checks, using rapid tests, and reporting in real time between nations now become crucial. Concurrently, creating local resilience, through engaging communities and insisting on sustainable city planning, assists in cushioning some of the danger that accompanies global travel (Allam et al., 2022). It is a dance: welcoming the advantage of globalization while instituting functional obstacles against biological dangers. Recognizing that diseases often hitch a ride on human movement, decision-makers must foster international teamwork and adopt holistic strategies that look beyond just the infections to include their wider effects on society. Ultimately, this layered approach is crucial if we're going to keep emerging and re-emerging diseases from running wild in our ever-connected world.

4.2.3. Urbanization and Population Density

Industrial changes and growing cities have reshaped our world in ways that touch both the environment and human health. Urban expansion means more folks living close together, and sometimes that creates odd little pockets where diseases seem to catch on more easily. People clustering in cities isn't just about quicker spread of well-known diseases, it also sets the stage for new microbes to appear. More often than not, fast-growing places find that rudimentary services trail behind exploding populations, and this only increases the health hazard. By the beginning of the 21st century, more humans were living in urban hubs than rural fields, and this brought a plethora of public health mysteries. And when lots of people concentrate in urban areas, our interactions with local pets and wildlife shift, at times making it more likely for viruses to jump between species (Doyle et al., 2020). Urbanization combined with overcrowding creates an entirely new level of sophistication in how infections catch on and flare up. Animals such as our domestic pets and even some that live in the wild but have become accustomed to urban living carry an unusually large burden of viruses that can be transmitted to humans. Their populations, growing with ours into their territories, increase those odds still further. That combination of urbanization and frequent contact often makes cities hotbeds for cross-species diseases. Furthermore, persistent activities such as hunting and wildlife trading simply introduce another variation, bringing individuals and animals closer—and sometimes filthier—together. To summarize, all this congregation not only accelerates disease transmission but also rearranges the behavior of infections, presenting new problems to old and reliable public health strategies (Doyle et al., 2020). In most rapidly growing cities, particularly in regions of Africa, the combination of sky-high population and hard living conditions makes populations more susceptible to both new and recurrent disease. Areas such as dense slums and informal settlements tend to have inadequate sanitation, clean water, or reliable healthcare services, which provide environments where infections can nearly run wild. When ecologic decline intersects with societal tension, it can induce resurgences of disease, particularly as humans move deeper into territory where mysterious bacteria are waiting. The speed and volume of city expansion influence not only where these diseases manifest but also how ready our health infrastructure is to combat them. Essentially, understanding these changes is important in shaping policies that can mitigate the health risks associated with exploding cities and high population densities (Songsore et al., 2005) (Figure 4.6).

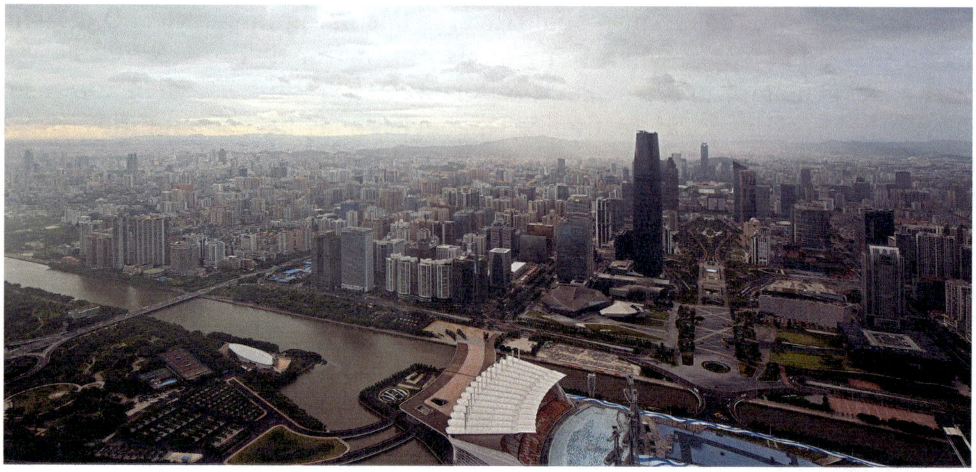

Figure 4.6. Urbanization and population density.

Source: By chensiyuan - Own work, CC BY-SA 4.0, https://commons.wikimedia.org/w/index.php?curid=15775341

4.3. Factors Contributing to Re-emerging Diseases

Population growth and movement in our world can spark a disease's resurgence when it appears to be contained. Cities expand rapidly, and continuous international travel propels bacteria across borders, occasionally depositing them in surprising places. Individuals who end up in more intimate contact with microbe carriers or wildlife, combined with dense populations and subpar sanitation, only exacerbate the problem. Economic development and wholesale deforestation discombobulate local ecosystems and tip that fine balance between man and nature, which in turn increases the odds of animal-to-human spillover. Dengue fever, West Nile fever, and other such infections really illustrate how these complex social and environmental fibers converge to trigger outbreaks (Chala & Hamde, 2021). Pathogens aren't standing still either. They mutate and evolve—a phenomenon that frequently goes hand in hand with human effects to allow old diseases to re-emerge. Mutations and genetic modifications enable these microbes to evade our immune systems and even dismiss medications. In most instances, overuse or even abuse of antibiotics and antivirals accelerates the development of resistant strains, which complicates the containment of infections even further. Animal reservoirs that naturally harbor these bacteria contribute an additional twist to the problem by maintaining a consistent reservoir available to fuel subsequent outbreaks. In general, the continuous evolution of these pathogens requires constant vigilance and flexible public health interventions to keep up (Chala & Hamde, 2021). Occasionally, the breakdown or interruption of health services amid crises provides one additional twist to the story. Consider COVID-19, dread of the virus and rigid movement restrictions kept many people from attending their routine vaccination appointments, which in turn paved the way for diseases such as polio to start re-emerging. With fewer medical professionals on hand and resources being diverted, the traditional protections failed at the moment they were most required. These care gaps and vaccine gaps make it that much harder to catch up and maintain hard-won gains in health. Supplemental immunization activities and catch-up campaigns are, hence, necessary if we are to prevent controlled infections from making a return and to safeguard our overall public health gains.

4.3.1. Antimicrobial Resistance (AMR)

Infectious diseases now are slightly more of a mystery with the increasing problem of AMR. Today, our tried-and-true treatments are losing their potency as microbes pick up new tricks to evade medicines, driving diseases from something you can work with into severe, at times critical, states. Longer disease episodes, increasing mortality rates, and continuously escalating healthcare costs have all emerged as these resistant microorganisms spread. Usually, whenever emerging or even back-from-the-dead diseases appear, AMR tends to make a usually managed epidemic a long-term headache. Our daily habits, environmental modifications, and even the smart means by which bacteria evolve all come together here, so combatting these persistent pests requires an active, worldwide, and collaborative effort. Overall, any good plan to combat infectious diseases must account for AMR (Onyebuchi et al., 2025). Contemporary research, in the majority of instances, burrows deep into the complex origins of AMR and the way it travels through human life, animals, and even our environment. Sophisticated genome research indicates that markers of resistance are exchanged more broadly than many anticipate, which only adds layers to an already complicated scenario. Consider, as an illustration, intensive antibiotic application in chicken agriculture—this appears to increase the number of types of different resistance genes, and occasionally these genes make a jump between groups of bacteria, stacking up the threats to public health. Such a horizontal gene transfer accelerates how rapidly harmful microbes evolve, so our normal remedies begin to cease being effective, particularly where there is not-so-good sanitation or infection control processes are subpar. Identifying these patterns highlights all the more why we require a One Health strategy—connecting surveillance and intervention across different sectors can assist in interrupting the transmission cycle (Napit et al., 2025).

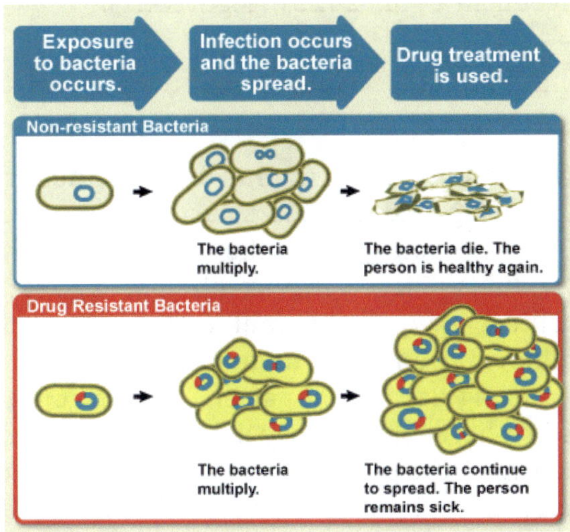

Figure 4.7. Antimicrobial resistance (AMR).

Source: By NIAID – NIH - http://www.niaid.nih.gov/topics/antimicrobialResistance/Understanding/Pages/drugResistanceDefinition.aspx, Public Domain, https://commons.wikimedia.org/w/index.php?curid=41858152

Addressing AMR requires our global health plan to transcend healthcare's traditional borders. Sure, there has been some progress with enhanced policies and better systems to monitor what's occurring. But much still falls through the cracks—such as sharing critical information, catching problems early, and ensuring resources get to those who need them most, especially in low-resource settings where both new and recurring diseases strike hardest. Efforts, overall, are now shifting toward refining antibiotic use, increasing infection prevention, and forging connections across borders to strengthen our defenses against

AMR-driven outbreaks. On top of that, ramping up investments in faster diagnostic tools and real-time monitoring systems would really help in catching problems sooner. In short, tying all these moves together into one robust global plan is key to keeping our antimicrobials effective and halting the comeback of resistant infections (Onyebuchi et al., 2025) (Figure 4.7).

4.3.2. Vaccine Hesitancy and Public Health Challenges

Diseases long held at bay by vaccines are reappearing, and it appears part of the problem is several biology and the way we behave. Individuals' increasing skepticism regarding vaccines, frequently fueled by suspicion, misinformation, and inequalities in society, are erasing decades of gains. There is genuine concern here, particularly if deadly viruses like Nipah enter the picture without reliable vaccines or medicines. Epidemics of such threats remind us that being slow to vaccinate will make things get out of hand, making it harder to prevent the spread. Overall, overcoming this problem isn't so much about scientific advancements—it's also about public health campaigns to repair trust in our immunization programs (Branda et al., 2025). The bigger picture isn't any easier either. Universal trends like fast-paced urbanization, climate change, and the intermingling of cultures have rendered it simpler than ever before to allow infections to traverse borders. In low- and middle-income countries, with limited resources to go around, vaccine hesitancy merely intensifies the situation, resulting in outbreaks of disease previously well-controlled. New technologies such as molecular diagnostics and new vaccines such as mRNA ones hold promise, but their advantages are not going to all corners, primarily because of gaps in healthcare systems. In most cases, re-establishing public trust and ensuring that all communities receive a fair deal with vaccines is totally imperative (Alsaeed, 2025). It's apparent that combating these health risks requires a combination of leading-edge technology and genuine consideration of the way individuals live and think. When there is ongoing vaccine skepticism, it's not merely sufficient to answer solely scientific or logistical questions—there needs to be actual community outreach and education as well. Global cooperation, with some combination of genomic surveillance, new vaccine research, and public messaging that resonates at the cultural level, can make an impact. Overall, breaking down vaccine hesitancy isn't just another task on the list; it's critical to maintaining our communities' health and resilience against dangers that still cast a large shadow today (Alsaeed, 2025; Branda et al., 2025).

4.3.3. Socioeconomic Factors and Healthcare Access

Access to healthcare isn't spread evenly, and social and economic forces have a giant role in that disparity; individuals on tight budgets tend to be holed up in crowded, unsanitary conditions where bacteria gain the upper hand. When things get scarce, basic protective care – from initial screenings to adequate treatments – has a way of falling away, letting infections start and build up with minimal check. In many places suffering from poverty, the local health systems struggle to do more than just keep pace, meaning outbreaks can persist and even worsen over time. The entire bargain is that social and economic hardships accumulate, with communities becoming more vulnerable to both new infections and old enemies returning; solving these root issues is typically the solution if we are ever going to witness equitable health outcomes among various groups (Matthew et al., 2021). Observing previous and current cases quite literally illustrates how economic disparities cause health threats to compound. Consider some African countries, say, a combination of high numbers and persistent poverty drives a cycle where infectious disease persists or merges, causing additional strain on already fragile health services (Nkengasong

& Mankoula, 2020). Despite advancements in medical science, it somehow appears that financial constraints prevent a lot of people from accessing life-saving vaccines, rapid testing, and treatments. The COVID-19 pandemic, in most instances, put these disparities into sharp relief as low-income populations tended to get caught in long wait times and increased rates of serious disease or mortality. It's apparent that incorporating social variables such as income levels, education levels, and work status into public health strategies is something we can no longer afford to disregard if we intend to effectively handle both new and ongoing outbreaks (Page et al., 2021). There's no magic bullet to address these inequalities, but a combination of measures could make an impact. Strengthening domestic health facilities, encouraging the manufacture of basic medical equipment at home, and improving the quality of healthcare staff all appear to be shrewd steps (Nkengasong & Mankoula, 2020). Engaging community health workers more tends to create a lifeline between services and underserved communities – enhancing the detection of hot spots, prevention activity, and the follow-through on treatments. Global initiatives that collaborate with local agendas can assist in channeling resources and technical expertise where they are needed. Unless seriously contemplating those underlying social and economic challenges, our worldwide efforts to contain emerging and recurring diseases are bound to be incomplete, and communities are likely to remain ensnared in a self-reinforcing loop of exposure and outbreaks (Nkengasong & Mankoula, 2020; Page et al., 2021) (Figure 4.8).

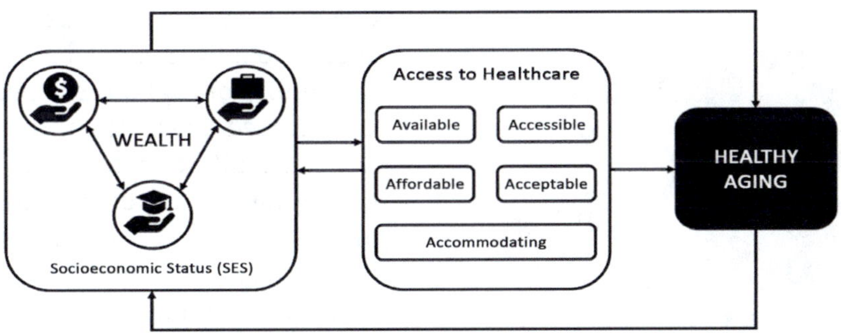

Figure 4.8. Socioeconomic factors and healthcare access.

Source: Frontiers in Public Health (2020). *Factors Affecting Healthcare Access Infographic.*

4.4. Case Studies of Emerging Diseases

The COVID-19 pandemic struck the globe in a hurry, illustrating for us firsthand just how chaotic new infections can become. It began in Wuhan, China – the virus was initially labeled 2019-nCoV and eventually SARS-CoV-2, finally igniting what we have come to refer to as COVID-19. The confusing names helped to make it more difficult for individuals and officials alike to gain a clear impression early on. By and large, this virus is not merely another member of the coronavirus clan; it has some strange biological uniqueness and changing patterns of spread that distinguish it from previous threats such as SARS-CoV. Sustained human-to-human transmission combined with symptoms that ping-pong between a mild cold and severe respiratory distress really tested health systems and demonstrated why rapid detection, simple naming, and straightforward messaging are so critical (Jiang et al., 2020). Looking closer at how COVID-19 unfolds inside the body gives us a peek into the virus's tricky dance with the immune system. It seems to work in three phases. At first, the virus multiplies quietly, causing vague, mild symptoms—this early phase is where antiviral treatments might work best. Then, things change as inflammation begins in the lungs and an overactive immune response is triggered, signaling the transition from direct viral damage to damage primarily fueled by our own body's defenses. In most instances, dividing the disease into these stages assists in personalizing treatment, allowing it to be simpler to determine more individualized care. Data from cases such as heart transplant patients even suggest that manipulating the immune system sometimes reverses the severity of the disease it becomes (Jiang et al., 2020).

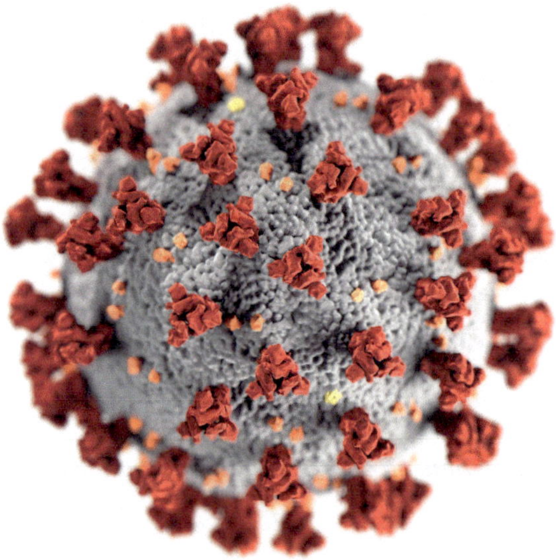

Figure 4.9. Scientists discover the opportunity to disrupt SARS-CoV-2.

Source: https://en.m.wikipedia.org/wiki/File:SARS-CoV-2_without_background.png

Meanwhile, the pandemic served as a reminder to everyone about how important it is to catch outbreaks early and activate public health interventions. Social distancing, proper hygiene, and even quarantines proved crucial to slowing the infection before useful medications were on hand. Still, things were a challenge – far too many were completely symptomless and immune systems were quite diverse, keeping everyone guessing. Divisions on the timing of use of treatments such as corticosteroids were only making matters more confusing to attempt to simply follow evidence while dealing with an ever-changing epidemic. Overall, this experience has driven us towards greater global cooperation, quicker sharing of data, and more responsive measures to combat these highly complex infectious threats (Siddiqi et al., 2020) (Figure 4.9).

4.4.1. COVID-19 Pandemic and Its Implications

Recent history has cast our global health landscape into grim chaos. COVID-19, appearing so rapidly, brought into focus how much of a complicated mess these diseases can be and how difficult it is to cope with their spread worldwide. It exposed vulnerabilities in our public health infrastructure and reminded us—nearly in repeat mode—that human existence, animal health, and the environment are strangely interconnected (this is what some refer to as the One Health concept). While all this was happening, though, it wasn't just our hospitals that were impacted; economies, schools, and our very social fabric were hit, exposing unequal levels of preparedness and gaps in resources. The rapid deployment of vaccines, for example, tended to demonstrate brilliant scientific acumen but also posed difficult questions regarding equity in access and the moving sands of public trust. In every sense, COVID-19 is a case study, a dramatic illustration of how new infections can spread and impact contemporary society, propelling us toward international collaboration and more adaptive strategies (Intergovernmental Panel on Climate Change, 2023). Burrowing into

COVID-19's deep-reaching impacts is to examine carefully how it combines with existing health challenges. Individuals already weighed down by long-term conditions such as chronic respiratory complications or compromised immune systems were worse off, adding further pressure on our already strained care systems. Not just physical wellbeing took a beating; mental wellbeing also suffered, with widespread bouts of depression, anxiety, and that all-too-common feeling of isolation becoming a routine part of the day-to-day. Such a fall-out, in a majority of cases, appears to mimic patterns associated with other ailments that keep recurring, where continuing issues within communities merely exacerbate issues daily. In addition, interventions like prolonged social distancing and mask mandates came with their own social and economic dilemmas, adding to the challenge of containing the disease. Overall, these intersecting problems demonstrate that pandemics do a whole lot more than inflict biological damage—they braid themselves into the heart of both personal and public health (Mullol et al., 2022). A closer inspection of COVID-19 in light of emerging compared to re-emerging diseases brings its peculiar features into sharp focus. Unlike with most re-emerging insects, they usually return on account of readily foreseeable changes to the environment or politics—COVID-19 presented as a new zoonotic spillover, driven chiefly by urban expansion and the non-stop pace of globalization. Its rapid mutations created a multitude of new variants, each of which added additional pressure on vaccine efficacy and other control efforts. In many respects, this rapid evolution reflects larger trends seen in emerging pathogens, where environmental pushes and the behaviors of humans both drive microbes to evolve and disseminate. One could argue that the pandemic has made it very clear: maintaining a close eye through ongoing monitoring, investing in strong healthcare, and tapping into knowledge from numerous disciplines are not only choices but necessities. This combination of strategies seems crucial to staying one step ahead of whatever is coming our way—whether that's some brand-new menace or some returning challenge coming back around—thereby strengthening our global resilience against continuously evolving microbial threats (Intergovernmental Panel on Climate Change, 2023).

4.4.2. Zika Virus Outbreak and Its Effects

They come on hard and suddenly, disturbing health systems across the world. Urbanization, global travel, and changes to the environment all thrust these diseases into the foreground. Consider Zika, for instance. First isolated all the way back in 1947 in Uganda, it largely flew below the radar until a sudden epidemic in the Americas revealed gaping holes in mosquito control and disease surveillance. Urban areas, where Aedes mosquitoes — those pesky insects that defy the use of outdated insecticides — breed, became breeding grounds for its proliferation. Obviously, new concepts such as releasing Wolbachia-infected insects or applying gene drive technology are being contemplated to combat these vectors, promising means of averting future crises (Wang et al., 2022). Examining where Zika originates also reveals a complex scenario that includes humans, animals, and nature. Overall, the combination of surprise viral mutations, humans encroaching on previously wild regions, and climate changes that benefit mosquito populations to explode provides perfect circumstances for diseases to leap from animals to humans. It's not merely a matter of infection totals; the repercussions have been extreme nervous system issues such as microcephaly and even Guillain–Barré syndrome. In general, comprehending these complex factors—with a little redundancy on how each component is important—is essential when designing effective control and prevention measures (Saba & Balwan, 2021). The Zika epidemic also cast an unflattering light on weaknesses in global health preparedness, particularly in areas with limited resources. The crisis revealed a clear need for more intelligent mosquito control programs, quicker diagnostic tests, and improved community outreach. It was not merely a health crisis; the social and economic consequences were also grave, from overflowing hospitals to travel restrictions and even stigmatization of the infected. This mad dash reoriented the public health agenda overnight and highlighted the value of coordinated global action. The continued thrust toward novel approaches such as symbiont-mediated or gene drive strategies may prove essential to future measures to combat Zika and other mosquito-borne threats (Wang et al., 2022) (Figure 4.10).

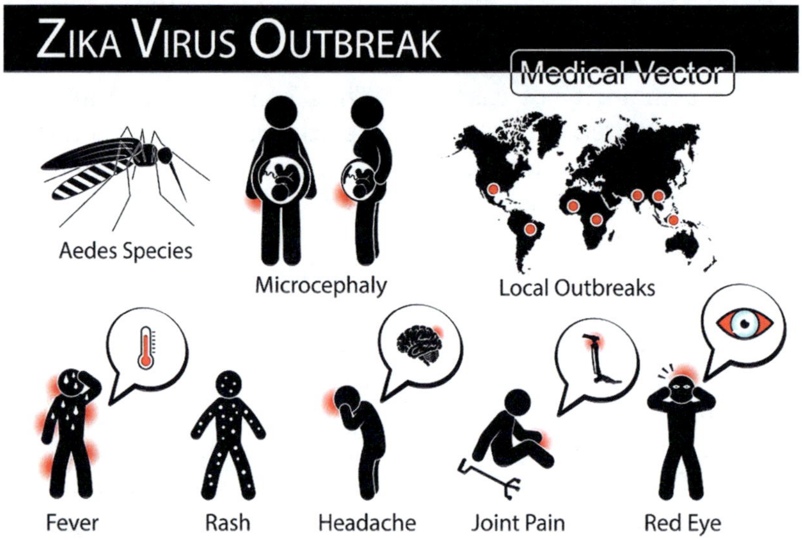

Figure 4.10. Zika virus outbreaks.

Source: iStock (n.d.). *Zika Virus Outbreaks Infographic.*

4.4.3. Ebola Virus and Lessons Learned

In 2014, West Africa was hit with full force by Ebola—a crisis that revealed vulnerabilities in local and global health systems. Severe poverty, widespread deforestation, and political instability in Liberia, Sierra Leone, and Guinea all contributed to accelerating the outbreak, with origins dating back to colonial days that left deep scars and enduring inequalities. Gender disparities, racism, and wider social divisions only made it more difficult for communities to come together, further complicating attempts to respond. Foreign aid arrived, but it soon became apparent that establishing enduring healthcare capacity in these vulnerable areas was no simple matter, particularly when climate change adds yet another stress layer. All these dirty socio-political and environmental problems, in the majority of situations, directed toward an immediate necessity to address the broader determinants that allowed new pathogens to get out of control (Kay et al., 2016). Infectious disease epidemiology has largely been changing how we manage outbreaks such as Ebola, moving away from past models of chronic diseases to more adaptive styles better adapted to new challenges. New technologies—everything from molecular diagnostics to electronic tracking systems—certainly assist us in identifying and even anticipating how disease spreads. Such developments have induced new ways to think about cause and effect and how pathogens behave, which has been essential to reconsidering how we assess vaccines and antimicrobial therapies. The Ebola outbreak highlighted that combining know-how from disparate disciplines is not only smart but essential when fast surveillance and speedy responses are warranted. Learning more about how diseases behave and how we engage with our environment is still central to controlling new as well as returning diseases, staying ahead of these scientific advances with public health education (Lewnard & Reingold, 2019). The Ebola lessons extend beyond the mere halting of an outbreak; they point to improved public health policy and wiser governance. Strengthening local health systems, gaining the trust of communities, and ensuring resources are equitably distributed all appear crucial to meeting future threats. The outbreak demonstrated—rather clearly—that established social inequalities and past marginalization can gravely weaken efforts at health, even prolonging an epidemic's reach at times. International and domestic partnerships premised on social justice and fairness proved to be central, particularly in light of Ebola's capacity to return. To that end, consistent investment in healthcare facilities and education, coupled with true concern for our ecosystem, continues to be important. In combating these interlinked challenges, we may well discover the keys required to tackle not just emerging but also re-emerging infectious diseases in the face of continuing societal and ecological changes (Kay et al., 2016).

4.5. Case Studies of Re-emerging Diseases

Diseases occasionally catch us unaware by reappearing when we believe they were kept in check, raising the red flag for public health. Consider how viral diseases, such as the various symptoms we experience with post-COVID-19 syndrome (PCS), surprisingly reappear. The syndrome presents itself in various guises: perpetual fatigue, respiratory issues, ongoing nerve problems, and chronic pain, all found through extensive clinical examinations. Gender differences, previous lung issues, and how bad the original infection was all insert their own variables into the equation. In most instances, early interventions using monoclonal antibodies and timely vaccination have a protective benefit—emphasizing the importance of rapid medical intervention. It's a reminder that re-emerging diseases rarely stick to neat definitions and require round-the-clock monitoring along with treatment plans tailored to the individual (Gentilotti et al., 2023). Looking back, bacterial issues like TB and diphtheria serve as clear warnings: if public health measures slack off, even diseases we once thought tamed can bounce back. Factors such as increasing antibiotic resistance, slumps in immunization levels, and even socio-economic turmoil all come together to make these infections crop up once more. When compared with what's occurring with viral trends presently, it is quite clear that our health systems could have some insidious vulnerabilities. The tug and push between a pathogen's capacity to adapt and the strength of our infrastructure to support us means there is a constant demand for flexible and resilient policies. Having examined in-depth case studies, it's apparent that prevention, rapid diagnosis, and thorough treatment are essential to balancing disease patterns over time. It's also noteworthy that managing these re-emergent diseases often requires a combination of perspectives—from the molecular level all the way up through clinical experience and epidemiological patterns. Recent breakthroughs in molecular diagnosis and how we classify disease, much as in oncology, imply that we might use similar strategies with great success for infectious diseases as well. For instance, by examining genetic or immunological markers, we would be able to diagnose and treat these recurring infections with greater accuracy. Such developments could lead the way to tailor-made treatments and more accurate prognoses of patient outcomes. Certain case studies, by integrating molecular discoveries with clinical presentations, guide us toward a personalized medicine solution—one that treats existing cases more effectively but also prepares our health systems for whatever future recurrences may appear (Oaknin et al., 2022) (Figure 4.11).

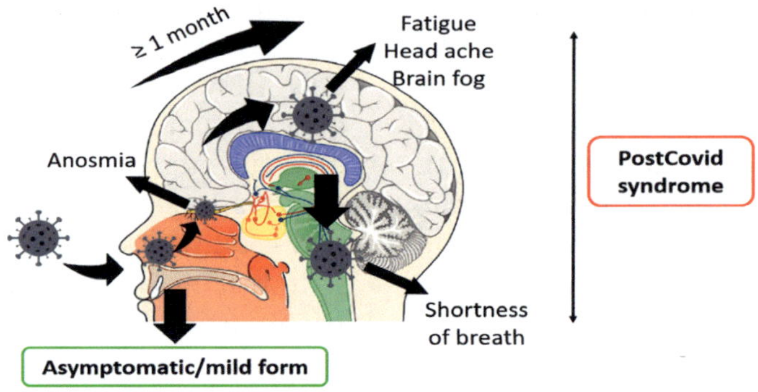

Figure 4.11. Post COVID-19 syndrome in asymptomatic patients.

Source: MDPI (n.d.). *Post-COVID Syndrome Illustration.*

4.5.1. Tuberculosis (TB) Resurgence and Treatment Challenges

Infectious diseases continue to evolve and mutate, it's a combination of biology, society, and environment in action. TB is a classic case; in spite of decades of attempting to eradicate it, it still persists. Urbanization, constant worldwide travel, and the development of drug-resistant strains all have their role, and yes, the intersection with conditions like diabetes mellitus only makes them more difficult. In most instances, the emergence of multidrug-resistant TB translates to our treatments simply not being enough anymore. New developments in materials science, such as aggregation-induced emission (AIE) biomaterials, suggest new avenues for catching and treating TB earlier, accentuating an intriguing intersection between disease control and biotech (Wang et al., 2024). Further there's the issue that TB frequently partners with chronic conditions such as diabetes mellitus (DM). Research typically indicates that individuals with TB are likely to develop diabetes much more often than the rest of us. Where both TB and DM are major problems, as they are in areas like India, then health initiatives have to stretch to encompass much, screening for additional conditions, early intervention, and integration of various models of care become imperatives. Considerations such as age, smoking, and even cardiovascular issues continue to emerge, prodding us into seeing treatment in terms of something greater than a war against bacteria (Singh et al., 2023).

TB's resurgence, with all its attendant complexities, truly demands a multi-layered public health approach that combines high-end research with practical care. All too frequently, our standard diagnostic equipment fails to detect drug resistance quickly enough, thereby slowing down treatment and increasing the danger of transmitting the infection. Emerging technology, based on sophisticated fluorescence magic and intelligent biomaterial science, appears promising in detecting the pathogen more quickly and providing specific treatment—thereby alleviating the burden on public health (Wang et al., 2024). Nevertheless, these advances have to come together with more robust healthcare infrastructures, improved adherence measurement, and increased public education to knock down the barriers from social and economic divides. To summarize, addressing TB's resurgence requires a unified effort that combines advanced science with practical clinical and community assistance (Figure 4.12).

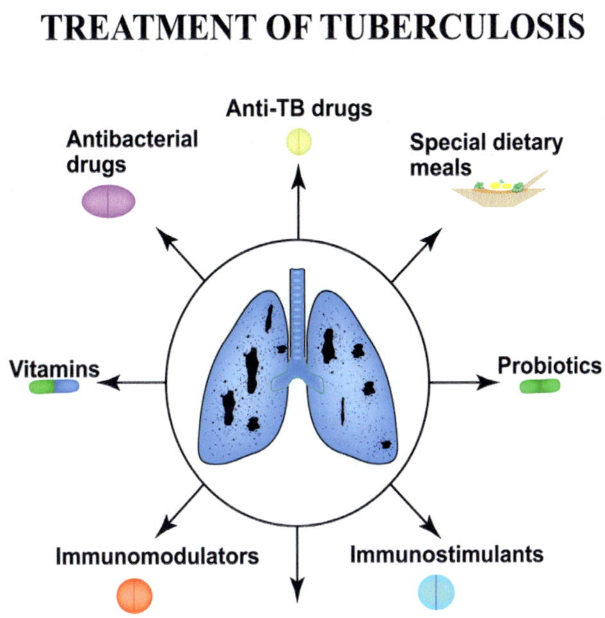

Figure 4.12. Treatment of tuberculosis (TB) world tuberculosis.

Source: VectorStock (n.d.). *Tuberculosis Treatment Awareness Design.*

4.5.2. Measles Outbreaks and Vaccination Rates

Occasionally public health policy shifts abruptly and, in the process, they reveal underlying issues that arise particularly with preventable diseases we have vaccines for—measles being a good example. In other places, you notice a ripple effect where vaccine hesitancy, lack of access to healthcare, and economic hardship combine and leave communities more vulnerable to outbreaks. Marginalized populations, more often than not, get hit harder because the local healthcare infrastructures and customized interventions simply don't quite target the problem. For example, during the COVID-19 pandemic, mandates to increase immunization not only drove up vaccination rates but also disrupted staffing for rural primary care clinics, suggesting larger systemic issues in our overall public health strategy (Brigit et al., 2023). Take the case of Romania, where things got particularly complicated. There, as vaccination rates fell below the threshold required for herd immunity, a measles outbreak went viral in 2016. This experience, primarily among young children and impacting the Roma community disproportionately, illustrates that cultural and demographic information counts—a good reminder that one size does not fit all. Clinical reports tend to reference the reality that children who miss out on vaccines risk severe complications, pneumonia, increased risk of death—further additional risk is introduced when you add in something like suboptimal nutrition or anemia. Age and ethnicity are typically involved, so any attempt at increasing vaccination will need to be both culturally sensitive and realistically inclusive (Turaiche et al., 2022). When you pull back and look at measles as part of the larger group of emerging or resurging diseases, it becomes apparent that good vaccination drives, not to mention educating local populations and monitoring closely, are essential. Below a 95% vaccination level, the door is open to rapid disease spread and quickly reversed years of achievement in keeping infections under control. It's not simply a matter of shots in arms, but ensuring that healthcare workers, particularly rural or underserved, can sustain the pace. Measles, in this context, truly illustrates how immunization gaps combined with economic and social barriers allow preventable diseases to rebound. Borrowing from recent mandates and outbreak research, public health officials can engage in adaptable policies that not only address outbreaks as they develop but also assist in maintaining the hard-earned advances of previous immunization campaigns (Hatch et al., 2023; Turaiche et al., 2022).

4.5.3. Dengue Fever and Its Increasing Prevalence

Human behavior and environmental changes have shaken things up in unforeseen ways—dengue fever is one very graphic example. Urbanization and constant travel have enabled the Aedes mosquito to roam further, accelerating the virus's transmission. Human water storage practices and overpopulated housing, incidentally, continue to provide additional areas for mosquitoes to breed, triggering outbreaks. A hospital in Chhattisgarh even conducted a study that caught up on several dengue virus types co-circulating, an indication that the entire scenario is quite complex and that staying on top of things is paramount. They registered DENV-2 as the predominant type alongside DENV-1, which really complicates matters for treating individuals who have been affected previously (Soni et al., 2025). Temperature increases and unusual patterns of rainfall also join in on the fun. When global heat increases and rain timing goes askew, Aedes mosquitoes begin to appear in areas that previously weren't on their radar. This is translating to dengue being a hot-button issue not just in tropical, warm corners but infiltrating milder climates as well. Scientists tend to articulate that climate changes are a primary catalyst for new and old epidemics of insect-borne diseases, with dengue at its core. Consider Venezuela, for example; its precarious dengue status with respect to changing weather is just one of the mounting challenges policymakers are dealing with.

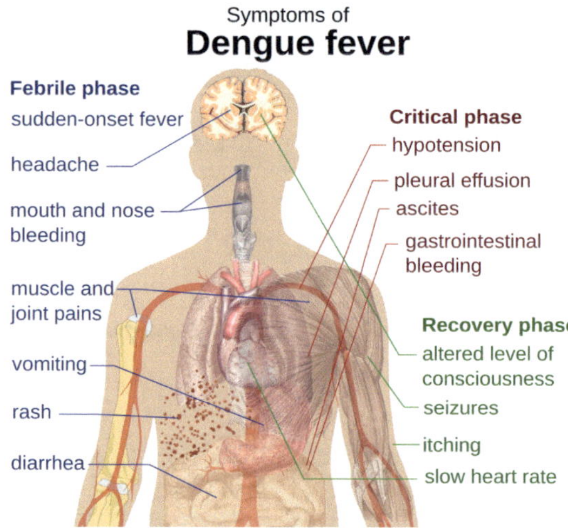

Figure 4.13. Dengue fever and its increasing prevalence.

Source: By Mikael Häggström - All used images are in public domain; references are found in Wikipedia article at Wikipedia:Dangue fever., Public Domain, https://commons.wikimedia.org/w/index.php?curid=12712988

Overall, our shifting climate appears to fuel the fire against dengue (Paz-Gañan et al., 2024). Dengue's increasing spread largely reflects the overall issues of diseases that continue to resurface. New diagnostic instruments such as NS1 antigen tests and RT-PCR serotyping now assist in charting out where the virus is lurking, allowing authorities to spring into action a little earlier. These tests, though not ideal, can identify when another bout of infection could develop into more serious problems such as dengue hemorrhagic fever. It's obvious that the management of dengue requires more than simply careful clinical care—ongoing monitoring of viral changes is involved as well. When health workers combine immediate patient care with constant monitoring of how the virus changes its trajectory, they are better positioned to predict outbreaks and direct resources to improved mosquito control and treatment protocols, ultimately attempting to keep dengue's resurgence at bay (Soni et al., 2025) (Figure 4.13).

4.6. Public Health Responses

Early detection and quick response are critical when fighting both emerging and re-emerging diseases, preserving our healthcare system and preventing the spread go hand in hand. Rather than a static checklist, early detection of outbreaks through daily monitoring allows health teams to observe how things are changing and intervene before issues blow up. For instance, in the case of COVID-19, employing RT-qPCR tests from respiratory samples was extremely crucial to validating cases and deciding on isolating individuals. Surprisingly, however, studies indicated that even when respiratory tests were negative, viral RNA still persisted in sputum and feces. This surprise caused most to reconsider how long an individual should be isolated and alter testing strategies accordingly. For the most part, having a combination of diagnostic approaches that consider various sample types appears to be the intelligent thing to disrupt transmission chains and reduce new cases—public health measures just have to remain adaptable and expand with evolving discoveries. If you expand beyond hospitals, the larger public health picture simply cannot help but account for the community aspect. Measures such as isolation guidelines, contact tracing, and promoting simple hygiene have long been standard practice. That said, pathogens are constantly evolving; they tend to surprise us in unexpected ways. The fact that SARS-CoV-2 RNA has been found in fecal matter hints at alternative routes, like fecal-oral or even aerosolized fecal particles—that our usual respiratory-based controls might miss. More broadly, this experience pushes against our usual protocols and inclines us toward more extensive testing practices, such as stool screening, particularly for those hospitalized with gastrointestinal problems (Livingston et al., 2020). In a sense, this sort of flexible adjustment demonstrates how integrating scientific research into public policy can facilitate engaging both new threats and revisited old enemies.

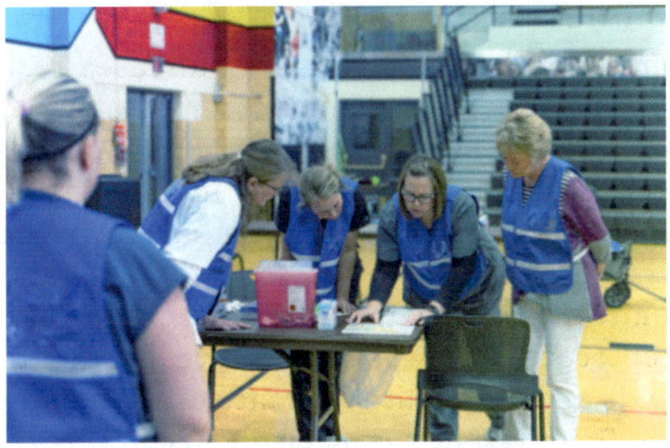

Figure 4.14. Public health response.

Source: https://external-content.duckduckgo.com/iu/?u=https%3A%2F%2Fclcpublichealth.org%2Fwp-content%2Fuploads%2F2022%2F06%2FCLCPH-PublicHealthResponse-Photo.jpg&f=1&nofb=1&ipt=9ba670f468fd62e36843ebd89f093070312d83ab856c1576f44dce11458e90d4.

On top of that, public health interventions must remember who is most at risk, individuals with comorbid conditions or compromised health, for instance. Older persons with dementia, for instance, can experience delirium and cognitive lapses that not only alter the trajectory of their disease but also shape how healthcare resources are allocated (Livingston et al., 2020). It turns out that models of care that emphasize prevention, rapid intervention, and a great deal of individualized support reduce hospital visits and improve overall health. When policymakers, clinicians, and researchers can work well together—even when things get a little complex along the way, it provides a setting where new ideas are quickly translated into action, and therefore fortify our public health defenses. Briefly, combining individualized care with more general epidemic control measures appears the most effective approach to managing infectious disease risk in heterogeneous populations (Figure 4.14).

4.6.1. Surveillance and Monitoring Strategies

Controlling new and recurring diseases really boils down to having robust surveillance and monitoring systems that can catch outbreaks quickly. These systems assist in catching the pathogens early enough so that responses can take hold when necessary. For instance, monitoring a constant lookout for group B streptococci in newborns has revealed that the trends and antibiotic resistance are dynamic—sometimes rather unexpectedly. When we draw in all the lab and clinical information, it becomes simpler to select multidrug-resistant strains, and that in turn compels us to reformulate our prevention strategies and treatment regimens. All these indications lead to round-the-clock real-time monitoring of pathogens to inform vaccine work and prepare for new threats or even old ones' resurgence (Creti et al., 2021). This active, hands-on surveillance enhances public health preparedness, reducing both deaths and total sickness from infections. Secondly, the addition of combined outbreak reporting systems is a major step, particularly when pathogens spread along mixed or uncertain pathways. In the US, the National Outbreak Reporting System (NORS) is an example, it aggregates reports on waterborne, foodborne, and acute gastroenteritis (AGE) outbreaks from as wide a range as direct contact to environmental spillovers, and even instances where we can't be 100% certain of the pathway. Reports from settings such as long-term care and childcare facilities have assisted in identifying seasonal patterns and usual suspects, such as norovirus, which appears in the majority of AGE outbreaks and unfortunately causes numerous fatalities. The increase in reporting over time suggests improved utilization of the system, providing us with a more comprehensive picture. That type of granular data allows public health people to home in on specific hygiene measures, more thorough cleaning procedures, and on-time isolation policies to enhance outbreak containment and lower disease effects (Wikswo et al., 2015). Surveillance does not end with addressing an outbreak immediately, it also channels into prevention and research activities on a wider level. Continuous data collection enables us to catch new drug-resistant bacterial clones in the making, such as with group B streptococci, where detecting these more resilient sub-groups leads the way for vaccine development and more specific use of antibiotics. Likewise, when NORS uncovers mysterious outbreaks, it exposes shortcomings in our capacity for identifying the perpetrators and prods us toward improvements in diagnostics. This cycle of back-and-forth activity between surveillance for outbreaks and refining our response strategies keeps us subtle as the infectious disease environment evolves. Ultimately, maintaining a wide, constantly evolving surveillance system is essentially the foundation of effective public health responses, lightening the burden of new and recurring infections by informing decisions with good, evidence-based information (Wikswo et al., 2015; Creti et al., 2021).

4.6.2. Vaccination Programs and Their Effectiveness

Vaccination campaigns have always been understood to reduce disease and mortality almost anywhere. They're one of the oldest weapons in our disease-fighting arsenal, but when new epidemics happen, it gets complicated because vaccines must race to keep pace with evolving microbes. Consider COVID-19, for example, vaccine distributions weren't even, with wealthier countries getting ahead while poorer countries fell behind, which really lays bare some long-standing global health disparities. Numerous African countries, especially, experience challenges such as weak infrastructure, the sudden introduction of new variants, and quite a lot of vaccine hesitancy. Everything indicates that the countries need to collaborate, strengthen cold chain mechanisms, and place emphasis on outreach at the community level so that more individuals receive vaccinations. For the most part, an understanding of the social, political, and cultural contexts is central to improving vaccine coverage and making sure that sudden infectious dangers do not affect those at greatest risk the most (Nachega et al., 2021). Accelerating access to vaccines is not only about logistics; it's also about adopting new scientific concepts that extend beyond conventional injections. Nanomedicine, for example, has some truly encouraging promise—working with teeny particles, it attempts to administer components of the vaccine right where they're required, perhaps reducing side effects. The nano-delivery systems have the potential to solve finicky challenges such as ensuring vaccines are stable and how to control the way they're released, something that's particularly important in low-resource areas. In most instances, combining these innovations with vaccination campaigns can make the immune response more acute and present more adaptable solutions as pathogens change. Generally, incorporating nanotechnology into vaccine development appears to be a visionary strategy in fighting infectious diseases more effectively and sustainably (Patra et al., 2018). Despite all these scientific updates, public trust remains a giant obstacle. Misinformation and a fundamental skepticism of big pharma tend to create vaccine hesitancy, particularly in communities with a track record of dodgy health projects. You can observe various levels of acceptance across African nations, which indicates just how important it is to engage in a manner that directly addresses local concerns. On the whole, straightforward health messages, when combined with the power of respected community leaders and healthcare providers, can build trust in vaccines and emphasize their role in avoiding disease outbreaks. In other words, effective vaccination campaigns depend not just on the latest science but also on public health practices that are attuned to each community's particular needs (Nachega et al., 2021).

4.6.3. International Collaboration and Response Efforts

Controlling new and resurgent diseases is a business that sometimes compels nations to join forces in ways not anticipated for global health security. Various parts of the world—for example, the WHO Eastern Mediterranean region—demonstrate how economic stress, political developments, and environmental shifts all combine to make disease transmission more serious. In most instances, nations have resorted to interventions such as the International Health Regulations (IHR) core capacities, which enable them to assess and fortify their health systems. Despite the advancement, gaps remain that remind us of the need for additional assistance, consistent advocacy, and additional capacity building. Strategies such as One Health, which unites human, animal, and environmental health, have been harnessed to promote multisectoral collaborations; when agencies pool resources, have loose oversight of surveillance and react in coordination, they can indeed master both emergent and re-emergent diseases (Elhakim et al., 2025). Looking back at past pandemics, it's clear that dealing with global health threats isn't just about solid plans within individual countries—it's about a patchwork of international efforts. Over time, our responses have shifted as more people recognize that sharing responsibilities across borders is key. Generally speaking, setting clear definitions for pandemics and leaning on evidence-based rules can kick-start more effective global mobilization and smoother coordination. When we delve into the social and biological aspects of outbreaks, we find that preventive actions such as wildlife protection and reducing zoonotic spillover require collaborative efforts across various sectors. A variety of actors—ranging from labs and health authorities to conservation societies and governments—have a role in increasing global surveillance and response. In addition, networks and biorepositories that enable data sharing and rapid responses truly highlight the need to work together to manage both emerging and recurring infectious diseases (Dias, 2024). It's difficult to deny that in our globalized world, diseases zip across borders with unnerving ease, which means coordinated international responses are absolutely necessary. All too often, individual national actions simply don't suffice against such rapid pathogen travel. That's why pressing for more robust global health regulations, investing in pandemic preparedness funds, and implementing comprehensive national action plans are all measures that nations have to address collectively. Also key is interweaving public health preparedness with policies that mitigate social and economic exposure—concerns too often exacerbated by war, displacement, or environmental degradation. By sharing the burden, by sharing capabilities, resources, and even some unpolished data, countries can move more quickly, shield communities better, and limit the mass disruptions from both new and recurring diseases. Ultimately, a real, though not entirely errorless, commitment to global collaboration is still at the center of fighting future health crises (Dias, 2024; Elhakim et al., 2025) (Figure 4.15).

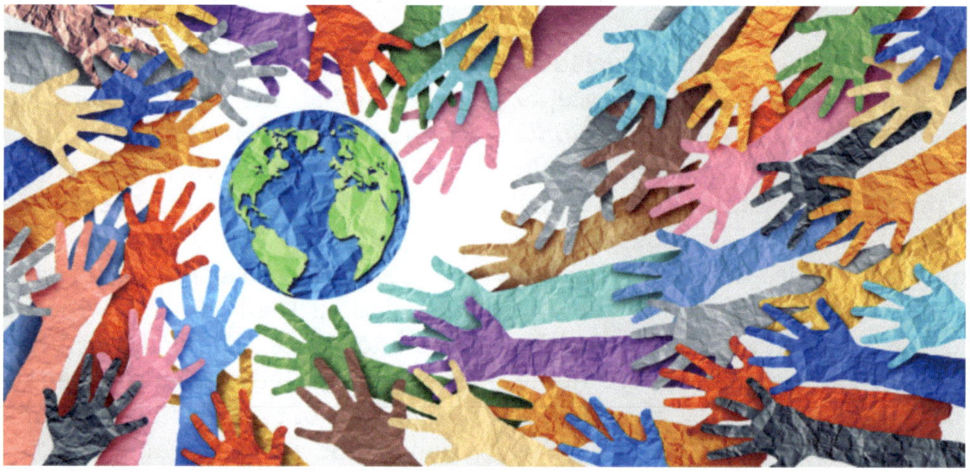

Figure 4.15. The international collaboration and response efforts.

Source: Level Up Village (n.d.). Shutterstock_1814911268 *Students Engaging in Virtual STEM Learning.*

CLOSER LOOK

ANTIMICROBIAL RESISTANCE IN RE-EMERGING INFECTIONS

Antimicrobial resistance (AMR) has become one of the greatest global health threats of the 21st century, playing a central role in the re-emergence of infectious diseases once thought to be under control. When bacteria, viruses, fungi, or parasites develop the ability to resist drugs that were previously effective, treatment becomes difficult, infections persist, and the risk of spread increases.

One of the most concerning examples is tuberculosis (TB). The emergence of multidrug-resistant (MDR-TB) and extensively drug-resistant (XDR-TB) strains has reversed decades of progress in TB control. Similarly, drug-resistant strains of malaria have reappeared in parts of Asia and Africa, undermining frontline therapies. Resistance in gonorrhea and typhoid fever has also re-established these as significant public health problems.

The drivers of AMR are multifactorial. Overuse and misuse of antibiotics, such as self-medication or incomplete treatment courses, accelerate resistance. Widespread use of antimicrobials in livestock and agriculture further contributes to the problem. Additionally, global travel and migration allow resistant strains to spread across borders, while weak healthcare systems in low-resource settings struggle to contain outbreaks.

The re-emergence of infections with resistant pathogens leads to higher mortality, prolonged hospital stays, and increased healthcare costs. Beyond the medical burden, AMR threatens modern medicine itself, making routine surgeries, cancer therapy, and organ transplantation riskier due to the danger of untreatable infections.

Addressing this crisis requires a multidimensional approach: developing new antibiotics and alternative therapies, strengthening infection prevention and control, implementing antimicrobial stewardship programs, and enhancing global surveillance. Public awareness and responsible antibiotic use are equally vital to slow down resistance.

Antimicrobial resistance is fueling the re-emergence of dangerous infections worldwide. Without urgent and coordinated action, even common illnesses could once again become life-threatening, reversing decades of medical progress.

Summary

Infectious diseases are always evolving, so we must remain vigilant and prepared with adaptive health plans. Pests, new and old, just won't go away—and conditions like environmental changes, urban density, and world travel just accelerate the process. Even when something like COVID-19 presents initially as mild, many people describe symptoms persisting a lot longer than they should. Most often, the evidence demonstrates that more than half of individuals with mild-to-moderate COVID-19 go on to be unwell for 12 months or longer (Boscolo et al., 2021). This type of long-term trouble makes it obvious that even infections that aren't fatal can still put a great strain on our healthcare systems. Public health initiatives, therefore, truly must broaden their focus to encompass follow-up treatment and rehabilitation as well as placing a focus on early prevention. It's also important to observe that older diseases, too often neglected while we concentrate on the new ones, continue to be a major headache. Such things as antibiotic resistance, vaccine skepticism, and even some political upheaval breathe new life into these diseases. Occasionally ailments we believed had been brought into check reassert themselves, making it more complex to address them. Consider how monitoring effectively lessened bullying via tried-and-true strategies , although settings are different, the message would appear to be this: vigilant, data-supported checks and well-designed strategies (Gaffney et al., 2021). By and large, addressing such re-emergent issues entails designing policies that rely on firm epidemiological information while taking in regional cultural nuances. So, in summing all this up, addressing both brand-new and recurring diseases truly demands a mixed bag of strategies. It's not sufficient to merely jump in and quash an outbreak; long-term treatment and comprehending the long-term effects, as well as addressing the social aspects, are just as crucial. Sustained investment in research, improved health systems, and public education are crucial, particularly in identifying vulnerable populations and implementing targeted interventions. Such a broad strategy strengthens our overall resilience against future pandemics or recurring local problems and keeps communities safe globally. Learning from the experiences of numerous public health interventions guarantees that our responses are effective and adaptable, capable of responding to both new and known infectious dangers (Boscolo et al., 2021; Gaffney et al., 2021).

Disease patterns also tend to present themselves as reflections of change in our environment and society—sometimes subtle, sometimes very dramatic. New diseases have a tendency to buzz onto the stage where they have not been before. They appear because of such things as animal-to-human transfers, spontaneous adjustments in their genetic makeup, or changes in the environment that allow them to spread. On the flip side, diseases we'd once nearly conquered sometimes come crawling back when public health measures lag when bacteria become unexpectedly tougher, or when everyday human behavior changes. In most cases, emerging conditions bring entirely fresh challenges while re-emerging ones reintroduce old problems in altered forms. Recognizing these nuances is generally essential for shaping effective monitoring and response strategies. Time and place have their own role to play here, as well. New diseases tend to erupt in regions that were not previously involved, so the local officials have to rush to identify the culprit. Very often, our current diagnostic techniques get outwitted by the paucity of initial information about these unknown pathogens. Around the same time, re-emerging threats usually strike populations with previous exposure to these infections, re-emerging as a consequence of factors such as rising microbial resistance, environmental alterations, or a decline in immunity due to less frequent vaccination.

Curiously, populations may sometimes dismiss such re-emerging threats as minor because they are accustomed to them, but that nonchalance can prove deadly. These trends tend to reflect more profound socio-political or economic failures, emphasizing that robust public health infrastructures and persistent prevention strategies are entirely essential. A look at the microscopic front line, and how pathogens engage with their hosts also delineates emerging and re-emerging diseases. Most in general, new infections tend to include insects that have either cross-leaped among species or adapted in ways confusing to the immune system, reorganizing the microbe-host equilibrium in some unforeseen way. Scientists have achieved significant mileage with "omics" technologies for sorting out the complicated interactions but in most situations, the particular roles of diverse microbial groups as well as chemical cues remain slightly opaque, compromising their practical applicability. On the other hand, re-emerging diseases could exploit compromised host defenses or environmental situations that enhance their virulence and resistance. This dynamic situation requires a balanced strategy that integrates microbiology, immunology, and strong public health strategies, even if at times the connections seem a little off.

References

1. Allam, Z., Nieuwenhuijsen, M., Chabaud, D., & Moreno, C. (2022). The 15-minute city offers a new framework for sustainability, livability, and health. *The Lancet Planetary Health, 6*(3), e181–e183. https://doi.org/10.1016/S2542-5196(22)00014-6.
2. Alsaeed, T. (2025). Emerging and re-emerging viral infections: A review of epidemiological trends, diagnostics, therapeutics, and public health interventions. *International Journal of Medicine in Developing Countries, 9(4)*. https://www.semanticscholar.org/paper/e198c60c61af425e364b4db59f013ceec5996b13 (accessed on 7 May 2025).
3. Appel, G., Grewal, L., Hadi, R., & Stephen, A. T. (2019). The future of social media in marketing. *Journal of the Academy of Marketing Science, 48*, 79–95. https://doi.org/10.1007/s11747-019-00695-1.
4. Boscolo-Rizzo, P., Guida, F., Polesel, J., Marcuzzo, A. V., Capriotti, V., D'Alessandro, A., Zanelli, E., et al. (2021). Sequelae in adults at 12 months after mild-to-moderate coronavirus disease 2019 (COVID-19). *International Forum of Allergy & Rhinology, 11*, 1685–1688. https://doi.org/10.1002/alr.22832.
5. Branda, F., Ceccarelli, G., Giovanetti, M., Albanese, M., Binetti, E., Ciccozzi, M., & Scarpa, F. (2025). Nipah virus: A zoonotic threat re-emerging in the wake of global public health challenges. *Microorganisms, 13*, 124. https://www.semanticscholar.org/paper/30004bbae09bcd41b74727f3ed3ed8e16dd69d18 (accessed on 7 May 2025).
6. Chala, B., & Hamde, F. (2021). Emerging and re-emerging vector-borne infectious diseases and the challenges for control: A review. *Frontiers in Public Health, 9*. https://doi.org/10.3389/fpubh.2021.715759.
7. Chen, C., Gao, G., Xu, Y., Pu, L., Wang, Q., Wang, L., Wang, W., et al. (2020). SARS-CoV-2–positive sputum and feces after conversion of pharyngeal samples in patients with COVID-19. *Annals of Internal Medicine, 172*, 832–834. https://doi.org/10.7326/m20-0991.
8. Creti, R., Imperi, M., Berardi, A., Lindh, E., Alfarone, G., Pataracchia, M., Recchia, S., et al. (2021). Invasive Group B Streptococcal disease in neonates and infants, Italy, years 2015–2019. *Microorganisms, 9*(1), Article 1. https://www.semanticscholar.org/paper/a9f04d5a3866069b60dd13978cac23766d69f5a3 (accessed on 7 May 2025).
9. de Oliveira Figueiredo, P., Stoffella-Dutra, A. G., Costa, G. B., de Oliveira, J. S., Amaral, C. D., Santos, J. D., Rocha, K. L. S., et al. (2020). Re-emergence of yellow fever in Brazil during 2016–2019: Challenges, lessons learned, and perspectives. *Viruses, 12*, 1233. https://doi.org/10.3390/v12111233.
10. Dias, R. A. (2024). Towards a comprehensive definition of pandemics and strategies for prevention: A historical review and future perspectives. *Microorganisms, 12*, Article 3456. https://www.semanticscholar.org/paper/944819660a2e19eb025b92fdcda9d3cf02816a18 (accessed on 7 May 2025).
11. Doyle, M. M., Evans, T. S., Hitchens, P. L., & Johnson, C. K. (2020). Global shifts in mammalian population trends reveal key predictors of virus spillover risk. *Proceedings of the Royal Society B: Biological Sciences, 287*(1924), 20192736. https://doi.org/10.1098/rspb.2019.2736.
12. Elhakim, M., Hamid, M., Elkholy, A., & Samhouri, D. (2025). Leveraging International Health Regulations (2005) to enhance health security in the Eastern Mediterranean Region: A

retrospective analysis from 2016 to 2023. *BMJ Public Health, 3, e001048*. https://www.semanticscholar.org/paper/f56a620a1a91c9cd73b11af65778803c26e72a37 (accessed on 7 May 2025).

13. Ernst, K. C., Fernandez, P., Diuk-Wasser, M., Enriquez, A. J., Berry, K., & Hayden, M. H. (2024). Contrasting perceptions, knowledge, and actions around Lyme disease in an urban area of emerging Lyme disease and an area of endemic Lyme disease in the Northeastern United States. *The American Journal of Tropical Medicine and Hygiene, 111*(4), 865–879. https://www.semanticscholar.org/paper/5ef37fdf4ce5c23f28cd7b14227c3b18da216c4d (accessed on 7 May 2025).
14. Gaffney, H., Ttofi, M. M., & Farrington, D. P. (2021). Effectiveness of school-based programs to reduce bullying perpetration and victimization: An updated systematic review and meta-analysis. *Campbell Systematic Reviews, 17*. https://doi.org/10.1002/cl2.1143.
15. Gainor, E., Harris, E., & LaBeaud, A. D. (2022). Uncovering the burden of dengue in Africa: Considerations on magnitude, misdiagnosis, and ancestry. *Viruses, 14*, 233. https://doi.org/10.3390/v14020233.
16. Gentilotti, E., Górska, A., Tami, A., Gusinow, R., Mirandola, M., Rodríguez-Baño, J., Palacios-Baena, Z. R., et al. (2023). Clinical phenotypes and quality of life to define post-COVID-19 syndrome: A cluster analysis of the multinational, prospective ORCHESTRA cohort. *EClinicalMedicine, 62*, 102107. https://doi.org/10.1016/j.eclinm.2023.102107.
17. Gorbalenya, A. E., Baker, S. C., Baric, R. S., de Groot, R. J., Drosten, C., Gulyaeva, A., Haagmans, B. L., et al. (2020). The species severe acute respiratory syndrome-related coronavirus: Classifying 2019-nCoV and naming it SARS-CoV-2. *Nature Microbiology, 5*, 536–544. https://doi.org/10.1038/s41564-020-0695-z.
18. Haider, N., Rothman-Ostrow, P., Osman, A. Y., Arruda, L. B., Macfarlane-Berry, L., Elton, L., Thomason, M. J., et al. (2020). COVID-19—Zoonosis or emerging infectious disease? *Frontiers in Public Health, 8*. https://doi.org/10.3389/fpubh.2020.596944.
19. Hatch, B. A., Kenzie, E. S., Ramalingam, N. P. S., Sullivan, E., Barnes, C., Elder, N., & Davis, M. M. (2023). Impact of the COVID-19 vaccination mandate on the primary care workforce and differences between rural and urban settings to inform future policy decision-making. *PLOS ONE, 18*(6), e0287553. https://www.semanticscholar.org/paper/888fb4e1977b082616ed704250ef56aaa6e6c0be (accessed on 7 May 2025).
20. Intergovernmental Panel on Climate Change. (2023). *Climate Change 2022–Impacts, Adaptation and Vulnerability*. https://doi.org/10.1017/9781009325844.
21. Jeger, M., Beresford, R. M., Bock, C. H., Brown, N., Fox, A., Newton, A. C., Vicent Civera, A., et al. (2021). Global challenges facing plant pathology: Multidisciplinary approaches to meet the food security and environmental challenges in the mid-twenty-first century. *CABI Agriculture and Bioscience, 2*. https://doi.org/10.1186/s43170-021-00042-x.
22. Jiang, S., Shi, Z. L., Shu, Y., Song, J., Gao, G. F., Tan, W., & Guo, D. (2020). A distinct name is needed for the new coronavirus. *The Lancet, 395*(10228), 949. https://doi.org/10.1016/S0140-6736(20)30419-0.
23. Kay, A., Mabin, A., Petherick, A., Saéz, A. M., Poteete, A. R., Price-Smith, A. T., Israel, B. A., et al. (2016). The social and political dimensions of the Ebola response: Global inequality,

climate change, and infectious disease. *Core.* https://core.ac.uk/download/287659558.pdf (accessed on 7 May 2025).

24. Lassi, Z. S., Naseem, R., Salam, R. A., Siddiqui, F., & Das, J. K. (2021). The impact of the COVID-19 pandemic on immunization campaigns and programs: A systematic review. *International Journal of Environmental Research and Public Health, 18*(3), 988. https://doi.org/10.3390/ijerph18030988.
25. Lewnard, J. A., & Reingold, A. L. (2019). Emerging challenges and opportunities in infectious disease epidemiology. *American Journal of Epidemiology, 188*(5), 873–882. https://doi.org/10.1093/aje/kwy264.
26. Lim, S., Yoon, H., Song, K. H., Kim, S. M., & Kim, H. B. (2020). Face masks and containment of COVID-19: Experience from South Korea. *Journal of Hospital Infection, 106*(1), 206–207. https://doi.org/10.1016/j.jhin.2020.06.017.
27. Livingston, G., Huntley, J., Sommerlad, A., Ames, D., Ballard, C., Banerjee, S., Brayne, C., et al. (2020). Dementia prevention, intervention, and care: 2020 report of the Lancet Commission. *The Lancet, 396*, 413–446. https://doi.org/10.1016/s0140-6736(20)30367-6.
28. Lu, Q., & Stappenbeck, T. (2022). Local barriers configure systemic communications between the host and microbiota. *Science, 376*(6590), 950–955. https://www.semanticscholar.org/paper/9fff569e76299a46a767f103924993f2e9cd564d (accessed on 7 May 2025).
29. Mousazadeh, M., Ashoori, R., Paital, B., Kabdaşlı, I., Frontistis, Z., Hashemi, M., Sandoval, M. A., et al. (2021). Wastewater-based epidemiology perspective as a faster protocol for detecting coronavirus RNA in human populations: A review with specific reference to SARS-CoV-2 virus. *Pathogens, 10*, 1008. https://doi.org/10.3390/pathogens10081008.
30. Mullol, J., Azar, A., Buchheit, K. M., Hopkins, C., & Bernstein, J. A. (2022). Chronic rhinosinusitis with nasal polyps: Quality of life in the biologic's era. *The Journal of Allergy and Clinical Immunology: In Practice, 10*, 1434–1453.e9. https://doi.org/10.1016/j.jaip.2022.03.002.
31. Nachega, J. B., Sam-Agudu, N. A., Masekela, R., van der Zalm, M. M., Nsanzimana, S., Condo, J., Ntoumi, F., et al. (2021). Addressing challenges to rolling out COVID-19 vaccines in African countries. *The Lancet Global Health, 9*, e746–e748. https://doi.org/10.1016/s2214-109x(21)00097-8.
32. Napit, R., Gurung, A., Poudel, A., Chaudhary, A. B., Manandhar, P., Sharma, A. N., Raut, S., et al. (2025). Metagenomic analysis of human, animal, and environmental samples identifies potential emerging pathogens, profiles antibiotic resistance genes, and reveals horizontal gene transfer dynamics. *Scientific Reports, 15*, Article 12345. https://www.semanticscholar.org/paper/93bbd25b334d7a40d5ae70859fa2a6ccca352610 (accessed on 7 May 2025).
33. Ng, K., Poon, B. H., Puar, T., Quah, J., Loh, W. J., Wong, Y. J., Tan, T. Y., et al. (2020). COVID-19 and the risk to health care workers: A case report. *Annals of Internal Medicine, 172*, 766–767. https://doi.org/10.7326/l20-0175.
34. Nkengasong, J. N., & Tessema, S. K. (2020). Africa needs a new public health order to tackle infectious disease threats. *Cell, 183*, 296–300. https://doi.org/10.1016/j.cell.2020.09.041.
35. Oaknin, A., Bosse, T., Creutzberg, C. L., Giornelli, G., Harter, P., Joly, F., Lorusso, D., et al. (2022). Endometrial cancer: ESMO clinical practice guideline for diagnosis, treatment and follow-up. *Annals of Oncology, 33*, 860–877. https://doi.org/10.1016/j.annonc.2022.05.009.
36. Onyebuchi, C., Okeke, H. N., Uzochukwu, O. H., Racheal, A. O., Kolade, E., Onyebuchi, A. O.,

Odekhe, E., et al. (2025). Emerging infectious diseases and global response strategies: A systematic review and meta-analysis. *International Journal of Research and Scientific Innovation*. https://www.semanticscholar.org/paper/278b7b6b2a3f4bbe997310e0677c4c9cbf456442 (accessed on 7 May 2025).

37. Oran, D. P., & Topol, E. J. (2021). Prevalence of asymptomatic SARS-CoV-2 infection. *Annals of Internal Medicine, 174*, 286–287. https://doi.org/10.7326/l20-1285.

38. Page, M. J., Moher, D., Bossuyt, P. M., Boutron, I., Hoffmann, T., Mulrow, C. D., Shamseer, L., et al. (2021). PRISMA 2020 explanation and elaboration: Updated guidance and exemplars for reporting systematic reviews. *BMJ, 2021, 372*. https://doi.org/10.1136/bmj.n160.

39. Patra, J. K., Das, G., Fraceto, L. F., Campos, E. V. R., Rodriguez-Torres, M. P., Acosta-Torres, L. S., Díaz-Torres, L. A., et al. (2018). Nano based drug delivery systems: Recent developments and future prospects. *Journal of Nanobiotechnology, 16*. https://doi.org/10.1186/s12951-018-0392-8.

40. Paz-Gañan, C., Aguiar, H., Coronado, H., Escalona, E., & Quintana, J. (2024). Emerging and re-emerging diseases in Venezuela as a consequence of climate change: A systematic review. *Health Leadership and Quality of Life, 3*. https://www.semanticscholar.org/paper/85643b9554c6574285c356ed0292ffb812c31708 (accessed on 7 May 2025).

41. Prüss-Üstün, A., Wolf, J., Bartram, J., Clasen, T., Cumming, O., Freeman, M. C., Gordon, B., et al. (2019). Burden of disease from inadequate water, sanitation and hygiene for selected adverse health outcomes: An updated analysis with a focus on low- and middle-income countries. *International Journal of Hygiene and Environmental Health, 222*, 765–777. https://doi.org/10.1016/j.ijheh.2019.05.004.

42. Saba, N., & Balwan, W. K. (2021). Potential threat of emerging and re-emerging zoonotic diseases. *Annals of the Romanian Society for Cell Biology, 25*(6), 29–36. http://annalsofrscb.ro/index.php/journal/article/view/4251 (accessed on 7 May 2025).

43. Santomauro, D., Mantilla Herrera, A. M., Shadid, J., Zheng, P., Ashbaugh, C., Pigott, D. M., Abbafati, C., et al. (2021). Global prevalence and burden of depressive and anxiety disorders in 204 countries and territories in 2020 due to the COVID-19 pandemic. *The Lancet, 398*, 1700–1712. https://doi.org/10.1016/s0140-6736(21)02143-7.

44. Siddiqi, H. K., & Mehra, M. R. (2020). COVID-19 disease in native and immunosuppressed states: A clinical–therapeutic staging proposal. *The Journal of Heart and Lung Transplantation, 39*, 405–407. https://doi.org/10.1016/j.healun.2020.03.012.

45. Singh, J., Punia, A., Jha, S. K., Narendran, M., Singh, S., & Kataria, D. (2023). Prevalence of diabetes mellitus and its associated risk factors among tuberculosis patients in Sonipat District, Haryana: A cross-sectional study. *Journal of Clinical and Diagnostic Research, 17(11), LC20–LC24*. https://www.semanticscholar.org/paper/e49a51549d7ef37e52f3da67d2d57620441b5184 (accessed on 7 May 2025).

46. Songsore, J. (2005). *Urbanization And Health in Africa: Exploring the Interconnections Between Poverty, Inequality and The Burden of Disease*. https://core.ac.uk/download/14504865.pdf (accessed on 7 May 2025).

47. Soni, R., Tandon, D., Hassan, S., Samal, D., & Sharma, D. (2025). Prevalence and circulating serotypes of dengue in Bastar, Chhattisgarh: A cross-sectional study. *The Canadian Journal of Infectious Diseases & Medical Microbiology, 2025*, Article 987654. https://www.semanticscholar.

org/paper/3acd14641c138013ae0a3fd0fd69548bfad43228 (accessed on 7 May 2025).

48. Turaiche, M., Grigoras, M., Bratosin, F., Bogdan, I., Bota, A. V., Cerbu, B., Gurban, C., et al. (2022). Disease progression, clinical features, and risk factors for pneumonia in unvaccinated children and adolescents with measles: A re-emerging disease in Romania. *International Journal of Environmental Research and Public Health, 19, 13165.* https://www.semanticscholar.org/paper/ed9d7b06bb3cea7f2db6bb928630264adfe5cc2e (accessed on 7 May 2025).

49. Wang, G. H., Du, J., Chu, C. Y., Madhav, M., Hughes, G. L., & Champer, J. (2022). Symbionts and gene drive: Two strategies to combat vector-borne disease. *Trends in Genetics, 38*, 708–723. https://doi.org/10.1016/j.tig.2022.02.013.

50. Wang, W., Wang, J., Hu, Z., Yan, X., Gao, Q., Li, X., Zheng, J., et al. (2024). Advancing aggregation-induced emission-derived biomaterials in viral, tuberculosis, and fungal infectious diseases. *Aggregate, 6(3), e715.* https://www.semanticscholar.org/paper/3d6d7fb0651fe6b8b36f1146decf0dcfb3398a53 (accessed on 7 May 2025).

51. Watson, O. J., Barnsley, G., Toor, J., Hogan, A. B., Winskill, P., & Ghani, A. C. (2022). Global impact of the first year of COVID-19 vaccination: A mathematical modelling study. *The Lancet Infectious Diseases, 22*, 1293–1302. https://doi.org/10.1016/s1473-3099(22)00320-6.

52. Wikswo, M., Kambhampati, A., Shioda, K., Walsh, K., Bowen, A., & Hall, A. (2015). Outbreaks of acute gastroenteritis transmitted by person-to-person contact, environmental contamination, and unknown modes of transmission—United States, 2009–2013. *Morbidity and Mortality Weekly Report. Surveillance Summaries, 64*(12), 1–16. https://www.semanticscholar.org/paper/9868b28f282814f8a8033b539f881cf5c265324a (accessed on 7 May 2025).

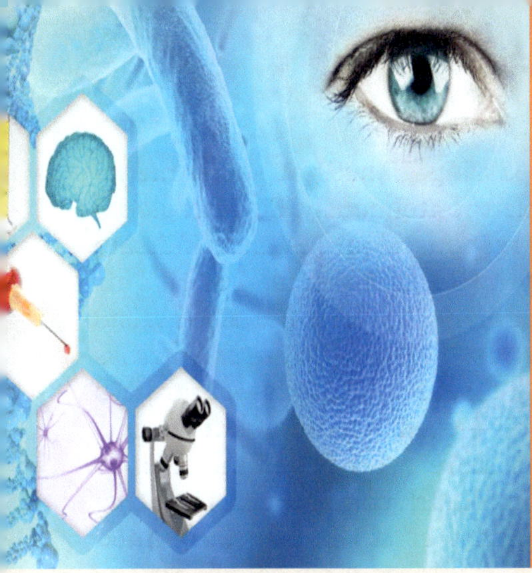

Chapter 5

GLOBAL HEALTH AND INFECTIOUS DISEASE SURVEILLANCE

Contents

Introduction

Now, in our globalized world, health problems don't belong to just one nation. Diseases that once only existed in some areas can now tend to become worldwide problems. World travel and computer connections make it simpler for diseases to shift locations, so gathering and verifying health information quickly becomes necessary. Surveillance systems essentially act as our lookout in our health system, detecting outbreaks early and pushing us in the direction of appropriate action. With advanced technology and improved methods of data sharing, we are often able to detect these hazards before they escalate into a crisis—this, in most instances, renders monitoring infections absolutely critical for public health (van Dalen et al., 1999). Knowing how infections cycle through populations requires combining knowledge from all kinds of disciplines, epidemiology, immunology, computer expertise, and even an examination of how human beings act. Surveillance today extends beyond the days of merely tabulating cases; it now incorporates predictive models, passing glances at social media buzz, and immediate feedback that enable officials to make decisions sponteneously. Current global initiatives and up-and-coming series of research on tropical disease responses, for instance, indicate that these methods have expanded significantly in breadth and depth (Bergquist et al., 2016). This hybrid perspective not only provides a more accurate portrait for following bacteria but also assists in assembling plans that harmonize local details with world trends. Also, collaboration across borders and idea-sharing play a big role in outsmarting infectious diseases. Nations—regardless of variations in resources and the type of outbreaks they encounter—exchange data, knowledge, and innovative techniques that build the global monitoring system more robust. Nations such as China, for example, have greatly spearheaded research and hosted landmark conferences, initiating discussions and disseminating good practices worldwide (Bergquist et al., 2016). Continued investment in surveillance infrastructures, capacity development, and intercountry collaborations all contribute to making our health systems subtle and poised to spring into action when new dangers arise. In the end, linking surveillance efforts to our global health strategy is key to keeping disease at bay and, one day, eradicating it (Figure 5.1).

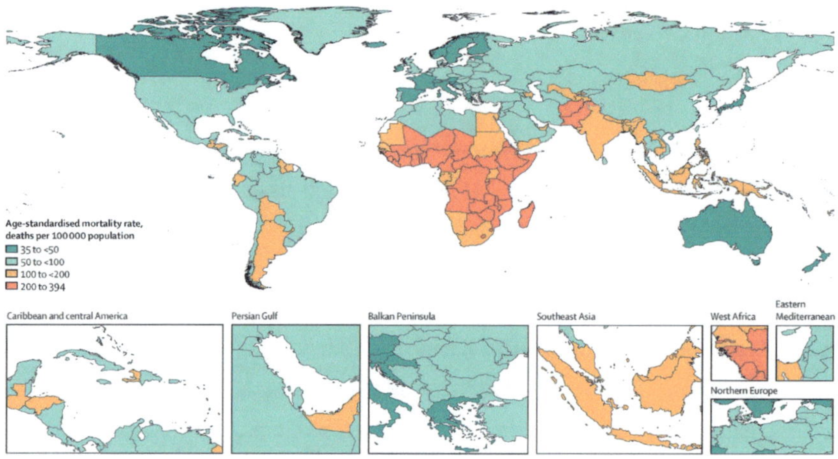

Figure 5.1. Global health and infectious disease.

Source: By Authors of the study: GBD 2019 Antimicrobial Resistance Collaborators - https://www.thelancet.com/journals/lancet/article/PIIS0140-6736(22)02185-7/fulltext, CC BY 4.0, https://commons.wikimedia.org/w/index.php?curid=127577221***Definition of Global Health***

Global health is not all about doctors and hospitals within defined boundaries—it's a combination of the way we care for our bodies, our minds, and even our social lives. In general, the concept goes far back: the WHO in 1948 defined health not only as freedom from disease, but as a complete condition of well-being. That initial vision, while seemingly simple on the surface, ultimately resulted in large, worldwide actions, such as the change observed in 1978 with the Alma Ata Declaration that ushered in concepts such as equity, community participation, and collaborating across many different areas. In most instances, this wider context reveals that our general health is inextricably linked to social conditions, so any successful intervention must address those as well (Rifkin et al., 2021). Meanwhile, when you go ahead and attempt to implement these concepts, things get complicated, particularly when it comes to monitoring and combating diseases that don't care about national borders. The pandemic due to COVID-19, however, served to highlight starkly just how interlinked everything is and how gaps in readiness even between those highly ranked on health security would emerge (Forman et al., 2021). The EU, for instance, has many members who, however great their rankings on paper, were unable to keep the virus out because coordination both locally and more broadly at the European level was out of balance. This hiccup highlights, in the majority of instances, the necessity to couple national control with collective action, establishing systems able to exchange real-time information, make decisions collaboratively, and allocate resources in a manner extending far beyond historic, rigid political borders. Picturing this, global health interweaves legal, institutional, and political strands that frame how emergencies are handled. The European experience, often characterized as being in some sense "constitutionally asymmetrical"—demonstrates that policies promoting market efficiency tend to receive more attention than policies aimed at social protection, detracting from effective governance at levels higher than the national (Forman et al., 2021). Addressing this lopsided arrangement typically involves taking a new glance at institutional functions and strengthening the authority bestowed upon agencies responsible for surveillance and emergency measures. Most experts currently recommend embracing a One Health strategy, which acknowledges the connected realities of human, animal, and environmental health. Effectively, when we widen the scope of what global health addresses to encompass governance, social determinants, and collaborative, cross-sector initiatives, the globe is in a better position to address infectious threats in our highly connected ecosystem (Forman et al., 2021; Rifkin et al., 2021).

Importance of Infectious Disease Surveillance

Control of infectious diseases truly depends on how fast one can determine whether an outbreak is a natural event or related to bioterrorism. It's not always an easy call, bioterrorist attacks can mimic a whole lot like the first signs of new infections. For the most part, this requires surveillance systems that are intelligent as well as fast enough to pick up on faint hints. Improving our detection techniques not only serves to minimize damage when real crises strike but also prepares nations for novel threats. Speedy solutions in detection and response can reduce the destruction wrought by outbreaks that otherwise go undetected. Essentially, staying watchful about infections is really the linchpin of national security as well as global health readiness (Chyba, 1998). Without these efforts, attempts at disease control would be greatly hampered. Not all places are keeping up in the same manner, and those disparities truly get in the way of our global capacity to manage diseases. Many developing regions are confronted with daunting challenges – underdeveloped infrastructure, weak reporting systems, and sometimes patchy inter-sectoral communication – which slow down the detection of outbreaks and allow diseases to get ahead. Overall, solving these problems involves focusing on endemic zoonotic issues in low-resource settings, as those challenges tend to coincide with threats from emerging infections. By investing in strengthening local capacities, we can create a more equitable, more efficient system for following outbreaks. This type of strategy not only enhances early warning initiatives but also facilitates longer-term health gains by combining local issues with wider international strategies (Barend et al., 2012). It's a change that's central to breaking down past barriers and improving our response to diseases as a whole. Ultimately, the true value of disease surveillance is in creating a responsive, adaptable public health system. Reliable and consistent reporting is critical; however, it tends to collapse for lack of solid incentives and weak regulatory guidelines - particularly in low-income areas. It's not merely a matter of new technology upgrading these systems; it also takes addressing cultural, social, and administrative barriers to free exchange of data among agencies. By promoting greater transparency and less structured communication between human and animal health communities, surveillance can transform into a more concerted practice—one that foresights and inhibits zoonotic threats. Such an integrated system is a closer-fitting global health architecture that provides fuller monitoring and quicker responses for new and underappreciated diseases alike. Finally, such surveillance is essential in safeguarding populations against the dynamic world of biologic threats (Barend et al., 2012) (Figure 5.2).

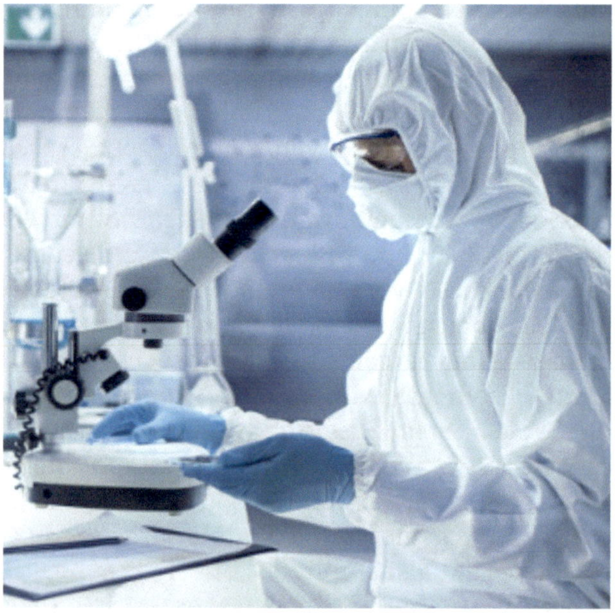

Figure 5.2. Genomic surveillance of infectious diseases.

Source: Illumina. (N.D.). *Genomic Surveillance of Infectious Diseases.*

5.1. Historical Context of Infectious Disease Surveillance

Human history's encounters with epidemics have curiously guided the way we monitor disease. During medieval times in Europe, when the bubonic plague raged, people started observing that recording even rough notes of outbreaks—however poorly executed—could in fact slow the spread. Early on, accumulating and disseminating scraps of information wasn't a refined practice; it was rather a coarse scratch at surviving during confusion. These improvised attempts improved over time, and by the 19th and early 20th centuries, public health authorities began to believe in organized, national methods of tracking disease. Large-scale incidents such as the Black Death and the Spanish flu, incidents that demonstrated just how quickly a crisis can propagate in our connected world, taught some important lessons (Bwanbale, 2024). By the 20th century, more travel and thriving urban life made it obvious that diseases truly don't mind crossing borders. The game-changer came with the establishment of organizations such as the World Health Organization, which, rather surprisingly, started bringing nations together under common reporting systems and real-time data sharing. Nevertheless, despite such advancements, unequal surveillance capacities were still an issue. For instance, during the COVID-19 pandemic, countries such as Kazakhstan faced tremendous challenges, made even more difficult by a steep decline in usual influenza cases, that highlighted residual vulnerabilities in national arrangements. In many respects, the complex intersection of traditional challenges and contemporary issues continues to influence a nation's ability to track health concerns effectively (Hujatullah et al., 2024). Emerging technological advances have transformed our method of identifying infectious threats. What was historically a world of manual records and primitive warnings has become an age of cyber platforms that quickly collect, analyze, and disseminate data, sometimes in nearly real-time. This shift, fueled by changing scientific understanding and altering political realities, highlights an unmistakable need for worldwide collaboration. In the majority of instances, the voids we observe currently in readiness can be traced to past limitations in global communication and resource distribution. Merging advanced technology with more resilient global alliances now appears downright necessary if we're to avoid future pandemics and enhance overall health security (Bwanbale, 2024).

5.1.1. Early Methods of Disease Tracking

As the years have gone by, individuals have been observing patterns of disease spread and attempting to track outbreaks as the needs of public health have changed. In the beginning, people generally kept records by merely recording who contracted the disease or even passed away, a fairly ad hoc system that tended to have holes and delays.

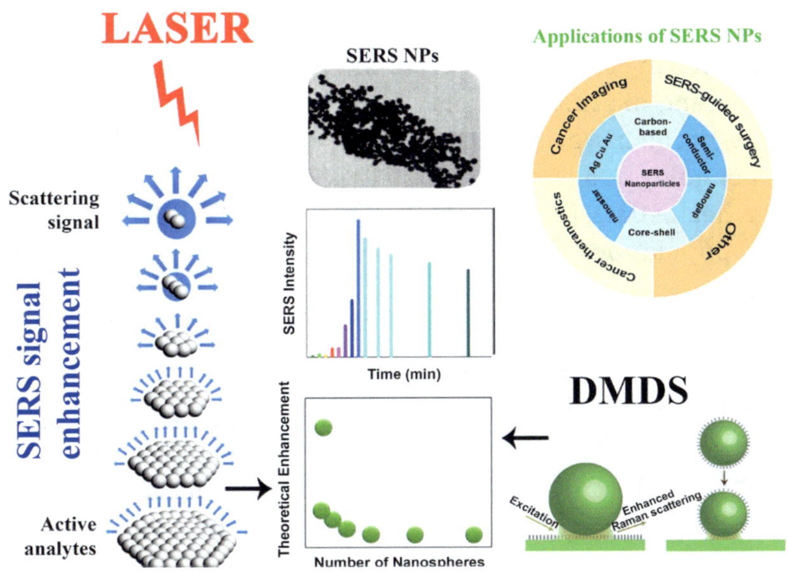

Figure 5.3. Methods of disease tracking.

Source: MDPI. (2023). *Methods of Disease Tracking.*

That loose-association system still managed to get the concept on the map—fast, accurate information is essential when battling infectious diseases. At that time, attributing animal or environmental causes to human disease was hardly on the horizon, although indications of those relationships were beginning to emerge. In a way, all those early attempts, though clumsy, ultimately laid the groundwork for a more integrated approach to doing things today, where we combination observations of humans, animals, and the environment into one big picture—something recent epidemics and the emergence of zoonotic cases have highlighted (Singh et al., 2024). Diseases today like to jump both borders and species, and that old-fashioned approach had to evolve quickly. Technology now plays a large part, with electronic health records and immense healthcare databases providing new perspectives without adding on top of added work. These new systems can alert, for example, health cases of flu-like by monitoring the speed and completeness of data. Research, some of it emanating from Brazil, for example, indicates that unless the information is good enough, the signals are lost, while good information enhances our capacity to act rapidly and intelligently (Florentino et al., 2024). Essentially, combining plain early monitoring with data-driven adjustments has made our overall strategy a great deal more agile. Nevertheless, transitioning from scribbled records to these fancy digital methods has not been all plain sailing. The change has its own attendant headaches, particularly in ensuring that all the data arrives on time and in full, which is essential for timely warnings. Research suggests the value of monitoring data quality in real time, catching delays and missing portions along the way prevents problems before they get out of control. This ongoing quality check is vital for keeping trust in health data, particularly across huge and varied populations. By setting standard quality benchmarks and leaning on new tech as needed, we're able to patch up older tracking ways, ultimately boosting global efforts to predict, monitor, and contain diseases before they spiral into full-blown pandemics (Florentino et al., 2024; Singh et al., 2024) (Figure 5.3).

5.1.2. Major Outbreaks and Their Impact on Surveillance Practices

Serious disease outbreaks have historically taken global health surveillance into unprecedented grounds. Consider the H1N1 flu outbreak of 2009–10, which truly brought home the need to exchange information in real time and identify problems early on to mitigate the far-reaching effects. That incident, and others, prompted many people to pay attention to systems such as the Global Public Health Intelligence Network (GPHIN) and HealthMap—systems that collect information from several sources to provide early warnings. When additional local outbreak reports were made available, these systems prompted a more concerted effort for readiness at home and overseas, increasing the speed at which responses could be initiated. Even with these advances, however, such networks inevitably highlight genuine gaps in surveillance capability and preparedness across countries, particularly when richer ones are contrasted with poorer ones, revealing established vulnerabilities in public health governance more broadly (Warren et al., 2010). Outbreaks have done more than simply prompt tech solutions; they've directed significant shifts in the way institutions and various fields manage disease surveillance. Take the case of the Disease Surveillance Networks (DSN) initiative, which on the whole illustrates how challenging outbreak experiences can compel communities to develop local expertise and collaborate more beyond borders. This project—intended to establish strong collaborations between several parties—ends up exchanging best practices as well as the expertise required for an accelerated response. Its emphasis on combinationincorporating what we understand of human, animal, and environmental health, traditionally labeled as a One Health strategy, reinforces that surveillance can't remain within traditional, narrow confines. By encouraging cross-disciplinary collaboration and even adjusting communication skills among local specialists, the DSN assists in constructing a stronger, more adaptable surveillance infrastructure, one that's prepared to address complex disease issues in our globalized world (Ekirapa et al., 2011). Simultaneously, large outbreaks have also spurred policy adjustments emphasizing collaboration on a global level and positioning surveillance networks as static components of public health strategies. Countries, increasingly, now deploy pandemic preparedness plans based on global surveillance information and informed by larger geopolitical and socio-economic dynamics. Mostly, these outbreaks uncover the fact that it's not enough to just depend on technology or data gathering; there's an actual need for diplomatic intervention and global collaboration to make information travel quickly and resources flow equitably. Overall, large infectious disease events have not just highlighted the vulnerability of existing systems but have also served as a powerful incentive for continued investment, new innovation, and a more sensitive type of diplomacy in global health surveillance activities (Warren et al., 2010).

5.1.3. Evolution of Technology in Disease Monitoring

Employing genomic sequencing in monitoring infectious diseases has truly revolutionized the way we monitor global health. It now provides us with a sort of precise understanding that wasn't quite possible previously. This technology, in simple terms, allows us to detect bacteria at the genetic level virtually in a flash, which in the majority of instances traces outbreaks and virus modifications in real time. In COVID-19, for instance, the readers of genetic codes were instrumental in selecting variations between Delta and Omicron strains—information later that scaled back vaccine strategies and public health responses. To that, these techniques are now directing personalized medicine by aligning treatments with one's own individual genetic profile, thereby improving how well drugs perform and even reducing side effects. In general, however, all of this really emphasizes how important continuous support for genomic research and facilities is to disease management worldwide (Wu et al., 2024). Analytics on data have progressed disease tracking from simply reacting to practically anticipating what's next. Large data integrated with artificial intelligence, particularly if viewed in light of the One Health concept bringing human, animal, and environmental health together—provides an innovative means to perceive risks differently. By accumulating portions of information from ecological scenes to socioeconomic tendencies, we have the ability to usually detect preliminary warning signs and strategize advance steps. This multi-disciplined combination hits the complex reality of zoonotic diseases to a point of reminding us that surveillance ought not to concentrate solely on humans but should also monitor for animal hosts and environmental factors. In the majority of cases, relying on these hybrid technologies makes our systems even more flexible and responsive to new threats (Singh et al., 2024). How we track disease just continues to advance, and that's evident in the manner that international collaboration and rapid information exchange through online platforms have increased. Improved connectivity now allows health collectives to disseminate information quickly, collaborate over reactions, and monitor outbreaks that span across borders. Devices such as mobile health applications, remote sensors, and cloud-based databases have expanded the surveillance net even where resources at times lack. And besides, combining disciplines such as genomics, artificial intelligence, and geospatial mapping has yielded a toolset that encodes the constantly changing landscape of infectious diseases with jaw-dropping precision. These technology combinations not only refine detection and response to outbreaks but also enable them to monitor how effective intervention strategies are, ultimately creating an even stronger health system. As technology evolves (sometimes in unexpected ways), it remains essential that our systems are inclusive and fair so that everyone can share in the benefits of these advances (Singh et al., 2024; Wu et al., 2024) (Figure 5.4).

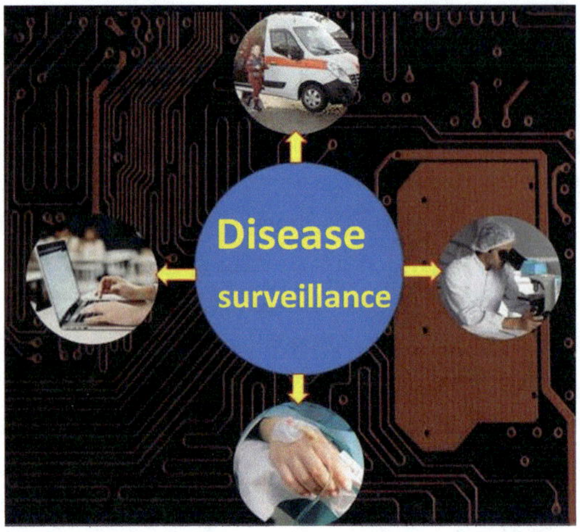

Figure 5.4. Technology in disease monitoring.

Source: https://blogger.googleusercontent.com/img/b/R29vZ2xl/AVvXsEgQdL6zDBEppKYQQMYkAkRkK0uQXLsVuuOcc3rATl3wm 66b86fK20MeHkJ3mpG9gDyCNxpLQZeBFylA7lNP0002pmSR2oagY9n_vKaYgcMDPNtIoVxc6DWatyYSkFuGccupiMJG1eTuED7E_lrhKCxiIVzQH-VMvWxS8Xk Dm-s2TcPloO0e0wrS2hkog/s548/12.jpg.

5.2. Current Global Health Frameworks

It has become rather tough to manage infectious diseases today, and healthcare systems worldwide are increasingly relying on advanced technology to assist. One such area is artificial intelligence, which is doing its part by advancing our methods of diagnosing, personalizing treatments, and monitoring disease trends more closely. You may be surprised to find that AI-based devices can identify problematic pathogens quite rapidly and even alert early when conditions such as sepsis begin to arise – which tends to result in improved patient outcomes. But translating these innovations from lab-like conditions into the real world isn't always a seamless process; there are very real issues of making sure data continues to hold up, ironing out difficult implementation problems, and ensuring that algorithmic decisions remain fair and accurate. In most cases, smoothing out these bumps will need clearer validation methods, a broader mix of voices from different sectors, and approaches that keep equity at their heart, so that AI truly helps control infections without widening existing gaps (Ibiam et al., 2025). New technology isn't standing still either. Current advances have led global health initiatives to shake things up by combining genomics, nano-immunotherapies, and AI into a single energetic combination. Consider the Next-Gen Global Health 6.0 initiative as an example; it's designed for precision medicine that combines live genomic monitoring with AI algorithms that can predict outbreaks and even create personalized treatment plans. Nano-immunotherapies, essentially adjusting the immune system with a remarkable degree of specificity, are putting a new spin on combating infections that have long defied conventional treatment. For the most part, this combination of early technologies is opening the way for flexible data-driven solutions that function in different healthcare environments, emphasizing the need for collaboration between disciplines and proactive policies that enhance access for all, particularly for communities that have been left behind (Anurogo, 2025). The true challenge for these global health strategies is whether they will remain adaptable in the presence of new infectious threats while at the same time manage historic social disparities. In other words, finding new tech isn't enough; policy efforts must be genuine and there must be international coordination to harmonize how surveillance is conducted and how it is shared. Rather than focusing primarily on detection and treatment, these systems are gradually moving to treat social determinants of health, closing the gap between innovative science and the day-to-day needs of the public. In the end, the success of these systems depends on mass participation from all sides, transparent (if occasionally a little inconsistent) communication, and training that empowers local health officials and workers. Overall, by remaining flexible and prioritizing equity, health strategies today can become far more inclusive and responsive, enhancing worldwide readiness and security in the process (Figure 5.5).

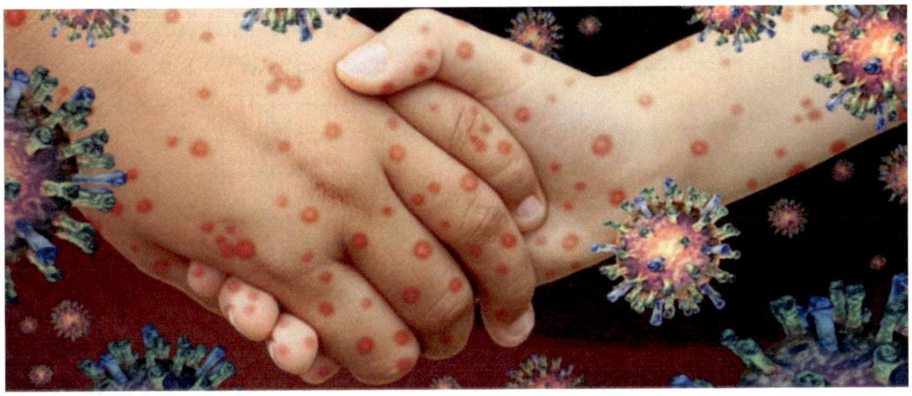

Figure 5.5. Infectious diseases.

Source: Care Insurance. (2023). *Most Communicable Diseases in India.*

5.2.1. Role of the World Health Organization (WHO)

Global health menaces today have become much more complicated, so it is no longer sufficient to operate within national boundaries. The WHO of course comes in to identify, monitor, and attempt to contain outbreaks worldwide. WHO, in its special position, brings together all sorts of actors—governments, public health authorities, even scientists, to create an informal yet functional network for monitoring diseases. They kind of cut back on reporting techniques and accelerate the dissemination of outbreak information, which in the majority of instances increases our worldwide preparedness and rapid reactions. Also, WHO provides technical assistance and capacity building to less resource-endowed countries, increasingly developing stronger health systems capable of intercepting and containing infectious agents early on. Monitoring infectious diseases isn't so much about tracking heat maps anymore either; there's been a significant change due to new methods and emerging tech that pinpoint where pathogens travel and who would be in danger. The WHO is keen to combination molecular testing with digital information streams and creative modeling sleights to know more about disease transmission. By and large, this type of progress belongs to a larger intellectual change in the study of disease—a transition that is based on thinner study designs and statistical techniques that are quite unlike the traditional techniques used for chronic diseases (Lewnard & Reingold, 2019). By advocating and disseminating these new methods, WHO ensures that our disease surveillance systems remain responsive but grounded in sound science, which subsequently informs improved public health decisions and more efficient interventions globally. Attention is not only given to the tech aspect; WHO also makes a big bet on collaboration that transcends politics and geography. Consider the Foundation's Disease Surveillance Networks program, for instance, it illustrates how cross-border, multi-layered collaborations are central to managing emerging health threats (Ekirapa et al., 2011). WHO encourages these types of networks, typically relying on the One Health concept, which integrates human, animal, and environmental health when designing surveillance or responses. This holistic perspective is rather critical in combating zoonotic diseases and other pesky infectious threats. Through ongoing efforts at better communication, exchange of information (albeit a little erratically sometimes), and coordination of policies among various global players, WHO consistently reinforces international health security and ensures responses to outbreaks appear timely and coordinated—keeping people safe nearly everywhere.

5.2.2. International Health Regulations (IHRs)

Initiatives to maintain our health in a secure position rely on frameworks that assist in detecting and managing outbreaks sponteneously. The IHRs play a significant role in engaging 196 nations in some informal agreement to monitor and inform the World Health Organization when something is amiss. This arrangement compels countries to be transparent about what is going on by setting out minimum standards for monitoring diseases and acting when problems arise. It also emphasizes the necessity of collaboration among various sectors and information sharing in a timely manner – something that is a requirement when every second matters. Nevertheless, despite its wide reach, most nations find it difficult to have their diverse health arrangements working together, and the IHR are adjusted over time to address new dangers and iron out global cooperation problems (MacFarlane et al., 2024). In fact, understanding how these components interact is the key to preventing the spread of diseases. Shifts in our surroundings and society have clouded the scenario when it comes to monitoring diseases, particularly those transmitted through insects. The IHR now guides both local and international efforts to contain infections that appear to be experiencing a resurgence – partly due to climate change and our increasingly smaller world. These are provided by early, warning instruments such as surveillance and epidemic intelligence, while travel restrictions and border screening emerge as crucial options to bring outbreaks under control. The experience of COVID, 19, say, exposed both the astute suggestions and the vulnerabilities in such plans – travel industries had to unite and intensify screening, demonstrating how vital it is for various groups to join in. In addition, when countries examine their essential capacities within the IHR, they can adjust their response to improve fit with the challenges they encounter, increasing readiness and resilience in most instances (Subtil et al., 2024).

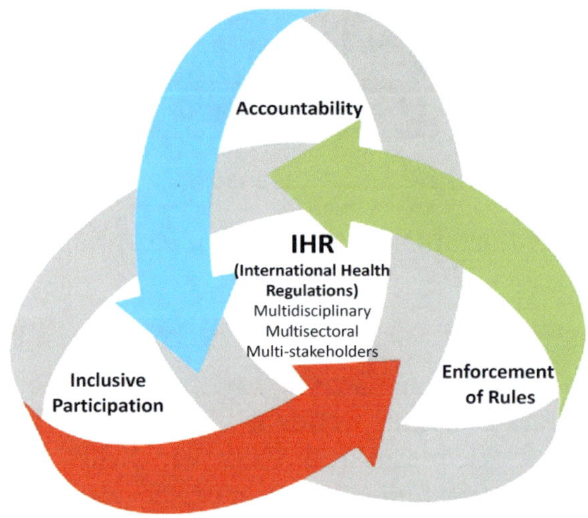

Figure 5.6. International health regulations (IHR).

Source: BMJ Global Health. (2020). *International Health Regulations.*

All of this demonstrates how the IHR is constantly evolving in a changing environment of infectious hazards. New and novel infectious threats continue to arise, and in turn, global health governance is compelled into a sort of subtle dance. The IHR continues to be a default framework for triggering rapid alerts and concerted action that assists in reducing cross-border health threats. The ongoing round of amendments – which is guided as much as anything by the stern lessons of more recent pandemics – seeks to smooth out reality-based challenges and get the IHR to work better locally as well as internationally. There's also a push to develop capacity, an imperative step because systems of surveillance are vastly different countries over, and many still struggle for equitable access to resources. This reinforcement of the initial pillars makes for a more solid network, one that identifies dangers earlier and can intervene with bolder actions. By facilitating a perception of mutual responsibility and innovative collaboration, the IHR continues to shape how we track disease and ensure our future global health (MacFarlane et al., 2024; Subtil et al., 2024) (Figure 5.6).

5.2.3. Collaboration Between Countries and Organizations

In the current battle against infectious diseases, it takes a lot to create durable networks across national boundaries and strict professional lines. Multiskilled groups take their expertise and resources and pool them together so that outbreaks get detected, reported, and resolved in record time—outbreaks that truly wait for no one. Several studies, in the majority of instances, identify that when various industries exchange technical knowledge and operate in coordination, surveillance is faster and more accurate. Such warmth of coordination not only facilitates functioning more smoothly but also fosters trust among all concerned—a key component for sincere info exchange and enduring relationships across cultures and continents (Kimball et al., 2011). In summary, addressing international health issues genuinely demands an infrastructure where nations and organizations combine capacities to minimize infectious threats. Regarding initiatives to strengthen global disease surveillance, attention normally turns towards bolstering local technical capacity as well as developing cross-border collaboration. These efforts focus on building capacity within countries and institutions so that information can be picked up by local specialists in new techniques for data collection and networking more organically. Too often, official information exchange and dissemination of best practices develop gradually out of discussions that combination disciplines together—an approach suited to the nonlinear ways that disease spreads. One Health concepts also come into play here; they remind us that human, animal, and environmental health are all interlinked, so a combination of sectors and countries need to keep vigil (Ekirapa et al., 2011). Essentially, these integrated strategies demonstrate how responses, stimulated by international partnerships, are central to addressing contemporary infectious disease control. Disease surveillance has come to rely on creating new and innovative alliances that destroy the conventional barriers between organizations, governments, and disciplines. Improvement in communications technology and information analysis has raised the stakes for global surveillance networks, but these technological advances must be supported by actual, credible partnerships. Network sustainability depends not only on that initial spurt of energy; it's also about sustained knowledge exchange and responsibility—something akin to a neverending, exchange that keeps everyone honest. Such cooperation requires coordination at all levels, from local corners to the global stage, so that surveillance information inform timely policies and concrete responses (Ekirapa et al., 2011). It appears that only by coming together in a considered, sometimes unclear, but real manner will we be able to achieve global health in our connected age.

5.3. Methods of Infectious Disease Surveillance

Accurate disease monitoring today results from the combination of traditional epidemiologic practices and a healthy dose of new technology.

Physicians and clinics continue to report cases in so, called passive surveillance, but the reports may get behind or lack information because of underreporting. In most circumstances, health authorities go out and look for cases in high, risk populations—a process we term active surveillance—and this process completes many of the gaps. Next, there are certain healthcare hotspots utilized as initial warning sites under sentinel surveillance; these are useful for detecting strange patterns before things spiral out of control. To add to this, new molecular techniques such as genomic sequencing allow us to identify the offending microbe and track its spread in real, time. To summarize, these diverse approaches improve both the accuracy and sensitivity of our surveillance system, establishing a strong foundation for rapid public health responses. This multi, faceted approach is particularly critical when working with diseases such as malaria, where maintaining a constant watch on drug efficacy is quasiessential (Lu, 2024). It's increasingly apparent that as disease threats become more multifaceted, we can't count on a single discipline, humans, animals, and their common environment all have a role to play. One Health surveillance is a new spin on old monitoring, combining hospital, veterinary clinic, and ecological study data. It's essential when working with zoonotic diseases that occasionally leap species barriers and induce pandemics. For the most part, sophisticated methods such as Big Data analysis and Artificial Intelligence assist us in evaluating risks in real-time, enabling speedier, better, coordinated public health action. Worldwide informationsharing systems, with their transnational collaborations, facilitate it to identify newly emerging risks and exchange successful response strategies. All this technology and collaboration lends the One Health model the potential to hone our surveillance and reduce the burden of infectious diseases globally (Singh et al., 2024). Technology continues to disrupt infectious disease surveillance by allowing us to gather and examine data in quicker, more accurate, and scalable manners. Mobile health programs and electronic reporting systems enable front, line workers to transmit reports virtually in real, time—avoiding the lags commonly associated with paper-based procedures. Remote sensing and geographic information systems make available the potential for environmental monitoring capable of suggesting when disease carriers can burst in size due to climate or land use changes. New diagnostics for detecting pathogens, such as point-of-care diagnostics and handheld sequencing machines—also assist local teams in probing outbreaks and responding on the ground. When you combine these new techniques with the more traditional surveillance methods, the outcome is a more acute system that detects hotspots and follows disease trends over time. In a way, these evidence-based reforms are central to guiding resources and planning interventions, as we persist in addressing emerging malaria challenges and enhancing our pandemic preparedness (Lu, 2024; Singh et al., 2024).

5.3.1. Passive versus Active Surveillance Systems

Monitoring infectious diseases isn't a one, note task—it really depends on the type of surveillance in play. You've got two main types here: passive and active. With passive surveillance, health providers and labs simply send in routine reports, and the system just gathers data without chasing down every case. This method is overall cost, effective and sustainable across massive populations, so it is convenient for monitoring long-term patterns in global health. Nevertheless, since it relies on voluntary reporting, there may be glitches such as underreporting or delay, which sometimes hinder the response when an outbreak arises. On the contrary, active surveillance involves a more proactive approach, experts get in touch directly with health facilities, communities, or certain populations to search for cases. Although this approach generates better and fuller data, it also takes a lot in terms of resources and labor, which can be an actual burden in low-resource environments struggling with challenges such as antimicrobial resistance (AMR) and chronic infections (Murray et al., 2022). When you begin contrasting passive and active methods, several significant differences emerge, particularly the speed at which information comes and how well the system detects signals. Active surveillance, for example, tends to excel by catching emerging threats—consider zoonotic coronaviruses like SARS, CoV, 2, where early discoveries can truly dictate intervention moves and containment efforts.

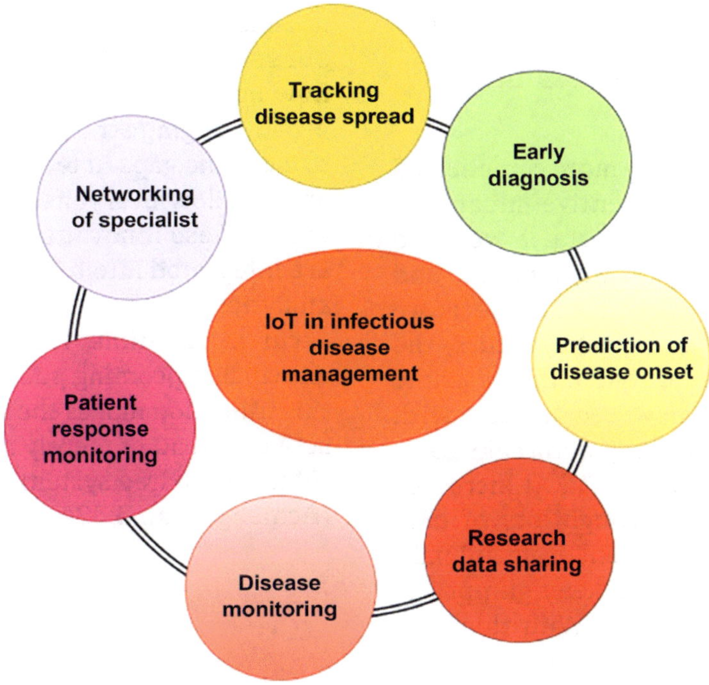

Figure 5.7. Monitoring infectious diseases.

Source: https://ars.els, cdn.com/content/image/3, s2.0, B9780128214725000120, f18, 01, 9780128214725.jpg.

In contrast, passive systems might miss the very first cases of a new microbe, as we've seen in past coronavirus episodes. It's important to note that nailing down a detailed molecular picture of these viruses, along with their spread, really depends on fast and precise data, something active surveillance is generally better at providing. Nevertheless, since active approaches are generally more costly to run, passive surveillance is still a mainstay in routine public health surveillance, with a mixed approach of the two strategies typically being the best option for effective disease control (V'kovski et al., 2020). Merging passive and active strategies appears to be a pragmatic means of enhancing our overall infectious disease surveillance on a worldwide basis. By combining the extensive, stable web of passive data with the targeted, high, speed edge of active approaches, you have a better picture that assists decision, making. This dual, barreled technique is especially essential when dealing with the growing flood of bacterial AMR, wherein detailed information about pathogens and drug performance is indispensable to designing informed public health strategies. In general, in most instances, increasing lab capacities and data infrastructures in low-resource areas continues to be necessary to close present information gaps. In general, by drawing on the respective strengths of each system, health officials can more closely predict changes in disease patterns, more efficiently prioritize resource allocation, and jump into action with timely interventions in response to new threats (Murray et al., 2022) (Figure 5.7).

5.3.2. Use of Data Analytics and Technology

Infectious diseases are getting more complicated to follow, so we need inventive means of combining varying types of data if we're to keep pace. Consider it: humans, animals, and nature are all interconnected, and the more disease that jumps across species occurs, the more this reality counts. One Health is a prime example, it combines new technology with global collaboration to identify outbreaks early on. Overall, coupling Big Data and AI increases our capacity to winnow through lots of data that comes from the environment, from animals, or from humans to provide a keen glimpse of what could cause an outbreak. With this type of combination, timely interventions become real, allowing the decision-makers to intervene as they should (Singh et al., 2024). In much of the world, such as sub-Saharan Africa, the impetus for data analysis and technological tools is accompanied by its own combination of obstacles and silver linings. Usually, the healthcare systems in place locally struggle with infrastructure challenges and blurry regulatory environments that complicate the ability to leverage the potential of big data to monitor disease. Nevertheless, the potential of these approaches is vast. By strengthening digital health systems and implementing more explicit rules, these systems can capture, disassemble, and respond to health data better. AI and analytics also enable the predicting of when outbreaks will strike, which in most scenarios means that resources can be distributed a little bit better. And, in addition, investing in the skills of people, no doubt a bit patchily from time to time, is essential if these technological instruments are to work their magic (Achieng et al., 2024). In addition to that, applying data analytics ethically in global health surveillance is a matter that requires a close examination of both the regulations and how data is handled. As digital health tools grow so rapidly, there is a dire need for shared policies that safeguard privacy but continue to allow important information to flow across borders. For the most part, smart, broad, ranging strategies need to be developed to close the gaps in technology between regions and to allow everyone an equal opportunity to access these innovations. When these concepts are integrated into our healthcare systems, data analytics do more than follow diseases as they occur in real-time, instead, they enable us to anticipate upcoming public health issues. Briefly, this transition makes the concept of surveillance active instead of merely reactive, creating more robust, prepared systems locally and worldwide (Achieng et al., 2024).

5.3.3. Community-based Surveillance Initiatives

Quick, reliable community-based data is essential when monitoring disease outbreaks. In most low, to middle-income communities, health services can be quite uneven—tending to lead to delays in detecting and managing crises. Locals end up playing an important part as they pick up on clusters of sickness and strange symptoms, reporting them promptly so that assistance can arrive earlier. This direct engagement not only fills gaps in healthcare access but also establishes a much-needed sense of trust and cultural acceptability. For example, early intervention is crucial for diseases such as tuberculosis (TB), where early detection and remaining on treatment are key to preventing drug-resistant strains (Gamon et al., 2013). Combining local day-to-day know, how and official health systems in the majority of instances increases our collective potential to track and suppress infectious hazards. Establishing a solid surveillance system is not necessarily about technology—it's about having a good understanding of local behavior and economic drivers that foster disease transmission. Too often, these kinds of programs combination in some education, which increases health literacy and makes people more likely to call out an issue when something's not right. This emphasis on education is important to break through misinformation and stigma that sometimes prevents people from accessing care. Meanwhile, these projects tend to unite partners from various disciplines, fitting into what can be described as a One Health approach that considers human, animal, and environmental health as interconnected (Aarestrup et al., 2015). Strategies here typically require adjusting to fit local politics and resources. By allowing information to flow from community levels all the way up to national agencies, these community-based efforts construct a responsive, evidence-based response, particularly important in places where resources are limited. Despite all their potential, community-based surveillance schemes encounter a fair amount of obstacles when it comes to remaining sustainable, providing good data, and integrating well with official health systems. Spontaneous training, consistent funding, and good tech support are all the things you have to maintain volunteers and keep reports on track. At times, a failure to follow up rapidly can chip away at the trust that community members have worked so hard to develop, decreasing their enthusiasm to participate over time. It's also difficult to merge locally collected data with national systems without some kind of standard framework and validation checks (Aarestrup et al., 2015). Building our evidence base through rigorous policy reviews can reveal cost, saving means to roll these out to multiple settings. Ultimately, though placing communities at the center of disease surveillance is promising for preventing and controlling outbreaks, it requires long-term commitment, intersector collaboration, and a seamless link with more comprehensive public health approaches (Aarestrup et al., 2015; Gamon et al., 2013) (Figure 5.8).

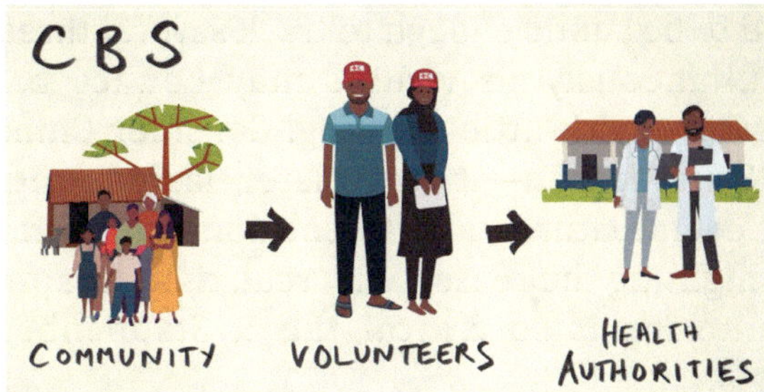

Figure 5.8. A community-based surveillance platform.

Source: Youtube. (N.D.). *Community-based Surveillance Platform.*

5.4. Challenges in Infectious Disease Surveillance

Global health is a moving target nowadays—quick city expansion and more people on the move make it really difficult to keep track of diseases. Traditional methods that rely on fixed population figures just don't work when pathogens spread so erratically. In most low-resource settings, the healthcare systems are in disarray; data get gathered patchily, and records are usually out of date. Critical intelligence winds up spread out among multiple agencies or regions, which makes it difficult to send speedy alerts and mobilize a coordinated response. South Korea, for example, has some robust systems but is still without the ability to combine data and bring diverse agencies to respond in crisis mode (Jang et al., 2025). terms, mending these weak links is critical if we hope for a smoother global defense against emerging infections. The problem only intensifies as bacteria continue to evolve. Respiratory pathogens exhibit all manner of behavioral spins—reversing which strains hold sway, according to shifts such as rates of vaccination and daily routines. The entire COVID, 19 experience quite compelled us to acknowledge that our surveillance mechanisms need to be subtle enough to track several threats simultaneously, as viruses may bounce back or evolve with little warning. Consider China's 2023 flu season—it came later, lasted longer, and even featured a different dominant strain, highlighting the reason why real, time, adaptive monitoring is so critical (Lu & Stappenbeck, 2024).

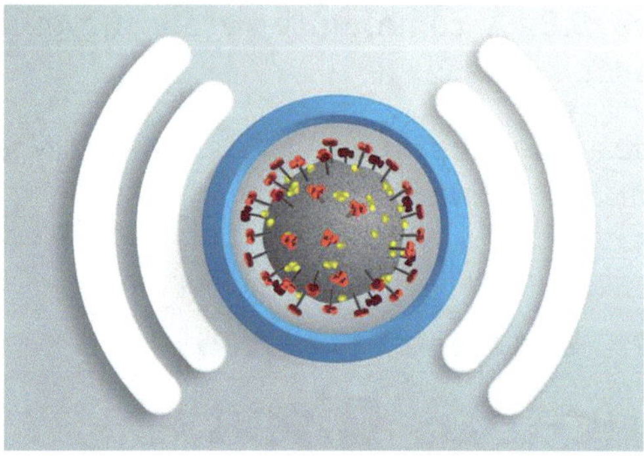

Figure 5.9. The challenges in infectious disease surveillance.

Source: The Hindu. (2021). *Challenges in Infectious Disease Surveillance.*

At times, getting a new or unusual disease before it gets out of hand is like attempting to strike a moving target. An increase in predictive technologies and multi, trigger warnings may just provide that early warning we require. Further there's the operational and tech end, which isn't a picnic either. Digital health has gone ahead in leaps and bounds, but several countries haven't yet figured out how to integrate AI and big data into everyday public health practice. Different tech capacity and data standards just confuse things further when information needs to be shared across borders. And further, many surveillance programs depend on uncertain variables such as political support or unpredictable funding. It typically requires a concerted international effort—one that establishes shared guidelines, improves system compatibility, and accelerates cross-border data transfer, to truly make an impact. The World Health Organization has observed, for example, that being part of a collaborative effort with standard reporting can break down these barriers (Jang et al., 2025). Finally, investing greater resources in smart tech and better governance holds the key to creating surveillance networks that are resilient enough to weather whatever future eruptions may eventuate (Figure 5.9).

5.4.1. Data Collection and Reporting Issues

Prompt collection and accurate reporting of health information is the essence of disease tracking, but issues arise everywhere in the world. Some areas have problems such as overcrowded labs and fragmented digital record systems that slow down and complicate the figures. Lowincome areas—where live data, sharing tools are usually absent—the lack of equipment makes reporting even more inconsistent. CombinationIncorporating disparate forms of inputs, like genetic information and environmental sensors, only exacerbates this problem because it requires sophisticated technologies and trained people. In short, if we do not solve these fundamental barriers, even intelligent AI and cutting, edge analytics cannot truly predict or resist outbreaks, which in most instances disempowers global health initiatives (Anurogo, 2025). Data reporting becomes even more complicated when you realize that the diseases themselves appear in a crazy assortment of times and locales. Anticipating how an outbreak may change requires you to have pipelines that can combine everything from population data to weather hints, but data tends to fall in disparate forms and at irregular frequencies. This patchwork complicates the operation of predictive models to function correctly since missing links in the chain rupture continuous insight. More recent platforms attempt to sew data together and present it in real-time across regions, suggesting how a more standardized method could assist officials in comprehending the built, in uncertainties within predicts (Keshavamurthy et al., 2024). Addressing data collection and reporting problems is not solely a matter of glitzy new technology—smart policies and actual global collaboration are also required. Next-generation frameworks combining genomic knowledge, nano, immunotherapies, and AI promise breaking through traditional surveillance boundaries; yet, their success is contingent on equitable access, particularly in regions most severely affected by outbreaks. Spurring open data habits and collaborations across disciplines could dismantle the info silos now partitioning us. Ultimately, developing flexible and sustainable surveillance systems that consider both speed and accuracy is essential to enhance health security across the globe in the context of dynamic disease threats (Anurogo, 2025).

5.4.2. Political and Economic Barriers

Global health and monitoring infectious disease rely heavily on nations working hand in hand, but politics can really interfere. There is tension and mistrust that creates tension between some nations and prevents them from sharing crucial information about emerging outbreaks, resulting in international response delays and complicating the management of diseases. National pride and sovereignty concerns tend to hold governments back from sharing vital information or from taking in foreign investigations even when openness could alleviate larger health threats. Political instability within nations can distort communication and infrastructure required for early detection, and sometimes leaders simply refuse to declare an outbreak for fear of damaging the economy or sparking a political backlash. Essentially, what is required is a push for more robust diplomatic relations and actual, binding international treaties that prioritize public health over short-term politics (Chu, 2025). Funding is another giant obstacle to effective infectious disease surveillance globally. Resources are too tight in most low and middle-income countries due to competing development priorities. This leads to under, resourced labs, weak data collection and analysis, and insufficiently trained staff to effectively identify and report disease. Economic disparities also ensure that sophisticated tools, such as AI, aren't universally accessible despite the potential for increasing the speed and accuracy with which outbreaks are identified. Under, investment results in haphazard, reactive surveillance instead of proactive, which makes it hard to anticipate outbreaks. Closing this gap requires innovative financing, global assistance, transfers of technology, and capacity development to enable even resource-poor countries to play their rightful role in international disease surveillance (Ibiam et al., 2025). Things only become more complicated when political and economic borders combine. Political choices tend to determine where funds go—frequently money for health facilities and monitoring gets slashed in the interest of immediate economic solutions, particularly when trade or tourism is at risk. Conversely, financial pressures will guide political decisions, rendering it far too easy to trade long-term health security for short-term fiscal relief. Then there is fragmented governance, where conflicting national interests and economic constraints render unifying strategies impracticable. What is essentially required is one that is integrating in nature, recognizing how economics and politics intersect—one that reinforces accountability, equitable sharing of resources, and good, faith communication among actors. In all but a minority of instances, developing robust surveillance systems involves giving space to political sensitivities and economic realities alike (Chu, 2025; Ibiam et al., 2025).

5.4.3. Ethical Considerations in Surveillance Practices

Global health monitoring is racing along at breakneck speed with the help of new technology that combines surprising amounts of innovation and a healthy dose of ethical concerns. Artificial intelligence and machine learning now sift through huge data streams to identify outbreaks even before they're fully grasped, but this speed bump also raises concerns about maintaining personal privacy and data security. Sensitive health information collected from every corner, sometimes without a second thought, could fall into the wrong hands, eroding public confidence in these systems. Biases buried in the algorithmic underbrush could inadvertently strike vulnerable communities disproportionately harder, exacerbating existing health disparities even further. Balancing rapid disease detection with minimal respect for individual rights isn't easy; it's a challenge we need to overcome to ensure fairness and promote global collaboration in times of health crises (Ekundayo, 2024; Ibiam et al., 2025). Transparency and accountability are not buzzwords in this case—they're the foundation of any reasonable health surveillance practice. Once AI begins calculating, it's important to be transparent about what's being done with the data, how it's being handled, and why particular conclusions emerge from the brew. Without some transparency, individuals may begin questioning public health initiatives just when cooperation is most critical. In most instances, ensuring algorithmic processes are transparent helps specialists identify mistakes or unjustified biases before causing harm. A degree of institutional control and actual, hands, on ethical analysis is required to balance these systems with human rights and public health objectives. Gathering together tech gurus, ethicists, and policymakers in an informal sort of roundtable can assist in shaping equitable regulations, even if the process is a little unfocused (Ibiam et al., 2025). Infectious diseases are not bound by national borders, so our moral fences must be equally adaptable, extending across boundaries to include equity and justice. Surveillance systems typically rely on data derived from a combination of various regions and socioeconomic backgrounds, posing difficult questions regarding consent and proper representation. Areas that are resource-poor may not have necessary protections, raising questions about who owns data and who ultimately benefits from it. To add to that, the digital divide can be such that only a few enjoy the full benefit of sophisticated monitoring, further entrenching already present inequalities. Ethical guidelines, then, have to be built on principles of inclusion and fairness to avoid unintentionally reinforcing old inequalities. Building trust means engaging communities in the process, giving due respect to local customs, and setting up data rules that are as equitable as they are practical (Ekundayo, 2024; Ibiam et al., 2025).

5.5. Case Studies of Successful Surveillance

Early warning systems that detect infectious threats operate in unexpected fashions. They combination all kinds of information, such as emergency room chief complaints and centralized public health records—to alert for outbreaks before they spiral out of control. Reviews have documented that when these systems bring together pre, diagnostic information, they can identify a potential pandemic even before widespread spread is seen. At times they operate independently; sometimes they provide a helpful supplement to traditional diagnostic techniques, particularly when data are standardized and rapidly transmitted across borders. Web, based sites, for instance, may allow remote health locations to report information quickly—accelerating responses where resources are limited. In most instances, the integration of multiple streams—from official health records to local staff reports—appears to be more effective than relying on a single source. Near real time monitoring on a daily basis, especially in the case of large events, tends to enable public health officials to respond more quickly, highlighting how important flexible, multisource systems have become for supporting international disease detection (Meckawy et al., 2022). Another illustrative example is the fight against AMR, an increasingly universal global health concern that requires pinpoint tracking to limit its effects. A large, crosscountry study covering 204 nations put more than 4.9 million deaths attributable to resistant bacterial infections in 2019, of which about 1.27 million were directly attributed to AMR. By collecting enormous datasets—from hospital files and microbiological isolates to epidemiological questionnaires—scientists were able to chart patterns of resistance by pathogen and drug combination. This holistic method even uncovered unambiguous geographic disparities, with western sub-Saharan Africa particularly severely affected. Overall, these results emphasize the necessity of strong data collection and surveillance infrastructures to inform targeted infection prevention, antibiotic stewardship programs, and policy decisions, particularly in low, income areas with limited laboratory capacity (Murray et al., 2022). A third example illustrates how predictive statistical modeling can be combined with surveillance data to inform public health responses. Scientists drew on millions of records from a range of sources to predict incidence, death rates, and even disability-adjusted life years attributed to infections such as AMR. This approach not only identifies disease burdens but also indicates which combinations of pathogens and drugs need to be targeted for intervention. Models were rigorously checked—adding in measures of uncertainty so that policymakers could generally balance risks realistically. The flexible, scalable character of these approaches allows them to function in a variety of healthcare environments irrespective of resource availability. In the majority of instances, such sophisticated surveillance and modeling platforms establish a strong base for anticipatory global health responses, and in the long run, increase readiness to meet upcoming infectious threats globally (Murray et al., 2022).

5.5.1. The Ebola Outbreak Response

Outbreaks of infectious diseases tend to reveal the public health system's weak points and its unseen strengths. The 2014 Ebola virus crisis in West Africa, for example, not only revealed serious weaknesses—but also unleashed surprising local and global responses that revolutionized epidemic control. Local communities, such as community leaders, religious groups, and even hospital facility committees, wound up taking a surprisingly central role in preventing the spread of the virus. They undertook activities like disseminating vital information and contact tracing, ensuring that the measures adopted were appropriate for the local culture and gained public confidence. Most often, this type of bottom, up engagement became critical for successful monitoring and the realignment of social behaviors—highlighting that forming alliances with community members is crucial for responding to epidemics (Gilmore et al., 2020). The obvious takeaway here appears to be that integrating community, driven efforts into the broader infectious disease surveillance web really maximizes response times and long-term outcomes. More broadly, the Ebola outbreak put Africa's requirement for a more robust public health infrastructure in sharp relief. Before and even throughout the crisis, the absence of firm national public health institutions frustrated rapid detection and containment—a circumstance that, in most respects, caused most efforts to stall. The crisis, however, hastened the formation of the Africa Centers for Disease Control and Prevention (Africa CDC), which is now the default point for coordination of responses across the continent—marshaling resources, sending epidemiologists, and even facilitating cross-border collaborations. The outbreak reminded everyone that having local capacity to make diagnostics and treatments is important, particularly when relying on external supplies can be perilous during global crises. This drive for self-sufficiency aligns with continuing efforts to build a new public health order in Africa that harmonizes workforce building, regional linkages, and broader resilience (Nkengasong et al., 2020). Further there is the broader socioeconomic effects picture that Ebola highlighted. In addition to its very tangible cost to health, outbreaks such as Ebola can derail economies, push already strained health systems to the limit, and even exacerbate social inequalities. The economic impact in West Africa demonstrated, quite prominently, that such epidemics can halt development plans, particularly in areas already struggling with endemic diseases and weak infrastructure. The response, which combined community outreach with lab networking and emergency operation centers, wasn't merely about addressing the virus immediately; it was a recognition of developing longer-term resilience. In most cases, this experience also served as a nudge for why steady investment in public health education and leadership training is so important to get future responders ready. Strengthening capabilities at local, national, and even continental levels remains a must if we're to manage future outbreaks in our interconnected world (Gilmore et al., 2020; Nkengasong et al., 2020) (Figure 5.10).

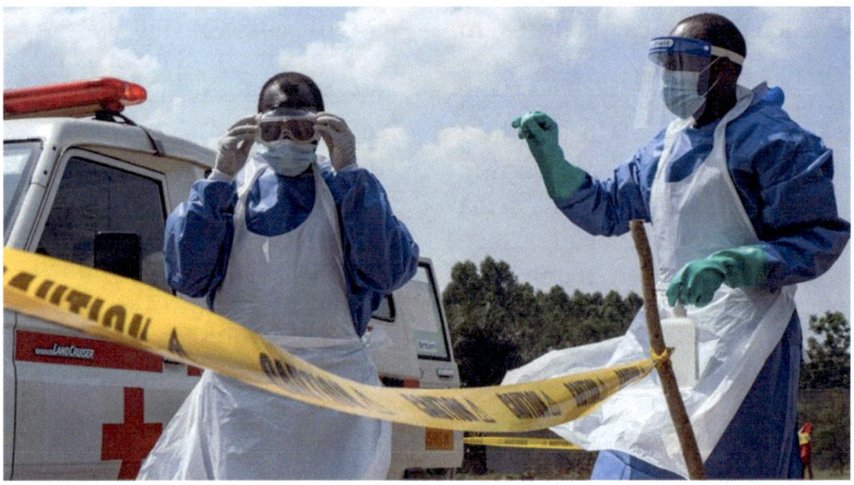

Figure 5.10. The Ebola outbreak response.

Source: International Federation Of Red Cross. (2025). *Uganda Red Cross Ebola Response.*

5.5.2. COVID, 19 Pandemic Tracking

Genomic sequencing turned the tables on COVID, public health personnel were able to detect new variants nearly in real-time as they emerged. Scientists pored over genetic information to track how the virus evolved and spread from host to host, frequently monitoring these developments in real-time. It wasn't merely signaling out the pathogen; the findings enabled them to fine, tune vaccines and modify treatments so they were able to match the virus's twists. In most instances, the entire process reminded us of just how important it is to step up our genomics labs across the globe—where some areas were finding it tough to sequence, detecting new variants became a race against time. Overall, deploying these methods improved not only crisis response urgently but also fueled health systems on a grand scale with a pinch of personalized medicine and acuter drug, response tactics. This advancement typically depicts how technology can be a strong partner for global health security against both existing and emerging infectious threats (Wu et al., 2024). Although COVID occupied our imagination, it did not leave other infections such as syphilis behind, which further complicated disease tracking. Consider Florida, for instance—surveillance data continued to point toward a sustained increase in cases of syphilis even as initial expectations were that pandemic lockdowns would quash other diseases. This increase was not restricted by gender, race, or age; , at-risk populations sometimes found themselves put at even higher risk when healthcare access was disrupted. In the majority of instances, this development shed light on the idea that one-size-fits-all solutions just can't fit all outbreaks (Niu et al., 2024). The repeating patterns in the data truly highlighted the necessity of dynamic, integral monitoring systems that can handle multiple threats simultaneously. The pandemic also accelerated significant changes in how we combination and exchange data, inspiring real, time reporting systems that spanned borders. Health organizations, governments, and researchers - all in coordination - established real, time dashboards, contact tracing applications, and online reporting systems to keep decision-makers informed as everything moved rapidly. Of course, these innovations had their own set of challenges, such as concerns about data fairness, privacy issues, and sometimes too much information without the appropriate analytical facilities. In some instances, satisfying both rapid reporting and responsible use of data was challenging, but COVID's lessons have laid the ground for an open, efficient global health surveillance system (Wu et al., 2024) (Figure 5.11).

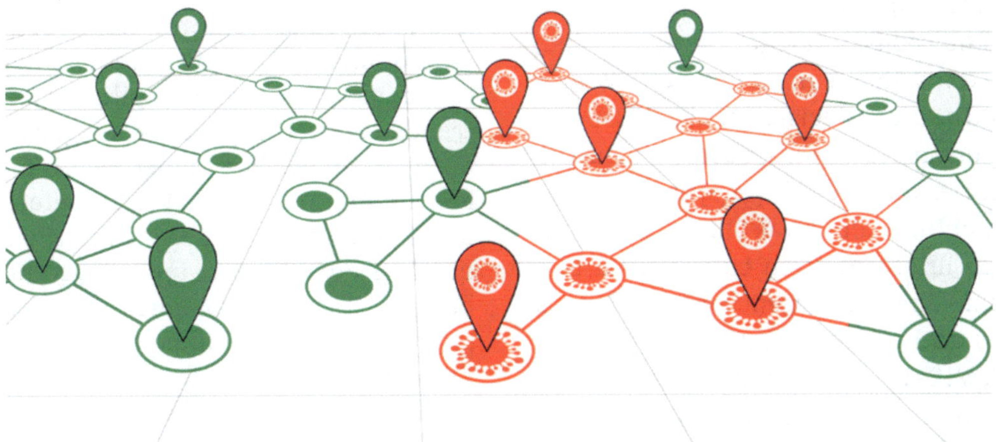

Figure 5.11. COVID, 19 pandemic tracking.

Source: https://www.pnas.org/cms/asset/2ebb3e4a, 201e, 45fb, b425, 2caac4e5bd1b/shutterstock_1752923663ct2.jpg.

5.5.3. Lessons Learned from Past Surveillance Efforts

Global outbreaks have demonstrated in the recent past that we just can't manage to live without efficient disease tracking systems. Consider African swine fever—neglected biosecurity in some areas and a weak early detection really illustrated how chaotic dispersed surveillance is. In the ASF episodes, factors such as sluggish diagnostic tests and inefficient controls on livestock movement contributed to disease dissemination and hurt small producers financially (Uwishema et al., 2021).

At the same time, when COVID, 19 hit, resources got stretched too thin, and routine monitoring for endemic diseases fell by the wayside. All of this generally speaks to the need for several local input, tech upgrades, and cross, field cooperation if we're going to keep infectious threats in check. Early on in the COVID-19 pandemic, fissures in regional coordination and legal authority served as a wake-up call—even with high-tech institutions, European Union member states could not coordinate their reactions and exchange information due to patchy governance and residual sovereignty concerns (Forman et al., 2021).

This lack of coordinated effort not only hindered early detection but also stalled quick response. There were issues with real-time data merging, uneven communication, and time wasted in receiving necessary supplies. To summarize, it's evident that simply possessing tech is not sufficient; you also need mandates that are transparent, robust interagency cooperation, and law systems that can handle quick info exchange and mutual decision-making. One of the most important lessons from these endeavors is the call for a One Health perspective, such that human, animal, and environmental health are viewed as interconnected components of a single system. The convergence of challenges presented by pathogens such as African swine fever and COVID-19 fully highlights the threat of gaps in surveillance (Forman et al., 2021; Uwishema et al., 2021). Viewing public health through a multidisciplinary lens allows to capture outbreaks near the point of origin and opens the door for wider, more successful responses. For example, the EU's shift toward creating a Health Emergency Preparedness and Response Authority hints at a trend toward consolidating control, increasing resources, and expanding mandates for pandemic preparedness. Generally, this history informs us that recurrent investments in the skills of the workforce, data standardization, and global cooperation are critical to developing robust surveillance systems for the threats of today as well as tomorrow.

5.6. Future Directions in Global Health Surveillance

The speed of technology's advancement has truly expanded the way we monitor the environment. Remote sensing, for example, captures enormous quantities of real-time information and detects minor changes that can be linked to disease epidemics or insect-borne diseases. We now monitor changes in climate, forest cover, air quality and even unexpected water-related catastrophes; all of these can be used as advance warnings for nature-influenced health threats. CombinationIncorporating the environmental specifics with health facts allows responses to be more agile—racing in when trends suggest impending danger from climate changes or habitat adjustments. Furthermore, identifying areas at risk well before outbreaks occur allows us to design interventions more quickly. For the most part, as these devices become increasingly fanciful and widespread, global health surveillance will rely more and more on such multi-layered surveillance and predictive models (Novikarany, 2025). Some of the lessons of blood safety and transfusion medicine reinforce some key lessons for future health monitoring, as well. There has been a shift away from waiting for things to go wrong and instead, getting in front of problems with active screening for infections passed through transfusions. Consider the West Nile virus incident; within almost the same time frame when the outbreak was identified, nucleic acid testing was implemented, indicating how cooperation among government agencies and private industry can successfully reduce risks of transmission. Of course, limitations such as tight budgets and complicated problems, consider *Babesia microti*, reiterate the difficulty of juggling costs, regional variation, and the pressures of test development. In most general terms, these challenges reiterate why our surveillance mechanisms must remain adaptable and agile, continually weighing efficiency, cost savings, and accessibility around the globe (Bloch et al., 2016). Gazing into the future, combining innovative technology with thorough cost-benefit analyses is destined to define global health surveillance and monitoring.

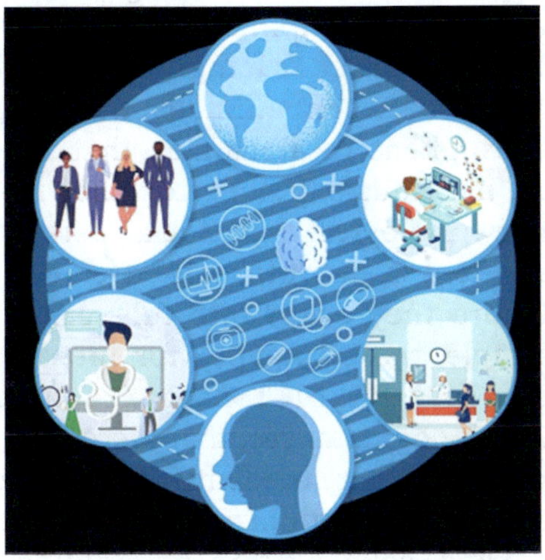

Figure 5.12. Global healthcare sector.

Source: Deloitte. (2022). *Global Healthcare Outlook.*

The trend towards technologies like pathogen inactivation and multiplex nucleic acid tests holds a type of broad-based protection against multiple infectious agents simultaneously—even if, occasionally, technical constraints and astronomically high prices cause the ride to be rough. Indeed, varying risk profiles between regions means we have to prioritize our resources judiciously, and having a strong hemovigilance framework would go a long way. Partnering between sectors and even incorporating mathematical modeling into the equation can truly make us better prepared for upcoming threats. In most instances, this integrated approach allows health systems to address both known and novel infections without going over budget. Finally, combining technological advancement with prudent economic planning and a culture of cooperation is the solution to establishing robust, responsive disease-surveillance systems worldwide (Bloch et al., 2016) (Figure 5.12).

5.6.1. Innovations in Technology and Data Sharing

Digital health technology has truly revolutionized the game of keeping an eye out for infectious disease. Apps, wearables, and online health records now provide us with nearly instant reporting on disease trends, alerting officials to outbreaks much earlier than ever before. In most instances, these tools enable remote care that reduces the number of risky in-person encounters, a feature that proved so invaluable during COVID-19. They also assist in closing the gap between health workers and the community, and spreading urgent news as well as quieting rumors more easily. Nonetheless, ensuring that our data remain secure and private is an incessant problem that cannot be glossed over if public trust is to persist. In general, combinationincorporating these digital tools into our pandemic response demonstrates that calm hands from both government and private stakeholders are required (Ezenwaji et al., 2024). The combination of human, animal, and environmental health sort of illustrates why data-sharing systems to support a One Health approach are necessary. These breakouts tend to emerge at the intersection of these worlds—zoonotic disease being a perfect example where observing animals and people together in real-time is absolutely essential. When veterinary, public health, and environmental surveillance individuals collaborate, it enhances the early warning systems and general perception of disease patterns. By and large, using these sources together not only aids in catching outbreaks sooner, but it also encourages cross-disciplinary inquiry to understand the numerous drivers of new infections. Ultimately, seamless data sharing between these fields is entirely at the heart of addressing global health challenges in a manner that honors the complex, interconnected world we inhabit. Tech advances continue to extend the envelope with advanced analytics, genomic surveillance, and even remote sensing—all of which provide added levels of detail to our knowledge of epidemics. Genomic sequencing, for example, can rapidly identify new variants of pathogens, informing more narrowly targeted public health action. In parallel, machine learning algorithms sort through vast amounts of data to identify trends and even predict paths of epidemics—albeit not always accurately. When such tools converge in adaptable digital platforms, they facilitate response coordination and resource deployment both domestically and internationally. Despite enduring challenges, embracing tech sharing and enhancing data management means that less-resourced locations can catch up as well. To summarize, the integration of these advanced methods with sustainable measures and community participation is a possible method to enhance infectious disease surveillance and resilience against future outbreaks (Ezenwaji et al., 2024).

5.6.2. Strengthening Global Health Partnerships

Disease detection worldwide depends on more than cutting-edge technology—it relies on effective, sometimes surprisingly haphazard, global collaborations that enable diverse groups to exchange information and resources quickly. Governments, international organizations, and research centers combine their knowledge in configurations that aren't always clear but are still effective in identifying emerging threats promptly. Scientists from different backgrounds combine forces—frequently more than once—in endeavors that attack pathogens without regard to national borders. Consider zoonotic viruses, for instance; staying ahead of them entails individuals from human health, animal husbandry, and even environmental agencies needing to work closely together. Spending on such kinds of models not only enhances local establishments, making warning systems perceptive and responsive to changing patterns of health but also mitigates risks from bioterrorism and agricultural problems, compelling nations to work towards cooperative, sometimes patchy, policies. The One Health approach is an unambiguous demonstration of the potential of combining skills from several different disciplines in revolutionizing infectious disease tracing. Essentially, it plugs gaps between animals, humans, and the environment in a manner that tends to astonish individuals, pulling together medical, veterinary, ecological, and social perspectives to the extent that outbreaks are identified even before they erupt into full-scale crises. For example, the US Agency for International Development's PREDICT program illustrates, in a majority of instances, that increasing local lab and field capacity to identify new pathogens at source can revolutionize the game. Through data sharing, collaboration on trainings, and coordination of efforts, it changes the paradigm from reacting to problems to attempting to prevent them from arising in the first place. Furthermore, the consistent stream of studies and collective knowledge that result from such endeavors gradually enhance our understanding of how viruses evolve and transmit—an understanding that eventually influences public health policies around the globe (Anthony et al., 2016). Maintaining and developing these international partnerships isn't a once-and-done transaction—it requires an extended, at times lopsided, commitment to equitable resource distribution, local capacity development, and adherence to open, if sometimes inconsistent, lines of communication among stakeholders. Aware that certain areas, particularly low- and middle-income nations, continue to struggle with outdated surveillance systems, global action in most cases must center on assisting these under-funded areas so that strong health systems can develop for early detection and containment. Mechanisms such as multilateral financing and collaborative governance serve to bind these efforts together so that everyone is collectively responsible for health security. Trust and data-sharing arrangements, while sometimes stymied by political or financial interests, still are necessary. By incorporating inclusivity and interdependence into the very fabric of these networks, we can more effectively make infectious disease surveillance—hopefully reducing the burden of pandemics and rendering our globalized world a safer place (Anthony et al., 2016).

5.6.3. Preparing for Emerging Infectious Diseases

In the early days of COVID-19, the crisis put our vulnerabilities in combating infectious diseases in harsh relief. It turned out that having resources and a built environment wasn't sufficient—what we required was astute leadership, effective teamwork, and adaptive decision-making at the moment it mattered. A good example is the way the EU's fragmented response—tied up by legal constraints and a division of power between continental institutions and national governments— ended up holding back vital measures and triggering a rush for much-needed equipment. This haphazard response made a bad situation worse. In a majority of instances, if we are really looking to prepare for emerging outbreaks, we need to rethink our functions, enhance cross-border collaborations, and establish governance layers that are capable of passing information rapidly, allocating resources equitably, and coordinating collectively (Forman et al., 2021). Monitoring systems for detection and diagnostic capabilities form a basis for the fight against emerging disease threats. When such pathogens as SARS-CoV-2 and influenza viruses appear with matching symptoms and spread in volatile patterns, increasing our guard against respiratory diseases is merely essential. Robust, one-stop tracking systems enable rapid detection, continuous monitoring, and more effective public health actions. Emerging technology tools such as telemedicine and digital contact tracing can be combined with traditional approaches to detect trends in real-time and expand our reach. And yes, distributing vaccines and antivirals to guard both vulnerable individuals and frontline workers is a significant factor in domesticating the effects when these two diseases co-occur. Overall, moving from reactive crisis solutions to consistent, long-term strategies anchored on robust surveillance is necessary to make the globe secure (Chotpitayasunondh et al., 2020). Our COVID-19 experience has demonstrated that there are specialized agencies that are crucial in spearheading preparedness. The establishment of organizations such as the European Health Emergency Preparedness and Response Authority (HERA) is a step towards centralized organization, one whose purpose is to scan upcoming threats, provide funding for significant research, and keep medical supplies stashed away in case of emergencies. Yet these organizations have their own challenges—legal entanglements, budget constraints, and jurisdictional battles—as they attempt to integrate with existing agencies like the European Centre for Disease Prevention and Control. Strengthening their mandate to incorporate improved monitoring capacity and honed workforce expertise can help them to be more agile when disaster strikes. A One Health strategy, acknowledging the intimate relationships among human, animal, and environmental health—is equally crucial to staying ahead of threats. Because epidemics disregard borders, being staunchly involved in worldwide activities such as the suggested Pandemic Treaty and equitable vaccine distribution isn't nice to have, it's a must (Forman et al., 2021) (Figure 5.13).

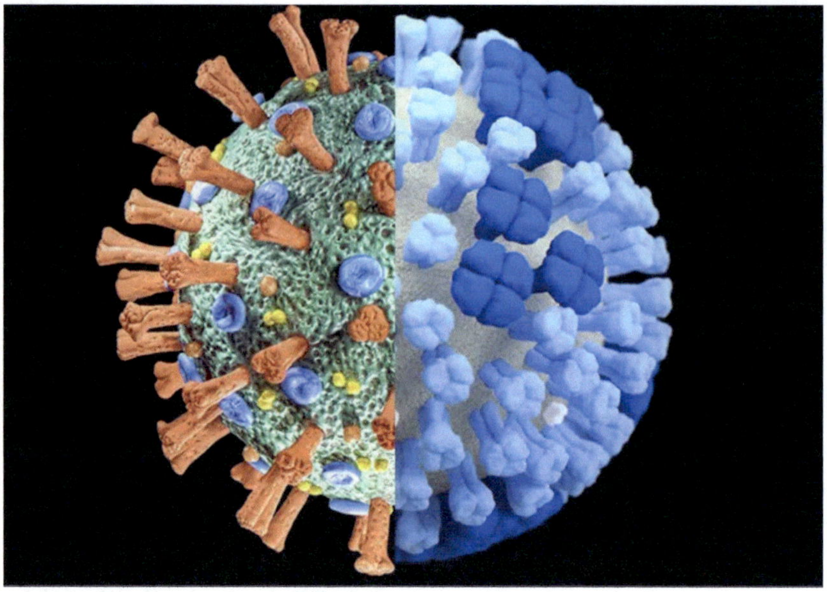

Figure 5.13. Preparing for emerging infectious diseases.

Source: https://assets.medpagetoday.net/media/images/88xxx/88684.jpg.

CLOSER LOOK

CHALLENGES IN SURVEILLANCE ACROSS LOW-RESOURCE SETTINGS

Disease surveillance is critical for early detection, monitoring, and response to outbreaks. However, in low-resource settings, several challenges hinder the establishment of strong and reliable surveillance systems, making populations more vulnerable to epidemics and re-emerging infections.

A primary challenge is the lack of infrastructure. Many regions face shortages of diagnostic laboratories, reliable internet access, and standardized data collection systems. Without these, identifying cases and tracking disease spread becomes slow and inaccurate. Furthermore, limited financial resources constrain investments in modern surveillance technologies, staff training, and sustained operations.

Human resource limitations are another major barrier. Skilled epidemiologists, laboratory technicians, and public health officers are often scarce in underserved areas. Even when trained personnel are available, retention is difficult due to low salaries and high workloads. This weakens the capacity to detect and respond quickly to health threats.

In addition, fragmented health information systems and inconsistent reporting practices lead to poor data quality. Many facilities rely on paper-based reporting, which delays information sharing and increases the risk of underreporting. Political instability, conflict, and poor governance in some regions further disrupt surveillance networks.

Cultural and social factors also play a role. Stigma, mistrust, and lack of community engagement can discourage individuals from reporting symptoms or seeking care, leading to hidden outbreaks. For example, during the Ebola crisis in West Africa, misinformation and fear severely hampered surveillance efforts.

Finally, global health inequities contribute to surveillance challenges. Wealthier nations often have advanced monitoring systems, while poorer regions depend heavily on external funding, creating vulnerabilities when donor priorities shift.

Addressing these challenges requires long-term investment in health infrastructure, workforce development, digital tools, and strong community participation. Strengthening surveillance in low-resource settings is not only vital for local populations but also for global health security.

SUMMARY

Strong infectious disease surveillance forms the center of our new world health landscape. Information from every type of source is combinationed together to identify trends and trigger timely responses, reducing disease and death. Consider cardiovascular disease, for example, it illustrates how infectious and noncommunicable diseases can combination and exacerbate public health, particularly in low- and middle-income areas where tracking systems sometimes lag behind (Roth et al., 2020). Early outbreak detection, intelligent resource allocation and low-cost, targeted health policies all rely on robust surveillance. Global objectives such as Sustainable Development Goal three can only be achieved if we continue to keep prevention and control at the center of attention. Precise, finely tuned epidemiological models are still the foundation of pandemic preparedness and disease surveillance. However, relying on a single model is dangerous, especially if regional details, time-series data glitches or reporting biases fall through the cracks (Jewell et al., 2020). The combination predictions we experienced during COVID-19, for instance, remind us to interpret model results with care. In general, combining several different modeling approaches and embracing their imprecision makes our systems more resilient. In the majority of cases, sharing these imprecisions with decision-makers, sometimes in a less-than-perfect form—guarantees plans to rely on genuine, context-dependent evidence instead of overly confident projections. Improving global health is a matter of adopting a multi-faceted approach that combines robust scientific approaches with equitable health policies. Surveillance data must be coupled with continued investment in the healthcare infrastructure, improved workforce training and clearer public health messaging so that responses play in multiple settings. Efforts truly must target areas with increasing disease burden where surveillance is constrained (Roth et al., 2020). Ethical sharing of data and open practices construct the sort of global trust required in times of health crises. By fostering an adaptive and well-supported surveillance system—with sophisticated analysis of data and well-balanced modeling—the world can more accurately predict and manage disease threats. Overall, this combined strategy is central to safeguarding public health and setting the stage for sustainable, long-term control of infectious diseases.

Decades have passed and infectious disease outbreaks seem to emerge more often and in unexpected, complex ways. Globalization, the rush of urban life, and shifts in climate all play a part, making it clear that keeping an eye out for new pathogens is a must if we're to ease their global impact. Surveillance installations that capture and verify epidemiologic data as it comes in are central to it—they inform the way public health reacts and fine-tune prevention strategies. Information collected from global epidemic watchers can identify abrupt hotspots and outline transmission routes, enabling health authorities to redirect resources and intervene fast. The increased threat posed by disease spread via vectors or directly transmitted from animals, for example, truly highlights the necessity for incessant refinement of our systems for surveillance to improve general global health performance (Sun et al., 2025). Public health preparedness is a second pillar in dealing with such infection risks across the globe. Current public health emergencies have brought into sharp relief severe fissures in current systems, and in the majority of instances, they indicate that strategies are needed that integrate real-time monitoring with transparent, practical plans. One can think of it as creating a clever, educated workforce, having labs that are capable of rapid identification of pathogens, and establishing networks that are early-warning beacons. All of these must also address day-to-day challenges, such as coordinating medical supply chains and establishing communication channels that can effectively disseminate news to decision-makers and the public alike—no matter if sometimes the details are a little complex. Takeaways from a combination of national and international readiness plans highlight the need for continued investments in these areas to remain resilient to future outbreaks (Saif-Ur-Rahman et al., 2025). When you put it all together, a multi-layered response is what's most evident: one that combines early threat detection, transparent but flexible communication, robust healthcare capacity, and dynamic policy architecture. Surveillance doesn't spit out data; it provides actual insights that support evidence-based decision-making and enable fast responses. Ongoing adjustment of these systems, maintaining stable funding, and coordinating with the international community can significantly enhance our capacity to manage high-impact diseases. Finally, strengthening global health security is really about a collaborative effort that fills the gap between detection, readiness, and response-even if that sometimes means that the process looks a little uneven-and makes sure that our health systems are still flexible and robust across the globe (Saif-Ur-Rahman et al., 2025; Sun et al., 2025).

REFERENCES

1. Aarestrup, F. M., Ahuja, S., Aidara-Kane, A., Zumla, A., Allegranzi, B., et al. (2016). Exploring the evidence base for national and regional policy interventions to combat resistance. *The Lancet, 387*(10015), 285–295. https://doi.org/10.1016/S0140-6736(15)00520-6.
2. Achieng, M., & Ogundaini, O. (2024). Big data analytics for integrated infectious disease surveillance in sub-Saharan Africa. *SA Journal of Information Management, 26(1), a1668.* https://www.semanticscholar.org/paper/cc2924577ee23919891f4de2899f44689b917931 (accessed on 7 May 2025).
3. Anthony, S. J., Ekiri, A. B., Gilardi, K. V. K., Goldstein, T., et al. (2017). One Health proof of concept: Bringing a transdisciplinary approach to surveillance for zoonotic viruses at the human–wild animal interface. *Preventive Veterinary Medicine, 137*(Part B), 112–118. https://doi.org/10.1016/j.prevetmed.2016.11.023 (accessed on 7 May 2025).
4. Anurogo, D. (2025). Next-gen global health 6.0: Integrative genomics, nano-immunotherapies, and AI for infectious and chronic disease convergence. *International Journal of Health and Medicine.* https://www.semanticscholar.org/paper/c90bd1c7266bdf43344b615ce022812acfc7bb57 (accessed on 7 May 2025).
5. Bergquist, R., Tanner, M., Utzinger, J., Yap, M., et al. (2016). Surveillance and response systems for elimination of tropical diseases: Summary of a thematic series in *Infectious Diseases of Poverty, 5*, 49. https://core.ac.uk/download/46605195.pdf.
6. Bloch, E., Simon, M., & Shaz, B. (2016). Emerging infections and blood safety in the 21st century. *Annals of Internal Medicine, 165*, 57–58. https://www.semanticscholar.org/paper/0f017b5ee18a78941b7a0bdfba9028d84d3bf4a1 (accessed on 7 May 2025).
7. Bwanbale, G. D. (2024). Global health security: Preparing for future pandemics. *Newport International Journal of Research in Medical Sciences, 5*(3), 42–45. https://www.semanticscholar.org/paper/c42766c88376912bc7ef26a1cf0723981b5d811c (accessed on 7 May 2025).
8. Chotpitayasunondh, T., Kølsen Fischer, T., Héraud, J. M., Hurt, A. C., Monto, A. S., Osterhaus, A. D. M. E., Shu, Y., et al. (2020). Influenza and COVID-19: What does co-existence mean? *Influenza and Other Respiratory Viruses, 15*(4), 407–412. https://doi.org/10.1111/irv.12824.
9. Chu, C. (2025). Global health security in the post-COVID-19 era: Threats, preparation, and response. *Osong Public Health and Research Perspectives.* https://www.semanticscholar.org/paper/0aa56f83548df17382b86f2be67d1eb9c62ac163 (accessed on 7 May 2025).
10. Chyba, C. F. (1998). Biological terrorism, emerging diseases, and national security. https://core.ac.uk/download/71349580.pdf (accessed on 7 May 2025).
11. Ekirapa, A., Matthys, B., Zinsstag, J., Crump, L., Yatich, N., & Ettarh, R. (2011). *Disease Surveillance Networks Initiative Africa: Final Evaluation.* https://core.ac.uk/download/86445038.pdf (accessed on 7 May 2025).
12. Ekundayo, F. (2024). Using machine learning to predict disease outbreaks and enhance public health surveillance. *World Journal of Advanced Research and Reviews, 24*(3), 794–811. https://www.semanticscholar.org/paper/96385980e95621272d83ac2303d1d073daaf17ff (accessed on 7 May 2025).
13. Ezenwaji, C., Alum, E., & Ugwu, O. P. C. (2024). The role of digital health in pandemic preparedness and response: Securing global health? *Global Health Action, 17*(1), 2419694.

https://www.semanticscholar.org/paper/b41a7012f6135a79e3b0294d01796a26100f12f1 (accessed on 7 May 2025).

14. Florentino, P., Bertoldo Junior, J., Barbosa, G. C. G., Cerqueira-Silva, T., Oliveira, V. A., Garcia, M. H. de O., Penna, G. O., et al. (2024). Impact of primary health care data quality on infectious disease surveillance in Brazil: Case study. *JMIR Public Health and Surveillance, 11, e67050.* https://www.semanticscholar.org/paper/1b80ead4b59baa72516d87b233a3f5d535fe06bc (accessed on 7 May 2025).

15. Forman, R., & Mossialos, E. (2021). The EU response to COVID-19: From reactive policies to strategic decision-making. *JCMS Journal of Common Market Studies, 59*(1), 56–68. https://doi.org/10.1111/jcms.13259.

16. Gamon, M. (2013). *Multidrug-resistant Tuberculosis in India: Solving A Problem by Reconstructing the Public Health Infrastructure* (Ronald E. McNair Scholars Program 2013, Book 12). https://core.ac.uk/download/67755957.pdf (accessed on 7 May 2025).

17. Gilmore, B., Ndejjo, R., Tchetchia, A., de Claro, V., Mago, E., Diallo, A., Lopes, C. A., et al. (2020). Community engagement for COVID-19 prevention and control: A rapid evidence synthesis. *BMJ Global Health, 5,* e003188. https://doi.org/10.1136/bmjgh-2020-003188.

18. Hale, T., Angrist, N., Goldszmidt, R., Kira, B., Petherick, A., Phillips, T., Webster, S., et al. (2021). A global panel database of pandemic policies (Oxford COVID-19 Government Response Tracker). *Nature Human Behavior, 5*(5), 529–538. https://doi.org/10.1038/s41562-021-01079-8.

19. Ibiam, V. A., Omale, L. E., & Taiwo, O. (2025). The role of artificial intelligence models in clinical decision support for infectious disease diagnosis and personalized treatment planning. *International Journal of Science and Research Archive.* https://www.semanticscholar.org/paper/2eb92ff69739febe03ab53228c14952fb2b7333f (accessed on 7 May 2025).

20. Jang, Y., Lee, H., & Park, H. (2025). Surveillance system for infectious disease prevention and management: Direction of Korea's infectious disease surveillance system. *Journal of Korean Medical Science, 40(8), e108.* https://www.semanticscholar.org/paper/a006fac0322c540deea32e8f419f63af9343297e (accessed on 7 May 2025).

21. Jewell, N. P., Lewnard, J. A., & Jewell, B. L. (2020). Caution warranted: Using the Institute for Health Metrics and Evaluation model for predicting the course of the COVID-19 pandemic. *Annals of Internal Medicine, 173*(3), 226, 227. https://doi.org/10.7326/m20-1565.

22. Keshavamurthy, R., Pazdernik, K. T., Ham, C., Dixon, S., Erwin, S., Charles, L. E., et al. (2024). Meeting global health needs via infectious disease predicting: Development of a reliable data-driven framework. *JMIR Public Health and Surveillance, 11, e59971.* https://www.semanticscholar.org/paper/f62f52e960601f6e9d97f0a894523576d45853b9 (accessed on 7 May 2025).

23. Kimball, A. M., Gugerty, M. K., Abernethy, N., & Curran, S. (2011). *Disease Surveillance Networks Initiative Global: Final Evaluation.* https://core.ac.uk/download/86445037.pdf (accessed on 7 May 2025).

24. Lewnard, J. A., & Reingold, A. L. (2019). Emerging challenges and opportunities in infectious disease epidemiology. *American Journal of Epidemiology, 188*(5), 873–882. https://doi.org/10.1093/aje/kwy264.

25. Lu, F. (2024). Biological threats to global malaria elimination I: Antimalarial drug resistance.

Zhongguo Xue Xi Chong Bing Fang Zhi Za Zhi (Chinese Journal of Schistosomiasis Control), 36(3), 233–238. https://www.semanticscholar.org/paper/54fc600e61be9a1c5885082ec2fa680d2b0495ae (accessed on 7 May 2025).

26. MacFarlane, A., Sá, R., & Silva, C. (2024). International Health Regulations–Role on disease control and global challenges. *The European Journal of Public Health, 34*. https://www.semanticscholar.org/paper/e467673f0d25f1029463a3807c9ac7c2635d76fa (accessed on 7 May 2025).
27. Meckawy, R., Stuckler, D., Mehta, A., AL-Ahdal, T. M. A., & Doebbeling, B. N. (2022). Effectiveness of early warning systems in the detection of infectious disease outbreaks: A systematic review. *BMC Public Health, 22*. https://doi.org/10.1186/s12889-022-14625-4.
28. Niu, E., Sareli, R., Eckardt, P. A., Sareli, C., & Niu, J. (2024). Disparities in syphilis trends and the impact of the COVID-19 pandemic: A join point analysis of Florida surveillance data (2013–2022). *Cureus, 16*(9), e69934. https://www.semanticscholar.org/paper/cec229f8db3bba17e025498e3d345cf9fdcd9730 (accessed on 7 May 2025).
29. Nkengasong, J. N., & Tessema, S. K. (2020). Africa needs a new public health order to tackle infectious disease threats. *Cell, 183*(2), 296–300. https://doi.org/10.1016/j.cell.2020.09.041.
30. Novikarany, R. (2025). Benefits of remote sensing for environmental monitoring. *International Journal of Integrative Sciences, 4(2)*. https://www.semanticscholar.org/paper/df5364f84b53f8a8bafbd8b9dccd48a9de2d0b6f (accessed on 7 May 2025).
31. Rifkin, S. B., Fort, M. P., Patcharanarumol, W., & Tangcharoensathien, V. (2021). Primary healthcare in the time of COVID-19: Breaking the silos of healthcare provision. *BMJ Global Health, 6*, e007721. https://doi.org/10.1136/bmjgh-2021-007721.
32. Roth, G. A., Mensah, G. A., Johnson, C. O., Addolorato, G., Ammirati, E., Baddour, L. M., Barengo, N. C., et al. (2020). Global burden of cardiovascular diseases and risk factors, 1990–2019. *Journal of the American College of Cardiology, 76*, 2982–3021. https://doi.org/10.1016/j.jacc.2020.11.010.
33. Saif-Ur-Rahman, K., Burke, N., Murphy, L., Parlour, R., Boland, M., Taneri, P., Reynolds, B., et al. (2025). Synthesizing public health preparedness mechanisms for high-impact infectious disease threats: A jurisdictional scan. *Journal of Evidence-based Medicine, 18*, Article 6228. https://www.semanticscholar.org/paper/6228f550ef1f20352b717108584183a36f2d18fb (accessed on 7 May 2025).
34. Singh, S., Sharma, P., Pal, N., Sarma, D., Tiwari, R., & Kumar, M. (2024). Holistic One Health surveillance framework: Synergizing environmental, animal, and human determinants for enhanced infectious disease management. *ACS Infectious Diseases, 10(3), 808–826*. https://www.semanticscholar.org/paper/6b9453e0c0a1c5682036d299f62a23f72ac170e8 (accessed on 7 May 2025).
35. Sun, Y., Liu, D., Wu, Y., Li, G., Luo, Y., Xiang, Q., Wu, Y., et al. (2025). Annual summary of global infectious diseases in 2024. *Zoonoses*. https://www.semanticscholar.org/paper/97089b35ecaa66b5d89ce979915311312bcb13d7 (accessed on 7 May 2025).
36. Uwishema, O., Chalhoub, E., Zahabioun, A., David, S., Khoury, C., AlSaraireh, T. H., Bekele, B. K., et al. (2021). The rising incidence of African swine fever during the COVID-19 pandemic in Africa: Efforts, challenges, and recommendations. *The International Journal of Health Planning and Management, 37*(3), 561–567. https://doi.org/10.1002/hpm.3357.

37. V'kovski, P., Kratzel, A., Steiner, S., Stalder, H., & Thiel, V. (2020). Coronavirus biology and replication: Implications for SARS-CoV-2. *Nature Reviews Microbiology, 19*(3), 155–170. https://doi.org/10.1038/s41579-020-00468-6.

38. van Dalen, P. (1999). Outbreaks of disease: Current European reporting. In *Maximizing the Security and Development Benefits from the Biological and Toxin Weapons Convention* (pp. 97–119).

39. Warren, A., Budd, L., & Bell, M. (2010). Surveillance networks and spaces of governance: Technological openness and international cooperation during the 2009 H1N1 pandemic. *AAG 2010, Annual Meeting of the Association of American Geographers*, Washington, DC. https://core.ac.uk/download/288387493.pdf (accessed on 7 May 2025).

40. Wu, G., & Wan, T. (2024). Leveraging genomic data for infectious disease surveillance and personalized medicine: Advances in public health genomics and COVID-19 pathway analysis. *Theoretical and Natural Science*. https://www.semanticscholar.org/paper/8c563f39f50265e137cd39af6b35e7065ea39dbb (accessed on 7 May 2025).

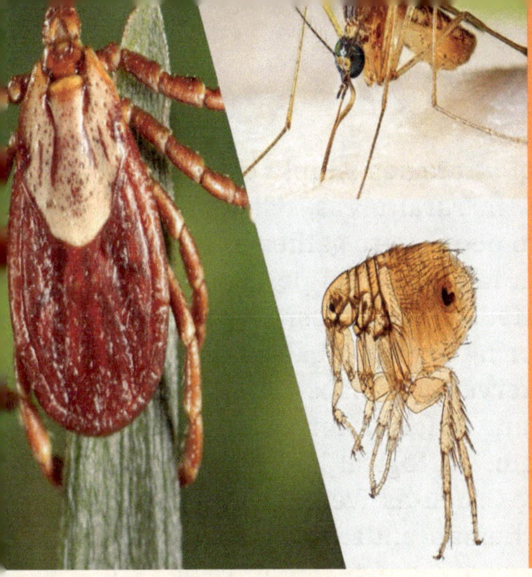

Chapter 6

ZOONOTIC AND VECTOR-BORNE DISEASES

Contents

Introduction

New infections are increasing, and this development destabilizes public health on a variety of levels. We observe that most of these diseases leap from animals or are borne on vectors, and they often result from an unclear interdependence of biological, environmental, and social forces. Researchers recently have been playing around with ecological niche modeling—an instrument that essentially examines where the hosts, the vectors, even local factors co-occur—to attempt to predict where epidemics will break out. It combines things like climate, geography, host travels, and even portions of human activity into something of a danger map. Most often, achieving the right balance in this combination is crucial if we hope to improve the prediction and mitigation of the effects of zoonotic or vector-borne disease (Lawrence et al., 2023). Let us consider the case of Plasmodium knowlesi malaria. Its history is a demonstration of just how well-complex the connections are between pathogen, insect, animal reservoir, and human population. It's apparent that disease control strategies simply can't adhere to rigid biomedical models; they must incorporate local contexts. In rural areas, where the risk typically is greater, methods of inquiry that include simply talking to people—to gather information through focus groups, interviews, or even pictorial narratives—can tap into local perceptions and daily realities that contribute to how these diseases are transmitted. These grassroots methods, rough around the edges though a few may be, are generally empowering to individuals and facilitate the development of more sustainable, more culturally attuned intervention plans (Naserrudin et al., 2022). Determining the reasons that these diseases occur so many different forms isn't an easy thing. It does require an interdisciplinary approach—a synthesis of ecological know-how, social observations, and old-fashioned epidemiology. While natural forces such as weather and terrain create some regions predisposed to vectors and reservoir hosts, human endeavors such as land use patterns and mobility trends put another spin on the exposure dynamics. Some reviews of the available studies tend to broadly indicate that social factors, while immensely impactful, tend to be overlooked in the models. Also, many of the tools that are used to predict outbreaks bypass tight testing and uncertainty tests—things, I suppose, that are occasionally neglected. In general, advancing in this field means we have to thread together disparate sources of data with a splash of methodological discipline, so that our predicts can halt outbreaks in their tracks (Lawrence et al., 2023).

Definition of Zoonotic Diseases

Humans and animals have a long, complex history together that determines how infections insidiously find their way into our lives. Through time, viruses, bacteria, parasites, and fungi creep their way from animal hosts into humans – zoonotic diseases, we call them. Our altering landscapes, driven by changing land use and growing human developments, disrupt the natural order and provide these bacteria with an opportunity to leap species. This is more than a clear scientific tidbit; it indicates that as wildlife habitats diminish, new possibilities of outbreaks and even pandemics begin to arise, a pattern seen in different studies (Plowright et al., 2021). Occasionally, the intersection between nature and human life merely ends up inviting these infections. Meanwhile, consider our daily interactions with animals. Dogs and cats as pets, initially viewed largely in terms of functionality, have today become bona fide companions. They sleep with people, are allowed to lick faces or even open sores – all behaviors that, overall, set the stage for a little bit more pathogen transmission. It is strange to say, but these more intimate connections, casually repeated over the years, outweigh the zoonotic risks. In a sense, our life choices are only making things more complicated, hence the One Health strategy – one that accounts for people, animals, and their environment simultaneously – keeps rearing its head in interactions (Overgaauw et al., 2020). But zoonotic diseases are not just about microbes changing hosts; they illustrate a larger narrative of how our behavior disrupts nature's balance. Urbanization, deforestation, and even fluctuations in wildlife populations all cooperate in a chain reaction: a reservoir host bears the pathogen, it's shed into the environment, overflows into humans, further cycles around people. It's understanding this process that is central to creating policies that preserve what some would term "landscape immunity" – those natural buffers that impede the transmission of infection. In all other instances, knowledge of this cascade of events is crucial for public health interventions for reducing the threat of emerging diseases (Plowright et al., 2021) (Figure 6.1).

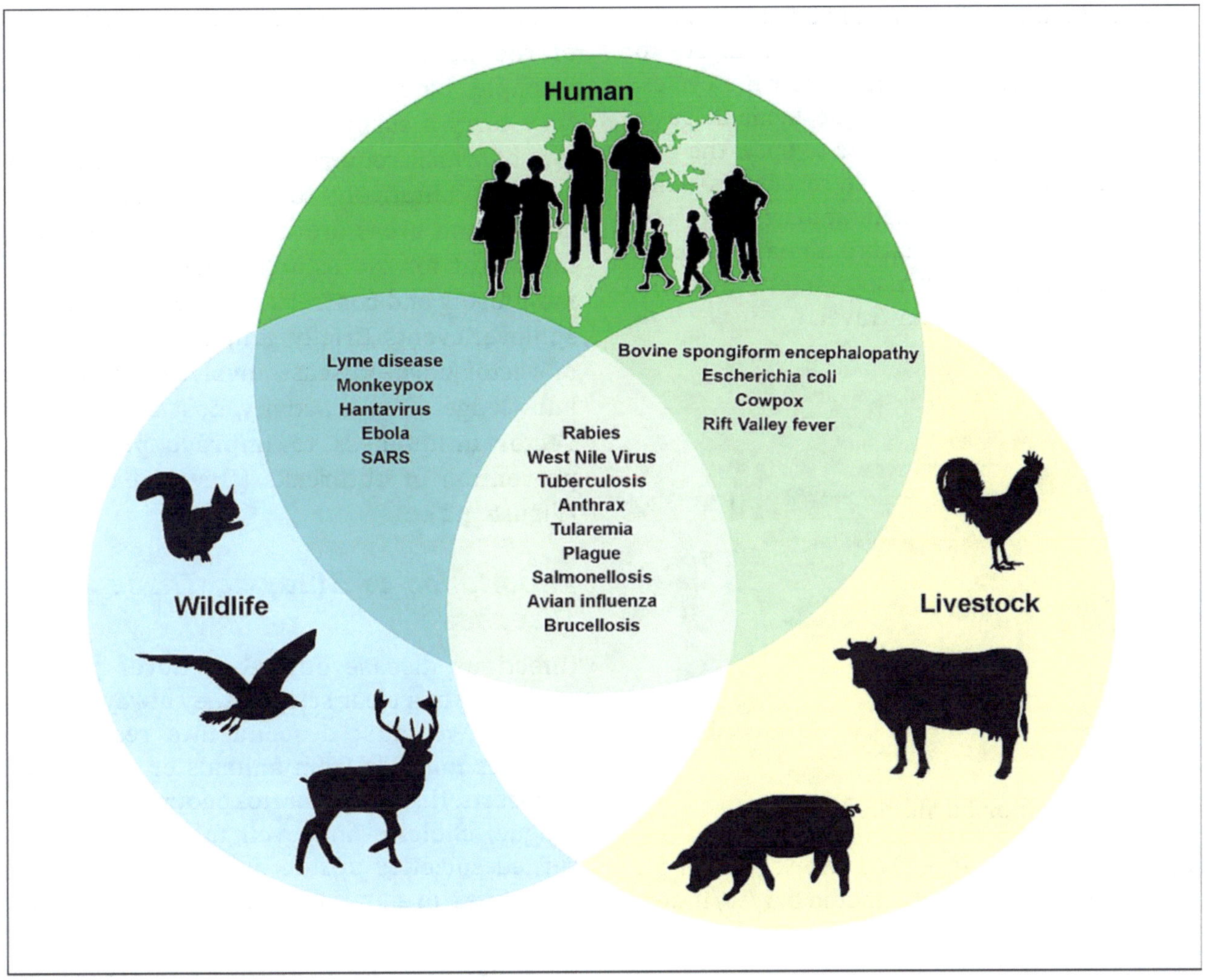

Figure 6.1. Understanding zoonotic diseases.

Source: By U.S. Government Accountability Office from Washington, DC, United States - Figure 3: Examples of Zoonotic Diseases and Their Affected Populations, Public Domain, https://commons.wikimedia.org/w/index.php?curid=65272231

Definition of Vector-borne Diseases

Animals, humans, and their habitats combine in a manner that makes it difficult for bacteria to travel. There is not only one path for bacteria to pass; several find their ride on small microbes—mosquitoes, ticks, or fleas, for example, that are natural messengers. These small carriers transport causative agents from the animal hosts to us, usually without being harmed themselves. Understanding how they operate is the most important thing about comprehending why diseases, which leap between species in unpredictable fashions, continue to resurface. They don't only transmit bacteria; they also influence how fast and where diseases appear, and that in turn determines general public health at the human-animal interface. Vector-borne diseases essentially depend on these living couriers to transfer pathogens throughout their life cycles. Diseases such as malaria, dengue, Lyme disease, and even Zika require a vector to span the gap between animals—usually wild reservoirs—and humans. Climate change, habitat disruption, and our own incursion into nature all have roles to play in determining how many vectors there are and how far diseases can travel.

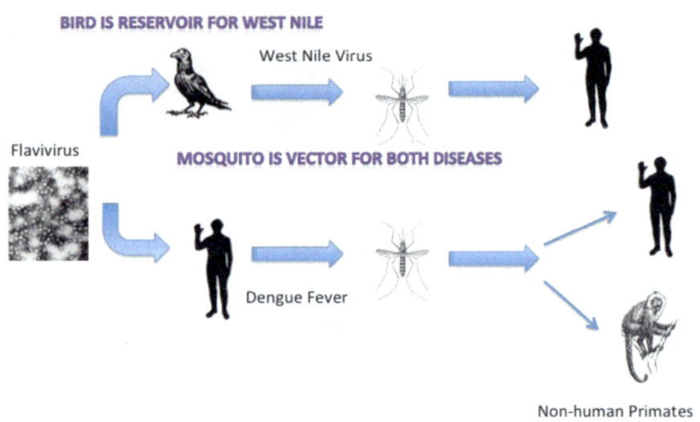

Figure 6.2. Vector borne diseases.

Source: By Kwasnyje - Own work, CC BY-SA 4.0, https://commons.wikimedia.org/w/index.php?curid=49676794

Agricultural practices that become increasingly intense due to more rapid land-use changes, and our contemporary global mobility all bubble up the interaction among people, vectors, and wildlife. Overall, this complex mix of vector biology and human-driven environmental modifications creates an elaborate puzzle of factors that drive disease emergence and persistence (Rohr et al., 2019). It's apparent that when disease jumps from animals to humans, our overall health is inextricably linked with that of wildlife and the ecosystem as a whole. Recently, scientists charting mammalian host-virus relationships have discovered that the composition of zoonotic viruses transmitted by arthropods largely relies on the characteristics of the host species and their habitat. For example, bats end up being big reservoirs—they carry a surprisingly high load of viruses, lots of which require a vector to find its way to us. Qualitatively, to identify which animal groups and areas are most vulnerable is very important for the establishment of successful monitoring and control strategies against these spillover events. Briefly, gaining a precise image of vector-borne disease involves merging our knowledge of viral activity, host behavior, and vector uniqueness to improve predict and prevention of outbreaks (Olival et al., 2017) (Figure 6.2).

Importance of Studying These Diseases

Infectious disease outbreaks never play out according to a clear script—they always remind us that we must descend into research on diseases jumping from animals or transmitted by insects. History generates enough examples—plague, cholera, and even influenza have all turned societies upside down while revealing fault lines in our public health arrangements. Our current COVID-19 drama, for example, demonstrates how zoonotic diseases can explode into worldwide crises, triggered by increasing animal–human interactions and our über-connected planet. Discovering how these pathogens cross over is essentially the starting point for developing astute prevention and control strategies. We've seen firsthand that quick moves, like isolating the sick, running quarantine measures, and even tightening border checks, can sometimes steer us clear of disaster. In most cases, early detection thanks to worldwide monitoring makes a huge difference. To summarize, this mixed bag of strategies proves that studying these infections is a key brick in keeping communities stable and building lasting health resilience (Naserrudin et al., 2022). Engaging local people in disease-spreading prevention is really what's needed when it comes to ending zoonotic and insect-borne diseases. Consider, say, studies based on community techniques in regions that are struggling with *Plasmodium knowlesi* malaria—it delves into the ways in which local customs and social uniqueness contribute to the spread of the disease. Operating side by side with the populations at risk provides information that isn't always evident from top-down research, showing both the obstacles and beneficial factors contributing to preventive action. By combining with ordinary views, policymakers can develop responses that are more attuned to local traditions and actual experience, which, in most instances, increases how well individuals comply with guidelines. This hands-on method assists in linking malaria control to wider, sustainable health objectives. It truly highlights the value that being immersed in social dynamics as well as a little bit of anthropology can bring when battling these diseases for the long term (Naserrudin et al., 2022). New tech tools are essential when grappling with the constant threat of animal-transmitted diseases as well as insect-borne ones. Rapid diagnostic tests, intelligent contact tracing devices, and biomarker detection all collaborate to raise alarms early—sometimes before they blow into full-fledged outbreaks. There are the innovative vaccine platforms and attempts to repurpose drugs already available; these measures aren't merely addressing familiar dangers but are our best hope against novel, volatile infections with pandemic potential. All these research-driven innovations help us avoid being caught unawares and respond quickly when public health is at stake. Investing in them strengthens our near-term response expertise as well as global health security—a double dividend. Ultimately, delving into zoonotic and vector-borne diseases is the pillar of scientific advancement that protects public health and prevents severe socio-economic upsets (Piret & Boivin, 2021).

6.1. Historical Context

These century-old diseases transmitted between animals and humans have formed part of our collective history with nature—far before the age of modern science. Early individuals had to swerve away from outbreaks that easily sneaked in on winged and crawling vehicles such as mosquitoes and ticks. Consider, for example, the Western Balkans, where accounts matter-of-factly mention that a combination of tick species (Ixodes, Hyalomma, etc.) was their role players in transmitting insects that sometimes affected people and at other times only pestered animals. Livestock were also not immune to these challenges, with diseases like *Theileria orientalis* and *Anaplasma marginale* sending old warnings about animal welfare and farm output. Alas, the patchwork nature of past data only indicates how difficult it was to follow these events, so we apparently still require a much steadier research agenda (Kapo et al., 2025). In Southeast Asia, Sulawesi island in Indonesia, in fact, the scene becomes even more complexed. Japanese encephalitis virus (JEV), which is typically transmitted by Culex mosquitoes, has been hanging on due to the island's seemingly infinite rice paddies and thriving populations of pigs and bats, who become unwitting hosts. Years of sporadic reports—documenting everything from human cases to infections in various animals—have gradually constructed a rich tapestry of how this disease is transmitted. In general, these historical indicators lead to an complex combination of nature, local economies, and routine cultural practices. While these indicators have generally guided today's disease control strategies, they also indicate the very real disconnects that still remain in monitoring and diagnosing such infections. It's a reminder that the fine line between our environment and these small insect carriers remains a significant component of public health initiatives today (Rahma et al., 2025). Delving into the history of these zoonotic and vector-borne diseases provides us with a kind of blueprint for today's disease wars. Previous attempts—usually characterized by patchy monitoring—show that stopping the spread from insects such as ticks and mosquitoes is not an easy feat. Retrospective narratives keep resurfacing, associating the origin of diseases with shifts in agriculture, urbanization, and animal husbandry practices; through time, these variables have continuously reconfigured how pathogens engage with their hosts. Both sets of stories, both from the Western Balkans and Sulawesi, indicate how local conditions and a combination of host animals have, interestingly enough, enabled these diseases to persist on and periodically reappear in sudden ways. Recognizing these age-old patterns is key if we're to devise practical, evidence-based solutions that combination lessons from back then with our modern tools, ultimately helping us keep zoonotic risks at bay (Kapo et al., 2025; Rahma et al., 2025) (Figure 6.3).

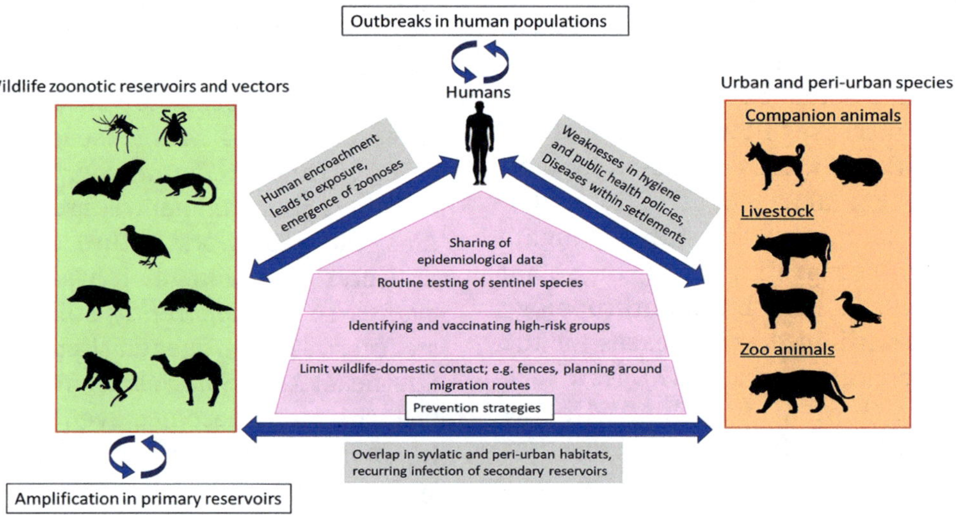

Figure 6.3. Zoonotic viruses.

Source: Springer Nature. (2022). *Zoonotic Viruses.*

6.1.1. Early Examples of Zoonotic Diseases

Humans and animals have coexisted across centuries—a reality that's produced bacteria jumping between them and about which history continues to remind us. Plagues such as plague, tuberculosis (TB), and even rabies emerged when people touched infected animals or made contact with small carriers like fleas. These early disease outbreaks ravaged communities, changed the way people traveled, and even transformed social hierarchies. Mostly, slobbly changes to the environment and normal human hustle simply made exactly the sorts of avenues for pathogen jump-poses to make them available. The seesaw in animals and people establishes the setting in which we recognize zoonotic diseases these days, all the way from bacteria through parasites and viruses (Rahman et al., 2020). Overall, it makes you think twice about how our everyday interactions with animals can lead to outbreaks. Farming took things to a whole new level when it came to animal contact—no wonder that it increased the odds for disease to arrive. The moment livestock became best buddies (or, you know, best buddies enough), bacteria discovered new ways to get across, with disease like brucellosis and anthrax cropping up out of nowhere. With fields growing larger and animals packed into small spaces, things deteriorated for disease transmission between animals further, unwittingly, to humans. These initial zoonotic incidents remind us, in a sort of ironic turn of events, that our pursuit of improved food sometimes invited unintended microbial visitors through the door. New studies indicate that combinationincorporating food production systems with wildlife habitats complicates matters a great deal when trying to monitor the spread of disease. Therefore, understanding how farming altered these exchanges is crucial to knowing where all these ancient disease epidemics originated and how they affect human health (Rohr et al., 2019). Weather fluctuations and how people were traversing the landscape introduced an extra level of danger during the early days. Seasonal fluxes tended to push people and animals into new areas, facilitating germ traffic—consider how anthrax and tularemia were able to disperse among certain pastoral populations. While doing that, climate shifts adjusted the quantities of irritating carriers like ticks and mosquitoes, who then transferred microbes like Rickettsia and other arboviruses. The function of these microbes, commingling with larger animal hosts, makes disease dynamics very complex and control much more difficult. In retrospect, these trends explain why incorporating our strategy, essentially the One Health concept, is important when addressing problems that interconnect our environment, animal life, and us. Even today, as zoonotic diseases keep recurring and reappearing, these early examples still provide insights on how to keep a closer watch and avoid outbreaks (Rahman et al., 2020).

6.1.2. Historical Outbreaks of Vector-borne Diseases

Diseases transmitted by vectors have plagued mankind for centuries, leaving profound scars on societies around the globe. Back in ancient times—early in the pre-mid-1900s period—humans needed to comprehend microbe habits and the nature of disease transmission to battle these diseases. In a particular instance, early malaria management entailed experimenting with mosquito breeding grounds, a decidedly local, do-it-yourself approach. Then, starting in the 1940s, everything changed as chemical pesticides became the answer, and little consideration was really given to nature's complex details. This switch, while at first it made the spread of most diseases dwindle, ultimately ignored the less obvious ways that insects act and bacteria are carried. Ultimately, the dependence on a one-size-fits-all strategy created problems such as resistance to insecticides, making it evident that incorporating a wider, more nuanced ecological perspective is needed (Wilson et al., 2020). Taking a closer look, the resurgence and recrudescence of these diseases also have connections to larger environmental and social changes, such as intensive agricultural expansion. As people required more food and there were more people, agricultural practices transformed the ground in ways that inadvertently increased the numbers of disease-carrying organisms. Such transformations ensured that humans increasingly came into contact with pests, a feat that only enhanced the transmission cycle. For the most part, since the 1940s, most of the new infectious diseases, particularly those jumping from animals—have been traced back to these tremendous changes in farming. It's an interconnected combination: extensive agriculture not only reshapes landscapes but also increases human-wildlife interactions, creating new pathways for disease to spill over (Rohr et al., 2019). It's a reminder that controlling vector-borne epidemics requires a combination of ecological, agricultural, and social knowledge. Looking at outbreaks such as malaria, dengue, and leishmaniasis, one finds that human activity, insect behavior, and germ transmission are interconnected. At first, chemical insecticides worked fairly well to control these vectors, but eventually resistance emerged and environmental changes made it clear that old methods required a rethink. The transition from nature-based interventions to over-reliance on pesticides, and now gradually back to more heterogeneous forms, echoes our changing understanding of disease patterns. Today's experts generally favor a balance: combining insecticide use with alternative, locally adjusted methods to bring down disease burdens sustainably. History tells us that lasting control isn't about relying solely on technological fixes; it requires ongoing research and strategies that dig into what truly drives transmission (Wilson et al., 2020).

6.1.3. Evolution of Public Health Responses

Public health has never been an easy case when it involves diseases that jump from animals to humans. The spread of pathogens is complicated – complex with how communities work, live, and even consume food. Officials used to simply lock things down with quarantine and increase sanitation in the olden days, but as new cases broke out more frequently, that easy solution just could not keep up. Live and wet markets, where animals are closely packed with humans, demonstrate how easy it is for these insects to slide across species boundaries (Naguib et al., 2021). Such markets aren't just the sites of spillovers but also embedded within local economies and food cultures, so attempting to close them or modify practices is not a straightforward decision. More recently, health systems have begun to lean into sweeping plans – combinationincorporating ecological brakes, stricter biosecurity and collaboration across experts , tilting the game from merely responding after issues have arisen to attempting to avoid them in the initial place. Crop expansion is accelerating to feed our increasing numbers, and with that, the dynamics of zoonotic disease dangers are becoming ever more complicated. When humans, domesticated animals, and wild animals get closer – sometimes in ways that baffle traditional control measures (Rohr et al., 2019) – it compels a rethink of how best to stay infection-free. Most times, it involves the combining of agricultural practices with infectious disease control, a mix that now manifests in policies promoting sustainable agriculture, prudent antibiotic use and even targeted vector control. One Health concepts have seeped into mainstream policy, stressing that the health of humans, animals, and the environment isn't distinct but closely intertwined. In general, this change isn't about mopping up a bad mess afterward; it's about disentangling the deep, frequently dirty, ecological and socio-economic causes that allowed these diseases to flourish. Now, the delicate balancing act between avoiding diseases but under the realities of genuine economic constraints is very much on center stage, particularly in those areas where smallholder agriculture and informal markets are still prevalent. Strides toward blocking the jump from animals to people tend to clash with tradition, scarce means and outdated facilities, and radical measures like shutting down markets or enforcing tight regulations on livestock prove difficult to execute (Naguib et al., 2021). In most cases, success has involved working with local stakeholders, taking clear but at times patchy risk communication and small, imperfect steps to build on market practice and animal trade standards. An increase in data-driven surveillance—that includes genomic sequencing and digital tracking—assists in catching things earlier, albeit with methods occasionally feeling a tad patchy. In all, this looser, context-dependent framework highlights how public health continues to adapt to fit around new zoonoses that threaten to evade it, while also safeguarding livelihoods and food security within an ever-changing world (Figure 6.4).

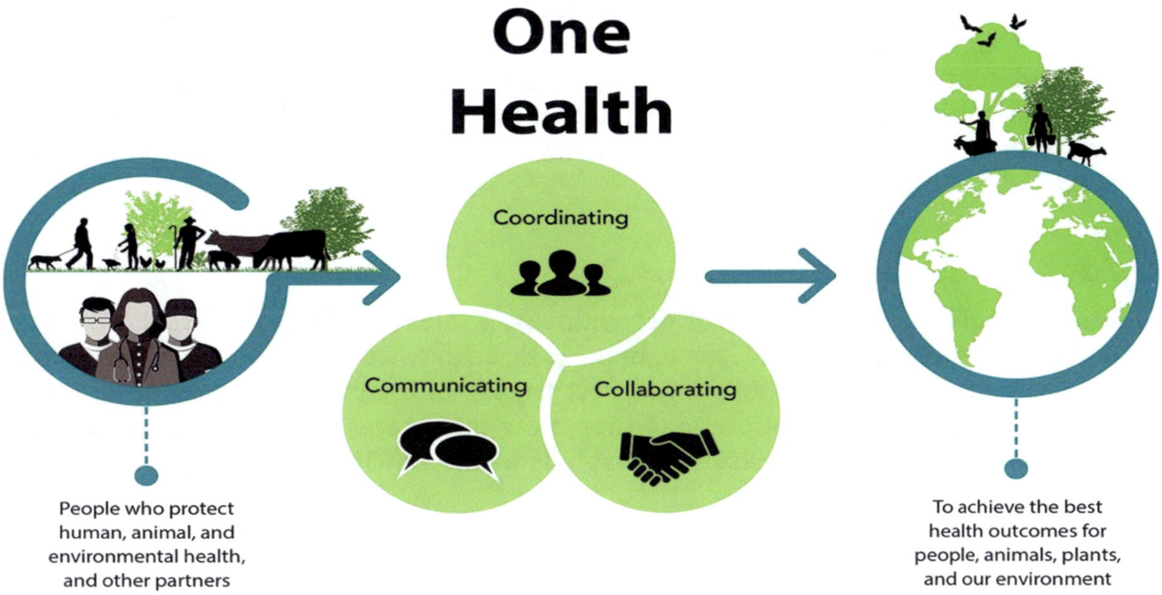

Figure 6.4. Public health has never been a straightforward matter when it comes to diseases that jump from animals to people.

Source: CDC. (2020). *One Health infographic.*

6.2. Mechanisms of Transmission

Determining how bacteria transmit from animals to humans isn't quite as easy as it appears. When humans come close to animals through activities such as breeding, hunting, or even the international animal trade, opportunity for spillovers increases—viruses, bacteria, and other small animals wind up crossing species lines. At times, bacteria are spread directly—bites or simply good old-fashioned touch, while at others, they creep in through areas contaminated by animal feces. It's a crazy combination of pathways that, if you take a closer look, makes sense for why zoonotic pathogens emerge and spread unpredictably. Traditional measures such as quarantine and isolation, for example, have largely managed to stifle outbreaks, highlighting why monitoring these transmission pathways is critical (Piret & Boivin, 2021). Environmental changes and human activities also determine how these diseases move. Climate change disrupts where vectors like mosquitoes, ticks, and fleas dwell which, in most instances, changes how well they can transmit bacteria. Urbanization and international travel take both the hosts and the vectors on unplanned journeys over borders. Further when animal migration or commerce re-mixes new contact between species that previously met but infrequently, disease re-emergence possibilities increase further. Overall, these interconnected ecological and human drivers make it difficult to predict outbreaks, a reminder that learning about these drivers is fairly critical to avoiding future spread (Rahman et al., 2020). Add in the fact that many different bacteria and modes of transmission make the picture even more complicated. Certain insects acquire disease organisms from ill animals further infect humans—a process influenced by the insects' own biology and behavior. Similarly, direct contact with body fluids or even consuming infected animal products can result in infection. The One Health concept unites human, animal, and environmental health, calling for combined monitoring and control techniques to interrupt these chains of transmission. Rapid diagnostic tools and global surveillance also have a significant role, identifying outbreaks early enough for timely, often suboptimal, interventions that can slow down widespread transmission (Rahman et al., 2020; Piret & Boivin, 2021).

6.2.1. Zoonotic Transmission Pathways

Humans and animals collide in ways that determine how infections begin and recur. Wild animals can harbor bacteria that subsequently leap to humans through twisting, sometimes bizarre, ecological pathways. Native vegetation and those tiny insect friends of theirs may be harboring viruses we never quite paid attention to until one day they blow into crops, such as when wild Asian rice transmitted a virus into cultivated rice, using aphids as the unwitting messengers.

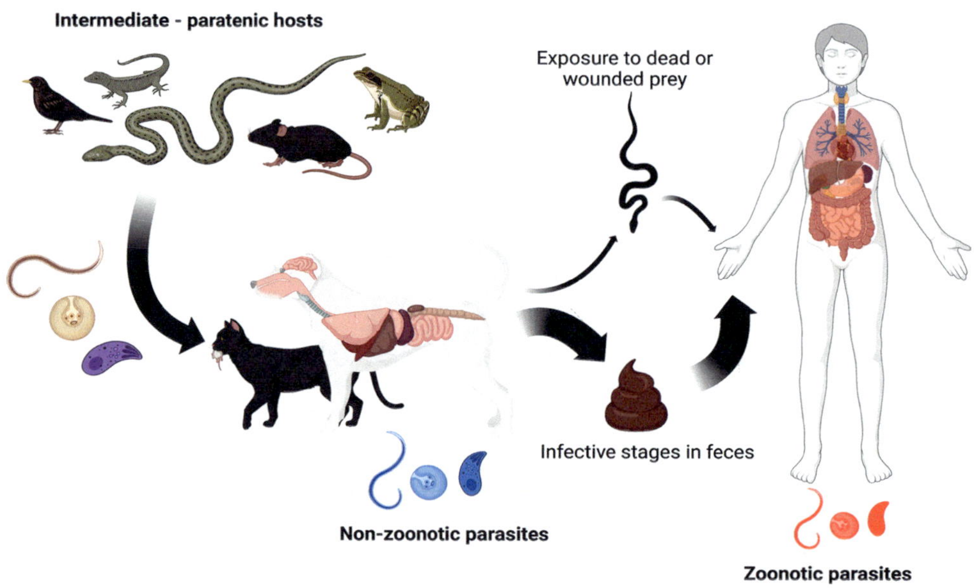

Figure 6.5. Zoonotic transmission pathways.

Source: Mendoza, J. (2023). *Transmission Routes of Zoonotic Parasites.*

This entire situation illustrates that natural viruses have the potential to become actual dangers if they happen to have the proper (or improper) link with a carrier, and it reminds us that wildlife, those little microbes, and human behavior all fit together in the transmission of disease (Yan et al., 2023). In most instances, such unforeseen spillovers can threaten food supplies and public health, so monitoring these pathways in nature matters. Numerous environmental factors act in unforeseen ways to influence disease-carrying microbe populations. Human activities, such as allowing plastic trash to accumulate—tend to create temporary habitats where mosquitoes, ticks, and the like can multiply. Plastic waste accumulate water and become a breeding ground for insects that disperse arboviruses like dengue, chikungunya, and Zika, typically riding on Aedes mosquitoes. With the onset of these novel, human-created pockets, the population of disease-transmitting vectors can grow rapidly, increasing the likelihood of infections. Add to that stagnant water in abandoned plastic bottles: not only does it harbor insects, but it is also a reservoir for disease-causing bacteria like leptospirosis, in which the biofilms end up preferring to settle on the plastic material. Evidently, when we do a bad job of taking care of our environment, we unintentionally create conducive conditions for the survival of vectors and the habitation of pathogens right near where we reside (Maquart et al., 2022). It's also fascinating the way plastic pollution distorts natural niches, facilitating the spread of bacteria. Plastic is not only a vector's safe haven; it also creates a sort of landing strip for microbes, allowing them to form biofilms and persist longer than they would otherwise. This type of contamination can even expand the range of pathogens, changing the typical patterns of how disease spreads between populations. Also, mountains of plastic clog drainage systems, leading to stagnant pools where vectors for schistosomiasis or malaria have all the room they require to thrive. Most often, the combination of environmental contamination, insect behavior, and germ interactions highlights just how complex zoonotic transmission can be, particularly in rapidly expanding tropical regions with uneven waste collection (Maquart et al., 2022) (Figure 6.5).

6.2.2. Vector-borne Transmission Mechanisms

Infectious disease travels in mechanisms that can become rather complicated, and vector-borne pathways certainly are distinct—even if they use an indirect ploy to transmit bacteria. Consider how small organisms such as mosquitoes, ticks, and fleas acquire bacteria from reservoir hosts and subsequently deliver them to human populations; they're more than just delivery vehicles. These small carriers also provide bacteria with an opportunity to remain for a while and even breed before leaping on to a new host. What they eat and where they like to hang out has a direct influence on the distance and effectiveness with which a disease can spread. As it happens, learning about these strange routes is most important when we lack sufficient pharmaceutical solutions. Public health measures, consequently, seek to attack both the populations of such vectors and the interfaces through which they come into contact with hosts, a notion that underlies the persistence of zoonotic diseases (Rahman et al., 2020; Piret & Boivin, 2021). Environmental changes—and, to be honest, our own endeavors—have been rewriting the narrative of vector-borne disease. Urban sprawl and global warming tend to spread the dwellings of these organisms, bringing new vectors and reservoirs to introduce bacteria into previously unexpected areas. When humans encroach upon wildlife habitats, they collide with new vectors and reservoirs, which in most instances can increase the likelihood of zoonotic spillover events. International travel and commerce, on the other hand, sometimes disperse these insects and their accompanying pathogens around the globe more rapidly than one might imagine. This mix of factors makes simple control measures rather tricky, demanding adaptive strategies that combination environmental oversight with public health planning. Generally speaking, getting a grip on these varied drivers is crucial if we're to predict when and where outbreaks might crop up (Rahman et al., 2020; Piret & Boivin, 2021). Zooming in even more to the microscopic, molecular, and cellular levels, the dynamic between vectors and pathogens truly sets the stage for disease transmission. Pathogens have to change and adapt just to survive inside of a vector, traversing sometimes tortuous developmental processes that ultimately allow them to infect vertebrate hosts. This biological symphony isn't uniform for all vectors or pathogens, it may alter such things as the time it takes symptoms to appear or how well the germ is transmitted.

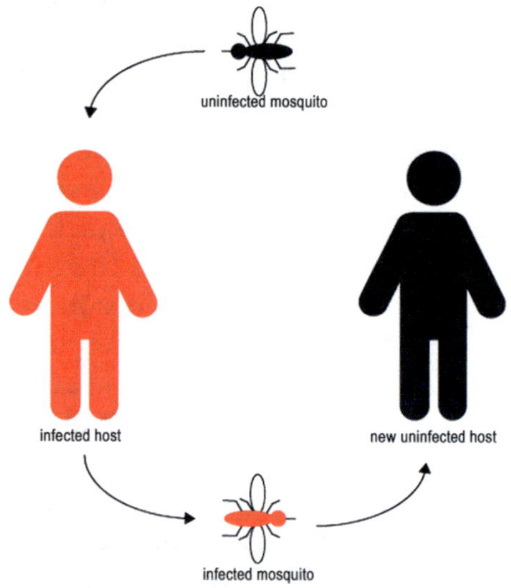

Figure 6.6. Vector-borne transmission mechanisms.

Source: ImmunoBites. (2018). *Mosquito Transmission.*

A vector's own immune response may sometimes even cut back the pathogen load, thereby modifying the overall outbreak scenario. Scientists must delve into these complex interactions to reveal potential vulnerabilities, perhaps through genetic manipulation or microbial interference. In addition, that novel diagnostic and surveillance technologies must collaborate with these measures to track both vector competence and the dynamic character of pathogens across different, sometimes volatile, ecological environments (Rahman et al., 2020; Piret et al., 2021) (Figure 6.6).

6.2.3. Role of Environmental Factors in Transmission

Environmental conditions dictate how diseases are spread between living organisms. Hosts, vectors, and pathogens all interact with each other in ways not always clearly understood—yet changes in the environment can change everything from the survival and reproduction of organisms to how they interact. Consider vector-borne diseases: ticks and fresh water snails, for instance, are heavily reliant on their location and local climate. In the eastern U.S., the Powassan virus, which is tick-borne, has been trending upward owing in part to alterations such as habitat fragmentation and climate shift. Even minute adjustments in the immediate landscape or microclimate may alter the population of ticks and how they encounter wildlife and humans, allowing the virus to appear in new locations (Hassett et al., 2021). Way up in highland regions, the challenge becomes even more singular, particularly when freshwater snail vectors are the case. Way over in the Northern Bolivian Altiplano, fascioliasis remains a problem despite preventive measures. Regional water conditions—temperature, pH, and water's resident time—take a major role in dictating the snail Galba truncatula's life cycle and population density. Even when temperatures appear too low overall for parasites to mature, the small pools of warmer water in microhabitats cause the parasites to continue maturing, extending the season of transmission. The difference between ephemeral and permanent water bodies usually results in seeing sometimes a single snail cycle a year and sometimes two (Bargues et al., 2021). Natural fluctuations and human-altered changes tend to get jumbled together, creating the perfect storm for vector-borne and zoonotic diseases. Temperature, humidity, and access to water naturally regulate vectors' life cycles and parasite maturation, but deforestation, agriculture, or urbanization can disrupt these balances, increasing opportunities for vectors to collide with hosts in areas they never have before. In most instances, these disturbances not only alter the frequency of contacts between vectors and hosts but also drive diseases into regions of the country that were not previously at risk. Multi-disciplinary, ecosystem-level strategy—one that integrates ongoing environmental surveillance with vector ecology studies—is usually essential for figuring out successful One Health strategies. These approaches target not just human health but also the environmental reservoirs and vector communities that underpin disease spread and new outbreaks (Bargues et al., 2021; Hassett et al., 2021).

6.3. Major Zoonotic Diseases

People are coming into contact with animals more than ever, either on farms, in growing cities, or just when we stray into the wild, which increases the risk of disease jumping between species. Zoonotic diseases, those diseases that can naturally spread from vertebrates to humans, now claim more than 60% of the microbes responsible for new diseases. You have bacteria, viruses, fungi, protozoa, and even parasites all hiding behind these epidemics. A mixture of circumstances—for example, changing climates, animal migrations, and our own hands in what is happening around us—determine how these diseases emerge on the scene and propagate. The COVID-19 pandemic, for instance, truly illustrated how a brand new zoonotic disease can wreak havoc in the world and highlighting the urgent need for enhanced tracking and control. Meeting these challenges involves coming together across disciplines because the One Health strategy reminds us that people's health, animals' health, and nature are all inextricably linked (Rahman et al., 2020). Some of the more concerning zoonotic concerns involve viruses such as rabies, Ebola, and coronaviruses that produce severe disease and death worldwide. Rabies, typically transmitted by bites from dogs, is still lethal if not treated quickly, particularly where resources are scarce. Outbreaks of Ebola, however, demonstrate how such animal-borne infections can trigger epidemics with high mortality rates, frequently originating from bats or primates. And it isn't just viruses at play; bacterial infections such as brucellosis and leptospirosis have also made a heavy mark on public health, hitting agricultural communities hard where people are in close contact with livestock. All of these examples drive home the idea that solid surveillance and proactive, everyday precautions are key to nipping these diseases in the bud (Rahman et al., 2020). Next, there's the tricky terrain of vector-borne zoonotic disease. In this case, animals such as mosquitoes, ticks, and sandflies harbor bacteria that infect humans. Diseases such as malaria, dengue fever, and leishmaniasis load disproportionately among poorer populations and are caused by a capricious combination of ecological and environmental factors that influence the behavior of these vectors. In most cases, local initiatives based on hands-on ecological expertise has reduced disease rates, but the intense use of insecticides today has introduced issues such as chemical resistance. That tells us we need to think more holistically, incorporating chemical, biological, and even environmental methods—to manage these risks safely. Ultimately, truly comprehending how insect life and disease transmission coexist is necessary to design long-term solutions that can adapt to our shifting climate and socio-economic conditions, and thereby reduce the overall burden of these vector-borne zoonoses.

6.3.1. Rabies

People and animals have coexisted for centuries, and that same confusion has many times induced the transmission of infections, particularly those transmitted by animals with diseases. Rabies, for example, makes us sit up and take notice because when its symptoms emerge, the result is nearly always fatal. A lyssavirus is responsible for this problem, generally entering by a bite from a diseased animal—most often a household dog. This disease, indeed, is such a textbook demonstration of just how unclear the entire cross-species transmission becomes; our ordinary contact with wildlife hosts continues it. For most situations, with cities spreading out and people walking into open territories, being able to decipher just how all this comes together and shifts patterns in the diseases matters. In practical terms, rabies reminds us—repeatedly—how inextricably intertwined the origins of human and animal health are, pushing humans toward the necessity of diverse methods to manage infections that transfer between species (Rahman et al., 2020).

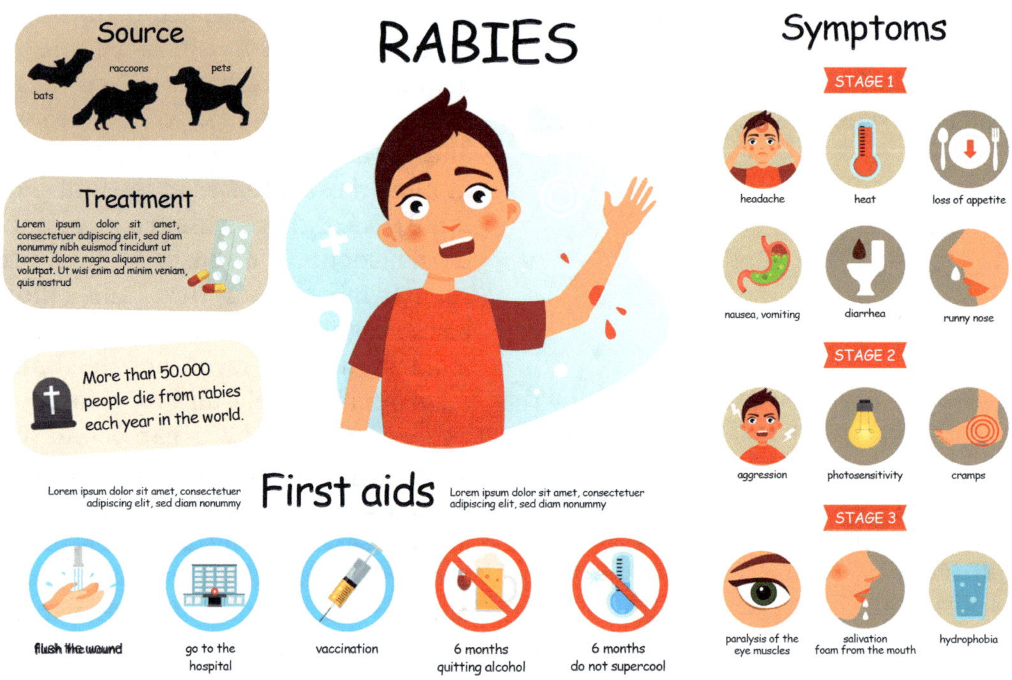

Figure 6.7. Rabies: Types, symptoms, causes, prevention, and treatments.

Source: Credihealth. (2024). *Rabies Disease Infographic.*

Throughout the history of the world, particularly among lower- and middle-income countries where healthy infrastructure and preventive tools tend to be lacking, rabies continues to be a significant burden. Despite the existence of effective post-exposure prophylaxis (PEP), most who require it never receive treatment in a timely manner, and this delay typically means a death sentence. Vaccination campaigns targeting animals used as carriers, most notably dogs, have been shown to erode the incidence of new cases—but the situation isn't wholly positive. Inequitable access to vaccines for both humans and animals means the issue persists in many areas. This gap in immunization often mirrors larger, global inequities in vaccine distribution, making it especially tough to control rabies alongside other diseases. Addressing these underlying challenges with improved vaccination efforts and targeted public health projects is fundamental if we're going to curb this threat (Rodrigues & Plotkin, 2020). Steering clear of hasty solutions to short-term authority, rabies is a sound argument for the adoption of One Health that binds together human, animal, and environmental health. It is only by combining sustainable control of this disease that really hinges on a combination of skills: veterinarians, health experts, and even wildlife experts must work together. This holistic perspective stems from an understanding that monitoring carriers of animals, disseminating community education, and providing decent healthcare to those who are at risk are all portions of the puzzle. Additionally, the role of habitat changes and changes in animal populations in the transmission of rabies is a factor and also needs to be considered in preparing interventions. Overall, by facilitating cooperation among the various disciplines and sectors, the One Health model presents what appears to be the greatest promise to mitigate the worldwide effect of rabies, addressing one of the most potent dangers spread by animals (Rahman et al., 2020) (Figure 6.7).

6.3.2. Hantavirus

Zoonotic diseases are on the increase, and our evolving world keeps demonstrating how our activities get complex with nature. Changes such as deforestation and urbanization tend to displace animal habitats, which consequently increases the likelihood that something like a virus escapes from animals to humans. Hantavirus, for instance, is largely transmitted through contact with rodents – its natural hosts – when people inhale small, unpredictable fragments of rodent feces. This danger is particularly evident in rural and proximate suburban areas. In the majority of instances, deciphering these environmental signs involves examining the complex dynamics between changed landscapes and animal behavior. There are even talks of "landscape immunity", essentially maintaining nature in a healthy equilibrium to reduce spillover threats – as one of the important concepts to maintain hantavirus and similar insects in check (Plowright et al., 2021). Getting into the molecular aspect, hantavirus operates in a quite unusual manner. It persists in rodent reservoirs while presenting serious risks to human health. In contrast to coronaviruses that have been the center of attention for their leaps from animals to humans, hantavirus falls under the category of Bunyaviridae and prefers to latch onto rodents exclusively instead of leaping from several hosts. It is this singular focus that complicates tracking and halting it because you genuinely need to know how local rodent populations and behaviors factor into transmitting the virus. Further, of course, the disease itself is all over the place – sometimes a mere fever, but sometimes it can get out of hand and cause dangerous complications to the kidneys or lungs. Veterinary and ecological studies of similar viruses continue to contribute portions of information on how these pathogens evolve and how they relate to their host, slowly developing a wider picture of disease emergence and what could work in controlling it (Decaro et al., 2020). Hantavirus control requires an interdisciplinary approach that combines ecology, virology, and even sociology. It's not only important to monitor rodents; we need to consider land use as well, particularly as settlements move closer to native areas. Communities that discover simple preventive measures and monitor their area do better against these outbreaks. At the same time, new molecular research throws light on how the virus evolves in time, knowledge that can ultimately guide us towards more effective vaccines and antiviral therapies if necessary. By and large, the interference with natural ecosystems appears to drive such animal-to-human jumps, and, in broad terms, science-informed policies that address ecosystem health as an integral component of disease prevention might be vital for comprehensive strategy against hantavirus and other dangers (Plowright et al., 2021).

6.3.3. Zika Virus

There has been a steady increase in infections

that sort of reveals just how knitted our existence is with nature and animals in recent years. Consider, for example, those diseases transmitted by insects—Zika virus, which arose so rapidly and disrupted public health protocols, reminds us that when the Aedes mosquito bites, chance doesn't necessarily rule. Urban sprawl and international travel have driven the virus into unprecedented territories, usually sending our health systems reeling. For the most part, Zika outbreaks have sent brutal realities such as birth defects and nerve conditions into sharp focus. This all points to a larger, more complicated truth: we truly need a more integrated, on-the-ground strategy for monitoring diseases that leap from animals to humans, one that considers how our surroundings and communities structure these risks (Lio et al., 2023). Looking deeper, climate appears to have a surprisingly complicated role with Zika and similar insects. Warmer days and additional rainfall promote the breeding of mosquitoes in terms that can prolong the season of virus transmission. It's almost as if the weather is revising the maps of both animal habitats and our neighborhoods, which has the result of bringing us more chance encounters with the carriers. In the majority of instances, even as we commonly associate antimicrobial resistance (AMR) with bacteria, the larger context, such as pollution or poorly treated wastewater, disrupts nature's equilibrium and can increase the transmission of such infections (Lio et al., 2023). In some sense, climate change is sort of a catalyst for diseases like Zika fever, pushing us toward more holistic, One Health-type approaches. It's not just about the virus, but also about the combination of social and natural influences involved when it comes to managing the Zika challenge. Population explosions, dense urban areas, and non-stop international travel have all created the context for repeated outbreaks, showcasing the complex dance between how viruses mutate, mosquito behaviors change, and human activities roll on together. Although a few vector-borne diseases appear to be being kept in check by diverse patches, Zika's frequent comebacks are a reminder that our global health bulwarks still have vast holes. By and large, getting different arms of the public sector to coordinate—enhancing mosquito control, and even duplicating public awareness campaigns (yes, occasionally more than a couple)—appears essential. Ultimately, the imprevisible propagation of Zika highlights the necessity for resilient, adaptive measures to respond to whatever the future holds (Chala & Hamde, 2021) (Figure 6.8).

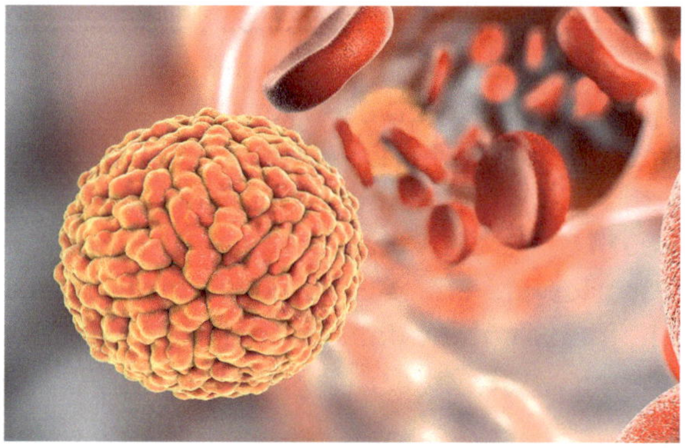

Figure 6.8. Zika virus.

Source: Science Photo Library. (2016). *Zika Virus in Blood.*

6.4. Major Vector-borne Diseases

Dense populations and mixed ecosystems bring humans and animals into close contact, which can stir up the spread of diseases carried by little microbes. Mosquitoes, ticks, and fleas, tiny, but mighty—carry bacteria that can leap from one species to another. In many cases, places where wildlife, pets, and people mingle (think live or wet markets) turn into unexpected hubs for zoonotic diseases. Live markets contribute significantly to local trade and food security, but they also have the potential to combine species in a manner that allows new pathogens to emerge. Areas with high densities of animals such as wild boars can experience vectors transferring infection between wildlife and humans. In general, understanding these complicated transmission patterns is central to developing solutions that both control the vectors and minimize human exposure (Altissimi et al., 2023; Naguib et al., 2021). Vector-borne viral diseases, including Crimean–Congo hemorrhagic fever, Rift Valley fever, and arboviruses, highlight an actual health concern in zoonotic situations. These viruses typically persist in animal reservoirs or hosts that amplify their numbers before being transmitted by ticks or mosquitoes to humans. Livestock and market environments can inadvertently amplify these risks when infected animals come too close to both vectors and human populations. And in most informal animal trading locations, poor biosecurity can amplify vector numbers—a factor that accelerates disease transmission. These viruses not only strike human health in a big way immediately, but they can also generate widespread economic and social distress, particularly in communities where the economy is heavily based on animal agriculture and trade (Naguib et al., 2021; Altissimi et al., 2023). Vector-borne parasitic diseases present another facet to the entire zoonotic scenario. Tick-transmitted insects like *Coxiella burnetii* and Borrelia species could creep into human society due to vectors that love market or farm environments. The interaction between wildlife reservoirs and domestic animals only increases the potential infection pool. Occasionally, food safety is compromised as well—meat could be contaminated with pathogens from such vectors, or wild animal meat is eaten without adequate screening. While some regulations attempt to control these risks, the dynamic combination of vector species, hosts, and environmental conditions ensures that management programs must be adaptable. For the majority of instances, continued surveillance combined with advances in food safety, vector control, and worker health practices continue to be essential for controlling outbreaks of these zoonoses (Naguib et al., 2021; Altissimi et al., 2023).

6.4.1. Malaria

Weather appears to pull along the path of most diseases transmitted by insects, and malaria – that pesky disease transmitted by Plasmodium parasites and primarily spread by Anopheles mosquitoes – is no exception. Temperature, humidity in the air, and even rainfall combine to affect both the insects and the bacteria; when conditions reach a sweet spot, parasites grow more quickly within mosquitoes while the insects bite more frequently, increasing the likelihood of an outbreak. But when temperatures deviate too far from optimal, parasite growth falters or mosquito populations decrease. Humidity quietly influences how long these insects persist and act, and heavy rain can produce all those small puddles of water that make an ideal breeding ground. In general, increasing heat and unstable rain patterns have pushed malaria areas to move outward and even change location around – a warning that climate information should make it into models used for anticipating and combating outbreaks efficiently (Zhang et al., 2024). Humans aren't necessarily being very nice to nature either, and our own-caused climate change only makes the malaria puzzle more complicated. Temperature and precipitation changes, courtesy of global warming, trigger cascade effects – not only do they modify the biology of these disease-vector insects but also the social environments in which transmission occurs. More heat weather can slowly drive Anopheles mosquitoes into new regions, sometimes into higher altitudes or greater latitudes, suddenly exposing people who previously had nothing to fear. At the same time, rainfall patterns that fall out of sync can upset mosquito breeding patterns, resulting in some instances in occasional surges or even a year-round hold on the disease in susceptible areas. Throw in human mobility, land use change, and occasionally weak public health infrastructure, and the problem becomes an authentic combination. terms, addressing it involves sewing together concepts in epidemiology, climatology, and public health – the latest studies recommend intensifying surveillance, improving prediction models, and being adaptable in controlling the added risk introduced by climatic variability (Ojeyinka & Omaghomi, 2024). Aside from weather concerns, social and economic factors contribute significantly to how malaria infects and how we treat it. Poverty, poor housing, restricted access to health care, and lack of access to preventive equipment such as bed nets treated with insecticides all increase the risk factor, particularly in districts where malaria is endemic.

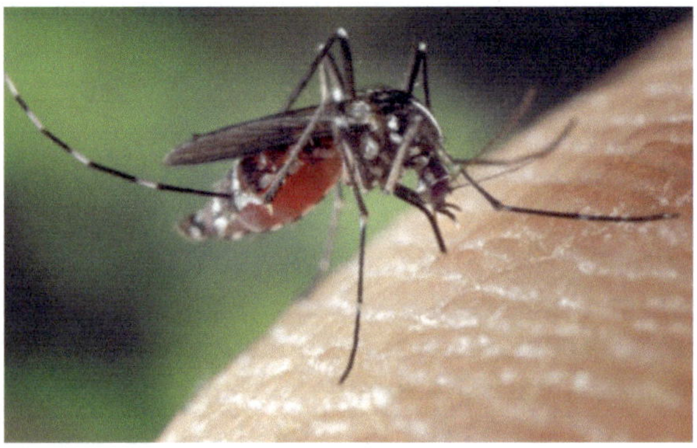

Figure 6.9. Tracking the global movement of malaria parasites and their variants.

Source: University of Melbourne. (2024). *Global Movement of Malaria Parasites.*

This compels vector control action to be adapted to local circumstances, combining pragmatic ecological understanding with community participation and good health education. The combination of biological, environmental, and social challenges demands an interdisciplinary consideration of malaria , one that views it as part of a larger world of zoonotic and vector-borne diseases. For the most part, increasing research on climate effects combined with improved health infrastructure and more intelligent mosquito control appears to be a good means of reducing the burden of malaria. Finally, encompassing approaches do more than address current public health concerns; they also create some level of resilience against the unpredictable fluctuations in disease risk driven by a changing climate (Ojeyinka & Omaghomi, 2024; Zhang et al., 2024) (Figure 6.9).

6.4.2. Lyme Disease

Humans and wildlife have been shaping disease trends for centuries, particularly when insects like ticks are involved. Lyme disease is a good example because it has become a genuine health concern since its transmission pattern is not simple, its scheme of transmission keeps evolving. The disease is caused by a spiral bacterium known as *Borrelia burgdorferi*, which typically makes its way to us after a tick bite from an infected tick, commonly referred to as a deer tick (or scientifically, Ixodes tick). These tiny organisms not only transmit the microbe but also act as their own little hideouts in the wild, hanging out with small mammals and birds. We're learning that, generally speaking, knowing how these tick populations and their animal hosts behave is key since shifts in the environment and even our own habits can nudge infection risks up. And with Lyme disease sometimes creeping in subtly and sticking around longer than expected, quick diagnosis and smart tick control measures become all the more crucial, fitting into our wider push for zoonotic disease oversight (Selzer & Epe, 2020). Keeping tick numbers in check is central if we're to control Lyme disease's reach. Recently, there has been some new development with animal parasiticides, namely a class called isoxazolines—that has shown potential, not only for the health of pets but for reducing the likelihood of these insects passing on diseases to humans as well. Most of the time, these medications, which began gaining popularity roughly a decade ago, prove effective in killing ticks by disrupting their lifecycle, which subsequently reduces the transmission of Borrelia. This new drug approach is a welcome development, particularly as compared to earlier therapies, which tended to get bogged down with resistance issues. Further, combining chemical control with less chemical intervention such as improved habitat control and even vaccination, would truly help to amplify Lyme prevention. And all this aligns nicely with the One Health concept that marries human, animal, and environmental health into one holistic strategy (Selzer & Epe, 2020). Lyme disease's propensity to bounce between wildlife, ticks, and people showcases the delicate challenges we have working with vector-borne diseases in a rapidly changing world. Climate change, sudden urban development, and changed land use have all created more fragmented environments where ticks appear to proliferate, increasing our risk exposure. Not to mention, with greater world travel and busier animal commerce, both ticks and the bacteria they spread find new methods of getting around, which further makes it hard to keep everything in check. This complex loop of wildlife reservoirs, advancing ticks, and human hosts demands greater vigilance, through enhanced field surveillance, public awareness, and organized health action. Addressing these challenges involves adopting a wide-angle perspective on all the variables involved and implementing multi-pronged control strategies that reflect the zoonotic management principles of the One Health approach (Rahman et al., 2020) (Figure 6.10).

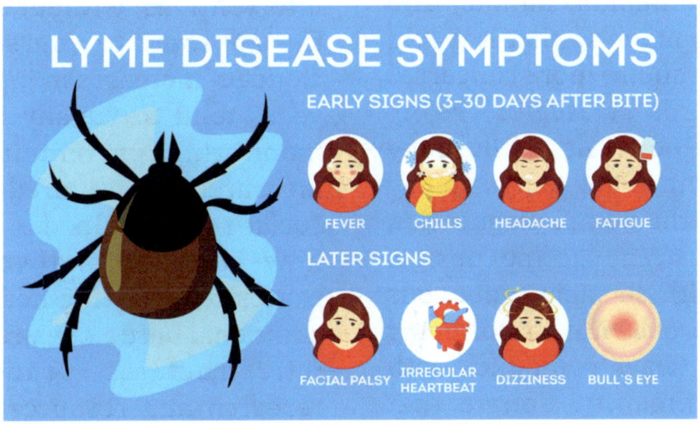

Figure 6.10. Lyme disease.

Source: https://www.thailandmedical.news/uploads/editor/files/Lyme-Disease.jpeg.

6.4.3. Dengue Fever

Vector-borne diseases affect us everywhere across the globe, particularly in hot, humid environments where insects have ample room to reproduce. Dengue fever, for example, has emerged as a cause of serious concern, spreading predominantly through Aedes mosquitoes. How human beings and such insects interact really drives the entire cycle of transmission—it demonstrates just how critical it is to examine both the local ecosystem and elementary biology. Urbanization and world trade have driven us in the direction of mosquito-infested regions, and consequently, dengue has spread in areas that did not expect to ever experience it. Controlling it gets complicated because the mosquitos are so adaptable and the virus in all its variants can create outbreaks that overwhelm at times our health infrastructures. More often than not, this problem requires greater than one approach, ranging from pest control and education among communities to systems of surveillance that can spring into operation when new dangers emerge (Piret & Boivin, 2021). Consider dengue fever, for example. You can observe the delicate balance between human behavior and the wildlife realm—even where the sole direct animal actors are the mosquitoes themselves. Yes, the dengue virus does not hide in a reservoir animal apart from its vector mosquitoes, yet we classify it with vector-borne zoonoses because it relies on both vertebrate and these arthropod hosts. Environmental changes such as deforestation, climate oscillations, and humans encroaching into uncultivated environments are altering mosquitoes' behavior and populations in non-predictive ways. In general, all this mix of human behaviors and nature's vagaries provides the perfect background for diseases to emerge and re-emerge. In effect, dengue fever illustrates the interdependence of human, animal, and environmental health so much so that it would be obvious now that we require more concerted surveillance and control strategies, really along the lines of the One Health philosophy (Rahman et al., 2020). Controlling dengue today involves thinking out of the box in diagnostics, mosquito biology, and even vaccine design. Difficulties still exist with so many infections asymptomatic and numerous viral strains being present simultaneously, which confounds both disease control and immunity. Couple that with the increasing insecticide resistance in mosquitoes and the burden of socioeconomic barriers, and control becomes that much more challenging to attain. In general, coming efforts will most probably rely on novel concepts, such as manipulating with mosquito DNA and deploying quicker tests—to catch problems early and ramp up our responses. Merging community participation, policy enforcement, and international collaboration into effective programs is crucial to alleviating dengue's burden. Such steps, with a generalization, solidify the imperative to have ongoing monitoring and preparedness for zoonotic and vector-borne diseases to keep future pandemics at bay (Rahman et al., 2020; Piret & Boivin, 2021).

6.5. Impact on Public Health

Healthcare in regions that have been torn apart by war and limited resources then becomes burdened with even greater stress when insects and wildlife spread disease. Groups trapped in instability—displacement, war, and shortfalls—then get exposed to such diseases in often not-so-clean-cut ways. Research has illustrated that diseases like leishmaniasis and dengue fever, to name two examples, strike hard at poorer males, with children and the elderly particularly vulnerable. It's difficult because the absence of firm, national data complicates planning focused interventions; without the figures, determining the appropriate course becomes even more clouded. Increases in infection rates over recent years tend to usually indicate that improved monitoring, prevention, and focused control measures are required to catch up with local social realities. In the end, this demonstrates how zoonotic and vector-borne infections exacerbate existing health disparities and add additional burden to already strained healthcare infrastructures, rendering more targeted research and resource distribution genuinely imperative (Koya et al., 2023). Public health interventions during the COVID-19 times didn't just set their sights on domesticating the virus—unintentionally, they ended up modifying the trajectories of other diseases in quite surprising manners. Lockdowns, quarantine, and distancing regulations, instituted to delay SARS-CoV-2, overlapped with a significant decline in many vaccine-preventable diseases, suggesting that reduced human contact and improved sanitation can indeed stem some spread. However, not all infection conformed to that model; some disease traveled by insects and some sexually transmitted diseases even saw a rise. In most situations, the effect of such policies appears to be highly variable based on a disease's pattern of circulation and the local socio-environmental context. This variable effect serves as a reminder that it is not easy to manage multiple infectious risks simultaneously – there must be flexible strategies that can accommodate a few unforeseen side effects here and there (Adegbija et al., 2021). When you step back from the immediacy of disease and death, the ripple effects of diseases that spread from animals or by insect bites really wreak havoc with social and economic life. Epidemics can interfere with work, overwhelm healthcare services and trap communities into poverty cycles, particularly in areas where money and resources are already short. All too frequently, the most disadvantaged are those communities already at the margins since restricted access to care and education slows down early diagnosis and treatment. Additionally, addressing host animals and improving our environments require a collaborative, inter-sectorial response that involves bringing together expertise from veterinary, environmental, and human health disciplines, albeit sometimes a little clunky. The ongoing rise and return of these pathogens clearly signal the need for strong surveillance systems and focused public health actions to smooth out long-term societal impacts. Embracing a broad One Health perspective that ties several fields together seems pretty crucial if we're going to protect public welfare and push for fairer health outcomes worldwide (Adegbija et al., 2021; Koya et al., 2023) (Figure 6.11).

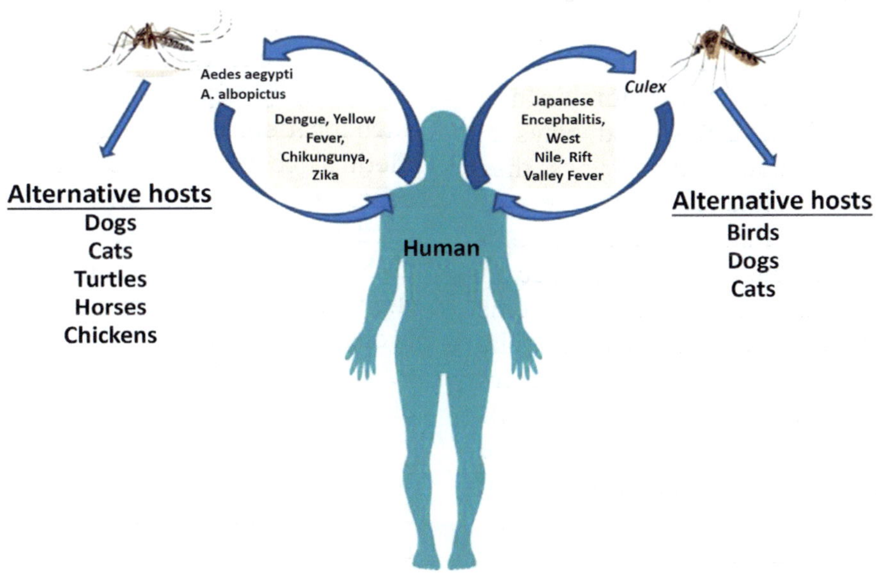

Figure 6.11. Zoonotic cycle of mosquito-borne arboviruses involving human.

Source: Sharma, P. (2018). *Zoonotic Cycle of Arboviruses.*

6.5.1. Global Health Implications

We exist in a more interconnected world than ever, and that proximity allows diseases , those that transmit from animals to humans and by annoying insects, travel across borders nearly at the speed of light. It's not just our own wellness that's at risk; animals and entire ecosystems are affected, and that, in turn, disrupts economies and communities worldwide. Consider canine babesiosis, for example. How it disrupts an animal's regular metabolism indicates how complicated and unruly host-pathogen conflicts become, with effects radiating to agriculture and livestock industries

(Kuleš et al., 2025). Such a situation makes it quite evident: we need mechanisms that do not merely confine themselves to one discipline but combine both veterinary and human health knowledge to detect outbreaks before they get out of control. And when you notice how mosquitoes rapidly evolve to fit changing circumstances, the task of containing disease only becomes more difficult, a reminder that we have to have a worldwide plan that examines all sides from biology all the way through to the environment. Environmental changes are spiking a wrench into the aged practices we knew disease. Climate changes, cities spreading into nature, and forests disappearing all bring humans closer to wild animals and the disease vectors that inhabit them. Mosquitoes are a prime example of this trend; as they migrate into new areas due to fluctuating temperatures and humidity, they spread their domain and keep us guessing (Bera, 2025). Old ways of combating these pests usually don't work, they sometimes result in resistance or hidden side effects in nature. A combination of a little old-fashioned ecological sense with more recent genetic and biological weapons usually seems to be the best route in most situations. The continuously changing context of both vectors and their environments means that public health regulation must be adaptable, prepared to respond to new, emerging pressures without becoming overly mired in inflexible planning. Health systems everywhere are creaking under the pressure as zoonotic and vector-borne diseases emerge and re-emerge in unexpected patterns our outdated infrastructures were not equipped to manage. The economic impact is wide-ranging, from rampant medical expenses and lost hours to significant disruptions in commerce and travel—problems that strike poor and middle-income nations even more severely, where disease surveillance isn't as comprehensive. Understanding how pathogens break down substances in hosts, like the insights we get from studying babesiosis, can help us craft targeted tests and treatments that not only ease the disease but also slow its spread (Kuleš et al., 2025). At the same time, weaving in lessons learned from examining insect carriers lets us better predict where the next outbreak might hit and fine-tune our defenses (Bera, 2025). Overall, adopting this sort of integrated, wide-ranging approach is critical to enhancing our preparedness and resilience in a world where these threats from disease are increasingly linked with our daily lives.

6.5.2. Economic Burden of Diseases

Zoonotic and vector-borne diseases affect not only community health—they play havoc with local economies. High hospital costs, lost workdays, and decreased tourism or even trade embargoes appear when outbreaks such as Oropouche fever occur in Latin America, occasionally crippling thousands. Individuals in such locations end up paying not only the direct medical costs but also the insidious indirect costs, lost income and compromised labor capacity. Spatial models even suggest as many as five million individuals could be exposed to the virus, a rather serious warning for tropical areas already on pins and needles (Romero et al., 2023). The economic implications of it all become even fuzzier when natural habitats contract, such as with declining vegetation; these changes remind us how intertwined our environment and healthcare loads are. Identifying these enmeshed economic impacts is essential for constructing prevention and response strategies that really do work. Once you drill into the figures, the disproportionate burden of disease expenses raises some severe questions regarding fairness and how we distribute our assets. In general, areas such as the WHO Eastern Mediterranean reflect a harder hit among those who are already in disadvantage—limited access to healthcare and poor living situations only expose them further to these diseases. It's a cycle of poverty; poor communities experience greater health issues further have fewer resources to pay for the costs.

Concurrently, the fact that some populations—let's say, children fighting leishmaniasis or elderly individuals fighting dengue fever, and even certain male populations—are disproportionately affected further clouds overall productivity and household budgets. Although cases of disease are clearly increasing, patchy studies and lacking socioeconomic information prevent us from comprehensively knowing the economic cost. Especially, investing in wide-ranging research that encompasses everybody is crucial to truly pin down and alleviate the additional burden placed on marginalized populations (Koya et al., 2023). Determining the complete financial burden of such diseases isn't a single-hemisphere endeavor—it requires an assortment of steady tracking, enhanced disease carrier management, and shrewd healthcare interventions. Direct expenses, such as treatment costs and managing emergencies, tend to rise in lockstep with the disease's ability to spread, so early diagnosis truly is important. Further there are the indirect expenses; the social upheaval and ongoing loss of productivity can persist long after the most obvious crisis appears to have passed, prolonging the path of recovery. To illustrate, models monitoring the Oropouche virus indicate environmental aspects, including the use and care of land, have a significant role in provoking outbreaks—implying the necessity of environmentally friendly management as a form of economic buffer. Failing to get sufficient attention from these factors does not only shoot up health threats, it also further exacerbates economic risks in hit areas. In the majority of instances, combining epidemiological knowledge with prudent economic planning proves to be the wisest decision to stretch resources and reduce the long-term effect of these health issues (Koya et al., 2023; Romero et al., 2023).

6.5.3. Challenges in Disease Control and Prevention

Controlling disease that leaps from animals to humans—and diseases carried by insects—is frequently hindered by a complex web of such factors as environmental changes, financial difficulties, and turbulent political landscapes. In areas like the Eastern Mediterranean, for instance, human interaction with animals, in tandem with weak health systems, combines to create a perfect storm of new and persistent infections. Warming climates, deforestation, urbanization, and population migration all combine to increase insect ranges and, honestly, increase our interaction with challenging pathogens. Predictions for outbreaks are damaged, particularly within crisis areas where health systems are already under strain. Despite having made observable improvements in surveillance and rapid response, chronic political turmoil and economic inequality oftentimes leave wholesale solutions beyond reach (Chughtai et al., 2023). Another hard nut to crack is that most of these bacteria are not only zoonotic but very flexibly accommodative to varying environments, such that total elimination is still more of a dream than a possibility. Consider *Trypanosoma cruzi*, the cause of Chagas disease, transmitted by more than 100 insect vectors throughout the Americas. This broad range of vectors, coupled with natural reservoir animals, makes transmission cycle interruption almost impossible. Yes, there have been achievements in preventing disease transmission through blood transfusions and organ transplantation, but combating the insect aspect of it is still a real challenge because the natural environments are simply too intricate. Consequently, public health measures have largely moved to the position of sustaining a level that is within our control as opposed to in pursuit of elimination, trusting that continuous surveillance and a catch-all group of control measures will keep transmission slowed (Rojas et al., 2022). Further there is the question of ensuring everyone receives health services, which only complicates matters when it comes to preventing and controlling disease. Screening initiatives for transmission of infections from mother to child, such as with Chagas—are commonly non-existent, particularly among pregnant women and of childbearing age, exposing glaring gaps in child and maternal care. Wherever these diseases are prevalent, there are scarce health facilities, economic barriers, and even social stigma that act as impediments to early diagnosis and effective, integrated treatment; all which weaken the effect of control programs. These systemic failures highlight the pressing demand for effective healthcare policies emphasizing affordable diagnostic testing, community awareness, and adaptable models of care. The resolution of these foundational problems is critical to translating scientific advancements into successful disease control and establishing a global resilience against zoonotic and vector-borne risks (Chughtai et al., 2023; Rojas et al., 2022) (Figure 6.12).

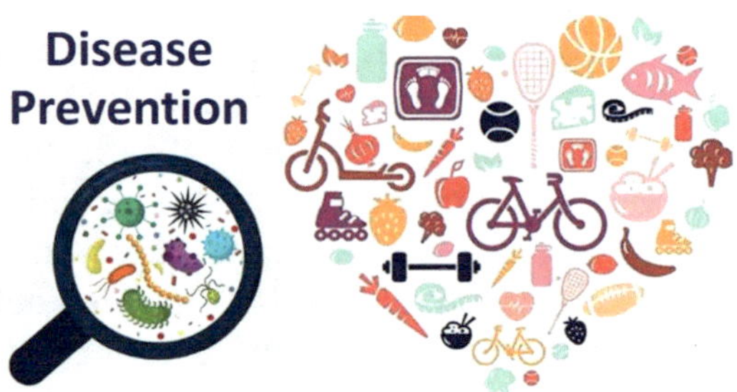

Figure 6.12. Challenges in disease control and prevention.

Source: Microbe Notes. (2021). *Disease Prevention Levels.*

6.6. Prevention and Control Strategies

Stopping animal-to-human diseases that jump and insect-borne diseases isn't solved by a quick fix. You have to target both the carriers and the bacteria. Cutting down on how many people get exposed to dangerous microbes—tampering with their environments, spraying pesticides, or even bed nets—is one sensible approach. Local knowledge is useful as well; reminding people to suit up with personal protection and steer clear of areas reputed to be high risk can be helpful. Early detection of symptoms and quick treatment is nearly as important. Consider Crimean–Congo Hemorrhagic Fever, for instance—medical professionals and individuals with those around livestock are severely at risk, so employing treatments such as Ribavirin with associated support measures illustrates the importance of combining medical treatment with outreach efforts among the public (Aslam et al., 2023). Determining precisely which insect species are at issue and understanding their habits is largely step number one to ending the cycle of infections such as filarial and nematode diseases related to it. Investigators frequently employ techniques such as PCR-based screening of mosquito samples to identify likely pathogens. In a Thai study, they found that certain Anopheles species were hosting Setaria parasites, something that indicated transmission routes nobody had looked closely at before. Observing how the evolutionary relationships between hosts and their insects sometimes mirror one another illustrates just how complicated these connections can become. This type of information allows us to customize control measures for microbes to suit particular groups of mosquitoes and their typical niches, assisting in better resource allocation and preventing outbreaks from getting out of hand in areas of endemicity (Siriyasatien et al., 2023). In most instances, monitoring the vectors along with targeted interventions constitutes the core of preventing disease transmission. Laws and cooperation across borders are fundamental building blocks when addressing diseases that migrate from animals or spread through insects. As a general rule, governments must implement policies that encourage public awareness, increase funding for research and vaccines, and establish clear plans for response to outbreaks. Just as crucial is to train health workers so they can treat infections safely and minimize the risk of contracting something in hospitals, particularly with hard diseases like

Crimean–Congo Hemorrhagic Fever. Combining veterinary and human medicine worlds—in what's sometimes referred to as a One Health strategy—assists in tracing animal carriers and our environments that trigger these problems. Because these diseases do not recognize borders, collaboration across the globe not only enhances the early warning system but also facilitates resource sharing. All these happenings together, even in their imperfectation, collaborate to contain the worldwide burden of zoonotic and vector-borne infections (Aslam et al., 2023).

6.6.1. Vaccination Efforts for Zoonotic Diseases

Working with outbreaks isn't as easy as using a checklist – sometimes you simply have to think outside the box. In most instances, combatting infectious disease involves seeing around corners, particularly when zoonotic diseases are the case; these are the diseases that bring with them animal carriers and dirty, challenging transmission chains. Vaccines, for example, come into view as an immediate answer: they're not only about preventing infections in humans but also about giving things time to slow down among animals, and that takes care of those dangerous spillover moments. Biotech advances have recently made it feasible to specifically design vaccines for home animals, wild animals, and us humans as well – targeting both the origin and the susceptible targets. If you snip the transmission chain at a few loose points, you assist public health in a very real, tangible manner, an idea that well suits the One Health philosophy bringing together people, animals, and the environment (Lio et al., 2023). Implementing these vaccination campaigns, however, is an entirely different ball game. It isn't only about figuring out the right bits of a pathogen to zero in on; you've also got to keep a watchful eye ensuring shots are safe across all sorts of species—what's effective for one group might not gel with another. Plus, getting vaccines to wildlife or livestock can be pretty tricky, and pathogens tend to shift over time so that regular surveillance and updates become almost inevitable. Combining vaccines with additional control measures, such as meticulous biosecurity measures and vector management—, an usually increase the overall outcome, particularly as climate change adjusts host and carrier patterns, increasing the chances of jumps from animals to humans. In most instances, continuous research and collaboration are the pillars for effectively adapting such programs to constantly fluctuating ecosystems (Lio et al., 2023).

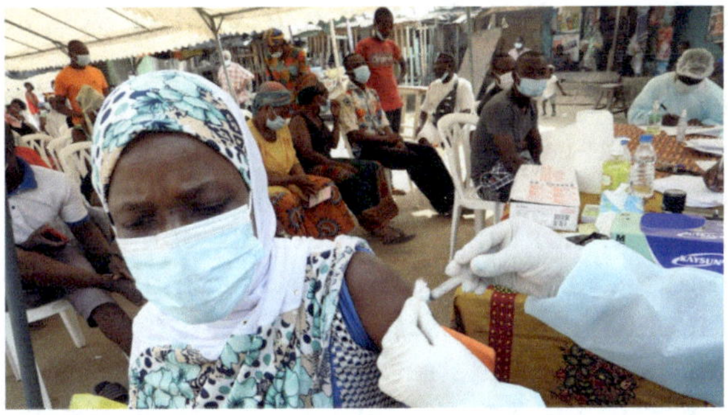

Figure 6.13. Vaccination efforts for zoonotic diseases.

Source: https://external-content.duckduckgo.com/iu/?u=https%3A%2F%2Fgdb.voanews.com%2Fcb700be9-2a32-4dc3-9f1b-343a860b90b9_w1200_r1.jpg&f=1&nofb=1&ipt=9c16d189cfed47bd29d7c3356382abcdedc8a32a502cb435217f7f9806fe8f89.

The need to nip zoonotic threats in the bud has never been so stark as in the COVID-19 experience. Emerging directly from animal reservoirs further racing quickly through human communities, it was, to be blunt, a wake-up call about the speed at which things can deteriorate. The rapid deployment of new vaccine technologies – mRNA and viral vector ones, for instance – demonstrated that rapid, creative action has the capacity to fundamentally alter the playing field when threats arrive. By and large, this adventure reinforces the imperative for close global observation, early warning systems, and vaccination work that crosses the animal-human gap, even when it sometimes seems like a puzzle with too many portions to solve. Improving vaccine infrastructure, whether in resource-rich areas or resource-poor areas, is critical to ensure equitable access and rapid response when new zoonotic or vector-borne threats emerge (Piret & Boivin, 2021) (Figure 6.13).

6.6.2. Vector Control Measures

Controlling animal-to-human jump diseases isn't so much a question of spraying microbe solution; it is largely a case of keeping parasites such as ticks, fleas, and mosquitoes under control. You had to observe the way these pests live—their habits, where they congregate, and what drives them—so you can determine an assortment of controls that break their life cycles. For example, removing any standing water can significantly reduce mosquitos, while cutting back overgrown underbrush may leave ticks fewer places to hide. Chemical controls, including the use of insecticides or acaricides, are frequently added to the arsenal as well, although they need to be used with caution to prevent the problem of developing resistance and causing collateral damage to the environment. It has been found, in most situations, that a combination of these strategies with persistent surveillance and grass-root participation helps to form an effective barrier to disease transmission. Recent advances in molecular biology have provided new means of monitoring such vectors with more accuracy. Conventional methods sometimes fail—species tend to resemble each other through minute overlaps, particularly in complex environments—so employing molecular hints now assists in identifying precisely which pests are at work and whether they carry any obnoxious pathogens. This is a refined strategy that enables the issuance of early warnings regarding new threats and assists in targeting interventions even when addressing wildlife, livestock, or people. In addition, molecular information not only explains patterns of distribution but also provides clues to any emerging resistance, informing modification of control measures in the majority of instances (Damian, 2024). Global health plans are more and more emphasizing that human, animal, and environmental health are interconnected. The One Health concept, for instance, promotes collaboration between veterinary, environmental, and medical professionals to address vector-borne and zoonotic disease in unison. In most endemic areas, strategies are crafted with a combination of meticulous policy planning, on-the-ground capacity development, and relentless vigilance—along with heavy reliance on outbreak responses, vector management, and community mobilization to have an impact. Not only does such an integrated strategy accelerate early detection, but it also enables the utilization of resources in a more intelligent manner. Broadly speaking, this comprehensive approach is an important ingredient in easing the world's burden of these diseases (Kodama et al., 2023).

6.6.3. Public Awareness and Education Initiatives

Controlling diseases that leap from animals or spread through insects begins by ensuring everyone is in the loop. In many densely populated developing areas, conventional myths and sheer misinformation tend to get in the way of real control. To illustrate, some Indians still utilize cow dung and urine as medication, even for COVID-19, which means there's an increased likelihood for diseases to make the leap across from animals. This tradition, rooted in age-old cultural and religious beliefs, continues partly because powerful actors support it and obvious, science-based information is not always present. Public health initiatives, therefore, must provide facts but also be mindful of local traditions and combating those false beliefs; influential actors such as religious leaders, healthcare professionals, and even media personalities can all assist in disseminating good information and preventing people from engaging in dangerous customs (Essar et al., 2021). Another significant perspective is how our relationship with animals, particularly our pets, is evolving. Nowadays, as increasingly individuals permit their beloved pets to share the bedroom or even the bed, there's a new risk of disease spread to contend with. Being a good pet owner now entails loving that intimate connection but also being clear and knowing that pets might be carriers of disease. The One Health principle, which interlinks the health of people, animals, and the environment, provides an effective means of transmitting this type of education. Vets and physicians, playing the role of facilitators, assist pet owners to identify means of enjoying their animal friends while reducing the likelihood of disease transmission (Overgaauw et al., 2020). To truly get the word out, awareness campaigns need to be specific to various populations who don't all enjoy equal access to healthcare or education. Rural areas, for instance, tend to struggle with poor testing and low health literacy, allowing diseases to fly under the radar. In most instances, the use of plain, simple language combined with culturally appropriate messages can make a difference. In addition, there has to be some amount of regulatory control so that misinformation is not spread—otherwise, media and political support could inadvertently be giving the thumbs-up to unsafe practices. Collaboration among the government, health professionals, educators, and community leaders is the solution to establishing trust and making these education initiatives sustainable. When accurate, respectful, and inclusive information is in focus, public health systems fare better at keeping outbreaks under control and promoting healthy habits globally (Figure 6.14) (Essar et al., 2021).

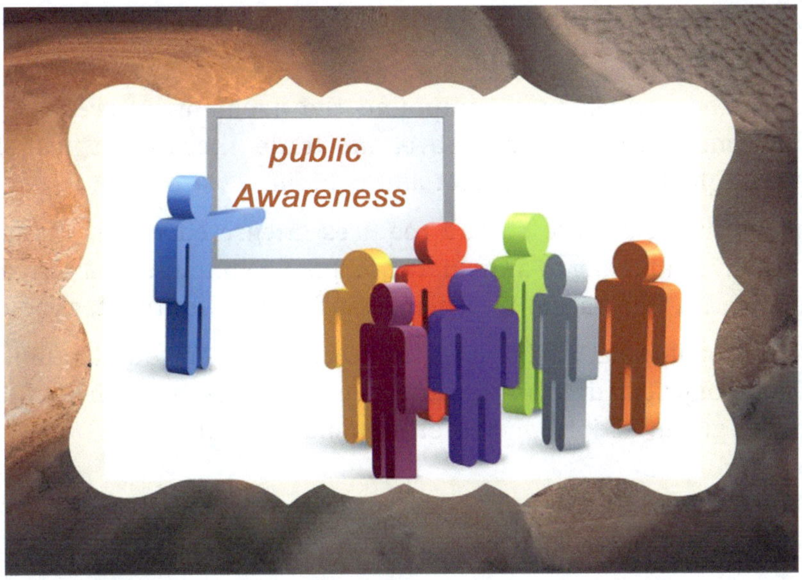

Figure 6.14. Public-awareness.

Source: National Public Trust. (2022). *Public Awareness.*

CLOSER LOOK

VECTOR ECOLOGY AND CLIMATE-DRIVEN DISEASE SPREAD

Vector ecology plays a pivotal role in the transmission of infectious diseases, particularly those spread by mosquitoes, ticks, and flies. Vectors act as carriers of pathogens between humans, animals, and the environment, and their survival, reproduction, and distribution are heavily influenced by ecological conditions. With climate change altering global ecosystems, the risk and range of vector-borne diseases are expanding at an unprecedented pace.

Temperature, rainfall, and humidity are key environmental factors affecting vector ecology. Warmer temperatures accelerate mosquito breeding cycles and pathogen replication within vectors. For instance, Aedes aegypti mosquitoes, responsible for dengue, Zika, and chikungunya, thrive in warmer and wetter conditions, enabling outbreaks in regions that were once unsuitable. Similarly, changing rainfall patterns create new breeding habitats, from stagnant water collections to seasonal flooding.

Climate-driven changes also extend the geographic range of vectors. Ticks that transmit Lyme disease are now found at higher latitudes and altitudes due to milder winters. Malaria, traditionally confined to tropical regions, has shown resurgence in highland areas of Africa and South America as temperatures rise. These shifts expose previously unexposed populations to new disease threats, straining fragile health systems.

Urbanization and land-use changes compound the problem by creating artificial habitats favorable to vectors. Combined with global travel and trade, these ecological shifts make vector-borne diseases increasingly difficult to predict and contain.

Addressing climate-driven disease spread requires integrated vector management, improved surveillance, and predictive modeling to anticipate hotspots. Community participation in eliminating breeding sites, coupled with innovation in vaccines and vector-control technologies, is essential.

Climate change is not just an environmental issue but a profound public health challenge. By reshaping vector ecology, it is driving the emergence and re-emergence of infectious diseases, demanding coordinated global action for prevention and control.

Summary

Human, animal, and environmental health all intersect in ways that make combating zoonotic and vector-borne disease a true knot to unravel. Evidence scattered here and there reveals that social, economic, and ecological enigmas all contribute to add up to make prevention difficult, and overall, those in vulnerable positions, particularly in areas experiencing humanitarian crises where firm disease data is difficult to obtain, tend to be most affected. Consider the Eastern Mediterranean Region for instance: much of the study homed in on just a few diseases and countries, so the larger picture is blurred and bespoke responses are unattainable. In the majority of instances, we must stretch out our gaze and delve deeper into population studies to truly gain an intuition of disease trends and distribute resources more equitably (Koya et al., 2023). It's only with that level of on-the-ground, intimate knowledge that we can cobble together strategies for each individual setting. Approaching matters from a One Health perspective also appears largely inevitable when combating these diseases. The notion that human health is intertwined with the welfare of animals and a healthful environment informs a combinationed, multidisciplinary effort—a reality reinforced by observations of waterborne insects in Florida's varied populations of microbes. As an example, the detection of pathogens such as Escherichia coli and Salmonellosis in marine mammals, fish, and even domestic livestock obviously suggests cross-species spillovers in the right (or wrong) circumstances. Such an approach prods veterinary, medical, and environmental professionals to collaborate, monitor disease hotspots, and predict outbreaks while attempting to nip the cause of these spillovers in the bud. With a holistic, cross-cutting perspective, public health systems are more able to anticipate emerging threats and safeguard human and animal health better (Jenkins et al., 2021). Overall, the intransigent challenges presented by vector-borne and zoonotic diseases require a multi-faceted, sustained effort in research, surveillance, and real-world intervention. Closing those existing gaps, particularly in those neglected areas—hinges on spending in high-quality, nationally representative research that engages socio-demographic and environmental dimensions. In addition, collaboration between sectors to implement One Health concepts can truly increase our capacity to identify, manage, and even prevent these conditions at a worldwide level. Ultimately, if we're going to see better health outcomes, we've got to accept the tangled nature of disease ecology and push for adaptive policies that keep up with the ever-changing dance between humans, animals, and their shared environment. Only by adopting this kind of sweeping, whole-of-cabinet strategy can we hope to make inroads into the mounting burden of zoonotic and vector-borne diseases in a manner that is both equitable and sustainable (Jenkins et al., 2021; Koya et al., 2023).

Reflecting back on the history of vector control is an interesting tale. In the past, local initiatives relied on a firm understanding of vector ecology and environmental adjustments unique to each location—initiatives that, overall, were reasonable for the given circumstance. Subsequently, about the middle of the 20th century, the focus essentially moved completely over to chemical controls. Such insecticides, hailed as a panacea, had a tendency to bypass the strict entomological and epidemiologic screening that might have provided them with a rock-solid foundation. Yes, all these strategies did reduce disease for a period of time, but relying so strenuously on chemistry ultimately led to annoying issues like insecticide-resistant insects, which necessitated reviewing long-term options (Wilson et al., 2020). Human activities, particularly agricultural, also have a significant part in the transmission of zoonotic and vector-borne diseases. Current research in Southeast Asia indicates that people working in or living near farms and plantations—consider oil palm, rubber, and even animal areas—have a higher risk of acquiring diseases such as malaria, hookworm, or scrub typhus. It appears the usage of these territories ultimately modifies the local habitat, creating a more hospitable dwelling for disease-spreading vectors. Notably, diseases which proceed along a faecal-oral pathway do not exhibit this phenomenon, showing the complex set of factors appearing to play out in a differing manner based on infection (Shah et al., 2019). Overall, these interlinked challenges, resulting from both historical vector control measures and current changing land-use practices—require a more holistic approach. Successful control today involves the integration of chemical and non-chemical methods, but only if supported by firm, ecology-conscious knowledge that takes local conditions into account. Concurrently, tackling how agricultural expansion reconfigures our landscapes is important, as such alterations can increase infection risks in unforeseen ways. In all probability, learning from past triumphs and missteps while acknowledging the complex effects of human endeavors may be our safest guess for a sustainable future in disease prevention (Shah et al., 2019; Wilson et al., 2020).

References

1. Adegbija, O., Walker, J., Smoll, N. R., Khan, A., Graham, J. E., & Khandaker, G. (2021). Notifiable diseases after implementation of COVID-19 public health prevention measures in Central Queensland, Australia. *Communicable Diseases Intelligence, 45*. https://doi.org/10.33321/cdi.2021.45.11.
2. Altissimi, C., Noé-Nordberg, C., Ranucci, D., & Paulsen, P. (2023). Presence of foodborne bacteria in wild boar and wild boar meat—A literature survey for the period 2012–2022. *Foods, 12*, 1689. https://doi.org/10.3390/foods12081689.
3. Aslam, M., Abbas, R. Z., & Alsayeqh, A. F. (2023). Distribution pattern of Crimean–Congo hemorrhagic fever in Asia and the Middle East. *Frontiers in Public Health, 11*, 1093817. https://doi.org/10.3389/fpubh.2023.1093817.
4. Bargues, M. D., Angles, R., Coello, J., Artigas, P., Funatsu, I. R., Cuervo, P., Buchón, P., et al. (2021). One Health initiative in the Bolivian Altiplano human fascioliasis hyperendemic area: Lymnaeid biology, population dynamics, microecology and climatic factor influences. *Revita Brasileira de Parasitology Veterinarian / Brazilian Journal of Veterinary Parasitology, 30*(2), e014. https://doi.org/10.1590/s1984-29612021014.
5. Bera, B. (2025). Mosquito ecology and disease transmission: Implications for global health and vector control. *Uttar Pradesh Journal of Zoology, 46*(8). https://www.semanticscholar.org/paper/bdafa99baf27722b6b43143130ad318c4e4270e0 (accessed on 7 May 2025).
6. Chala, B., & Hamde, F. (2021). Emerging and re-emerging vector-borne infectious diseases and the challenges for control: A review. *Frontiers in Public Health, 9*, Article 715759. https://doi.org/10.3389/fpubh.2021.715759.
7. Chughtai, A. A., Kodama, C., Joshi, R., Tayyab, M., Paiman, M. A., & Abubakar, A. (2023). Control of emerging and re-emerging zoonotic and vector-borne diseases in countries of the Eastern Mediterranean Region. *Frontiers in Tropical Diseases, 4*, Article 1240420. https://doi.org/10.3389/fitd.2023.1240420.
8. Crump, L., Martinoli, D., & Zinsstag, J. (2021). Links between biodiversity and human infectious and non-communicable diseases: A review. *Swiss Medical Weekly, 151*, w20485. https://core.ac.uk/download/551516193.pdf (accessed on 7 May 2025).
9. Damian, D. (2024). Navigating the landscape of tick diversity: Integrating molecular approaches for enhanced control measures. *Vector Borne and Zoonotic Diseases, 25*(1), 1–13. https://www.semanticscholar.org/paper/f14411e1b5dc7d585b994dcd61fbc5bee369c38e (accessed on 7 May 2025).
10. Decaro, N., & Lorusso, A. (2020). Novel human coronavirus (SARS-CoV-2): A lesson from animal coronaviruses. *Veterinary Microbiology, 244*, 108693. https://doi.org/10.1016/j.vetmic.2020.108693.
11. Essar, M. Y., Kazmi, S. K., Hasan, M. M., Costa, A. C. S., & Ahmad, S. (2021). The rampant use of cow dung to treat COVID-19: Is India at the brink of a zoonotic disease outbreak? *Journal of Medical Virology, 93*(12), 6471–6473. https://doi.org/10.1002/jmv.27258.
12. Hassett, E., & Thangamani, S. (2021). Ecology of Powassan virus in the United States. *Microorganisms, 9*, 2317. https://doi.org/10.3390/microorganisms9112317.

13. Hawkes, C., & Ruel, M. T. (2025). *Understanding The Links Between Agriculture and Health.* https://core.ac.uk/download/pdf/6288827.pdf (accessed on 7 May 2025).

14. Jenkins, M., Ahmed, S. A. S., & Barnes, A. N. (2021). A systematic review of waterborne and water-related disease in animal populations of Florida from 1999–2019. *PLOS ONE, 16*(8), e0255025. https://doi.org/10.1371/journal.pone.0255025.

15. Kapo, N., Zuber Bogdanović, I., Gagović, E., Jurković Žilić, D., Sukara, R., Adzic, B., Kadriaj, P., et al. (2025). Non-zoonotic tick-borne pathogens in Western Balkan. *Parasites & Vectors, 18*, 107. https://www.semanticscholar.org/paper/d457de875552e90a1b8c0f711cc9bf86c2b9564e (accessed on 7 May 2025).

16. Kodama, C., El Rifay, A. S., Badra, R., Abu Salbi, R., Abubakar, A., & Kayali, G. (2023). Operationalizing One Health: Strategic guidance for prevention and control of emerging and re-emerging vector-borne and zoonotic diseases in the Eastern Mediterranean Region. *Frontiers in Tropical Diseases, 4*. https://www.semanticscholar.org/paper/b03c695eeffa6d5ed82ede75e3ae21f59900d096 (accessed on 7 May 2025).

17. Koya, S. F., Abdalla, S. M., Kodama, C., Keïta, M., & Abubakar, A. (2023). Vector-borne and zoonotic diseases in the Eastern Mediterranean Region: A systematic review. *Journal of Epidemiology and Global Health, 13*(1), 91–107. https://doi.org/10.1007/s44197-023-00091-7.

18. Kuleš, J., Rubić, I., Rešetar Maslov, D., Efendić, M., Martinković, K., Pongrac, E., Šmit, I., et al. (2025). Metabolomics insights into salivary profile in dogs with *Babesia canis* infection. *Biomolecules, 15*, 520. https://www.semanticscholar.org/paper/5f24018092928c5a94ea3c71fff213df61287efe (accessed on 7 May 2025).

19. Lawrence, T., Takenaka, B. P., Garg, A., Tao, D., Deem, S. L., Fèvre, E. M., Gluecks, I., et al. (2023). A global examination of ecological niche modeling to predict emerging infectious diseases: A systematic review. *Frontiers in Public Health, 11*, 1244084. https://doi.org/10.3389/fpubh.2023.1244084.

20. Maquart, P. O., Froehlich, Y., & Boyer, S. (2022). Plastic pollution and infectious diseases. *The Lancet Planetary Health, 6*(10), e842–e845. https://doi.org/10.1016/S2542-5196(22)00198-X.

21. Naguib, M. M., Li, R., Ling, J., Grace, D., Nguyen-Viet, H., & Lindahl, J. F. (2021). Live and wet markets: Food access versus the risk of disease emergence. *Trends in Microbiology, 29*(7), 573–581. https://doi.org/10.1016/j.tim.2021.02.007.

22. Naserrudin, N. A., Culleton, R., Hod, R., Jeffree, M. S., Ahmed, K., & Hassan, M. R. (2022). Exploring the key anthropological drivers of and barriers to zoonotic malaria preventative behaviour in a community exposed to *Plasmodium knowlesi* infection in Malaysia: Protocol for a qualitative study with a participatory research design. *BMJ Open, 12*(6), e060866. https://doi.org/10.1136/bmjopen-2022-060866.

23. Ojeyinka, O. T., & Omaghomi, T. T. (2024). Climate change and zoonotic diseases: A conceptual framework for predicting and managing health risks in the USA. *GSC Biological and Pharmaceutical Sciences, 18*(3), 001–010. https://www.semanticscholar.org/paper/1825507ee0a7298d75e46077c6f61de73cf6d6ca (accessed on 7 May 2025).

24. Olival, K. J., Hosseini, P. R., Zambrana-Torrelio, C., Ross, N., Bogich, T. L., & Daszak, P. (2017). Host and viral traits predict zoonotic spillover from mammals. *Nature, 546*, 646–650. https://doi.org/10.1038/nature22975.

25. Piret, J., & Boivin, G. (2021). Pandemics throughout history. *Frontiers in Microbiology, 11*. https://doi.org/10.3389/fmicb.2020.631736.

26. Plowright, R. K., Reaser, J. K., Locke, H., Woodley, S., Patz, J. A., Becker, D. J., Oppler, G., et al. (2021). Land use-induced spillover: A call to action to safeguard environmental, animal, and human health. *The Lancet Planetary Health, 5*(4), e237–e245. https://doi.org/10.1016/S2542-5196(21)00031-0.

27. Rahma, N., Nuradji, H., Dharmayanti, N., Sendow, I., Adji, R. S., Saepulloh, M., Rusdiyah, R., et al. (2025). Historical and current perspectives on Japanese encephalitis in Sulawesi, Indonesia. *Veterinary World, 18*(2), 419–439. https://www.semanticscholar.org/paper/7db47dd12dc57b890591c5742c71947a86175945 (accessed on 7 May 2025).

28. Rahman, M. T., Sobur, M. A., Islam, M. S., Ievy, S., Hossain, M. J., El Zowalaty, M. E., Rahman, A. T., et al. (2020). Zoonotic diseases: Etiology, impact, and control. *Microorganisms, 8*(9), 1405. https://doi.org/10.3390/microorganisms8091405.

29. Rodrigues, C. M. C., & Plotkin, S. A. (2020). Impact of vaccines: Health, economic, and social perspectives. *Frontiers in Microbiology, 11*. https://doi.org/10.3389/fmicb.2020.01526.

30. Rohr, J. R., Barrett, C. B., Civitello, D. J., Craft, M. E., Delius, B. K., De Leo, G. A., Hudson, P. J., et al. (2019). Emerging human infectious diseases and the links to global food production. *Nature Sustainability, 2*, 445–456. https://doi.org/10.1038/s41893-019-0293-3.

31. Rojas de Árias, A., Monroy, C., Guhl, F., Sosa-Estáni, S., Souza Santos, W., & Abad-Franch, F. (2022). Chagas disease control-surveillance in the Americas: The multinational initiatives and the practical impossibility of interrupting vector-borne *Trypanosoma cruzi* transmission. *Memoria's do Instituto Oswaldo Cruz, 117*. https://doi.org/10.1590/0074-02760210130.

32. Romero-Álvarez, D., Escobar, L. E., Auguste, A. J., Del Valle, S. Y., & Manore, C. A. (2023). Transmission risk of Oropouche fever across the Americas. *Infectious Diseases of Poverty, 12*. https://doi.org/10.1186/s40249-023-01091-2.

33. San Lio, R. M., Favara, G., Maugeri, A., Barchitta, M., & Agodi, A. (2023). How antimicrobial resistance is linked to climate change: An overview of two intertwined global challenges. *International Journal of Environmental Research and Public Health, 20*(3), 1681. https://doi.org/10.3390/ijerph20031681.

34. Selzer, P. M., & Epe, C. (2020). Antiparasitics in animal health: Quo vadis? *Trends in Parasitology, 36*(1), 77–89. https://doi.org/10.1016/j.pt.2020.09.004.

35. Shah, H., Huxley, P., Elmes, J., & Murray, K. A. (2019). Agricultural land-uses consistently exacerbate infectious disease risks in Southeast Asia. *Nature Communications, 10*. https://doi.org/10.1038/s41467-019-12333-z.

36. Siriyasatien, P., Intayot, P., Sawaswong, V., Preativatanyou, K., Wacharapluesadee, S., Boonserm, R., Sor-suwan, S., et al. (2023). Description of potential vectors of zoonotic filarial nematodes, *Brugia pahangi*, *Setaria digitata*, and *Setaria labiatopapillosa* in Thai mosquitoes. *Heliyon, 9*(4), e13255. https://doi.org/10.1016/j.heliyon.2023.e13255.

37. Wilson, A. L., Courtenay, O., Kelly-Hope, L. A., Scott, T. W., Takken, W., Torr, S. J., & Lindsay, S. W. (2020). The importance of vector control for the control and elimination of vector-borne diseases. *PLoS Neglected Tropical Diseases, 14*, e0007831. https://doi.org/10.1371/journal.pntd.0007831.

38. Yan, W., Zhu, Y., Liu, W. C., Zou, C., Jia, B., Chen, Z. Q., Han, Y., et al. (2023). Discovery of aphid-transmitted rice tiller inhibition virus from native plants through metagenomic sequencing. *PLOS Pathogens, 19*(3), e1011238. https://doi.org/10.1371/journal.ppat.1011238.

39. Zhang, L., Lv, C., Guo, W., & Li, Z. (2024). Temperature and humidity as drivers for the transmission of zoonotic diseases. *Animal Research and One Health, 2*(3), 323–336. https://www.semanticscholar.org/paper/e588630b164e5d4ae8ca2f6fcf1dfa88a012b20c (accessed on 7 May 2025).

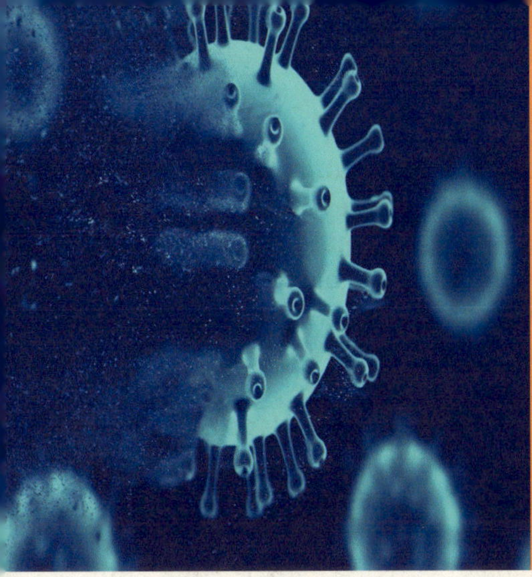

Chapter 7

ANTIMICROBIAL RESISTANCE (AMR)

Contents

Introduction

Modern medicine has been running in high gear, saving thousands of lives by killing off most infectious diseases—but now there's a twist called antimicrobial resistance (AMR). It's when microbes, in a rather sneaky twist, figure out how to evade the drugs we target at them. It's not merely an individual health glitch; it overflows into global health security, food safety, and even our general sustainability. As our usual treatments start to lose their oomph, infections begin persisting longer and are harder to deal with, which can unfortunately translate to more persistent diseases and increased mortality rates. Essentially, this problem requires an amalgam of expertise—not just from physicians but also from environmental and agricultural experts—to sort out and address all that drives resistance to work (Angelos et al., 2017). Recognizing these interrelated factors is usually the initial step towards creating strategies that succeed both locally and globally. Much of addressing AMR involves understanding that it's based on problems such as unequal healthcare access and environmental challenges. In certain remote locations—consider certain Cambodian rural regions where contemporary medical centers are not so much in pace—individuals resort to misusing or abusing antibiotics just because quality care is not easily available. Maladies like malaria, HIV, and tuberculosis (TB) subsequently become even more challenging to treat when drug-resistant strains surface (DeHart et al., 2020). This truly emphasizes the necessity of improving local healthcare facilities and implementing management systems appropriate to the region. And the domino effects on food security and the environment imply we require a collaborative effort in multiple areas. The One Health concept, which connects human, animal, and environmental health, is a clear illustration of this type of thinking (Angelos et al., 2017). Addressing all these intertwined issues appears to be paramount if we're to retard the growth of resistance. Getting a little deeper, the complexity of AMR arises from its numerous sources, not just from clinical overuse but also from how we produce and even contaminate our environment. The intensive use of antibiotics in agriculture has, in the majority of instances, facilitated resistant genes leap through the food chain and permeate natural environments. This situation requires more than a medical solution; it necessitates the establishment of educational and policy initiatives that bridge disparate scientific and social fields. Education and research, all driven by a One Health philosophy, are important to equip future professionals and policymakers with the expertise to balance food security with the maintenance of our medicines' efficacy (Angelos et al., 2017). Ultimately, only through collective, cross-sector efforts that lean into sustainable practice can we expect to stem the implacable tide of AMR.

Definition of Antimicrobial Resistance (AMR)

AMR poses an increasing public health threat. Microbes, bacteria, viruses, fungi, and parasites, can rapidly become adept at evading treatments that are intended to halt them. For the most part, our conventional drugs become ineffective because these bacteria adjust while in the presence of the chemicals intended to kill or hinder them. This isn't nature's oddity; our overuse and abuse of antimicrobials in medicine, agriculture, and even more general environmental circumstances puts these mechanisms into overdrive. The result? Increased periods of disease, increased health care expenses, and, in most instances, increased mortality rates—a complex network of results that demands new examination. At its core, AMR occurs when bacteria learn tricks to counter or simply bypass drugs meant to stem their growth. Sometimes, it takes a mere small genetic adjustment; other times, resistance genes—stolen from nearby cells via horizontal gene transfer—are involved. These changes reduce a drug's capacity to function effectively, which in turn disrupts treatment regimens and inadvertently facilitates the spread of resistant strains. Most importantly, these problems aren't limited to hospitals—veterinary clinics and public spaces experience this spread as well. Utilizing genomic technology, for example, presents a promising, if still nascent, means of detecting these resistance patterns ahead of time and adapting interventions accordingly (Jauneikaite et al., 2023). In most instances, this tech-facilitated surveillance is an optimistic but convoluted frontier in addressing a moving target. Though we've made strides in monitoring resistant bacteria in clinical and animal settings, the environmental side still remains a bit of a blind spot. Soil, water, and other natural reservoirs often become hotspots for antibiotic residues and chemical byproducts that help resistant microbes thrive. However, our knowledge of baseline levels of resistance in these natural environments, the perilous pathways along which these genes move, or even the transmission beyond recognized pathogens is at best patchy. In most cases, reconstructing a complete picture of AMR involves filling gaps between human, animal, and environmental health. Coordinated monitoring in these areas isn't simply a good idea—it's an imperative to be able to more effectively contain the international spread of AMR (Bengtsson et al., 2023) (Figure 7.1).

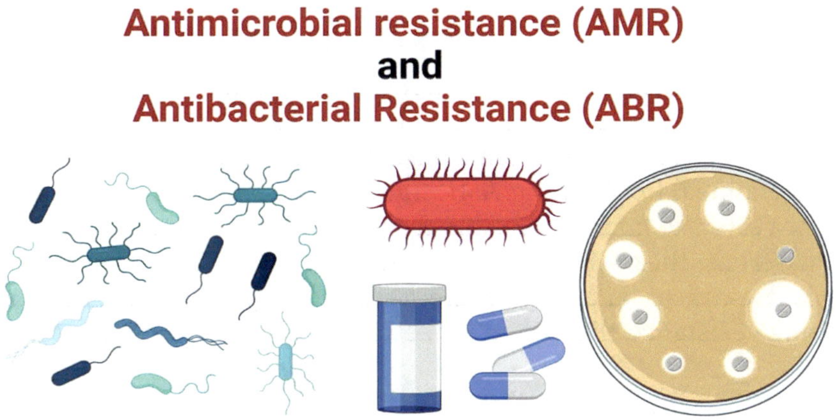

Figure 7.1. Antimicrobial-resistance (AMR).

Source: Microbe Notes. (2022, October). *Antimicrobial Resistance (AMR) and Antibacterial Resistance (ABR).*

Historical Context of Antimicrobial Resistance (AMR)

AMR has long roots extending nearly a century. Consider how the introduction of salvarsan in 1910 triggered antimicrobial therapy, shortly thereafter, Fleming's discovery of penicillin in 1928 revolutionized the picture, initiating what many people refer to as the golden age of natural antibiotics. During that whirlwind of time, with big categories of drugs emerging left and right, clinical practice dramatically shifted and fatalities due to infection fell appreciably. But paradoxically, this same breakthrough also pushed bacteria into evolving, gradually, as antibiotics spread, microbes learned to sidestep them (Hutchings et al., 2019). terms, the very success in preserving lives created a shaky ground for the emergence of resistance. Peeling some more layers, the tale of AMR isn't merely about medicines—it's also about genes and molecules. Contemporary resources such as the Comprehensive Antibiotic Resistance Database (CARD) have become essential for charting how resistance genes evolve over time. CARD, for instance, isn't just an archive; it's a living record that monitors unexpected patterns of gene behavior utilizing a combination of controlled vocabulary and detection tools. This tool, by mapping the constantly shifting resistome at the microscopic level, provides us with a glimpse into how pathogens continue to evolve as a response to antibiotic pressure (Alcock et al., 2019). In most instances, combining history data with contemporary genetic knowledge teaches us just how dynamic bacterial adaptation can be. Looking back on the mid-century optimism, the steady drop in fresh antibiotic discoveries and the rise of sturdier, resistant microbes show us the other side of the coin. That early burst of innovation eventually ran headlong into the fact that microbes are incredibly adept at adapting. Recent advances in genome mining and gene editing suggest a potential renaissance in antimicrobial discovery, nearly as if contemporary science is attempting to catch up with nature's own adroit ploys.

Nevertheless, completely addressing the AMR crisis involves keeping one eye on the past, from the early successes in antibiotic breakthroughs to the current complicated genetic databases (Alcock et al., 2019; Hutchings et al., 2019). In general, our future as drug developers and stewards will be one of reconciling celebrating previous achievement with preparing for continuing challenges.

Importance of Addressing Antimicrobial Resistance (AMR)

Antimicrobial treatments old school just aren't doing the trick anymore, disrupting contemporary medicine and shaking health systems around the globe. What were once-contained infections are now returning stronger and more resilient—often translating into longer hospital stays, higher medical costs, and more lives claimed. Confronting AMR now is the priority if we hope to keep antibiotics effective and prevent resistant microorganisms from getting even more formidable. Consider, for instance, bio-nanomaterials; these green, sustainable materials are based on natural material such as biowaste and plant extracts, and they could potentially provide the new, multi-dimensional approach to outpacing resistance that we need better than our current approaches.

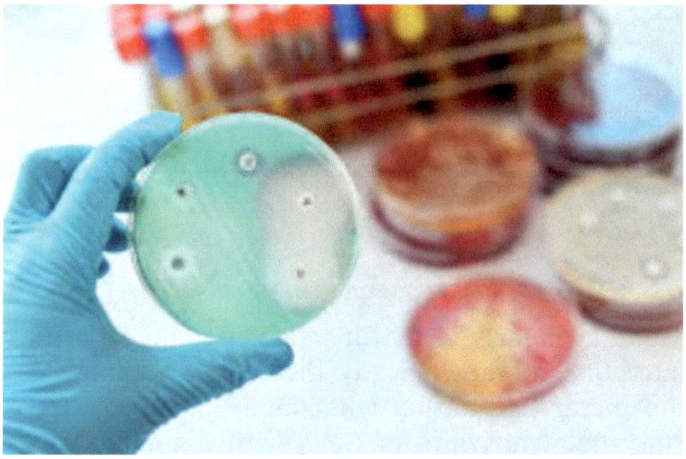

Figure 7.2. Antimicrobial treatments.

Source: https://encrypted-tbn0.gstatic.com/images?q=tbn:ANd9GcQAZcrcTO1gdrT9vyn0UUZPTKNe3 msymd5FZA&s.

Incorporating these cutting-edge materials into our treatment regimen could turn the tide on managing AMR, highlighting the necessity to experiment with new approaches (Barsola et al., 2024). Rapid, accurate tests are a big part of this fight—detecting drug-resistant microbes early can turn treatment around in a big way. Technologies such as surface-enhanced Raman spectroscopy (SERS), when combined with AI, emerge as surprisingly effective at detecting these dangers quickly. They allow us to look inside bacterial strains at the molecular level so that physicians can tailor antibiotics with a precision that is difficult to beat. In the majority of instances, the inclusion of machine learning and even deep learning enhances the validity and future-directed ability of such diagnostic processes. With such quick decision-support, we can also reduce unnecessary antibiotics use—a primary contributor to resistance accrual. In short, investment in these frontier detection technologies aligns squarely with public health objectives to curb the progression and reduce AMR's effect (Al-Shaebi et al., 2023). Beyond cutting-edge technology, combatting AMR is simply linked to our wider aspirations of sustainable development and public health security. If we allow AMR to get out of control, it might upset progress in surgery, cancer treatment, intensive care—you name it—where combatting infections is simply essential. And besides, the uncontrolled transmission of resistant bacteria literally jeopardizes the One Health concept, the one that connects human, animal, and environmental health. Adopting a more integrated, even patch-work style that includes eco-friendly strategies such as bio-nanomaterials is good for a healthier, more sustainable health system. Not only do they reduce toxic impacts and environmental contamination, but even save money by converting waste into a resource. In most instances, fighting AMR by collaboration between various disciplines and astute, agile regulations is the method to guarantee long-term health gains while pursuing our international sustainability objectives (Barsola et al., 2024) (Figure 7.2).

7.1. Causes of Antimicrobial Resistance (AMR)

AMR is increasing, and a great deal of that has to do with the way we use antibiotics, both in clinics, but also on farms. Too many people get too many scripts, take too little, or quit too soon, and that's just leaving some of the bacteria hanging around, developing resistance. In animals, antibiotics are hurled at animals to enhance growth and ward off disease, and this additional use contributes to resistance genes being disseminated among different bacteria. It's as if the drugs are selecting out the strong cookies—the survivors are the resistant ones. You can observe this in pathogens such as the ESKAPE bacteria (i.e., *Enterococcus faecium, Staphylococcus aureus, Klebsiella pneumoniae, Acinetobacter baumannii, Pseudomonas aeruginosa*, and *Enterobacter* spp.), which in most instances become huge pests in hospitals because they can withstand several antibiotics (Aruwa et al., 2024). Such a tendency gravely undermines what our drugs are capable of doing today, allowing these resilient strains to propagate and spread across the world. It's not just about abuse, however; bacteria get clever too. Most of them create these protective clumps known as biofilms—a sort of a communal shield that renders antibiotic therapy much less effective. Further, their quorum sensing, such as a whispery discussion among bacteria about how to construct these biofilms and escalate their defenses, enables them to remain robust even when the environment is unforgiving. Overall, all this bacterial "talk" translates to surviving in conditions that would otherwise kill them, even higher doses of antibiotics and evading our immune systems (Aruwa et al., 2024). When you combine genes with these DIY refuges and chemical discussion, you have a recipe for the rapid rise of multidrug resistance. All of this speaks to the necessity of new, creative methods rather than relying completely on our old antibiotics. The global cost of AMR becomes even more dire when you look at how badly many areas are at tracking it. In resource-poor areas, such as much of sub-Saharan Africa, missing data and poor lab facilities result in excessive deaths due to resistant infections. In most instances, the lack of robust infection control, the shortage of efficacious antibiotics, and the shortages in diagnostic centers all contribute to this self-perpetuating cycle—ongoing infections increase healthcare expenditure, which in turn discourages effective treatment. By and large, augmenting data gathering and microbiological capabilities is central to grasping these patterns of resistance and firming up brighter interventions. Without tackling these broader issues, our efforts to slow down AMR will keep missing the mark, leaving resistant infections as a major global health threat (Figure 7.3).

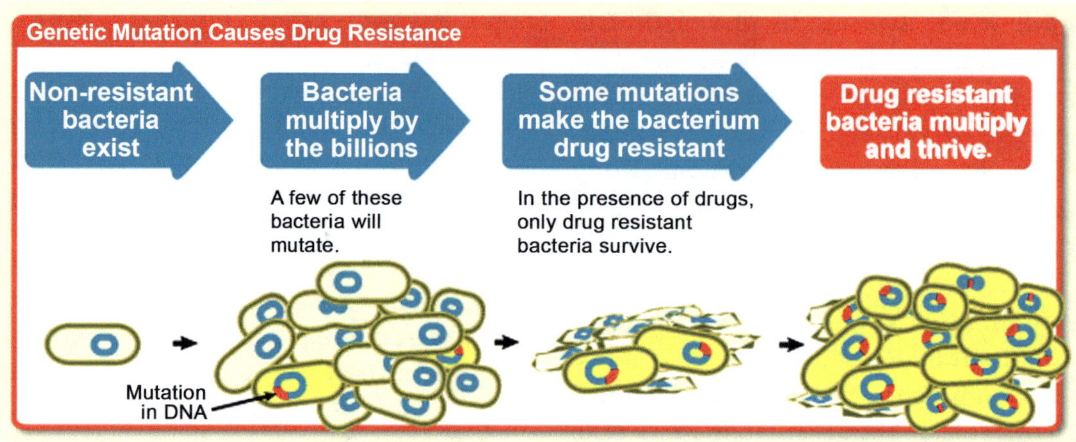

Figure 7.3. Causes of antimicrobial resistance (AMR).

Source: National Institute of Allergy and Infectious Diseases (NIAID). (n.d.). *Antimicrobial Resistance, Genetic Mutation.*

7.1.1. Overuse of Antibiotics in Healthcare

AMR is an increasing concern that leads us to reconsider how we use antibiotics, particularly in facilities such as hospitals and clinics where overuse is fairly prevalent. Physicians occasionally turn to these medications when they are not entirely certain of the diagnosis or feel pressure from patients' expectations, especially in high-volume outpatient practices. This excessive reliance on antibiotics not only exhausts their strength, but also accelerates the development of resistant bacteria. Numerous attempts have attempted to raise awareness among patients and healthcare practitioners about improved practices, but the outcomes prove to be all over the map. In most instances, merely increasing patient awareness does change attitudes toward antibiotic use, but without complementing those changes with targeted efforts on clinicians, prescription rates hardly decline (Aarestrup et al., 2015). Altering these ingrained practices in both the medical community and the public at large is a persistent problem, which makes long-term stewardship plans very difficult. International and national efforts to curb antibiotic use tend to run into roadblocks because healthcare systems and regulations are so diverse. The One Health concept—putting human, animal, and environmental health together, essentially says that combating resistance involves collaborating across many disciplines. terms, each policy measure requires a judicious test for cost-benefit and local feasibility, particularly in areas with low resources and a heavy disease burden. Monitoring antibiotic use and resistance trends does assist, but such systems cannot be independent without concrete infection prevention measures. All of these combined indicate that reducing antibiotic overuse requires a combination of strategies, each designed to its own social and economic context (Aarestrup et al., 2015). Depending on education initiatives or policy adjustments alone won't correct the overuse of antibiotics if the underlying issues, such as questionable diagnostic methods and unequal access to healthcare, aren't also being addressed. Quick tests that can differentiate between bacteria and viruses are still not utilized as much as they might be, forcing physicians to err on the side of caution with antibiotics. Cultural attitudes and long-standing beliefs about the efficacy of antibiotics persist among both patients and providers; too often, a quick clinic interaction isn't sufficient to dispel these myths. While numerous programs succeed in altering patient perceptions, these alterations don't consistently reduce prescriptions unless physicians are also educated and engaged (Bell et al., 2019). Simply put, combining better diagnostic techniques, widespread education campaigns, and stricter policy regulations is necessary to slow down AMR, even if it involves addressing a complex, multi-layered issue.

7.1.2. Agricultural Practices and Antibiotic Use

Organic material has been incorporated into fields for centuries to provide soil with a shot and assist plants in really performing. Manure, compost, and even sewage sludge, take important nutrients with them while helping the soil retain water and be more resilient as a whole. This additional organic contribution typically sets off a busy, diverse mix of microbes that assist in transferring nutrients around, leaving the soil in good shape. Yet things aren't always smooth; sometimes, unwanted contaminants like leftover antibiotics and stubborn bacteria tag along. These residues can, in most cases, open a door for AMR to spread, letting resistant genes sneak into food chains and affect human health. Smart, balanced management and treatment methods are needed to keep these upsides while preventing extra AMR worries (Alekhya et al., 2024). In recent times, alarm over surging AMR compelled most to reconsider overuse of antibiotics on the farm. Historically, antibiotics have been married to agricultural practice for quicker growth and agile disease management but in doing so also set the stage for resistant strains of bacteria to emerge in animal microbiomes further transfer into soils and water via manure. More recently, however, a change in direction towards probiotics is gaining notice as a more organic solution. Producers like *Lactobacillus fermentum* and *Bacillus subtilis* have, as a whole, proven to encourage an animal's immunity and even optimize nutrient uptake—keeping animals healthier and weaning them away from constant usage of antibiotics. To summarize, relying on these helpful microbes presents a promising pathway to stem the trend of antibiotic misuse, aligning nicely with worldwide efforts to address AMR (Uzoka et al., 2024). Despite these heartening shifts, the network of agricultural practices and antibiotic application still requires a wide-ranging, measured response to the threat of AMR. While organic matter addition does wonders for soil, they must be treated properly to reduce any remaining antibiotics and pathogen burdens before they are applied to the land. Simple methods such as composting or even anaerobic digestion can reduce the levels of harmful contaminants and slow the advance of resistance genes. Simultaneously, combining probiotic approaches to animal husbandry naturally enhances disease resilience, thereby reducing the dependence on antibiotics. terms, an integrative approach—one that balances safe waste disposal with sound antibiotic policies and new biological options—is necessary. When such strategies converge with continuous oversight and realistic policy steps, farming is in a better position to weaken its potential contribution towards advancing AMR ultimately for safeguarding both our nature and public wellbeing (Alekhya et al., 2024; Uzoka et al., 2024).

7.1.3. Poor Infection Prevention and Control Measures

Slippages in infection control in health care facilities drive the development of AMR. Clinics and hospitals, which are meant to be safe havens of cure, sometimes become unsuspected hotspots for nosy, multidrug-resistant microbes—often because they are overcrowded and have patchy hygiene habits. Inadequate sanitation, dubious sterilization of instruments, and poor isolation procedures allow bacteria such as methicillin-resistant Staphylococcus aureus and carbapenem-resistant Enterobacteriaceae to spread with surpriseful ease. In most instances, such conditions do not only accelerate infection rates but also facilitate survival and propagation of resistant strains of bacteria, thereby making treatment increasingly difficult. Increased interventions and hospital stays over long periods then mount additional pressure on healthcare resources and economic stability (Sharma et al., 2024). Indisputably, such inconsistencies in infection control make clinical challenges even harder while mounting increased public health impact. In low-resource settings, things still get more complicated. Inadequate infrastructure, absence of proper clean water, or reliable sanitation provide an optimal setting for resilient microorganisms, which further spoils efforts on a larger level to manage AMR. All things considered the glaring disparity between the well-stocked facilities in better-off parts of the world and poorly endowed ones in the developing world truly puts into perspective just how uneven AMR's effects can be—those locations with the highest fatality rates also struggle the most with infection control challenges. Such disparity suggests a need for immediate investments that enhance hygiene levels, accelerate all-encompassing surveillance, and implement stricter sterilization measures (Murray et al., 2022). Without those system changes, even novel antibiotics or vaccines could have their impact undercut by uncontrolled, rampant spread. Closing these gaps in infection prevention is really at the heart of global efforts against AMR. Fundamental measures, such as thorough hand hygiene, cleanliness of environments, and good wound care—can take a big bite out of hospital-acquired infections that then fuel resistance. There is also a requirement for continuous staff training, regular enforcement of policies, and smooth coordination with antimicrobial stewardship programs to ensure responsible antibiotic use. With the multi-factorial nature of AMR, prevention will have to exceed individual facilities and must be addressed by coordinated public health interventions with strategic resource management (Sharma et al., 2024). If infection control is not prioritized, we risk not only worse patient outcomes but also the ongoing degradation of antibiotic effectiveness, triggering a chain reaction that emphasizes the urgent need for systemic reform of infection control measures globally (Figure 7.4).

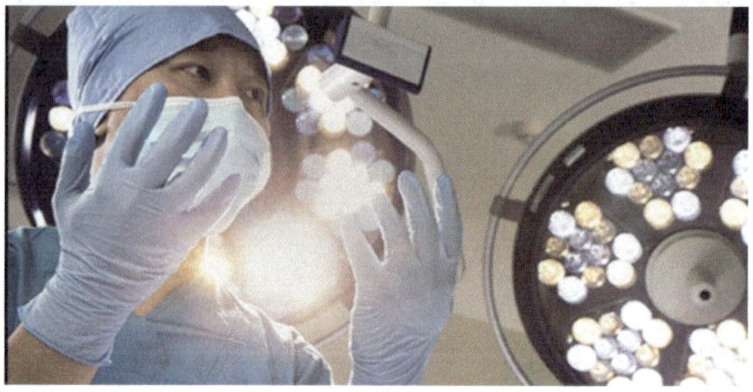

Figure 7.4. Poor infection prevention and control measures.

Source: https://cdn.who.int/media/images/default-source/temporary/ipc_hero.tmb-479v.jpg?sfvrsn=b9906ad0_3%20479w.

7.2. Mechanisms of Antimicrobial Resistance (AMR)

Microbes thriving against antimicrobials isn't a single-trick act, it's a complicated combination of genetic changes and molecular tricks. Bacteria, for example, tend to produce enzymes that degrade medicines; consider beta-lactamases as an example—they break down the beta-lactam ring of penicillin and cephalosporins, so the antibiotics simply lose their oomph. Further there's the strategy of modifying the very spot where drugs are meant to bind, a maneuver that's often triggered by mutations in the genes encoding those targets. These mutations tend to decrease the grip of the drug, allowing the bacteria to remain present even when subjected to antimicrobials. In addition to these intracellular modifications, mobile genetic components, plasmids, transposons, and integrons, silently transport resistance characteristics from one set of bacteria to another (Bha & Altınok, 2023). This relaxed gene swapping, horizontal gene transfer, can quickly spread resistance in a manner that treatment becomes a real headache. Another sneaky thing up the bacterial sleeve is efflux pumps, essentially integrated into the cell membranes. These pumps actively eject antibiotics, maintaining drug levels within the cell far below what is required to be effective. Very frequently, such membrane proteins turn out to be versatile, metabolizing more than a single class of antibiotic and doing so at the same time to promote multidrug resistance.

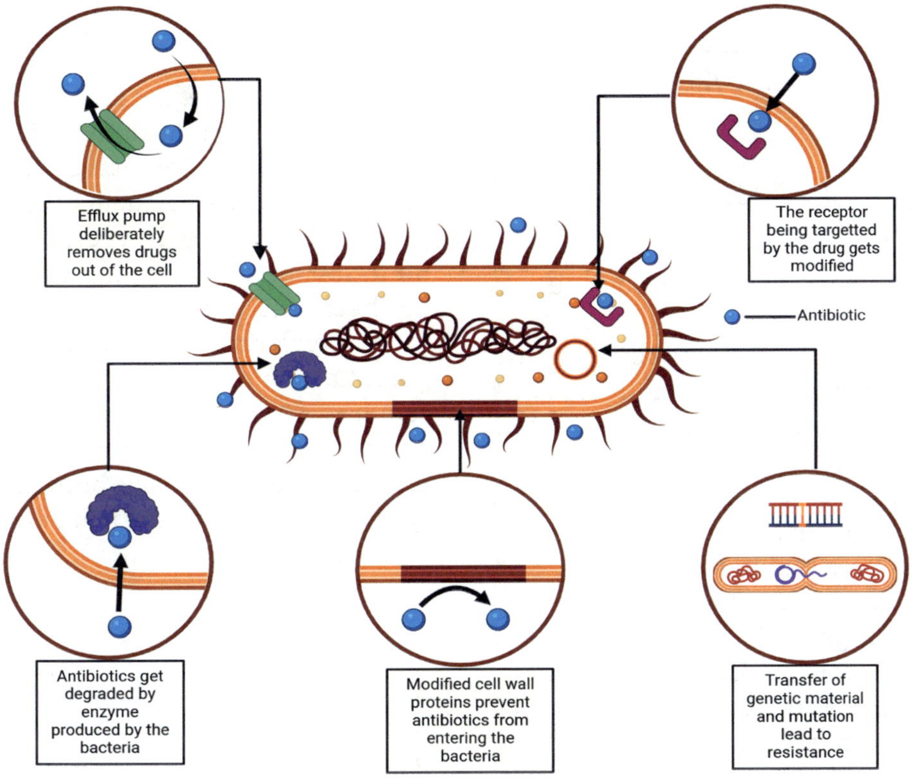

Figure 7.5. Mechanisms of antimicrobial resistance (AMR).

Source: https://cdn.prod.website-files.com/621e95f9ac30687a56e4297e/66718721791a19e491bd 4a53_V2_1718693601965_798b5e56-d953-47ac-b872-4a32724abb5b_HIGH_RES.png.

While this goes on, bacteria will also modulate their cell membranes—modifications in porin channels, say, will limit the proportion of drug entering in, an occurrence particularly prevalent among most Gram-negative organisms. Broadly speaking, the misuse and abuse of antibiotics—either in hospitals or on the farm—escalates the pressure on these microbes to master these resistance stunts. Uncontrolled use in animal feed is a telling example, since it inadvertently selects and disseminates the resistant strains (Salam et al., 2023). All of these resistance tactics, cumulatively stacked together, threaten the world's health very seriously. The genetic flexibility of microbes, fueled by spontaneous mutations as well as by gene exchange of resistance determinants through horizontal transfer, makes them able to respond quickly to antimicrobial exposure. In all but a few instances, this translates into the necessity for constant surveillance of resistance patterns as much as it does to create new strategies to outwit these microbes. Exploring the molecular basis of resistance not only helps to devise novel therapies, such as inhibitors targeting resistance enzymes or efflux pumps—but also highlights the critical importance of effective antibiotic stewardship and novel disease control strategies in both clinical and environmental contexts (Bhat & Altınok, 2023; Salam et al., 2023) (Figure 7.5).

7.2.1. Genetic Mutations in Microorganisms

Microbes can modify their character due to random changes that occur while copying DNA; these random genetic adjustments power AMR. Some of these modifications may be benign or even deleterious, but a few provide bacteria with that extra boost when drugs are present—essentially, a survival tip. The combination of various microbes within a host, as well as how our immune system and the external environment interact, ultimately forms a kind of playground for these mutations. For the most part, the handshake between our typical microbiota and our body's defenses can modify how frequently these mutations persist, rendering it a complex dance between microbe genetics and host responses (Hou et al., 2022). Occasionally, these genetic mutations play havoc with critical cellular functions, such as modifying drug targets, activating efflux pumps, or turning on enzymes that destroy antibiotics. See, these mutations tend to appear in the genes of important bacterial enzymes or membrane proteins, thereby making drugs less effective. Further, mutations in the gene control centers turn up the resistance systems so that bacteria can withstand doses that would otherwise kill them. And let's not forget the microbiome itself—it can bias the immune response so as to inadvertently support the accumulation of mutation, particularly in chronic infections where extended use of drugs allows such changes time to accumulate. This mix of microbe genetics and immune modifications is the secret to understanding why resistant strains continue to emerge at different body sites (Zheng et al., 2020). To truly get a handle on AMR, we must get into the details of how these genetic changes not only occur but spread among different microbe communities. Examining mutation rates in hotspots such as the gut or the respiratory tract can typically indicate how local host and microbes influence the development of resistance. In most instances, practices such as balancing the microbiota can potentially mitigate the pressure that fuels these mutation events. Merging strategies focusing on both the microbes' genetic aspect and their interfacing with the host holds genuine potential for addressing AMR. In general, this requires a holistic perspective that takes into account genetic alterations in that continuous, less-than-perfect dance between our immune system and microbiome (Hou et al., 2022; Zheng et al., 2020).

7.2.2. Horizontal Gene Transfer

AMR is now a genuine nightmare, compelling us to examine more closely how microbes exchange their resistance characteristics. Horizontal gene transfer leaps in, allowing bacteria to pass on genetic traits directly without adhering to the traditional parent-to-offspring channel. This clever trick facilitates the exchange of antibiotic resistance genes among a variety of species and environments, accelerating the emergence of pathogens that can ignore several drugs. It's not purely a hospital issue either—farms and fields, where plant care uses antimicrobials and pesticides, may inadvertently give these robust strains an advantage. Environmental microbes, animal-related microbes, and plant enemies usually find themselves caught up in HGT in most situations, and it just adds to the challenge of dealing with AMR beyond human medicine alone (Miller et al., 2022). Investigating where antibiotic resistance lurks reveals some surprising places, not only clinics, but also wastewater zones, wildlife ecosystems, and even oceanic environments. These are the zones usually overlooked, yet they prove to be the very transfer points and safe houses for resistance genes. Plasmids and bacteriophages, those traveling genetic hitchhikers, facilitate the transfer of these genes and aid bacteria in their adaptation under stress. In many cases, this gene shuffling boosts bacterial survival in all sorts of settings. Generally speaking, seeing how much the environment matters here opens our eyes to the full picture of AMR dynamics and points to the need for several surveillance and control strategies that look at both natural and human factors (Jian et al., 2021). Addressing the turns of horizontal gene transfer truly demands a combination of strategies to combat AMR effectively. It's essential to understand how co-resistance, cross-resistance, and gene control all work off of each other, oftentimes, resistance to one medication comes with the baggage of resistance to another, courtesy of interdependent genetic factors disseminated through HGT. This complicates treatment strategies and can cause prevalent multidrug resistance. Farm practices, such as intensive use of chemicals, also set off the pot, reminding us to handle pesticides and antibiotics carefully across industries. Having in mind the strong connection among human, animal, and environmental health, the so-called One Health approach, could be our safest bet in retarding the increase in resistance and preserving our antimicrobials for the future (Miller et al., 2022) (Figure 7.6).

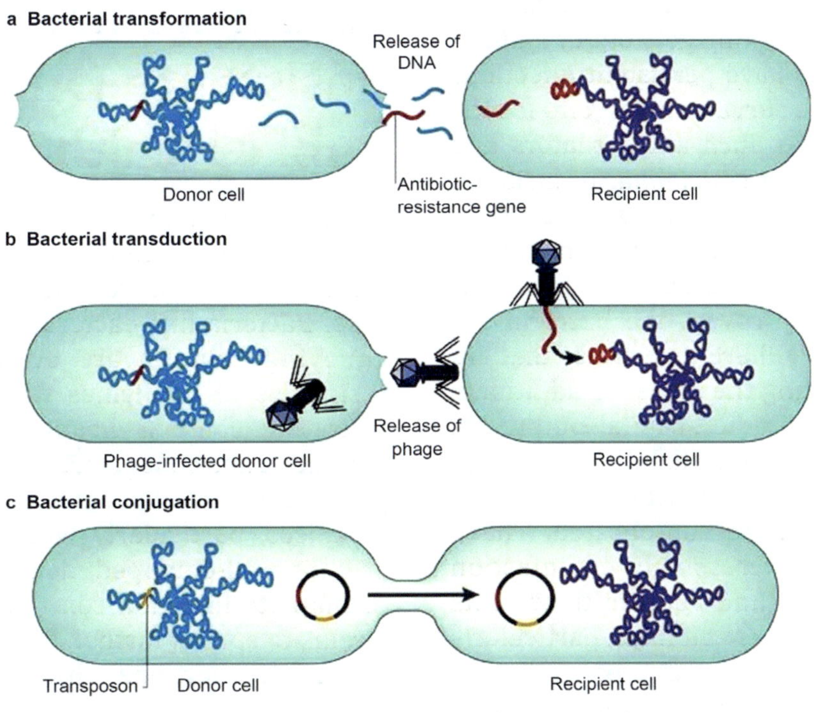

Figure 7.6. Horizontal gene transfer.

Source: Microbe Online. (2013, September). *Horizontal Gene Transfer Mechanism.*

7.2.3. Biofilm Formation and Its Role in Resistance

Bacteria have learned some smart tricks to weather extreme conditions. Occasionally they cluster together in so-called biofilms—small communities of cells encased in a self-produced goo that behaves like a shield. The slimy coating effectively prevents drugs from penetrating, so the bacteria have a cozy little lodging within. When times get tough, they flip from free-floating existence to adhering to surfaces, reducing their energy consumption while increasing their team defense. You can even observe them discussing through quorum sensing, a type of cell-to-cell interaction, and activating multi-drug pumps to eject unwanted chemicals, so antibiotics are less effective. Overall, constructing these groups provides them with a definite leg up over both drugs and the immune system (Singh et al., 2021). In hospitals, this biofilm thing gets out of hand. It is not uncommon to have persistent infections because the biofilms serve as reservoirs for the microbes on surfaces such as ventilators and catheters. *Acinetobacter baumannii,* for instance, is notorious for being able to produce dense biofilms and resist numerous drugs, making it difficult to treat and jeopardizing patient care. The biofilm not only covers the bacteria but also allows them to adhere to surfaces that are not even living, setting the stage for additional colonization and sporadic hospital outbreaks. Even conditions like the availability of glucose can fine-tune the amount of biofilm produced, so control is even more complicated. That's why hospitals rely increasingly on infection prevention measures and specific treatments intended to dislodge these biofilms, particularly in intensive care units (Gedefie et al., 2021). At a more specific, molecular level, the sweet exopolysaccharides that constitute the biofilm are central to both maintaining the structure's cohesion and fending off antibiotics. These molecules form the physical barrier that retards drug progression while also interfering with the signaling networks that govern biofilm activity. With quorum sensing, the bacteria choreograph activities such as activating resistance genes or ripening the biofilm, and in the background, small efflux pumps in the membranes strive to throw off antimicrobial compounds. This constant complex interaction among exopolysaccharides, cell-signaling, and drug pumps creates a layered barrier that truly challenges traditional methods of battling bacterial infection. It is in understanding these relationships that it is usually considered imperative to come up with new treatments to ultimately knock off those recalcitrant biofilms and address mounting resistance on a worldwide scale (Singh et al., 2021).

7.3. Impact of Antimicrobial Resistance (AMR) on Public Health

AMR is becoming more than a challenge these days, undermining our capacity to cure infections that were once approached with ease. Bacteria like bacteria, viruses, and other annoying bacteria are evolving, developing resistance to medicines that once worked, a shift that compels hospitals to have longer patient admissions, more complicated medical procedures, and heavier prices. In most instances, particularly where health facilities are not well-equipped, delayed diagnoses and incomplete infection controls enable resistant strains to spread further. It is shocking to know that as our first-line antimicrobials disappear, decades of medical advances may be undone, rendering routine surgeries and treatments that depend on these agents much more dangerous. Overall, according to experts, we require new medical advances as well as more effective infection prevention strategies to truly get ahead of this epidemic. In the absence of concerted international cooperation, routine infections can develop into diseases that simply cannot be cured, further overwhelming healthcare resources and leading to more unnecessary deaths. Farming habits and the environment also contribute a significant share to how AMR is transmitted. Overuse of antimicrobials in food animals, to drive growth or ward off disease—can push bacteria to adapt, and these resistant microbes often end up on humans through food or environmental channels. This complicated connection ensures that viewing human, animal, and environmental health as components of the whole—what some have termed the One Health strategy—is relatively essential for combating AMR. In several places, governments have already started to rein in antimicrobial use in livestock, hoping to slow resistance and its jump into human populations. To summarize, untangling these intertwined pathways is key if we're going to stop resistant bacteria from taking over and to preserve effective treatments for future generations (Almansour et al., 2023). Basic necessities such as good water, sanitation, and hygiene (WASH) matter more than we realize in mitigating AMR's effects, particularly in low-resource settings. To illustrate, in Nigeria, a shortage of good WASH facilities allows infections to spread without control, which usually translates to more antimicrobials being utilized—and that, consequently, fuels resistance. Conversely, areas that have stronger WASH systems, like the United Kingdom, experience tangible gains; fewer infection rates logically translate into fewer dependents on these drugs. This simple dichotomy reinforces why investment in robust WASH policies and infrastructure is crucial to breaking the vicious cycle of infection and resistance. In the end, all of us, from policymakers to the general population, must chip in, raising awareness, addressing sanitation problems, and promoting prudent use of antimicrobials to successfully halt the emergence of AMR (Ezugwu et al., 2024) (Figure 7.7).

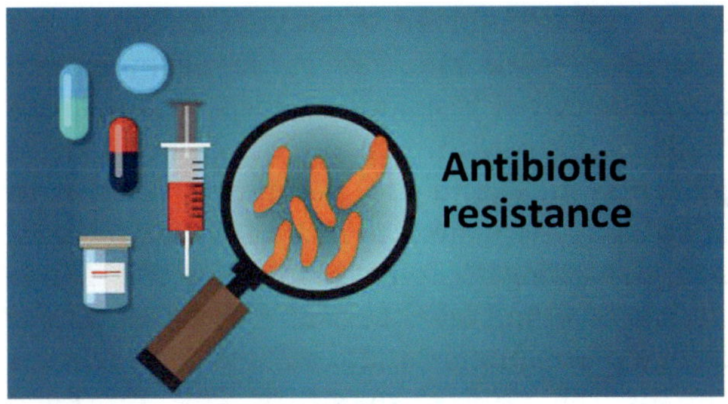

Figure 7.7. Antimicrobial resistance (AMR) on public health.

Source: https://encrypted-tbn2.gstatic.com/images?q=tbn:ANd9GcSo0vFUDP-2uJj7qzn-_5ifppK8kmNYbIc4LySrqf-k7SPB68H9.

7.3.1. Increased Morbidity and Mortality Rates

AMR is making it more difficult to treat these days, particularly in nations where there is already a strained health system. In most instances, once easy-to-control microbes now resist not only usual but also last-resort antibiotics. You understand, pathogens evolve rapidly, and bacteria such as Klebsiella and Pseudomonas are now resistant to medications like colistin, a drug previously depended upon to maintain infections at bay. This increasing obduracy between microbes is correlating with greater disease spread and an increase in severe cases, with few additional alternative treatments beyond just exacerbating the issue. In general, what begins as a minor infection or wound will become a lengthy struggle, rising mortality rates to those of AMR and warranting new thoughts on treatment along with more astute intervention policies (Garvey, 2023). In most regions of the world, including the Middle East, hospitals are seeing a concerning increase in the prescription of antibiotics. Evidence indicates that over half of inpatients receive antibiotic therapy; in Jordan, rates could even be as high as approximately 98.1%. Frequently, antibiotics are retained on board longer than they need to be after surgery, a procedure intended to prevent infection but one that, ironically, serves to promote the development of resistant bacteria. The overuse leads to more difficult-to-treat infections, so patients may end up persisting longer in hospitals, experience more complications, and, according to some reports, face a higher chance of dying from resistant bacteria. These trends place an inordinate burden on resources and overall tend to illustrate why improved antibiotic stewardship programs and strong national action plans are so vital (Haseeb et al., 2023). The cost of disease and mortality from AMR forces us to consider on a large scale. The creation of new treatments and a review of healthcare policies are not merely possibilities; they are necessities. Antimicrobial peptides are a case in point. They provide a multi-pronged approach to targeting bacteria and appear to act quickly, having the potential to lower the chances of resistance accumulation. But their introduction into daily clinical practice remains hindered by issues such as high cost of production, complicated pharmacokinetics, and even the innate susceptibility to protease degradation. If we were able to surmount these barriers, the global burden of resistant infections would decrease, and additional lives may be saved. For the most part, strengthening research on other agents, enhancing infection control and surveillance measures, and increasing stewardship activities appear to be the only feasible means of containing the soaring threats posed by AMR. These strategies combined hold the promise of reversing harmful trends and re-establishing effective means of controlling and treating infections (Garvey, 2023).

7.3.2. Economic Burden on Healthcare Systems

AMR's emergence is disrupting our healthcare systems globally, putting a huge economic burden that nobody anticipated. What was once a fast solution for infections now translates to longer hospital stays, more complex tests, and the requirement for expensive, last-resort antibiotics. Expenses skyrocket as hospitals rush to hire additional staff and increase infection controls—elements that add to the pressure, particularly in areas with limited resources. When the treatments fail to perform as anticipated, further interventions are required, which in turn redirects limited funds away from other essential services. In most instances, this resultant burden compromises the overall capacity to deal with both infectious and chronic diseases, as an indication of the imperative need for keen, strategic investment in combating AMR (Ahmed et al., 2024). Aside from the glaring medical expenses, AMR silently accumulates indirect expenses by lengthening recovery times and lowering labor productivity. Patients with resistant infections tend to experience prolonged recoveries and even permanent disability, which detracts from total economic production—national economies take the hit, especially in low- and middle-income countries. With more money pouring into combating these hardy infections, less funds are available for prevention and health promotion. And if all that's not enough, the extensive use of antimicrobials in agriculture and animal husbandry only complicates the problem further, making cost management even more challenging. This complex network of issues truly warrants an integrated One Health approach that addresses the socioeconomic origins of AMR and its far-reaching consequences (Ahmed et al., 2024). Not only are resistant infections a pest for general medicine, they're also undermining oral health. Dental procedures that previously functioned well now falter against infections that are resistant to standard antibiotics, increasing the prices for sophisticated therapies and complication treatment. The Global Oral Health Status Report consistently points out that oral diseases alone accumulate billions in direct and indirect costs annually. As dental infections become more difficult to treat, healthcare systems have to invest more in specialized treatments, an issue exacerbated in low-income communities where dental professionals are not easily accessible. Furthermore, the regular exclusion of oral health from universal coverage schemes postpones timely treatment, which only inflates the overall cost as conditions become more severe. Overall, integrating oral health into overall antimicrobial stewardship programs—and increasing resources correspondingly—appears necessary to mitigate these rising economic burdens (Figure 7.8).

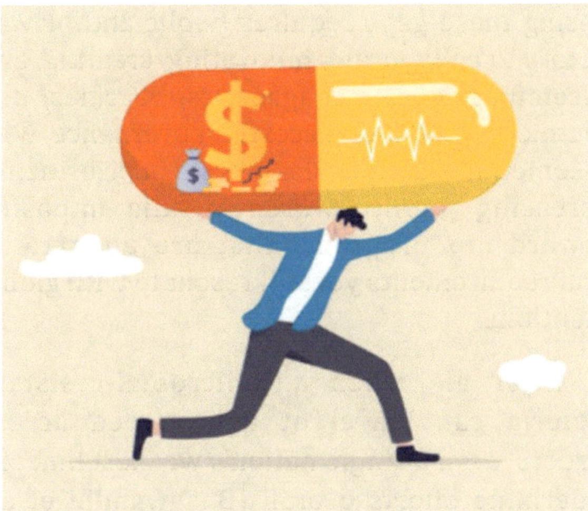

Figure 7.8. The economic burden on healthcare systems.

Source: https://external-content.duckduckgo.com/iu/?u=https%3A%2F%2Fwww.denefits.com%2Fwp-content%2Fuploads%2F2022%2F03%2FHealthcare-is-a-Growing-Financial-Burden-for-Patients.png&f=1&nofb=1&ipt=defa335e9cde90a6772ab1ee64ce4a938374d516fb3ef615125f505747b0536e.

7.3.3. Challenges in Treating Common Infections

Infectious disease control has become a literal headache recently as AMR slowly devours our first-line treatments. Physicians are now fighting infections caused by bacteria that simply disregard our standard antibiotics, and thus the old standards no longer work in the same way. Not only is this trend prolonging the duration of sickness but also increasing death rates—merely because we have fewer choices to treat them. It's also evident that not all parts of the globe bear this burden equally; low-resource regions tend to incur much larger death tolls associated with these resistant insects. In most such locales, labs and surveillance systems aren't adequate, complicating it that much more to get a timely, accurate diagnosis. Thus, clinicians are frequently left to settle for guesswork-based treatments that may fall short with these recalcitrant strains, exacerbating infection spread and increasing healthcare expenses (Murray et al., 2022). All this essentially amounts to a call for improved diagnostic equipment and more stable data gathering to inform treatments that truly fit the issue. Consider surgical site infections, for example, they reveal the extent to which resistant bacteria can destroy the consistency of our care. Previously, routine antibiotic therapy before surgery was a safe wager, but those times appear to be in the rearview mirror as resistant organisms multiply and lead to more post-operative complications. With these types of infections, patients can end up spending more time in hospitals, incurring additional surgeries, and, in the worst-case scenario, a greater chance of dying. The changing scenery of these resilient pests compels us to reconsider the way we approach surgical care, compelling us to adapt antibiotic use based on local patterns of resistance and specific patient risk. Hospitals now possess this tightrope act: they must effectively prevent infection while staying aligned with antimicrobial stewardship in order not to aggravate the resistance issue further. In the meantime, our own data at present aren't sufficient to unambiguously inform these modifications and leave a glaring gap in our knowledge of how to best treat these operating room infections (Menz et al., 2021). Outside of the operating room, routine infections are becoming a complicated labyrinth due to a broad spectrum of resistant microbes. Microbes such as *Escherichia coli, Staphylococcus aureus, Klebsiella pneumoniae* and some others have now become quite obstinate by being resistant to several broad classes of antibiotics. This process compels physicians to deal with complicated treatment schedules, particularly for prevalent conditions like lower respiratory infections, which, on their own, were responsible for over 1.5 million deaths in 2019 due to resistance. When treatments flounder under the weight of resistance, it not only makes things worse for the patients but also puts a heavy burden on our healthcare systems with longer therapies, extended hospital stays, and the need for costly backup medications. All these challenges reinforce the necessity for region-specific policies that advocate for good infection control, judicious use of antibiotics, and the promotion of new treatment and vaccine development to combat these stubborn pathogens (Murray et al., 2022).

7.4. Global Perspectives on Antimicrobial Resistance (AMR)

AMR isn't merely an issue of discrete patients or discrete health environments, it compels us to consider the big picture. Previously, antimicrobials were assessed primarily on their direct impact on a single body, but nowadays there is increasing pressure to value a wider context. Resistance mechanisms now extend far beyond single boundaries, combining human health with environmental considerations, agriculture, and animal husbandry. Consider, for example, the way antibiotic application in our agriculture sometimes triggers resistance that ultimately affects human lives, a complex, ecological web that needs to be addressed. Specialists in fields such as engineering, ecology, and veterinary medicine now find themselves working together in new and unexpected ways, as local decisions can have far-reaching effects worldwide. More often than not, addressing this challenge involves embracing integrated, global measures that combine wisdom from ecology, medicine, and agriculture (Bandura et al., 2018). Struggles with combating AMR become even more complicated due to how resources are disproportionately distributed. In many parts of the world, misuse and overuse of antibiotics in humans and animals exist in tandem with glaring deficits of essential treatments. In general, this gap accelerates resistance in some regions while depriving others of sufficient life-saving drugs. Closing these gaps requires public and private sectors to collaborate, innovating, creating, and disseminating new diagnostics, vaccines, and treatments globally. Successful governance, with its sometimes uniqueness, assists in prioritizing, increasing public awareness, and imposing stewardship programs that are adapted to local requirements yet still resonate with global intentions.

After all, when antimicrobial-resistant bacteria can travel at light speed across borders, even a single nation's weakest link can undermine efforts overall (Bhagwandin et al., 2017). Innovation in combatting AMR also has its own market challenges, frequently smothering new methods of treatments and diagnostics. Critics have suggested that existing research and development tends to fall short when it comes to triggering sufficient investment in AMR-specific solutions, largely because economic uncertainties and muddled regulation get in the way. For the most part, then, the way forward requires a global framework that combines extensive political support with active grassroots implementation. It could perhaps also assist in the utilization of intellectual property rights in innovative manners, perhaps integrating them within reward or prize schemes to stimulate new ideas. Furthermore, when all of the various stakeholders get together and exchange their knowledge, stewardship and access efforts can be greatly enhanced, ensuring that new tools come into practice. Addressing these challenges of markets and governance is central to opening the way for a sustainable, effective global response to resistance (Bhagwandin et al., 2017) (Figure 7.9).

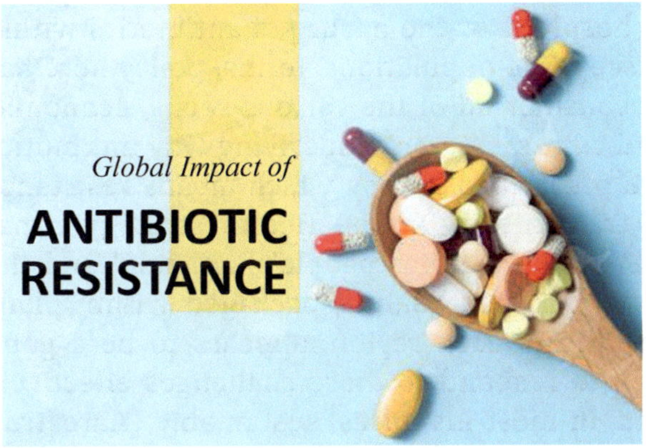

Figure 7.9. Global impact of antibiotic resistance (AMR).

Source: GoEdu. (2022, February). *Global Impact of Antibiotic Resistance.*

7.4.1. Antimicrobial Resistance (AMR) as a Global Health Threat

Antibiotics turned the tables in the 20th century. They cured millions and altered the way we deal with infection, but their triumph has ironically created a new threat—AMR. The use of these medications in excess, both in human treatment and agriculture, has pushed bacteria to evolve in surprising forms, allowing drug-resistant organisms to flourish. In hospitals and daily life, resistant microbes just keep coming back, weakening treatments and making diseases harder to defeat. Fewer available drugs, more virulent diseases, and exploding healthcare costs indicate just how bad it has become across the globe. We can lose decades of research into a postantibiotic world if we don't act quickly and collectively (Salam et al., 2023). It only gets more complicated when you look at how biology, society, and the economy all sort of swirl together to drive resistance. For instance, in animal farming, antibiotics are used not only to treat but also to enhance growth and keep future infections at bay, which allows resistant bacteria to grow and ultimately get a free ride to humans via food or the environment. Addressing this complex problem requires close monitoring under surveillance, following prudent antibiotic use, and exerting pressure toward innovative drug development. Brighter horizons such as bacteriophage therapy may be in store, but they must undergo a great deal of lab testing and new regulations before they can be applied en masse. Because various areas confront fantastically disparate problems from resistant pests, research agendas and policies must be both locally adjusted and globally aligned (Edwards et al., 2024). Stepping back to see the larger picture, AMR requires all of us to do our part, whether in public health, agriculture, or regulation—to slow and even reverse its growth. This involves establishing strict surveillance, restricting easy availability of antibiotics, and providing people with access to good medicines, vaccines, and fast diagnostics. Strict laws regulating the use of antibiotics in all sectors are important as well. Governments, physicians, scientists, and farmers really need to work together, despite the different issues they face in each location. Without sustained efforts and consistent investment, the acceleration of AMR could not only jeopardize effective therapies but also destabilize economies through increased health expenses and reduced productivity. Obviously, AMR poses a serious threat that necessitates urgent, cross-cutting efforts to make antibiotics effective for coming generations (Edwards et al., 2024; Salam et al., 2023).

7.4.2. Variations In Antimicrobial Resistance (AMR) Prevalence Across Regions

AMR doesn't appear the same in every place. Local practices in medicine, government regulations, and even the overall health of the economy all combine to create the differences.

In most places where health care is less robust, infections take hold and AMR appears more readily because fighting off infections is a challenge in the first place. Further there's the use of how and when antibiotics are applied, whether it's in treating humans or in agriculture. In general, in most low- and middle-income countries, the regulations on antibiotics are a little more relaxed, which can drive bacteria to become resistant in some surprising ways. And also, the infrastructure available to monitor AMR may be very variable, so the data tend to emerge mixed, making it more difficult to craft policies that are right on target. In general, these challenges require very locally attuned strategies, achieving equitable and efficient control of AMR worldwide (Aarestrup et al., 2015). The agricultural and food production world introduces an additional complexity into the narrative. Local practices and standards of safety contribute significantly to how resistant microbes are spread. For instance, food animals at times are a primary source for these persistent pathogens, and they may find their way into our diets through the food chain. More often than not, research has established that even minimal variations in the genetics of ubiquitous bacteria , e.g., different types of Salmonella present in pork , contribute to the asymmetry we observe in AMR from region to region. These genetic uniqueness influence not just how bacteria adapt and how bad they are, but also how easily they acquire resistance, frequently with the assistance of factors such as plasmids and phages. When you add in the various ways antibiotics are used in animal husbandry, what you are left with are local AMR patterns that render global solutions much more difficult. In short, knowing these molecular and ecological details is pretty crucial if we're going to develop measures that really fit the needs of each region (Barrett et al., 2019). Social and economic factors are another big player in creating these AMR gaps. In many poorer areas , where access to proper health care is tricky , people might turn to self-medication or grab antibiotics over the counter. This usually results in their misuse and can, in fact, accelerate resistance. Alternatively, whilst richer areas hold tighter to rigid controls, they have their own issues such as infections acquired in hospitals or the misuse of antibiotics within susceptible populations. terms, policy here has to consider all of the various social, economic, and cultural factors underlying why antibiotics are prescribed and by which means resistance is transmitted. A One Health strategy , that essentially marries people's, animals,' and the environment's health , packaged within plans specific to each region, appears to be a good way to respond to these challenges effectively and, in most instances, sustainably (Aarestrup et al., 2015).

7.4.3. International Efforts to Combat Antimicrobial Resistance (AMR)

AMR is a global headache that makes us abandon the customary lines of demarcation between public health, academia, and policy. Large organizations such as the World Health Organization, the U.S. CDC, and even the European Centre for Disease Prevention and Control have stepped in, announcing collaborative initiatives to strengthen infection prevention across the world. They attempt, in most instances, to put together disparate IPC efforts with AMR control strategies and make it unmistakable that the reduction of drug-resistant microbes is not only a medical concern—it's also a significant patient safety priority. Consider the WHO SAVE LIVES: Clean Your Hands campaign, for instance; it's a good reminder of how combined efforts across different regions and sectors can create a robust barrier against threats from AMR (Abbas et al., 2019). AMR's complicated nature compels us to create policy guidelines that can adapt to various political and economic contexts, addressing human, animal, and environmental health simultaneously. Existing plans emphasize judicious antimicrobial use, strict surveillance, and improved infection control practices, although the outcomes can be slightly different from nation to nation. This patchy success compels us to really rely on complete, evidence-based reviews. By introducing a standardized approach to testing policies and a One Health perspective, interventions that target the particular challenges of less-resourced countries can be revealed. In most instances, these considerate, context-informed strategies are the key to delineating stable policies that truly maintain AMR under control (Aarestrup et al., 2015).

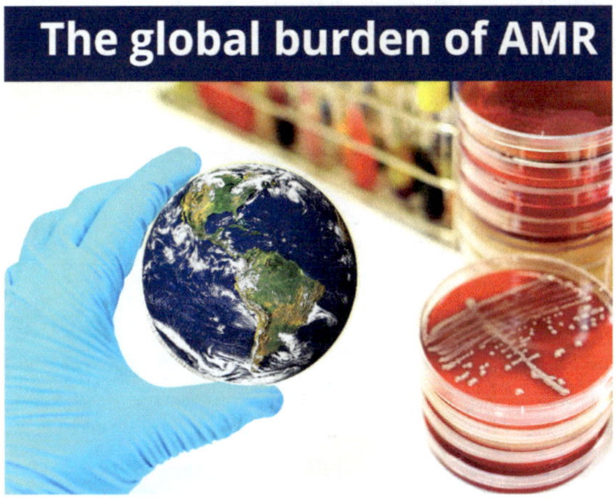

Figure 7.10. The global burden of antimicrobial resistance (AMR).

Source: AMR Vet Collective. (n.d.). *The Global Burden of AMR.*

When moving forward with international AMR initiatives, it is essential to shake up current networks and encourage fresh partnerships between scholars, policymakers, and health professionals. Extending the scope of IPC networks, and integrating antimicrobial care into wider public health strategies, could well result in concerted tactics for monitoring, researching, and battling over AMR. Granting research and development equal importance to prevention promotes the development of an equally weighted game plan—one that addresses the issues of today while watching the threat of tomorrow from emerging resistant microbes. Ultimately, strong global leadership continues to be essential because resistant bacteria do not respond to borders or remain isolated in one particular healthcare environment; they propagate about, requiring an ongoing, unified response (Abbas et al., 2019) (Figure 7.10).

7.5. Strategies to Combat Antimicrobial Resistance (AMR)

AMR is an issue that's worsening and needs a combination of strategies—you require active surveillance, new thinking, and some good policy shifts. Worldwide and nationwide, various programs are monitoring resistant microbes, sometimes quite innovatively. They employ technologies such as whole genome sequencing and bioinformatics to detect even subtle genetic changes that can generate resistance. All of that information presents health professionals an opportunity to tighten their antibiotic decisions and even see what is perhaps yet to follow. See, if you spot organized efforts like the US National Strategy for combating antimicrobial-resistant bacteria, then you are reminded that persistent political support and stable financing are integral. Without these rudimentary systems, our efforts might well be everywhere and nowhere, illustrating just how critical coordinated surveillance and collaboration across fields really are (Bristow et al., 2019). Concurrently, pursuing new treatments is categorically crucial to remaining one step ahead of these recalcitrant microbes. Scientists are looking to alternatives such as monoclonal antibodies, bacteriophage treatment, and even newer drug classes—topoisomerase inhibitors and fluoroketolides, for instance, which attempt to avoid the typical resistance pitfalls. These new approaches seek to attack pathogens directly, without further advancing resistance.

Vaccines and peptide mimics also appear as proactive measures that can reduce infection rates and reduce the use of antibiotics. Generally speaking, these advances lean heavily on continuous research support and require a kind of team effort that spans academia, industry, and public health to turn lab ideas into treatments (Bristow et al., 2019). Then there's the crucial matter of using antibiotics wisely. Overusing these drugs, both in healthcare and farming, is a big driver of resistance. Educating doctors and the general public on mindful, prudent antibiotic use can put less pressure on bacteria and break their momentum towards adaptation. Having rapid diagnostic instruments provides additional support, allowing clinicians to determine soon enough whether the infection is bacterial or not, which means there are fewer ineffective treatments. Overall, this combination of wiser behavior and improved technology demonstrates that fighting AMR is not only a science issue but also about effective communication and wise policy changes (Figure 7.11).

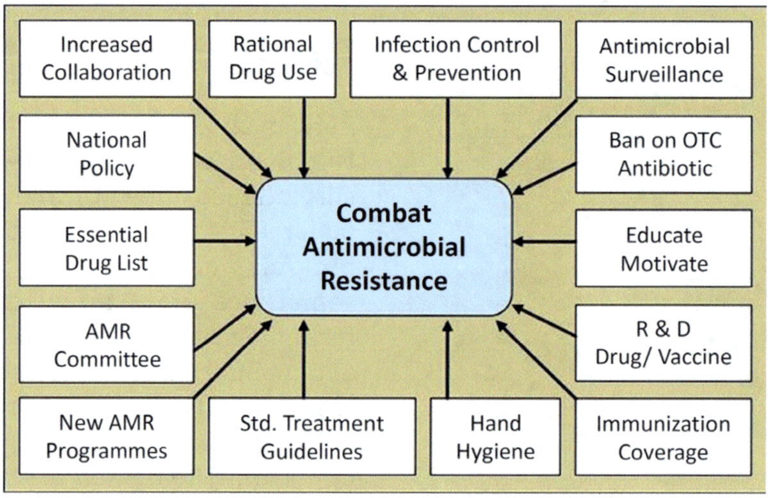

Figure 7.11. Combat antimicrobial resistance (AMR).

Source: Europe PMC. (n.d.). *Combat Antimicrobial Resistance.*

7.5.1. Development of New Antibiotics

New advances in the field of material science are rattling the battle against antibiotic resistance. Today, new hopefuls such as antimicrobial hydrogels are emerging to assist in coping with recalcitrant infections in hospitals and other healthcare facilities. They can be engineered to release various forms of antimicrobial agents—sometimes antibiotics, sometimes metal nanoparticles or even peptides, providing a type of multi-layered protection against resistant bacteria. In most instances, these gels are also CRISPR-Cas9 carriers, allowing us to target and edit genes that make bacteria resistant to treatment. Their inherent characteristics, including being biocompatible and releasing drugs in a controlled manner, allow treatments to be targeted exactly where treatment is needed and side effects kept low. Combining nanotech with conventional antibiotics, by and large, adds to our treatment arsenal and highlights how combining disparate areas of research can give rise to novel antibiotic concepts (Carpa et al., 2022). New classes of antibiotics are shrinking, and with growing numbers of multidrug-resistant microbes, we're truly compelled to think anew about treating infections. Lipid nanoparticles, for instance, are filling in by producing delivery systems that encase antibiotics within small liposomes. These systems not only serve to maintain the stability of the drugs and increase their bioavailability but also facilitate improved drug accumulation at the site of infection, reduce total toxicity, and protect against premature breakdown of the drug. It is fascinating that these liposomes can sometimes be specifically designed to penetrate recalcitrant biofilms and even merge with bacterial membranes, thus being effective against resilient infections such as MRSA. On the whole, by enhancing targeting and pharmacokinetics, these small carriers are a step in the right direction to revive our war against resistant bacteria (Ferreira et al., 2021). In today's war against AMR, looking for new molecules alone is not sufficient anymore. Now, we must adopt smarter delivery mechanisms that get the best out of the drugs we already possess. Technologies like hydrogel-based delivery systems and nanotech encapsulation methods are pointing us towards a new direction, a one that not only enhances drug targeting and delivery but also lays the ground for employing gene-editing technologies like CRISPR-Cas9 to switch off resistance genes. In the majority of instances, this fusion of pharmaceutical progress with genetics and materials science insights has the potential to produce treatments that are stronger, sustainable, and eventually successful. Overall, the future of antibiotic development seems to lie in this multidisciplinary mix, offering hope for better solutions to the global AMR crisis (Carpa et al., 2022; Ferreira et al., 2021) (Figure 7.12).

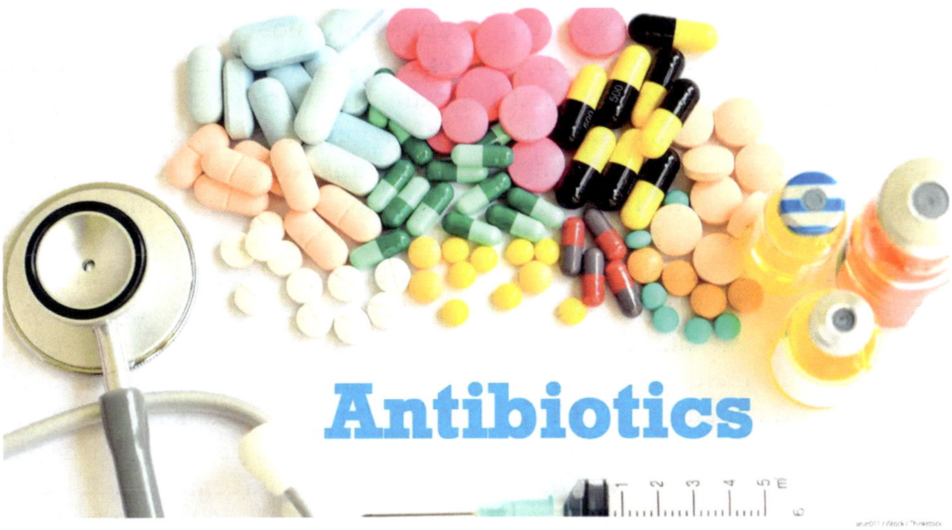

Figure 7.12. Development of new antibiotics.

Source: https://external-content.duckduckgo.com/iu/?u=https%3A%2F%2Ftse1.mm.bing.net%2Fth%3Fid%3DOIP.w4Ax-Q4pFQaGL85oGjHCEQHaEK%26pid%3DApi&f=1&ipt=2e8c23030e1f2a33d993a26c79a3ab058fda4353b1965668baf40977ed7d8dbb.

7.5.2. Implementation of Stewardship Programs

Tackling AMR is not merely about ad hoc solutions—it requires efforts that are dispersed far wider than the individual clinics. Stewardship programs, for example, have an important role to play by refining the way that antimicrobials are prescribed. They work to ensure the right drug, in the right dose, for the right duration of time, which tends to avoid resistance levels escalating. In reality, this results in physicians, pharmacists, laboratory specialists, and infection control staff all converging, haphazardly at times, to develop guidelines appropriate to the local context. Today, new technologies such as machine learning even contribute by predicting resistance patterns in real-time-like fashion, thus driving clinicians toward improved decision-making. These advance warnings have the ability to influence antibiotic selections and forestall abuse, combining clinical intelligence and technology to safeguard antibiotics and enhance patient care amid increasingly pervasive AMR pressures (Sakagianni et al., 2023). All the while, stewardship activities must be integrated into a bigger context wherein AMR is viewed as a totality—linking human, animal, and environmental well-being through a One Health framework. Global and national strategies generally emphasize that there has to be a broad-scale strategy, through coordinated policies, enhanced surveillance, and strengthened capacity in various sectors. There are, however, ample obstacles, such as limited resources, incomplete lab facilities, and insufficient trained personnel that generally hamper such initiatives. Most often, this implies scaling up financing, education, and leadership to establish long-term programs capable of adapting to local requirements. In brief, stewardship is only one of the important tiles in the mosaic of activities that connect data, rational drug use, and behavior change among healthcare workers and the general public (Mudenda et al., 2023). In the long term, success with such programs does not depend on technical fixes alone. It also depends on fostering a culture of responsibility and continued improvement in healthcare facilities. Monitoring on a regular basis how antibiotics are being prescribed, providing direct feedback to prescribers, and keeping this consistent with resistance surveillance are all involved. In addition, it is helpful to the greatest extent possible if these efforts can coordinate with regulatory guidelines, such as the AWaRe classification system, which classifies antibiotics according to their potential to drive resistance—so that antimicrobial access is stringently managed. Where science innovation intersects with company policy and consistent education, stewardship programs can reduce the misuse of antibiotics and stem the progress of resistant insects. These measures eventually serve as a cornerstone in curbing AMR globally and safeguarding public health (Mudenda et al., 2023; Sakagianni et al., 2023).

7.5.3. Public Awareness and Education Initiatives

Individuals are fighting hard against antibiotic resistance, and a significant portion of that battle relies on informing the public. And yet, strangely enough, much of the healthcare universe appears to be falling short when it comes to education. Local chemists, for example, have a rather important role in informing the use of antibiotics among patients, though apparently not everyone is clamoring to lead by example. In most instances, only a minority have maintained up-to-date training or incorporated fresh guidelines into daily practice, leaving something to be desired in patient consultations. Although pharmacists might function as go-to teachers, there is a recognizable imbalance in how they give tips on self-care or double-check antibiotic orders – a disparity that appears differently in standalone stores than in larger chains. Notably, most people surveyed appear fine with pharmacists taking a glance at medical records and speaking with patients about prescription information. All of this suggests a two-pronged challenge: to increase training among pharmacists regarding stewardship resources and to develop public awareness regarding sharing data, confidentiality, and cooperative care procedures (Hancock et al., 2015). Public education initiatives become even more complicated when it comes to initiating them since standardized stewardship programs aren't implemented consistently. Throughout community centers, though most know of national toolkits such as TARGET and SSTF , aimed at informing governance, policies, and even detailed clinical action plans – their implementation differs. In most cases, only around half of the participating organizations have functioning stewardship committees, and even fewer have allocated special staff to these programs. Sporadic review and unequal implementation of these toolkits tend to disperse the stewardship message, and thus induce uneven public communication regarding antibiotic usage; this, in turn, erodes attempts at curbing irrational prescribing and patient non-adherence (Ahmad et al., 2018). Simply put, an even stronger, more concerted drive for stewardship policies appears necessary to clarify and expand the ambit of these public awareness campaigns. Simultaneously, good public awareness can't just be left to healthcare professionals; it's also about creating communities that really understand the risks and consequences associated with AMR. Educational efforts must venture out of the clinical environment, extending to reach out with community-oriented, accessible methods that connect with people across the board. These initiatives ought to deconstruct why it's so crucial to use antibiotics properly, address typical misconceptions (and repeat important points occasionally to hammer them home), and emphasize that both patients and society are accountable in preventing resistance. And in most instances, having an open dialogue regarding data sharing and patient confidentiality is essential if we wish to instill trust. With both professional expertise and public know-how increasing, such educational strategies are capable of synchronizing local behaviors with international agendas for managing AMR, creating a more sustainable approach to managing antibiotics at all levels (Hancock et al., 2015; Ahmad et al., 2018).

7.6. Role of Research and Innovation in Addressing Antimicrobial Resistance (AMR)

AMR is not a puzzle you solve in one move—it requires a combination of new thinking that reaches way beyond typical healthcare solutions. Research and innovation power the initiative, igniting strategies and solutions that are as creative as they are practical. In India, for instance, the National Alliance of Medical Professionals on Antimicrobial Resistance (NAMP-AMR) illustrates how assembling specialists from various disciplines—and even opening up to policy contributions—makes for a more adaptable defense. Strong surveillance systems, complemented by enhanced laboratory work, enable new discoveries to be converted into practical approaches to infection management and the judicious use of antimicrobials. In the majority of instances, these initiatives do not only refine existing practices but also establish a configuration that can immediately mobilize the moment new trends in resistance arise (Karthikeyan et al., 2024). At the molecular level, scientists are discovering classes of antimicrobial agents that could potentially revolutionize the treatment of infections. Consider amidine-containing compounds, for example, they raise eyebrows with their peculiar structures and broad-spectrum attack against microbes. It's a reminder, truly, that small adjustments can give a kick to the efficacy of these drugs against resistant pests. As researchers sort out exactly how these drugs play havoc on bacteria, fungi, and even parasites, they're setting the stage for new-generation drugs that surpass the bounds of current therapies. For the most part, these advances indicate that continued innovation can hold promise for surmounting resistance as well as breathing new life into our global antimicrobial arsenal (Abidin et al., 2024). And it doesn't end with new medications. The ethos of innovation also appears in how we control and direct antimicrobial use through wiser policy and education. Evidence-based changes, such as refining stewardship programs, revising regulations, and even increasing public education, can shift patterns of prescribing and using antimicrobials in a way that slows down the development of resistance. Science is now intertwined with decision-making at both the national and global levels. Global cooperation and collective knowledge even ensure that best practices are continuously evolving, responding to new challenges as they arise. Overall, this dynamic combination of research, innovative thinking, and policy adjustments not only induces new scientific discoveries but also ensures those discoveries have practical applications in combating AMR (Karthikeyan et al., 2024) (Figure 7.13).

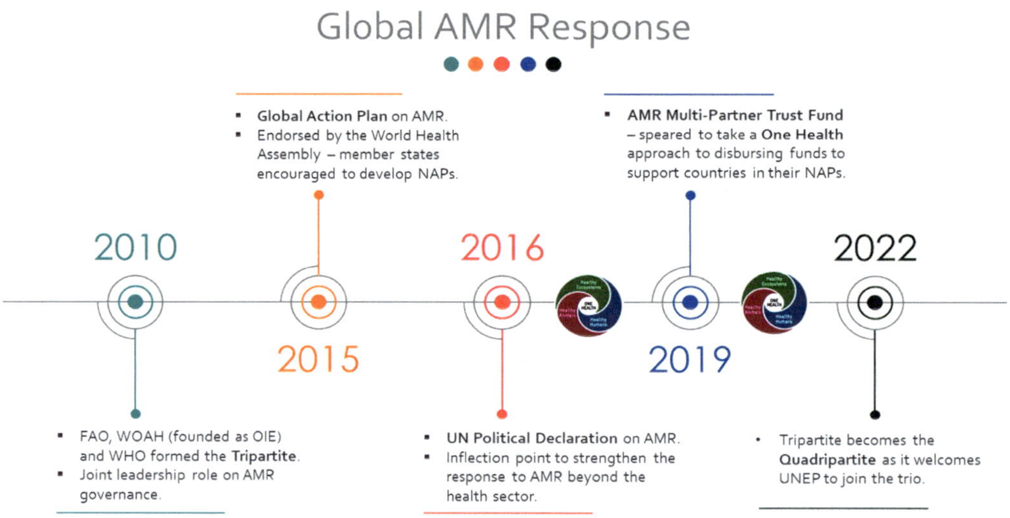

Figure 7.13. Role of research and innovation in addressing antimicrobial resistance (AMR).

Source: BMZ Health. (n.d.). *Timeline: Historical Aspects of the AMR Response.*

7.6.1. Advances in Diagnostic Technologies

Diagnostic technology has progressed a great deal recently, it's really transformed how we detect AMR both quickly and precisely. Rather than waiting on those slow, outdated culture-based techniques, we now depend more on molecular tests that detect resistance genes directly from a patient's specimen. With technologies such as PCR, Next-generation sequencing and even microarray analysis, clinicians can view resistance markers in hours instead of days. This rapid feedback usually serves to guide the right application of antibiotics, which in a majority of situations curbs those unnecessary scripts that drive resistance. And when such molecular techniques are married with clinical decision support systems, what happens is that the result is a shot in the arm for actionable insights to doctors. Generally, the velocity and accuracy of such breakthroughs represent a significant stride toward early treatment and tailored treatment protocols that, simply put, improve results while curbing the dissemination of resistant microorganisms. Not much on the molecular trail, biosensor technologies have now started emerging as a potential substitute for addressing AMR. These clever gadgets operate by sensing biological signals, such as bacterial toxins or resistance-associated enzymes—using biochemical processes that set off electronic impulses. That translates to point-of-care testing potentially occurring with virtually no additional lab equipment, which is particularly worth it in resource-scarce environments. By being able to identify resistant strains where they happen, biosensors assist in reducing lag time between diagnosis and treatment, ultimately keeping those pesky bacteria at bay. Technological progress in nanotech and materials science has, in the majority of instances, refined the sensitivity and specificity of such sensors, even permitting simultaneous detection of multiple resistance factors in a single test. This move toward decentralizing diagnosis gives clinicians the ability to make educated and timely decisions, a critical component in preventing the spread of resistance (Buhr et al., 2025). Placing these diagnostic advances within a One Health model truly emphasizes their widespread relevance to human, animal, and environmental health. Because antimicrobials are used so extensively in veterinary medicine and agriculture, it is equally important to be able to rapidly identify resistant pathogens in animals as well. The veterinary profession is now experiencing a change, with quick tests like in human medicine becoming more common, which supports early intervention in the management of livestock. The information from these tests also helps to feed global surveillance systems, monitoring patterns of resistance and guiding policy as well as stewardship programs. All of these, collectively, constitute an integrated method required to address the multi-faceted problem of AMR, as indicated in recent industry and academic discourse (Buhr et al., 2025).

7.6.2. Research on Alternative Therapies

AMR is accelerating these days, forcing scientists to look beyond our familiar antibiotics for new, creative remedies. Essential oils, for example, are under the spotlight because humans have been aware of their germ-killing ability for centuries. New research indicates that the oils can strike bacteria on multiple fronts simultaneously, a strategy that could stall how rapidly microbes can adapt to evade treatments. Lab tests often paint an encouraging picture, yet putting these results into practice is tricky—method differences and a lack of solid safety/dosing data in real-life settings stand in the way. In most cases, sorting out these hurdles is key if we're to use essential oils as helpful add-ons or even alternatives, especially for those stubborn, high-threat microbes flagged by global health experts (Romanescu et al., 2023). CombinationIncorporating them with our existing treatments could very well provide antimicrobial management with the boost it needs. In the meantime, apart from plant extracts, small proteins known as bacteriocins are emerging as heavy hitters in combating resistant microbes. Produced by ribosomes and primarily churned out by lactic acid bacteria (LAB), these peptides have an affinity for homing in on multidrug-resistant strains. You tend to hear strains such as Lactobacillus plantarum and Enterococcus faecalis mentioned more often—they're understood to be producing good quantities of bacteriocins, which can be utilized both for curing infections and making food safer. For instance, incorporating these peptides in dairy products like cheeses has reduced harmful and spoilage bacteria, which consequently reduces our dependency on chemical preservatives and daily antibiotics. Whether used as undiluted peptides or by infusing bacteriocin-producing microorganisms into a product, such compounds provide an adaptable pathway which might be employed both as defenders of foodstuffs and medicinal agents. More investigation into what they do, which insects they target, and how to optimize delivery is necessary to fully explore their potential (Aljohani et al., 2023). Reconsidering our entire treatment strategy now appears prudent as resistance mechanisms double and compound, rendering single-drug treatments increasingly suspect. Mixing various strategies, such as essential oils, bacteriocins, and conventional antibiotics—may very well produce a combination that outwits bacteria while maintaining toxicity at bay. These combinations are dense with diverse active ingredients that interfere with bacterial gossip and biofilm accumulation, both of which have roles in how resistance arises and persists. That said, rigorous clinical testing and clear protocols are still crucial to verify safety, nail down optimal dosages, and understand long-term outcomes. A multidisciplinary effort, combinationincorporating insights from microbiology, pharmacology, and clinical work, is generally speaking essential if we're to turn these exciting lab findings into real-world fixes against the AMR challenge (Aljohani et al., 2023; Romanescu et al., 2023).

7.6.3. Collaboration Between Public and Private Sectors

AMR is not another buzzword but rather a complex labyrinth that demands new, cohesive strategies and not sporadic, isolated quick fixes. Previously, patchy remedies have simply failed to do enough to stem the increasing spread of resistant infections, and it is certain that we must get together our strength. When government agencies and private firms pool resources, expertise, and the infrastructure to set it up, they establish a sort of shared space that's particularly worthwhile in regions where health care is thin. You can almost envision how the agile energy of private actors combined with the stable regulation of government agencies can rev up antimicrobial care, monitoring, and research. Joint ventures, such as those for vaccine development and launching new vaccines, demonstrate in the majority of instances how such collaboration can address a problem as complex and global as AMR to promote more sustainable access even in populations with significant health system issues (Akegbe et al., 2023).

Simply put, establishing these alliances is a grassroots approach to bolstering our collective response. Harking back to public–private partnerships is a defining step in assembling coordinated efforts against AMR. These partnerships engage government institutions, private companies, and even neighborhood social entities into an frequently unpredictable yet vibrant combination that sharpens resolution-making and sets projects in motion. For example, consider Colombia's multi-sectoral activities—various stakeholders, ranging from animal protein industries to regulatory centers, have collaborated in quite an unplanned manner to facilitate wiser antimicrobial utilization and mitigate risks associated with day-to-day farming. Sometimes these public–private initiatives have also provided the platform for global experts to exchange experiences, thereby strengthening the country's response infrastructure and increasing public awareness as well. Evidently, as resources are combined and stakeholders remain actively involved, the effect of national AMR plans receives an added fillip, providing implementable models that other low- and middle-income areas could well follow (Rodríguez et al., 2023). Augmenting local production of vaccines in areas where resources are limited further points towards the importance of public–private collaborations. In Africa, say, over-reliance on imported vaccines makes the population exposed to risk from supply bottlenecks and lagged outbreak response—ones which again can again exacerbate AMR issues. By having public institutions and private investors contribute investments into local R&D and even manufacturing systems, such gaps can be reduced significantly. Generically, developing innovation centers and providing incentives to the private sector with parallel government monitoring can assist in constructing vaccine systems that don't rely so heavily on outsiders. These arrangements not only maintain a form of health care sovereignty but also assist in providing timely immunization coverage, which is crucial in preventing infections that tend to require antimicrobial treatment. These collective efforts collectively ensure a combination of policy expertise with hands-on manufacturing know-how, accelerating sustainable response to AMR (Akegbe et al., 2023) (Figure 7.14).

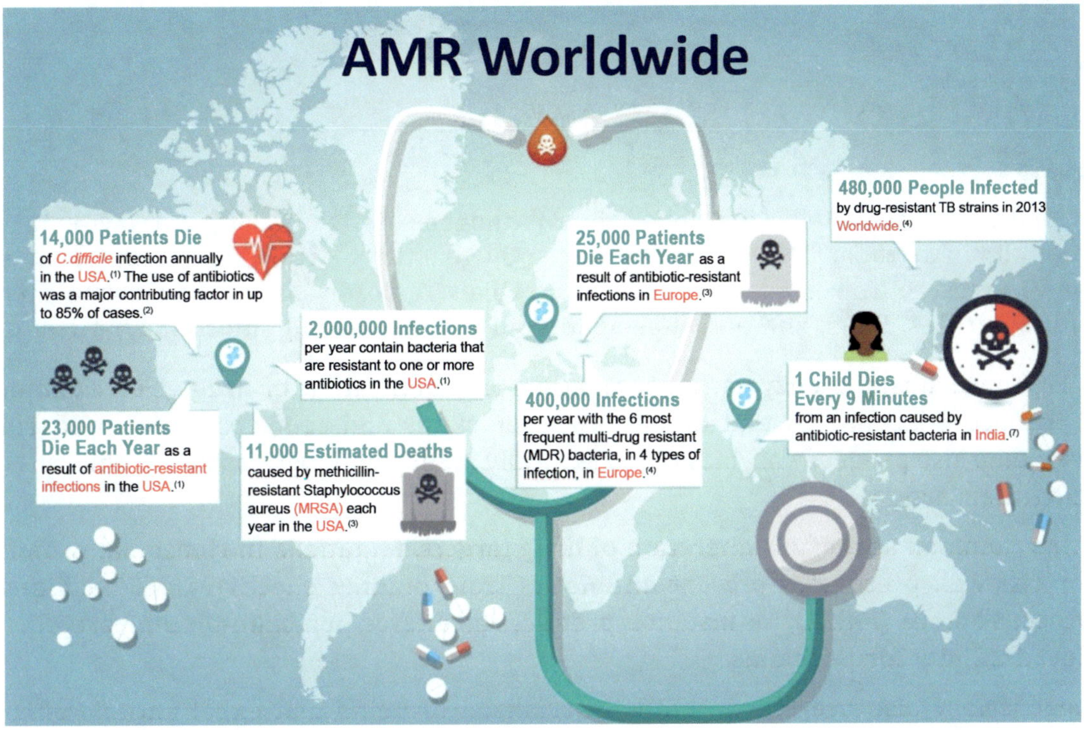

Figure 7.14. Public and private sectors of antimicrobial resistance (AMR).

Source: bioMérieux Connection. (2018, March). *AMR Worldwide Infographic.*

CLOSER LOOK

MECHANISMS OF ANTIMICROBIAL RESISTANCE IN PATHOGENS

Antimicrobial resistance (AMR) develops when pathogens evolve strategies to withstand drugs designed to eliminate them. This process is driven by genetic mutations, horizontal gene transfer, and selective pressure from the misuse of antimicrobials. A closer look at the mechanisms reveals how bacteria, viruses, fungi, and parasites adapt and persist, making infections harder to treat.

One key mechanism is enzymatic degradation or modification of drugs. For example, many bacteria produce β-lactamases that break down penicillins and cephalosporins, rendering them ineffective. Some also produce enzymes that chemically modify aminoglycosides or chloramphenicol, neutralizing their action.

Another common strategy is alteration of drug targets. Mutations in ribosomal proteins, DNA gyrase, or cell wall precursors prevent antibiotics from binding effectively. Methicillin-resistant Staphylococcus aureus (MRSA), for instance, produces an altered penicillin-binding protein (PBP2a) with reduced affinity for β-lactams.

Pathogens may also use efflux pumps, specialized proteins that expel antimicrobial agents before they can reach toxic concentrations inside the cell. Multidrug efflux systems in Pseudomonas aeruginosa and E. coli contribute to resistance against several antibiotic classes simultaneously.

Additionally, reduced permeability of cell membranes limits drug entry. Gram-negative bacteria often modify their porins, decreasing uptake of β-lactams and fluoroquinolones. In some cases, pathogens adopt metabolic bypass pathways, producing alternative enzymes that perform essential functions despite drug inhibition, as seen in sulfonamide-resistant bacteria.

Horizontal gene transfer through plasmids, transposons, and bacteriophages accelerates the spread of resistance genes across microbial communities. This allows even non-pathogenic bacteria to act as reservoirs of resistance.

Antimicrobial resistance is a multifaceted defense system in pathogens. By degrading drugs, altering targets, pumping out toxins, and sharing resistance genes, microbes adapt rapidly. Understanding these mechanisms is critical for developing novel therapies and preserving the effectiveness of existing treatments.

Summary

AMR is rapidly on its way to becoming one of our biggest issues—one that challenges us to reimagine the way we typically deal with infections. Treating repeated cases of urinary tract infection, for example, illustrates that keeping antibiotic use closely monitored, in tandem with cautious diagnostic measures, really slows the advance of resistant strains. Local treatment options, which rely on local antibiogram results, and emphasis on avoiding excessive use of antibiotics, go hand in hand with continuous education for patients and healthcare providers. In most instances, although alternatives such as non-antibiotic prevention are fascinating, the present research informs us that more hands-on, stringent work is necessary to pin down safety and efficacy. Overall, the changing jigsaw puzzle of AMR is one of tug-of-war between microbes' adaptation and our attempts to match up with current guidelines and policy that is well-informed (Anger et al., 2019). In addition to tightening up antibiotic management, there is a critical role for developing stronger health systems, particularly where care just isn't living up to potential. In low- and middle-income communities, where unsuitable treatments and misdiagnoses and damaged chains of care too often do more harm than good, a reliable system that always provides respectful and competent care supports patient trust (and that patient trust, in turn, increases treatment compliance). Equal access to the proper medicines and accurate diagnostics must be complemented by robust data systems that monitor resistance patterns and results. Spending on workforce development, good governance, and infrastructure upgrading isn't an add-on nicety—it's the core of a sustainable response to AMR (Kruk et al., 2018). The struggle to counter AMR isn't solely about laboratory tests or clinics—it's equally a social and political battle as it is scientific. National officials and international allies, in short, must collaborate with a combination of wise use of antibiotics, renewed health systems, and a dash of community participation. Policy should promote new studies on new treatments and diagnostics and support those research projects that design interventions for the needs of the world. Public education campaigns, however repetitive at times, reduce misuse and raise support for high-quality care. Ultimately, only a constant combination of responsive, evidence-led policies and collective action can control AMR and keep antibiotics working for generations to come (Anger et al., 2019; Kruk et al., 2018).

Surveillance efforts recently demonstrate that AMR differs significantly from one bacterium to the next and across different parts of the world and, therefore, is a international problem. Both food animals and human isolate data frequently indict resistance to antibiotics we typically trust, Salmonella and Campylobacter, for example, are typical offenders. It appears that, in most instances, certain key drugs are experiencing increasing resistance, particularly in poultry-associated strains, although overall multi-drug resistance is still not very prevalent. Detection of carbapenemase-producing isolates in a few nations certainly raises eyebrows due to their robust resistance patterns and the potential for them to spread far and wide. And, overall, longer-term studies throughout much of Europe have revealed some decreases in resistance levels, probably due to concerted monitoring and intervention strategies. The inclusion of pathogens in veterinary medicine introduces a further complexity to the tale. Studies on usual mastitis suspects such as *Staphylococcus aureus* and *Streptococcus uberis*, microbes that are known to produce robust biofilms, illustrate that they persist longer and are more pathogenic. These microbes tend to be resistant to multiple classes of antimicrobials, like penicillin, ampicillin, and tetracycline, reminding us that resistance is as much an animal-health concern as it is a human one. Interestingly, high biofilm production and AMR do not seem to always be in concert, which indicates that multiple, perhaps separate, factors are involved when therapies fail and infections persist. This finding, in the majority of instances, suggests more focused studies to sort out all these various threads and modulate treatments accordingly (Fidelis et al., 2024). Overall, a summary of these findings provides us with a general perspective of the present AMR landscape, which is replete with challenges and guarded advances. The continuing battle with resistant bacteria in human patients, food animals, and veterinary clients is evidence enough why concerted approaches are necessary. Better surveillance systems have been important for detecting new patterns of resistance, guiding considered antimicrobial use, and establishing preventive measures. Furthermore, more insight into the numerous factors contributing to resistance, such as how formation of biofilms occasionally but not invariably relates to drug action—will be important in crafting more successful control measures. Combining epidemiological surveillance, molecular research, and intelligent antimicrobial prescribing, in some sort of partnership fashion, appears to be the best hope for slowing down the growth of resistance and safeguarding future therapy (Fidelis et al., 2024).

References

1. Aarestrup, F. M., Ahuja, S., Aidara-Kane, A., Zumla, A., & Allegranzi, B. (2016). Exploring the evidence base for national and regional policy interventions to combat resistance. *The Lancet, 387*(10015), 285–295. https://doi.org/10.1016/S0140-6736(15)00520-6.

2. Abbas, M., Ahmad, R., Allegranzi, B., Bagheri Nejad, S., Harrington, R. A., Mathai, E., & Pittet, D. (2019). Broadening the infection prevention and control network globally: 2017 Geneva IPC-think tank (Part 3). *Antimicrobial Resistance and Infection Control, 8*, 74. https://doi.org/10.1186/s13756-019-0539-1.

3. Abdul Haseeb, M., Saleem, Z., Maqadmi, A. F., Allehyani, R. A., Mahrous, A. J., Elrggal, M. E., Kamran, S. H., et al. (2023). Ongoing strategies to improve antimicrobial utilization in hospitals across the Middle East and North Africa (MENA): Findings and implications. *Antibiotics, 12*(5), 827. https://doi.org/10.3390/antibiotics12050827.

4. Abidin, A. Z., Norrrahim, M. N. F., Mohamed Shakrin, N. N. S., Ibrahim, B., Abdullah, N., Abdul Rashid, J. I., Mohd Kasim, N. A., et al. (2024). Amidine-containing compounds: Antimicrobial activity and its potential in combating antimicrobial resistance. *Helion, 10*, e32010. https://doi.org/10.1016/j.heliyon.2024.e32010.

5. Ahmad, R., Akpan, M. R., Ashiru-Oredope, D., Doble, A., & Patel, M. (2018). Antimicrobial stewardship programmers in community healthcare organizations in England: A cross-sectional survey to assess implementation of programmers and national toolkits. *Antibiotics, 7*(4), 97. https://doi.org/10.3390/antibiotics7040097.

6. Ahmed, S. K., Hussein, S., Qurbani, K., Ibrahim, R. H., Fareeq, A., Mahmood, K. A., Mohamed, M. G., et al. (2024). Antimicrobial resistance: Impacts, challenges, and future prospects. *Journal of Medicine Surgery and Public Health, 2*, 100081. https://doi.org/10.1016/j.glmedi.2024.100081.

7. Akegbe, H., Onyeaka, H., Mazi, I. M., Olowolafe, O. A., Omotosho, A. D., Oladunjoye, I. O., Tajudeen, Y. A., et al. (2023). The need for Africa to develop capacity for vaccinology as a means of curbing antimicrobial resistance. *Vaccine X, 14*, 100320. https://doi.org/10.1016/j.jvacx.2023.100320.

8. Alcalde, R. E., Alvarez, P. J. J., Ashbolt, N., Bischel, H. N., Halden, R. U., Gu, A. Z., & Vikesland, P. J. (2018). An environmental science and engineering framework for combating antimicrobial resistance. *Environmental Engineering Science, 35*(10), 951–964. https://doi.org/10.1089/ees.2018.0224.

9. Alcock, B., Raphenya, A. R., Lau, T. T. Y., Tsang, K. K., Bouchard, M., Edalatmand, A., Huynh, W., et al. (2019). CARD 2020: Antibiotic resistome surveillance with the comprehensive antibiotic resistance database. *Nucleic Acids Research, 48*(D1), D517–D525. https://doi.org/10.1093/nar/gkz935.

10. Alekhya, G., Sudarshan, S., Darjee, S., Rajareddy, G., Kumar, A. A., St., Kadapa Sreenivasa Reddy, et al. (2024). Organic boost or health risk? The dual impact of organic amendments in agriculture. *International Journal of Research in Agronomy, 7(8), 844–853*. https://www.semanticscholar.org/paper/9db6598d0bc0a2c8f7ed452810237f316e04d258 (accessed on 7 May 2025).

11. Aljohani, A. B., Al-Hejin, A. M., & Shori, A. B. (2023). Bacteriocins as promising antimicrobial peptides: Definition, classification, and their potential applications in cheeses. *Food Science and Technology, 43*. https://doi.org/10.1590/fst.118021.

12. Almansour, A., Alhadlaq, M., Alzahrani, K. O., Mukhtar, L. E., Alharbi, A. L., & Alajel, S. M. (2023). The silent threat: Antimicrobial-resistant pathogens in food-producing animals and their impact on public health. *Microorganisms, 11,* 2127. https://www.semanticscholar.org/paper/aa2b0480ce18efc92be8e5609924d28a009aaa38 (accessed on 7 May 2025).

13. Al-Shaebi, Z., Akdeniz, M., Ahmed, A. O., Altunbek, M., & Aydın, Ö. (2023). Breakthrough solution for antimicrobial resistance detection: Surface-enhanced Raman spectroscopy-based on artificial intelligence. *Advanced Materials Interfaces*. https://doi.org/10.1002/admi.202300664.

14. Angelos, J. A., Arens, A. L., Cadriel, J. L., Johnson, R., & Fossler, C. P. (2017). One Health in food safety and security education: Subject matter outline for a curricular framework. *One Health, 3*, 56–65. https://doi.org/10.1016/j.onehlt.2017.04.001.

15. Anger, J. T., Lee, U., Ackerman, A. L., Chou, R., Chughtai, B., Clemens, J. Q., Hickling, D., et al. (2019). Recurrent uncomplicated urinary tract infections in women: AUA/CUA/SUFU guideline. *The Journal of Urology, 202*, 282–289. https://doi.org/10.1097/ju.0000000000000296.

16. Aruwa, C. E., Chellan, T., S'thebe, N. W., Dweba, Y., & Sabiu, S. (2024). ESKAPE pathogens and associated quorum sensing systems: New targets for novel antimicrobial development. *Health Sciences Review, 11*, 100155. https://doi.org/10.1016/j.hsr.2024.100155.

17. Bandura, A., Fishbein, M., MacPherson, D., Cabinet Office, Department of Health, Public Health England, Department for Environment, Food & Rural Affairs, & World Health Organization. (2018). Antimicrobial resistance: A biopsychosocial problem requiring innovative interdisciplinary and imaginative interventions. *Journal of Infection Prevention, 19*(4), 170–175. https://doi.org/10.1177/1757177418771182.

18. Barrett, J. B., Frye, J. G., Gupta, S. K., Hiott, A. E., Rhodes, N. J., & Jackson, C. R. (2019). Genomic comparison of diverse *Salmonella* serovars isolated from swine. *PLOS ONE, 14*(11), e0224518. https://doi.org/10.1371/journal.pone.0224518.

19. Barsola, B., Saklani, S., Pathania, D., Kumari, P., Sonu, S., Rustagi, S., Singh, P., et al. (2024). Exploring bio-nanomaterials as antibiotic allies to combat antimicrobial resistance. *Bio Fabrication, 16*, 042007. https://doi.org/10.1088/1758-5090/ad6b45.

20. Bell, R. A., Burstein, V. R., Kravitz, R. L., May, L., & McFadden, R. (2019). Communication interventions to promote the public's awareness of antibiotics: A systematic review. *BMC Public Health, 19*(1), 899. https://doi.org/10.1186/s12889-019-7258-3.

21. Bengtsson-Palme, J., Abramova, A., Berendonk, T. U., Coelho, L. P., Forslund, S. K., Gschwind, R., Heikinheimo, A., et al. (2023). Towards monitoring of antimicrobial resistance in the environment: For what reasons, how to implement it, and what are the data needs? *Environment International, 178*, 108089. https://doi.org/10.1016/j.envint.2023.108089.

22. Bhagwandin, N., Jenner, A., & Kowalski, S. P. (2017). *Antimicrobial Resistance (AMR) and Multidrug Resistance (MDR): Overview of Current Approaches, Consortia and Intellectual Property Issues*. https://core.ac.uk/download/215505935.pdf (accessed on 7 May 2025).

23. Bhat, R. A. H., & Altınok, İ. (2023). Antimicrobial resistance (AMR) and alternative strategies for combating AMR in aquaculture. *Turkish Journal of Fisheries and Aquatic Sciences, 23.*

https://doi.org/10.4194/trjfas24068.

24. Błaszczyński, G., Nojek, P., Nowotarska, A., Pawlik, K., & Kwiatkowska, D. (2024). The impact of prolonged antibiotic use on the development of bacterial resistance: A literature review. *Journal of Education, Health and Sport, 71*, 56137. https://doi.org/10.12775/jehs.2024.56137 (accessed on 7 May 2025).

25. Bristow, C. C., Cristillo, A. D., Dillon, J. A., Dong, K., & Kirkcaldy, R. D. (2019). Antimicrobial resistance in *Neisseria gonorrhoeae*: Proceedings of the STAR Sexually Transmitted Infection-Clinical Trial Group programmatic meeting. *Sexually Transmitted Diseases, 46*(3), e18–e25. https://doi.org/10.1097/OLQ.0000000000000929.

26. Buhr, B. L., Holtkamp, D., & Sornsen, S. (2025). Healthy competition in the animal health industry. *CORE*. https://core.ac.uk/download/pdf/6546489.pdf (accessed on 7 May 2025).

27. Carpa, R., Remizovschi, A., Culda, C. A., & Butiuc-Keul, A. (2022). Inherent and composite hydrogels as promising materials to limit antimicrobial resistance. *Gels, 8*(1), 70. https://doi.org/10.3390/gels8020070.

28. DeHart, C. (2020). Health concerns in Cambodia compounded by historical and rural setbacks. *Senior Honors Theses, 967*. https://core.ac.uk/download/322850889.pdf (accessed on 7 May 2025).

29. Edwards, S. J. L., Tao, Y., Elias, R., & Schooley, R. T. (2024). Considerations for prioritizing clinical research using bacteriophage. *Essays in Biochemistry, 68*, 679–686. https://www.semanticscholar.org/paper/76afb9f0efe559677050463aa0f6c62251b427df (accessed on 7 May 2025).

30. Ezugwu, N. V., Gayle, A., & Anyamene, C. (2024). Epidemiology of antimicrobial resistance and the Wash project: Averting a potential public health crisis in Nigeria using the United Kingdom as a case study. *International Journal of Tropical Disease & Health, 45(6), 87–104*. https://www.semanticscholar.org/paper/a06ef1e72d73da5309d8f33117f7004d2cc3c034 (accessed on 7 May 2025).

31. Ferreira, M., Ogren, M., Dias, J., Silva, M., Gil, S., Tavares, L., Aires-da-Silva, F., et al. (2021). Liposomes as antibiotic delivery systems: A promising nanotechnological strategy against antimicrobial resistance. *Molecules, 26*(7), 2047. https://doi.org/10.3390/molecules26072047.

32. Fidelis, C. E., Orsi, A. M., Freu, G., Gonçalves, J. L., & Santos, M. V. D. (2024). Biofilm formation and antimicrobial resistance of *Staphylococcus aureus* and *Streptococcus uberis* isolates from bovine mastitis. *Veterinary Sciences, 11*(1), 170. https://www.semanticscholar.org/paper/142afb1cc3c6463c5fb41842385ea4c0371d09ad (accessed on 7 May 2025).

33. Garvey, M. (2023). Antimicrobial peptides demonstrate activity against resistant bacterial pathogens. *Infectious Disease Reports, 15*, 454–469. https://doi.org/10.3390/idr15040046.

34. Gedefie, A., Demsiss, W., Belete, M. A., Kassa, Y., Tesfaye, M., Tilahun, M., Bisetegn, H., et al. (2021). Acinetobacter baumannii biofilm formation and its role in disease pathogenesis: A review. *Infection and Drug Resistance, 14*, 3711–3719. https://doi.org/10.2147/idr.s332051.

35. Hancock, L. J., & Mellor, C. (2015). An evaluation of antimicrobial stewardship in community pharmacy. *Fields: Journal of Huddersfield Student Research, 2*(1), e23. https://core.ac.uk/download/30734256.pdf (accessed on 7 May 2025).

36. Hou, K., Wu, Z. X., Chen, X. Y., Wang, J. Q., Zhang, D., Xiao, C., Zhu, D., et al. (2022). Microbiota in health and diseases. *Signal Transduction and Targeted Therapy, 7.* https://doi.org/10.1038/s41392-022-00974-4.

37. Hutchings, M. I., Truman, A. W., & Wilkinson, B. (2019). Antibiotics: Past, present, and future. *Current Opinion in Microbiology, 51*, 72–80. https://doi.org/10.1016/j.mib.2019.10.008.

38. Jain, N., Dutt, U., Radenkov, I., & Jain, S. (2023). WHO's global oral health status report 2022: Actions, discussion, and implementation. *Oral Diseases, 30*, 73–79. https://doi.org/10.1111/odi.14516.

39. Jauneikaite, E., Baker, K. S., Nunn, J. G., Midega, J., Hsu, L. Y., Singh, S., Halpin, A. L., et al. (2023). Genomics for antimicrobial resistance surveillance to support infection prevention and control in healthcare facilities. *The Lancet Microbe, 4*, e1040–e1046. https://doi.org/10.1016/s2666-5247(23)00282-3.

40. Jian, Z., Zeng, L., Xu, T., Sun, S., Yan, S., Yang, L., Huang, Y., et al. (2021). Antibiotic resistance genes in bacteria: Occurrence, spread, and control. *Journal of Basic Microbiology, 61*, 1049–1070. https://doi.org/10.1002/jobm.202100201.

41. Karthikeyan, V., Saini, N., Nadarajan, R., Gopimohan, M., & Roy, P. (2024). Multidisciplinary collaboration in combatting antimicrobial resistance: Insights and outcomes from the National Alliance of Medical Professionals on Antimicrobial Resistance (NAMP-AMR) initiative. *Cureus, 16(9), e68932.* https://doi.org/10.7759/cureus.68932.

42. Kruk, M. E., Gage, A., Arsenault, C., Jordan, K., Leslie, H. H., Roder-DeWan, S., Adeyi, O., et al. (2018). High-quality health systems in the Sustainable Development Goals era: Time for a revolution. *The Lancet Global Health, 6*, e1196–e1252. https://doi.org/10.1016/s2214-109x(18)30386-3.

43. Menz, B. D., Charani, E., Gordon, D., Leather, A., Moonesinghe, R., & Phillips, C. (2021). Surgical antibiotic prophylaxis in an era of antibiotic resistance: Common resistant bacteria and wider considerations for practice. *Infection and Drug Resistance, 14*, 5235–5252. https://doi.org/10.2147/idr.s319780.

44. Miller, S. A., Ferreira, J. P., & LeJeune, J. T. (2022). Antimicrobial use and resistance in plant agriculture: A One Health perspective. *Agriculture, 12*(2), 289. https://doi.org/10.3390/agriculture12020289.

45. Mudenda, S., Chabalenge, B., Daka, V., Mfune, R. L., Salachi, K. I., Mohamed, S., Mufwambi, W., et al. (2023). Global strategies to combat antimicrobial resistance: A One Health perspective. *Pharmacology & Pharmacy, 14*, 271–328. https://doi.org/10.4236/pp.2023.148020.

46. Murray, C. J. L., Ikuta, K. S., Sharara, F., Swetschinski, L. R., Robles Aguilar, G., Gray, A. P., Han, C., et al. (2022). Global burden of bacterial antimicrobial resistance in 2019: A systematic analysis. *The Lancet, 399*, 629–655. https://doi.org/10.1016/s0140-6736(21)02724-0.

47. Panwar, D. (2024). Role of biotechnology in combating antibiotic resistance. *Journal for Research in Applied Sciences and Biotechnology, 3*(6), 173–183. https://core.ac.uk/download/636456668.pdf (accessed on 7 May 2025).

48. Rodríguez, M., Vásquez, G., & Cediel, N. (2023). Alianzas públicas, privadas y público-privadas para implementar Una Salud como acción contra la resistencia antimicrobiana en Colombia. *Revita Panamericana de Salud Pública, 47*, 1–1. https://doi.org/10.26633/rpsp.2023.64.

49. Sakagianni, A., Koufopoulou, C., Feretzakis, G., Kalles, D., Verykios, V. S., Myrianthefs, P., & Fildisis, G. (2023). Using machine learning to predict antimicrobial resistance—A literature review. *Antibiotics, 12*(3), 452. https://doi.org/10.3390/antibiotics12030452.

50. Salam, M. A., Al-Amin, M. Y., Salam, M. T., Pawar, J., Akhter, N., Rabaan, A., & Alqumber, M. (2023). Antimicrobial resistance: A growing serious threat for global public health. *Healthcare, 11, 1946*. https://www.semanticscholar.org/paper/c407db18ae42c799c2cd400c86ffc1c0d41fb7a1 (accessed on 7 May 2025).

51. Sharma, S., Chauhan, A., Ranjan, A., Mathkor, D. M., Haque, S., Ramniwas, S., Tuli, H. S., et al. (2024). Emerging challenges in antimicrobial resistance: Implications for pathogenic microorganisms, novel antibiotics, and their impact on sustainability. *Frontiers in Microbiology, 15*. https://doi.org/10.3389/fmicb.2024.1403168.

52. Singh, S., Datta, S., Narayanan, K. B., & Narayanan, R. (2021). Bacterial exo-polysaccharides in biofilms: Role in antimicrobial resistance and treatments. *Journal of Genetic Engineering and Biotechnology, 19*, 140. https://doi.org/10.1186/s43141-021-00242-y.

53. Uzoka, U. H., Abimbola, O. G., Isiaka, A. B., Bolawa, O. P., Ugwor, E., Ani, N. V., Anakwenze, V. N., et al. (2024). The role of novel probiotic strains in enhancing immunity and preventing infections in livestock: A comprehensive review. *Revista Foco, 17(11)*. https://www.semanticscholar.org/paper/91051a0b1f2bc53bfff6318e73fc5605b8f0e737 (accessed on 7 May 2025).

54. Zheng, D., Liwinski, T., & Elinav, E. (2020). Interaction between microbiota and immunity in health and disease. *Cell Research, 30*(5), 492–506. https://doi.org/10.1038/s41422-020-0332-7.

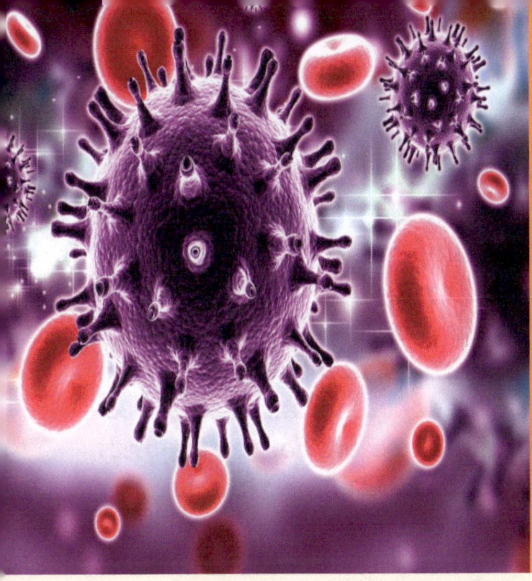

Chapter 8

HIV/AIDS

Contents

Introduction

In the later decades of the 20th century, a brutal new disease started causing havoc with health systems and leaving researchers grasping for answers. HIV, a virus that gradually develops into what we know as AIDS by weakening the immune system, made us all redefine the way that we confront disease. Rather than a single, uniform appearance, scientists soon had to factor in more complex variables—how our immune defenses and genes interact, for example, to determine why some individuals appear to keep it at bay. Recent genome-wide analyses, for instance, have revealed clues that certain genetic markers within the MHC may enable some individuals to better manage HIV, opening up surprising avenues for treatment and even vaccine concepts (Rahmouni et al., 2025). HIV isnt afraid to come out swinging; it targets CD4+ T cells, disabling the bodys own defenses against infection and causing all sorts of ugly side effects. That weakening doesnt just make individuals vulnerable to opportunistic microbes but also confuses matters when attempting to diagnose other diseases, such as, for example, sarcoidosis, which remains fairly uncommon in association with HIV. In an interesting twist, some HIV-positive patients, especially those on highly active antiretroviral therapy (HAART), have demonstrated features of sarcoidosis. In a general sense, this ironic phenomenon reflects how recovery of immune function can at times cause unforeseen inflammatory reactions, further complicating things for clinicians (Su et al., 2024). Analyzing the situation from a bigger perspective, HIV/AIDS has never been simply a biological enigma. Since it was first detected, the epidemic has worked its way through countless communities, frequently affecting marginalized populations the hardest because of socioeconomic difficulties and unequal access to healthcare.

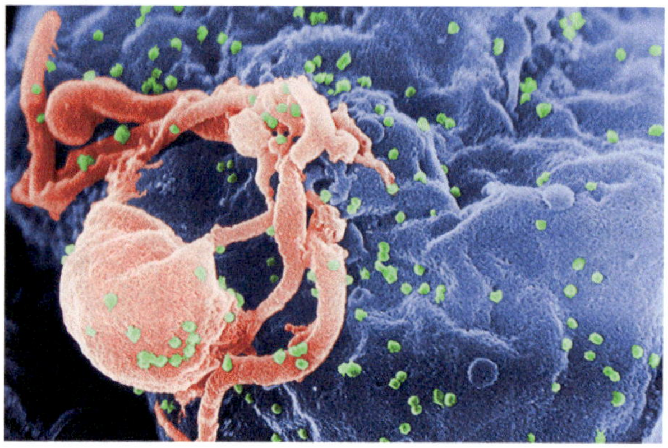

Figure 8.1. HIV/AIDS.

Source: By Photo Credit: C. GoldsmithContent Providers: CDC/ C. Goldsmith, P. Feorino, E. L. Palmer, W. R. McManus - This media comes from the Centers for Disease Control and Prevention's Public Health Image Library (PHIL), with identification number #10000.Note: Not all PHIL images are public domain; be sure to check copyright status and credit authors and content providers. | Deutsch | English | македонски | slovenščina | +/−, Public Domain, https://commons.wikimedia.org/w/index.php?curid=3909584

With time, the international response evolved from crisis management to long-term approaches, combining prevention, education, and routine access to antiretroviral therapies in an attempt to improve quality of life. Despite all the advancements, issues such as stigma, fluctuating treatment compliance, and co-infection risk continue to exist. For the majority, integrating our genetic findings with feasible clinical and public health interventions seems to be the promising next step toward long-term remission—or perhaps even a cure, toward a cautiously optimistic future in the battle against this disease (Su et al., 2024; Rahmouni et al., 2025) (Figure 8.1).

Definition of HIV and AIDS

Learning about HIV and AIDS begins with a fundamental examination of virology and immunology. HIV is a retrovirus that targets CD4+ T cells , those very defenders that prevent infections from getting the better of us. When these cells are depleted, the body's defense system weakens and the individual is left vulnerable to opportunistic diseases and even certain types of cancer. Overall, to have HIV is for the virus to exist, but for the levels of CD4+ T cells to fall below some point or AIDS-related diseases to arise is when the condition is considered AIDS (James et al., 2018). In other words, what differentiates the two is how severely the immune system has been damaged and what symptoms appear in the body. The trajectory of an HIV infection can be unpredictable. At first, you might experience an acute retroviral syndrome that is a kind of nasty flu, followed by a long period in which no symptoms seem apparent as the virus secretly multiplies. Even when you're feeling fine, though, the gradual breaking down of immune defenses is happening. If left untreated, opportunistic diseases such as tuberculosis (TB) or some forms of cancer may eventually occur, signaling the transition into

AIDS. This turning point is significant because it changes treatment regimens and changes the patient's prognosis. In most instances, since HIV inserts itself into the host DNA and evades the immune system, constant medical care is still a necessity (Jeffrey et al., 2018). Globally, it's not always easy to define HIV versus AIDS. Diagnostic standards continue to evolve, and advances in laboratory tests, either antibody tests or nucleic acid tests, are making detection earlier possible, which can assist in stopping the development toward AIDS. This sharp distinction is key to formulating public health policy and to determining how resources are prioritized to counteract the epidemic. Research focusing on disease transmission, its frequency, and cumulative burden still emphasizes the need for these distinctions (James et al., 2018). Finally, this understanding not only benefits individual clinical care but also informs public health initiatives aimed at limiting transmission and increasing life expectancy in those who are infected.

Historical Context of the Epidemic

In the early 1980s, HIV/AIDS entered the public eye and rearranged everything about the way we conceptualize health. Before HIV being pinned as the etiology of AIDS, people were still referencing earlier epidemics—smallpox, cholera, TB—that had long guided medical practice and social opinion. That history made it fairly evident that this new crisis was not merely another disease issue; it entwined with the way people perceived and treated each other, particularly about who received care and who got left behind. It demonstrated, in a very concrete manner, that problems such as stigma, inequality, and access to health care have been there all along. So to summarize, this was not an isolated success of science but a reminder that social factors have a large play as well (Snowden, 2019). Meanwhile, the early years of HIV/AIDS were also characterized by established ideas about drug users and people already living on the edges. Don't forget, the crack cocaine epidemic of the 1980s only made things more complicated. Harm reduction concepts, such as syringe exchange programs that were necessary to slow the virus among people who injected drugs—encountered hard pushback driven by time-worn biases, particularly against racial and ethnic minorities. In most cases, these steps toward life-saving measures were delayed longer than necessary, gaining traction only later in the decade due to local initiatives and some new research about their effectiveness. This lag wasn't all about slow science; rather, it was more about a society mired in old perceptions that made progress difficult (Don, 2017). Considering where we are today with HIV/AIDS, it appears that the old problems still reappear when we attempt to create improved health systems. Even with solid evidence supporting measures like methadone, buprenorphine treatments, and syringe exchange programs, political and social hang-ups have kept these strategies from spreading as widely as needed. In many suburban and rural spots, the lack of proper harm reduction resources shows just how much we've not fully learned from the past. And, more importantly, the current opioid crisis demonstrates unequivocally that people judging individuals for experimenting with psychoactive substances is still a significant barrier. The history of harm reduction in the last 40 years unveils to what extent our public health triumphs and setbacks are reliant on both solving medical challenges and daily prejudices (Don, 2017).

Importance of Studying HIV/AIDS

Addressing issues in public health, particularly those as serious as HIV/AIDS with its serious medical and social impacts, requires that we continue researching and educating constantly. Many times, when we explore HIV/AIDS, it not only explains to us how the disease travels from person to person but also illuminates the circumstances that expose individuals to the disease and how to prevent new occurrences. For example, information on dual protection - consider in which circumstances use of a female condom could be a good alternative when a male condom is not going well, can widen options for prevention. It's interesting how incorporating these alternatives into existing initiatives, such as projects aimed at halting mother-to-child transmission or promoting voluntary male circumcision, serves to show how research tends to flow back and help shape policy as well as routine practice. Yet, gaps still persist in how these programs are put into action, underlining, in most cases, a need for more targeted studies that help smooth over the delivery of these protective measures; all in the hope that evidence-based innovations will tailor interventions to the varied needs of different populations. Beyond the medical realities, it is easy to notice that HIV/AIDS research also puts the spotlight on the important role of community participation and social support networks. NGOs, for instance, tend to fill in the gaps in areas most affected—these institutions, with their combination of social capital, community involvement and youth participation, are likely to be key to getting interventions to work. If we glance at grassroots movements that induce political energy within communities and link individuals in unexpected networks, we realize that treating HIV/AIDS isn't merely a health issue, but incorporating sound social strategies as well. In most instances, knowing how such community forces collaborate facilitates the creation of models that can scale up and enhance NGO efficiency, while at the same time developing local groups committed to prevention as well as assistance (Neff et al., 2009). More broadly, HIV/AIDS research has a significant function in reconfiguring public health systems and informing policy. Overall, the findings gleaned from current studies form a foundation for training campaigns that address stigma and misinformation—obstacles that can prove particularly recalcitrant to prevention and treatment. Additionally, through its inducement of some interdisciplinarity—where medicine, social science, and behavioral science converge—the research yields methods that more closely approximate the complexities of living with HIV/AIDS in actual practice. This holistic perspective not only improves individual health outcomes, but also creates a sort of community resilience by making disease interaction less stigmatized and by encouraging people to test and remain on treatment. Overall, maintaining a consistent academic interest in HIV/AIDS is nearly indispensable for driving forward global health equity and ensuring that interventions, designed with cultural sensitivity in mind, reach most-at-risk individuals (Figure 8.2).

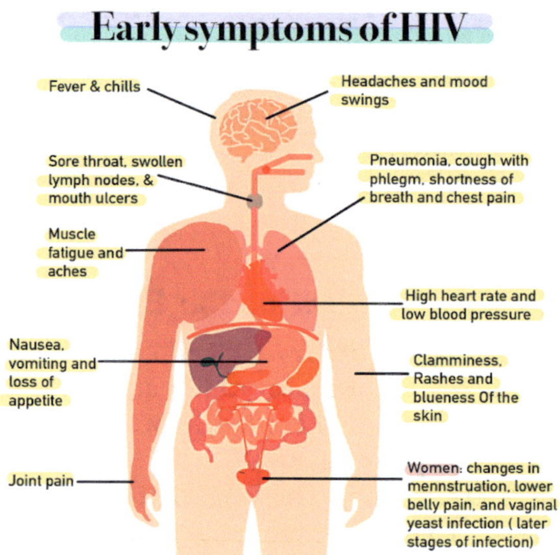

Figure 8.2. HIV symptoms.

Source: By Nicolearyanne - Own work, CC BY-SA 4.0, https://commons.wikimedia.org/w/index.php?curid=90646674

8.1. Transmission of HIV

We need to know how HIV travels from individual to individual to address its spread across the globe. The virus primarily finds a hold when bodily fluids such as blood, semen, vaginal secretions, and even breast milk are involved. Sexual encounter, particularly if anal sex occurs without a condom, usually ends up being the primary method HIV is transmitted, largely due to the efficiency with which the virus travels through mucosal tissues (Timmons-Vendryes et al., 2025). However, there is more to it: also sharing unclean needles, receiving contaminated blood products, or a mother transmitting the disease to her child at birth or through lactation can also initiate things. Quite often, the combination of these confused perceptions, social stigma, and yay-ngo misinformation obfuscates the vision and ultimately hinders prevention while reinforcing discrimination against vulnerable people such as women and other oppressed groups. In the majority of instances, increasing public awareness regarding these pathways is essential for charting effective prevention strategies that combine both medical and behavioral interventions (Timmons-Vendryes et al., 2025). Biomedical advances have transformed how we perceive HIV risk. With the advent of treatments like pre-exposure prophylaxis (PrEP), post-exposure prophylaxis (PEP), and antiretroviral therapy (ART), the risk of contracting or transmitting the virus has declined significantly (Bhandari & Giri, 2025). Further there's that game-changing concept, "Undetectable equals Untransmittable" (U=U), which emphasizes that if one maintains their viral load under control, they're really not a threat to others sexually. But somehow there still appear to be gaps—access to these tools and their ideal use are still unequal, especially for those who most need them. And though these advances certainly reduce HIV risk, there's been a strange increase in other sexually transmitted diseases, adding another complication to the overall aims of sexual health management. In general, a balanced prevention strategy must weave together clever medical strategies with ongoing education, attempts to reduce stigma, and an equitable allocation of health care (Timmons-Vendryes et al., 2025). Social and structural determinants combination into the formula as well, making it difficult to understand exactly how HIV spreads. Cultural bias, economic hardship, and even changing migration patterns all bring levels of risk, particularly where health care is in short supply (Bhandari & Giri, 2025).

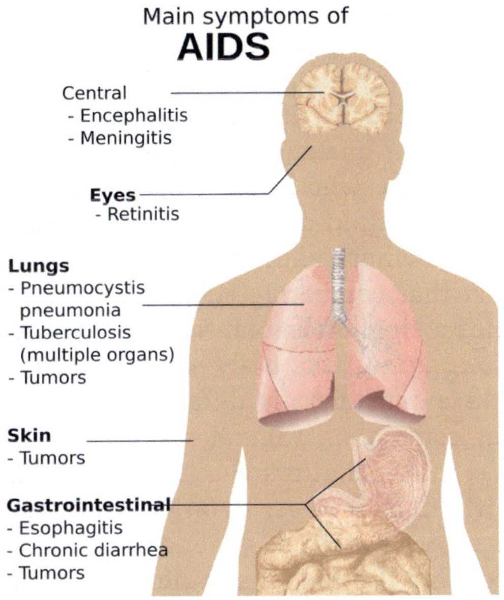

Figure 8.3. Transmission, symptoms, and signs of AIDS.

Source:By Mikael Häggström.When using this image in external works, it may be cited as:Häggström, Mikael (2014). "Medical gallery of Mikael Häggström 2014". WikiJournal of Medicine 1 (2). DOI:10.15347/wjm/2014.008. ISSN 2002-4436. Public Domain.orBy Mikael Häggström, used with permission. - All used images are in public domain., CC0, https://commons.wikimedia.org/w/index.php?curid=5425813

Women, for instance, may have an added burden through gender-based discrimination and less power to negotiate safe practices. Discrimination can even be present from families or healthcare workers, further excluding those in need. In most instances, combating these issues isn't necessarily about medicine. It's about seeing the big picture—supporting education, nudging economic stability, and relaxing societal stigma. Empowering individuals living with HIV/AIDS through supportive policies and grassroots efforts (coupled with local initiatives) can go a long way toward breaking the transmission cycle and enhancing the quality of life (Bhandari & Giri, 2025) (Figure 8.3).

8.1.1. Modes of Transmission

HIV finds its way into the body through a handful of routes, and knowing these paths is key if we're going to control its spread. The virus usually moves along when specific body fluids, like blood, semen, vaginal fluids, or even breast milk, are exchanged. Sex, particularly unprotected sex, is far and away the most prevalent method it passes from one person to another; in much of sub-Saharan Africa, for instance, young women tend to bear a disproportionate brunt. The virus can pass through mucous membranes or compromised skin during those times, and needle-sharing among people who inject drugs produces a direct blood-to-blood threat. Even transmission from a mother to child during pregnancy, childbirth, or breastfeeding continues to be a large concern in regions where antiretroviral therapy is not immediately available. All these different channels suggest that combating HIV may require approaches that are specific to regional circumstances and not a single formula. Not only does risk involve how a person becomes exposed, but also on the condition of the body when the virus comes into contact with it. For example, some sexual acts have substantially different risks; receptive anal sex tends to have a greater per-act risk of transmission than vaginal sex. Very often, being infected with a different sexually transmitted disease makes matters worse by interfering with natural barriers or attracting additional immune cells HIV finds it easier to target (Haynes & Mascola, 2017). The virus, being a chameleon in reality, flaunts a vast array of genetic diversities and changes its guise perpetually, thus becoming more difficult for the immune system to identify. In the majority of instances, as soon as HIV comes into contact with CD4+ T cells, with the help of its envelope protein, it primes the infection—a process scientists are hoping to prevent with novel vaccine approaches (Haynes & Mascola, 2017). Social causes contribute immensely to the transmission of HIV, as well. In sub-Saharan Africa, for example, young women aged 15 to 24 see their infection rate as much as eight times that of their male counterparts (Haynes & Mascola, 2017). This is not merely a function of biology but rather because of restricted exposure to preventive strategies, gender and sex in relationships, and economic constraints that make them more susceptible. Stigma and discrimination, occasionally emerging in testing and treatment, can also feed the epidemic indirectly by deterring individuals from necessary health services. In general, public health strategies must combine biomedical interventions such as antiretroviral therapy and pre-exposure prophylaxis with measures that address behavior and community organization. For the most part, tacking the complex mess of these social and medical problems is our best bet for cutting back on the epidemic and maintaining new infections in retreat (Haynes & Mascola, 2017).

8.1.2. Risk Factors Associated with Transmission

Risk factors for HIV transmission originate from numerous sources. Mother-to-child transmission, for example, continues to be particularly concerning where antenatal care isn't universally accessible. Studies in Eastern Europe indicate that complications such as maternal anemia and compromised immune system, as evidenced by low CD4 values, can increase the risk for HIV transmission from mother to child. At times, when HIV has progressed in a pregnant woman, the risk increases even more, even if antiretroviral therapy is ongoing. In general, though these medicines reduce transmission, persisting health issues in mothers require additional, specialized care to safeguard infants (Cambrea et al., 2022). All things considered, maternal health focus is a significant component of diminishing perinatal HIV infections. Risk behaviors also propel HIV transmission. Unprotected sex with various or unknown partners predisposes to HIV exposure, and concurrent infections, such as other sexually transmitted infections—may compromise the body's natural barriers, facilitating viral entry. Furthermore, injecting drug users have a direct pathway for HIV transmission when sharing needles - a case of direct blood-to-blood transfer. On top of that, co-infections like hepatitis B and C tend to complicate treatment and accelerate disease progression, so managing these cases usually requires an integrated clinical response (Terrault et al., 2015). In the majority of instances, integrating harm reduction, simple safe-sex education, and regular screening appears downright necessary to curb further spread. Then there's the larger context of social and environmental factors. Economic inequality, restricted access to good health care, and the stigma of HIV testing all contribute to delayed diagnosis and silently drive uncontrolled transmission. For groups in areas such as sub-Saharan Africa or among marginalized communities elsewhere, these structural barriers strike even more forcefully. In the meantime, variables such as an individual's viral load or genetic profile combine with these social factors to modify the risk of transmission. Although antiretroviral therapy has turned HIV from a fatal disease into a manageable chronic condition, uneven treatment access still leaves open transmission chains (Cambrea et al., 2022; Terrault et al., 2015). Generally speaking, addressing these wider structural challenges is absolutely vital if we're to control the epidemic and move toward global health equity (Figure 8.4).

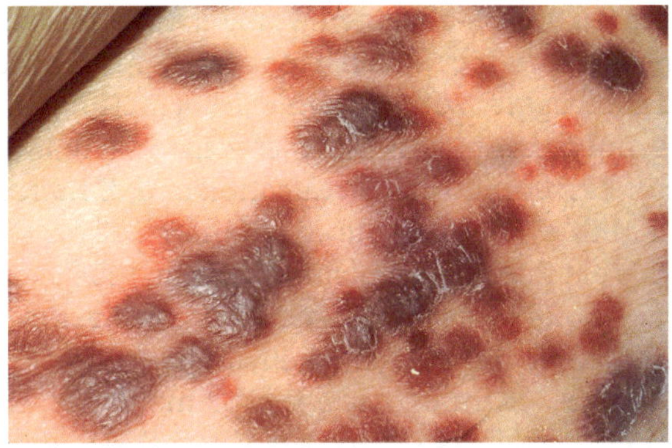

Figure 8.4. HIV infection.

Source: By Unknown author - National Cancer Institute, AV-8500-3620, Public Domain, https://commons.wikimedia.org/w/index.php?curid=859393

8.1.3. Myths and Misconceptions About Transmission

Misconceptions regarding the mode of transmission of HIV still stand in the way of effective prevention and treatment. Individuals tend to hold on to the notion that the virus gets transmitted through casual contact, eating a meal together or even a mosquito bite, and contribute to stigma and unnecessary fear. Primarily, such false notions arise due to lacunae in education and cultural practices which prevent frank discussions about the virus. In most developing countries, particularly among women of reproductive age, such beliefs increase their risk by bypassing prevention measures. Because these misconceptions have a direct influence on whether individuals choose testing and prevention, clear-cut, community-level education becomes imperative (Yimer et al., 2024). Where you reside and how much education you've received can influence your perception of HIV. Research indicates that people in rural or low-income communities are more likely to cling to these false concepts than city dwellers. For instance, studies from Ethiopia typically conclude that better-educated women grasp the facts much better than less-educated or non-educated women. Affluence also appears to affect beliefs; poorer communities often struggle with credible information, and this only complicates the confusion. In most instances, empowering education and enhanced availability of good sources of information will do a great deal in diminishing such myths (Yimer et al., 2024). Mother-to-child transmission is still a sensitive area where such misperceptions germinate. Although it's the primary method through which children aged below 15 years acquire HIV, there's still much misunderstanding regarding whether the virus is transmitted during pregnancy, at delivery, or during lactation. Many pregnant women aren't entirely in the know when it comes to essential prevention methods such as antiretroviral therapy or complementary feeding, which results in lost opportunities for interrupting transmission. In The Gambia, for example, there are those who still believe HIV can be transmitted through a mosquito bite or food sharing, again highlighting the necessity of enhanced counseling during pregnancy. Correcting these confusion with explicit policies and timely communications is, in the majority of instances, imperative to scaling up prevention services and safeguarding newborns (Yimer et al., 2024).

8.2. Symptoms and Stages of HIV

HIV infection occurs in a number of stages that aren't linear. Initially, after having been exposed, the individual may experience about something that feels a great deal like the flu—fever, exhaustion, inflamed glands, and an occasional rash. It is simple to overlook these indications since they are similar to regular viral microbes. Through this period, the virus reproduces rapidly while the immune system begins to respond, even if the symptoms are apparently slight. Afterward, mysteriously, the disease comes into a period of lesser disturbance when HIV remains present but barely in evidence. This time, in which the symptoms are perhaps only imperceptible, is the crucial period for identifying the disease in its early stages, even as the virus insidiously continues to deplete the body's defenses. Then, years could go by before the transition happens again. For the most part, if the infection is not treated, individuals eventually arrive at a stage characterized by obvious manifestations such as recurring fever, loss of weight, long-term diarrhea, and a variety of secondary infections. The immune system is now gradually weakened—oral thrush, shingles, or certain types of pneumonia begin to occur because the body is unable to defend itself against even small attackers. There may also be issues in mental functions and other neurologic conditions, which only further complicates patient care (Livingston et al., 2020).

This stage of the process is a grim reminder of how important it is to pay attention to the way HIV progresses, as well as initiating therapies that slow the deterioration of the immune system. Lastly, this can become extreme to the point of reaching an acute stage of Acquired Immunodeficiency Syndrome, or AIDS, where immune system weakening gets to be dire. By this time, what was perhaps once a controllable condition can make an individual vulnerable to life-threatening infections and cancers that would otherwise be held at bay. Patients can experience extreme weight loss, persistent fevers, debilitating fatigue, and a range of neurological issues. A diagnosis is usually made when specific opportunistic infections appear or when the CD4 cell count plummets dramatically—obvious signs that the immune system is collapsing. While medicine has made great strides in making HIV a more manageable disease, the overall effect still resonates loudly throughout public health, considering the intricate interplay between the virus and the body's immune defenses (James et al., 2018) (Figure 8.5).

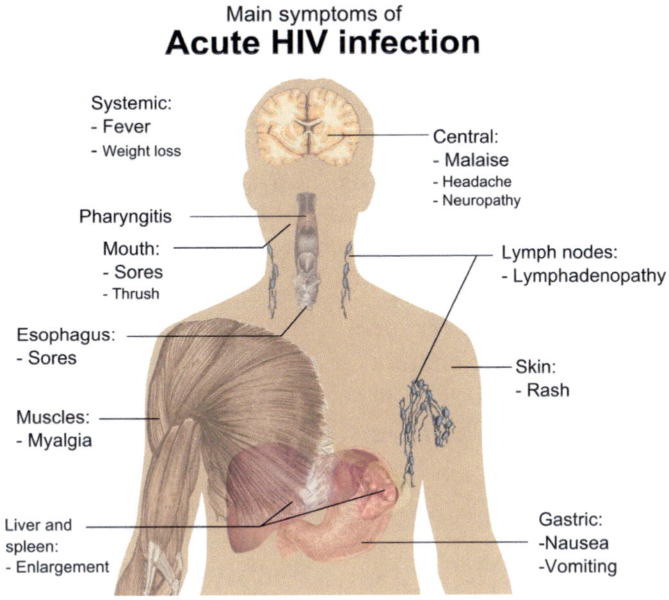

Figure 8.5. HIV/AIDS symptoms, diagnosis, and treatment.

Source: By Mikael Häggström.When using this image in external works, it may be cited as:Häggström, Mikael (2014). "Medical gallery of Mikael Häggström 2014". WikiJournal of Medicine 1 (2). DOI:10.15347/wjm/2014.008. ISSN 2002-4436. Public Domain.orBy Mikael Häggström, used with permission. - All used images are in public domain., Public Domain, https://commons.wikimedia.org/w/index.php?curid=5622996

8.2.1. Acute HIV Infection Symptoms

Immediately following HIV infection, there is this baffling set of symptoms that can seem exactly like some other viral flu, so getting it early becomes very difficult. Individuals usually initially begin to feel like they've come down with the flu – fever, simple fatigue, sore throat, even swollen glands in some cases. This is so because our own immune system quite abruptly jumps into gear, fighting off a virus that's replicating at full speed in mere minutes. Notably, the viral load increases to extremely high levels at this initial stage, thereby increasing the likelihood of transmitting it. Despite the fact that the body is resisting with everything it has, it can't keep the virus entirely at bay , slowly but surely, those precious immune cells begin to decrease. This disorganized combination of signals frequently causes misdiagnosis or delay in testing, so it's definitely worth paying attention to these early warning signs; catching them is essential for prompt treatment and may prevent the virus from becoming established in long-term reservoirs. Boring deeper down, you begin to notice that acute HIV infection has some significant changes in how our immune system works. The virus prefers to target CD4+ T cells – particularly those that have CCR5 receptors which are found largely in our gut-associated lymphoid tissue. To lose them early on causes mucosal defense to go haywire, and that can lead to a larger, more general immune overresponse. Most studies indicate that, by and large, the more actively the virus multiplies in this window of time, the worse the disease gets. Early ART might be a promising strategy; it seems to help shrink viral hideouts while giving the immune system a fighting chance. The constant tug-of-war between the virus spreading and the body's desperate counterattack likely explains why many patients also go through rashes, muscle aches, and gastrointestinal troubles during these early days (Ananworanich et al., 2012). From a public health perspective, these initial HIV warnings represent a critical point for intervention. Because at this point, people tend to be super contagious due to explosive viral loads, catching the problem early and leaping onto treatment can make an enormous impact on preventing transmission. Indeed, models of mathematics suggest initiating treatment earlier in the context of acute infection might change trends in epidemics on a wider level, specifically in high-risk populations such as men who have sex with men.

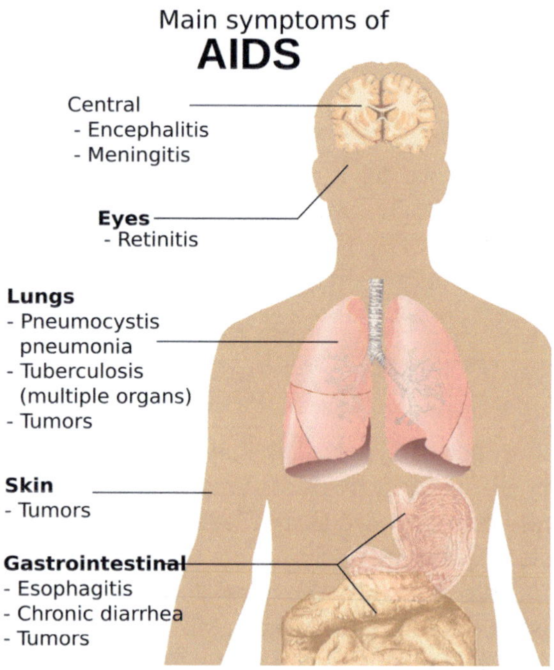

Figure 8.6. Acute HIV infection symptoms.

Source: By Mikael Häggström.When using this image in external works, it may be cited as:Häggström, Mikael (2014). "Medical gallery of Mikael Häggström 2014". WikiJournal of Medicine 1 (2). DOI:10.15347/wjm/2014.008. ISSN 2002-4436. Public Domain.orBy Mikael Häggström, used with permission. - All used images are in public domain., CC0, https://commons.wikimedia.org/w/index.php?curid=5425813

Additionally, reducing the intensity of symptoms using rapid therapy might allow for the maintenance of immune capacity and improved outcomes for patients. Overall, raising awareness of these initial symptoms among health professionals and the general public is essential; early diagnosis and timely treatment not only protect personal health but are also instrumental in stemming the epidemic (Cumberland et al., 2013) (Figure 8.6).

8.2.2. Clinical Latency Stage

Following the initial explosive outbreak of infection, HIV enters a long, silent phase that individuals tend to refer to as the clinical latency stage. During this stage, the virus continues to replicate, though slowly—and most people feel almost normal in spite of this covert activity; this can create a false impression of well-being. This stage, which can last for years, is influenced by factors such as how robust one's immune system is and whether or not ART is accessible. It's a sobering moment since the virus creeps into and damages the immune system, most importantly the CD4+ T cells that serve as chief sentinels. Unless treated on time, such slow degradation opens one up for increasing susceptibility to opportunistic infection and ultimately to AIDS. Rolling out access to ART during this period becomes essential for prolonging life and enhancing general health, although health worker shortages in some areas create universal coverage a serious problem (Bloom et al., 2025). Understanding how this quiet phase functions is important for informing improved HIV/AIDS therapies. During latency, HIV retreats into reservoirs, avoiding both immune surveillance and the activities of antiretroviral therapies, making it difficult to eradicate entirely. Certain new studies are attempting to turn the page by reviving the latent virus so that it is susceptible to targeted treatments or immune clearance. For instance, drugs such as histone deacetylase inhibitors, such as vorinostat, are being investigated for inducing viral expression from latent reservoirs without significantly rising viral loads or disrupting immune cell counts, as seen in trials for HIV-associated lymphomas (Aboulafia et al., 2018). These strategies suggest the potential for functional cures through targeting those silent infections that current therapies overlook. The clinical latency phase thus offers both a significant challenge and also a potential for novel treatment strategies for sustainable viral suppression and potentially even viral eradication. HIV persistence during this latent phase has a large bearing on public health interventions to manage the epidemic. Since most people are asymptomatic, early detection of the infection and adherence to therapy are crucial to avert disease development and minimize the risk of transmission. Concurrently, the prolonged duration of clinical latency translates to more untreated cases eventually needing lifelong treatment, putting more pressure on health systems, particularly where medical services are limited by fewer medical practitioners available to scale up ART efforts (Bloom et al., 2025). The cycle demands policy intervention that addresses not just the health issues but the infrastructural and human resource problems in the care of HIV. Initiation of new treatment protocols incorporating wake-up agents for the latent virus can potentially reduce the viral reservoirs and ultimately reduce the long-term treatment burden (Aboulafia et al., 2018). Ultimately, successful management of the clinical latency phase is crucial if we hope to stem HIV/AIDS globally, enhance the well-being of patients, and ensure that there is no re-emergence in viral transmission.

8.2.3. Progression to AIDS

When HIV first comes on the scene, you literally have to excavate how the virus and our immune system become complex. Initially, the virus primarily targets the CD4+ T cells—those critical players in our defense mechanism—and, with time, slowly grinds them down, bit by bit, rendering the body weaker at fending off infections that would otherwise not be problematic. Even with HAART in the wings to slow down the pace by keeping viral counts low, there are still challenges like drug resistance and the long-term toxic side effects that continue to raise their heads. These challenges drive researchers to seek new drugs that target not just the typical viral enzymes, like reverse transcriptase and RNase H, but also to mitigate unwanted side effects and protect against resistance. One such promising concept is the design of drugs that can interfere with multiple phases of the life cycle of the virus, a tactic which, in a majority of instances, would provide more long-term management of the disease and redirect its course away from complete AIDS development (Tratrat et al., 2025). As the disease approaches AIDS, patients find themselves confronting all kinds of challenges—not only the traditional infections, but brain fog and mood swings that scramble their everyday lives. For instance, a lot of them complain about fighting insomnia, but the reasons appear to be an assortment of factors; it is not one thing. The virus upsetting the immune system, side effects of the meds, and even stress all appear to interfere with sleep, making individuals more susceptible. Studies have established some associations between memory loss, other health issues related to AIDS, and some treatments such as efavirenz with an increase in risk of insomnia, which sometimes even exacerbates immunosuppression and erodes quality of life. In general, addressing some of these non-immunological problems is a necessity for holistic care, particularly when mental stress proves to be a significant contributor to sleep disorders in this population (Reid & Dwyer, 2005). When the disease eventually becomes full-blown AIDS, the additive damage to the immune system renders individuals highly vulnerable to opportunistic infections and cancers that are central to diagnosing AIDS. It's really at this tipping point that the body just can't keep the hidden bacteria or new invaders at bay, often leading to serious disease or even death. Once the count of CD4+ T cells falls to really low levels, the body loses one of its main defenses, opening the door to life-threatening infections like *Pneumocystis jirovecii* pneumonia and even Kaposi's sarcoma. Monitoring tight viral load and immune markers closely is crucial so that initial measures can occasionally restore a degree of immune activity and delay the appearance of AIDS. In the future, combining targeted antiviral drugs with methods addressing more general concerns, such as neuropsychiatric complications and sleeping disorders, may well turn the tide for HIV/AIDS patients (Reid & Dwyer, 2005; Tratrat et al., 2025) (Figure 8.7).

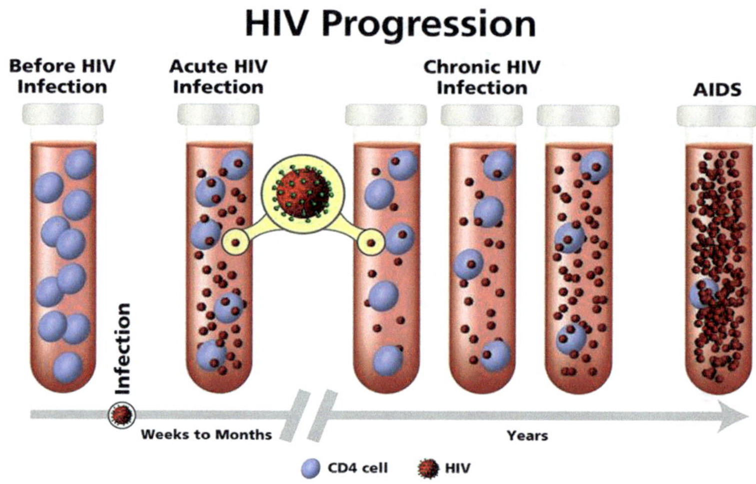

Figure 8.7. HIV progression.

Source: Clinicalinfo.HIV.gov. (n.d.). *HIV Progression.*

8.3. Diagnosis of HIV

Early HIV detection is crucial for patient management and will assist in reducing virus transmission. Diagnostic methods have improved dramatically—remember when tests tested for the presence of antibodies through means such as ELISA, followed by confirmation with Western blot. Those methods are good, but they typically require a lag before antibodies appear, which slows down the entire process. More recent molecular methods, such as virus RNA testing, leap in shortly after exposure, alleviating that lag. This combination of methods holds a prominent position in the clinic and in public health, as an immediate initiation of antiretroviral therapy reduces both severity of disease and risk of transmission. Apart from standard laboratory procedures, computer modeling has entered the fray to enhance early HIV detection through symptom analysis. For example, computer programs like the Naïve Bayes classifier employ what is reported by patients along with epidemiological information to calculate the probability of an infection, essentially performing number crunching and symptom counts and comparing these to stored data banks. It's not a catch-all, however; rather, model-based systems like the online variety provide a rapid, low-cost method for flagging potential cases to undergo confirmatory testing (Aisah et al., 2024). They are a convenient addition to the old tests in the face of our quickly evolving diagnostic technology. Comprehending HIV's effects is not merely about diagnosing the virus early—there's also the larger context of how it crosses over with other disease conditions. Studies have explored links between HIV parameters and conditions such as hypertension, and by and large, there is no direct correlation between HIV's distinct characteristics and elevated blood pressure. Rather, general cardiovascular risk indicators like advanced age, increased body mass index, and other chronic conditions like diabetes or hyperlipidemia often play a greater role in blood pressure issues. This subtlety illustrates just how complicated it can be to treat HIV when other chronic diseases are part of the equation. In the majority of instances, pinning down an HIV diagnosis is hand in hand with maintaining a keen eye on other health issues, all collectively contributing to enhancing patient outcomes and quality of life (Denu et al., 2024) (Figure 8.8).

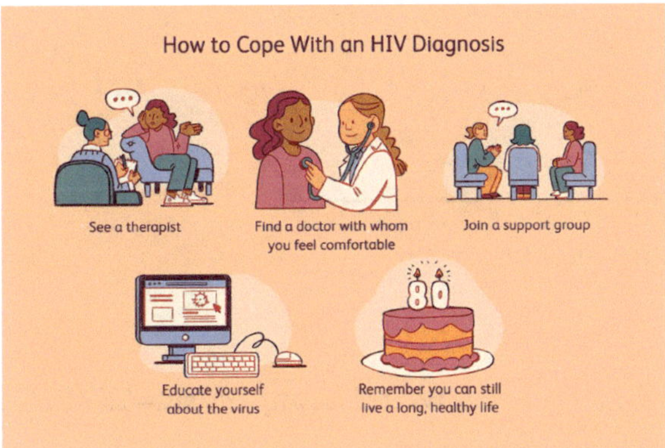

Figure 8.8. HIV diagnosis.

Source: https://external-content.duckduckgo.com/iu/?u=https%3A%2F%2Fwww.verywellhealth.com%2Fthmb%2FWiC9OV5CxAiJJvpjK7k0FeM1xUQ%3D%2F1500x1000%2Ffilters%3Ano_upscale()%3Amax_bytes(150000)%3Astrip_icc()%2Fhiv-diagnosis-5194292-Final-9c7e2ec491ed4ba48f669f5494c10503.jpg&f=1&nofb=1&ipt=97b73a29464667dc7963d68e24d906d00076ebc1599af1c3b1cb177f1ee29fb85.

8.3.1. Types of HIV Tests

Early, accurate diagnosis is very important in the management of HIV/AIDS—it launches our battle with the virus by stopping its replication and initiating early treatment. Various tests are done, each performed differently, has varying waiting time before results can be obtained, and has distinctive markers they check for. Take a sample example – most begin with an antibody test that detects the body's natural response, tending to come positive after some weeks from when the person became infected. Next, there is the fourth-generation, or antigen/antibody combination test; it detects both antibodies as well as the p24 protein (a protein of HIV, which shows earlier), and thereby reduces waiting time. Nucleic acid tests (or NATs) start right out to identify HIV RNA, providing the quickest results following exposure, but they're frequently more expensive and not necessarily found everywhere. At the end of the day, the best test is determined by clinical necessity, what's readily available, and the necessity of early detection of the virus. Rapid HIV tests, a staff favorite in numerous screening programs, spit out results in minutes, facilitating getting people into care more rapidly. These tests primarily detect HIV antibodies in blood or oral fluid and are thus a success with outreach groups, they're easy and provide instant results, although a subsequent test may be necessary to confirm any reactive result. Laboratory-based testing such as ELISAs are often still the norm in many instances because they provide high levels of accuracy through identifying both antibodies and antigens simultaneously. Improved testing methods of recent times have driven up sensitivity in the acute phase of HIV infection, a vital step in controlling transmission. Providing a range of options for testing appears to go a long way in adapting approaches to particular groups in different settings, driving up early detection and rapid treatment initiations (Haberer et al., 2015). In addition to these conventional strategies, research is underway to find new diagnostic devices such as self-test kits and point-of-care NATs—potentially marrying fast testing with earlier diagnosis. Self-testing provides an opportunity for people to test for HIV in private, an attractive way of cutting stigma and perhaps even persuading additional people to test. Conversely, making sure that a positive self-test is followed by a confirmatory test and appropriate care continues to be challenging. Point-of-care NATs hold promise with the potential to combine rapid results with early detection capability, extending the frontiers of antibody-based tests. For the most part, knowing the various tests and employing them correctly is the secret to making prevention and treatment programs function effectively. Considering HIV risk behaviors and prevention concepts continuously change, test guidelines must evolve as well—to achieve results not only precise and rapid but also available in actual settings (Haberer et al., 2015) (Figure 8.9).

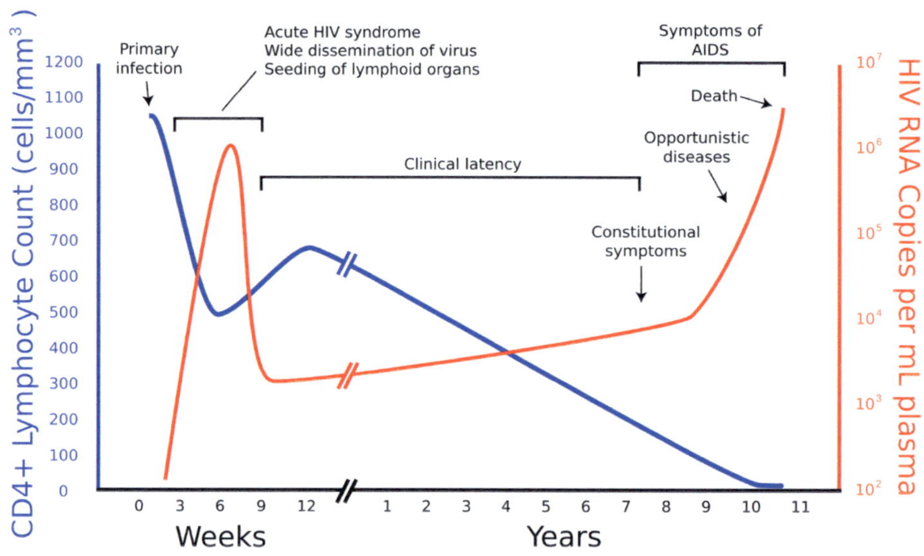

Figure 8.9. HIV tests.

Source: By Sigve - Own work, CC0, https://commons.wikimedia.org/w/index.php?curid=15383502

8.3.2. Importance of Early Diagnosis

HIV can creep up on a person so subtly that many don't realize what's going on until the infection has taken hold. Frequently, people may not even be aware of issues such as opportunistic infections or unusual lesions that suggest an impaired immune system. Take Kaposi's sarcoma lesions in the mouth, for example – in several clinical cases, these marks were the first hint of HIV, and early detection meant quick treatment could start (Silveira et al., 2025). Spotting these subtle clues early is key because it lets doctors start Highly Active Antiretroviral Therapy (HAART), which in many cases slows the disease's progress and cuts down on complications. Seeing these symptoms not only results in better treatment but also has a tendency to enhance the overall prognosis and quality of life for the afflicted. Missing the early diagnosis of HIV also leaves an individual more susceptible to a variety of other infections, which both cause and advance the disease. In untreated individuals, conditions such as pulmonary tuberculosis (PTB), pneumocystis pneumonia, and candidiasis tend to appear suddenly (Das et al., 2024). Such infections interact with each other to further compromise the immune system, and hence treatments become complex for HIV-positive individuals.

Early diagnosis opens up a treatment plan that addresses both HIV and these secondary conditions simultaneously, and this tends to enhance survival possibilities. Initiating antiretroviral therapy earlier than later also serves to safeguard the immune system, reducing the chances for serious complications. Realizing how HIV and such opportunistic infections seem to go hand-in-hand truly highlights the value of early detection, particularly when resources are scarce. Early detection of HIV through consistent testing can alter the course of the disease by providing access to both medical care and some much-needed emotional support. Regular screening for those in high-risk groups implies the virus can be detected before the immune system is seriously compromised. This approach is indeed good for the patient - it saves them from the worst-case scenario - but also for society as a whole by reducing viral loads and subsequent spread (Das et al., 2024). Early diagnosis usually encourages patients to get more involved in their care and stick with their antiretroviral regimen, which is crucial for keeping the virus at bay and avoiding serious conditions like Kaposi's sarcoma (Silveira et al., 2025). Spending broadly on initial testing proves to be a good decision for handling an individual's well-being as well as handling HIV on a broader level, showing that early detection is vitally crucial.

8.3.3. Challenges in HIV Testing

Policy communication is a significant force in implementing HIV testing strategies, but it hits a lot of roadblocks. In Zambia, for instance, the implementation of the test-and-treat-all strategy utilized both formal and informal channels to communicate information to healthcare workers; oddly enough, many frontline providers never got it—despite the fact that the policy was clearly embedded in the National HIV/AIDS Strategic Framework. Verbal orders and brief text messages confused matters further, making it difficult for providers to adhere to the guidelines consistently, and even broadcast media did not always reach the target with each segment of the community. Overall, this confusing means of conveying information diminished the capacity of healthcare workers to provide prompt, accurate HIV testing. Overall, closing such gaps requires concerted efforts to enhance training, enhance the dissemination of messages, and eventually empower providers as well as patients (Simooya et al., 2023). The COVID-19 pandemic added another hurdle, causing additional barriers in the implementation of HIV testing globally. Regular healthcare services were severely impacted, and interventions such as quarantine and social distancing rendered it much more difficult for individuals to access testing in person. Even when self-testing kits became available in certain regions, their distribution remained patchy, particularly in disadvantaged communities—enlarging the testing uptake disparity. As a result of the pandemic, many people now avoid going to health facilities to access care, while health facilities redirect their efforts toward managing COVID-19. The early detection has thus become delayed more than before, and connecting patients with care has been even more challenging. In all the instances, all these added pressures have heaped on pre-existing challenges of HIV testing, prompting new and innovative solutions (Jiang et al., 2020). Maintaining HIV testing during such crisis times evidently demands adaptable healthcare provision and resourceful allocation. When COVID-19 struck, treatment facilities immediately became swamped, which resulted in delayed initiation of antiretroviral therapy and disrupted regular follow-ups. A few nations—at least partially—countered with innovative steps such as decentralized drug delivery, extended prescription durations, and even telemedicine consultations to assist in alleviating the burden. Nevertheless, these solutions rely heavily on the availability of sufficient infrastructure and financing, which is not always present in low-resource environments. Additionally, residual stigma and reluctance among patients, particularly those who are not yet ready for immediate treatment—still hinder testing uptake. For all intents and purposes, overcoming the obstacles in HIV testing truly necessitates a combination of approaches: adaptable service delivery, strong communication, and meaningful community involvement are all most important in maintaining the process of care on track and establishing trust over time (Jiang et al., 2020; Simooya et al., 2023) (Figure 8.10).

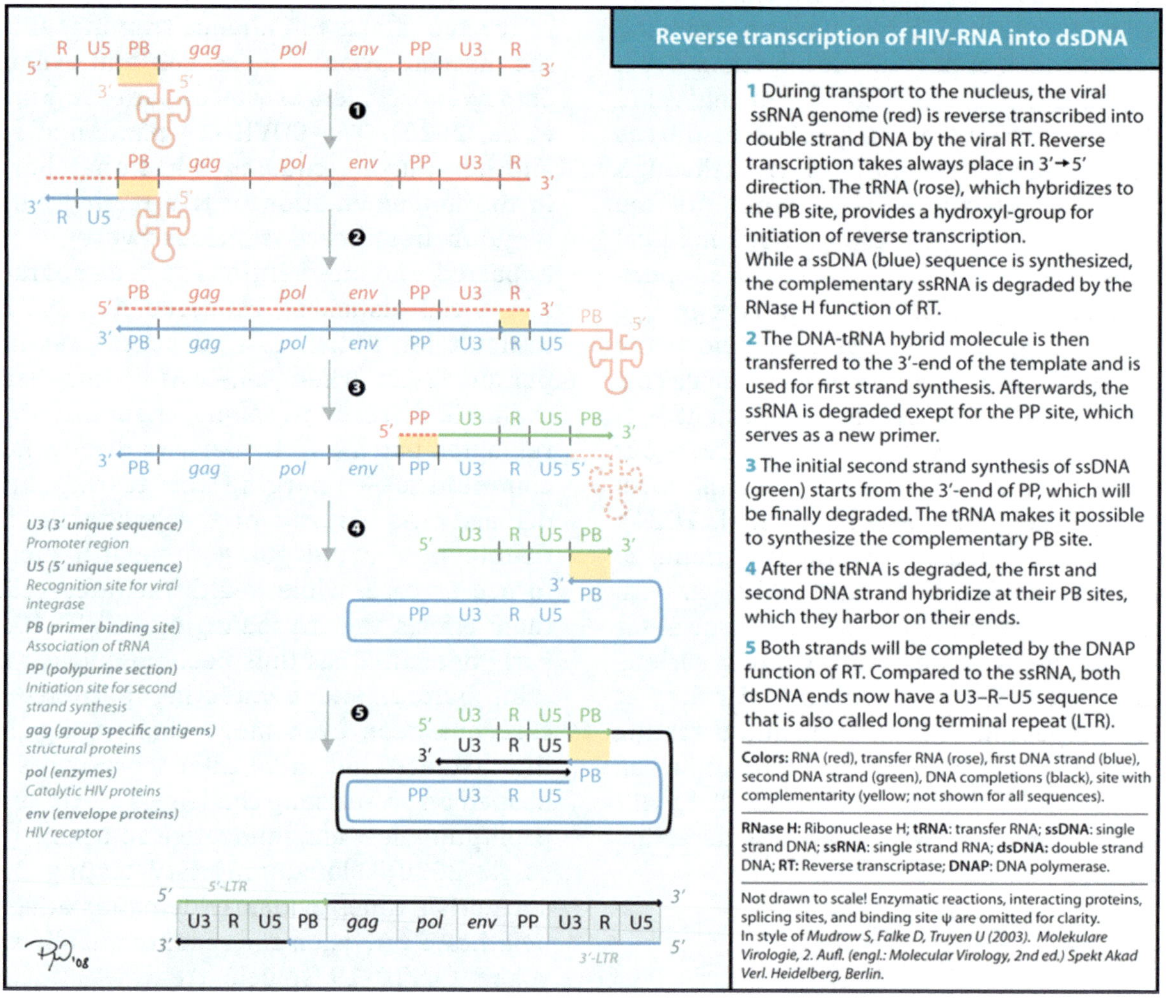

Figure 8.10. Challenges in HIV testing.

8.4. Treatment Options

Medical advancement has truly transformed how we perceive HIV/AIDS. What was once a death warrant now frequently becomes a chronic condition, owing principally to ART. ART, the therapy that reduces the levels of the virus in individuals, prevents the disease from advancing and also reduces the likelihood that it spreads. But the therapy isn't without its glitches. There are side effect issues, instances of the virus becoming resistant to the drugs, and, quite simply, gaining access to everybody, particularly in areas where there is less resources—is still a hard nut to crack. These issues have led scientists to experiment with new concepts such as stem cell transplants or gene modifications that are designed to either stimulate the immune system or target reservoirs of the virus that are hidden.

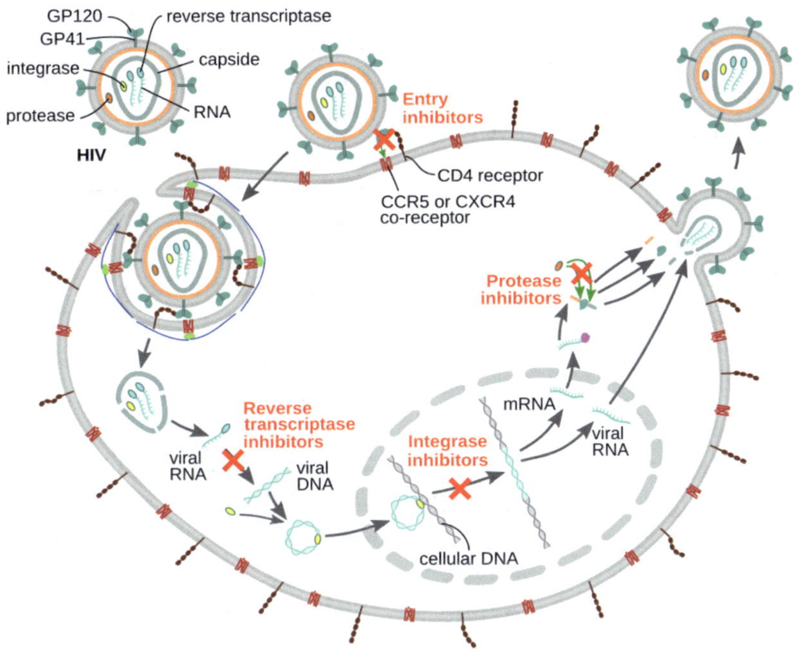

Figure 8.11. Treatment options for HIV.

Source: By Thomas Splettstoesser (www.scistyle.com) - Own work, CC BY 3.0, https://commons.wikimedia.org/w/index.php?curid=29443283

There's also been enthusiasm for using agents that wake up dormant HIV cells, thereby making them more vulnerable to the immune system or assisting ART in doing its work. Overall, these new strategies are contributing to an expanding toolkit that's meant to bypass the boundaries of traditional treatment and get us one step closer to a functional cure (Alum et al., 2024). Despite all these advancements, much is still not even on the earth. Although science has brought along these new treatment models, lots of areas, especially in developing and middle-income countries, continue to struggle. Cost barriers, weak healthcare infrastructures, and persistent social HIV stigmatism keep treatment distant from many. These obstacles interfere with both the routine deployment of ART and the launch of newer forms such as long-lasting injectables or test therapeutic vaccines that are currently undergoing clinical trials. For the most part, it is apparent that simply having better treatments is insufficient; we must confront the very real-world impediments that stand in the way of individuals' access to care. Older issues, including drug resistance or lack of testing and diagnosis, and stigmata that never lose their grip entirely, make it even more difficult. A smart combination of biomedical breakthrough with initiatives that address structural and behavioral problems – even tolerating a little bit of messiness in how fixes are assembled – appears downright essential to fill that gap between success in the lab and everyday life (Mami et al., 2024). Ahead, there's a concrete sense of optimism in the changing treatment landscape. Gene-editing technologies such as CRISPR, for instance, promise to retool our own cells to resist HIV, and novel therapeutic vaccines could enable the immune system to attack the virus more effectively. In addition, continuous advancements in PrEP are likely to reduce numbers of new infections even further, reinforcing the message that prevention does indeed go hand-in-hand with treatment. But sustained progress will depend on solving the underlying social problems, such as poverty, unequal access to education, and gender disparities that determine how the virus is transmitted. In most instances, making sure medical advances reach everyone will require sustained investment in research, improving health systems, and promoting partnerships that heavily factor in human rights and equity. This multi-faceted strategy is central to gradually turning HIV/AIDS from a prevailing epidemic into a disease that, hopefully, we will eventually be able to leave completely behind us (Alum et al., 2024; Mami et al., 2024) (Figure 8.11).

8.4.1. Antiretroviral Therapy (ART)

HIV/AIDS management isn't what it once was. New antiretroviral therapies are now reaching deep into the virus's replication cycle, knocking it down and improving patient results. Recently, new drug combinations have appeared that not only keep individuals on schedule with their medications but also reduce the burden of side effects—a true victory for daily life. Consider the case of Uganda: they've implemented community-based care that combines single-dose fixed treatments with longer-acting ones, making it easier for people to remain consistent with their regimens. Meanwhile, offloading some responsibilities onto non-specialist health workers has helped redistribute the burden and address resource constraints. Obviously, it's not merely a matter of the drug; how you administer it is important too (Kato, 2024). On a second front, there's constant pressure to develop novel antiretroviral agents to expand treatment options and transcend drug resistance challenges. Most often, this type of innovation is what propels the field ahead. In China, for example, the recent registration of Ainuovirine, a novel non-nucleoside reverse transcriptase inhibitor, demonstrates the drive to innovate. Certain retrospective clinical trials suggest that regimens constructed with Ainuovirine work about as well as previous treatments for viral suppression but have more tolerant safety profiles, particularly with lipid metabolism and liver enzymes. This less harsh side-effect profile would then permit patients to remain on their treatment longer, which is essential when side effects occasionally interfere. Overall, these new drugs appear to unlock the potential for more individualized treatment regimens that could better address diverse patient needs (Guo et al., 2024). But it's not just a matter of the drugs—those are only part of the equation. Scaling up ART on a wider basis relies on how well health systems can respond to regional issues and remain focused on patients. In most resource-constrained environments, innovative strategies such as task-shifting and community-based care have become critical for expanding coverage and maintaining patient engagement. These methods enable the reduction of stigma, travel, and fragile infrastructure-related problems by optimizing local community networks. When innovative medicines are combined with adaptive, responsive care models, the aggregate outcomes are impressive—improved adherence, reduced transmission, and an overall smoother care experience. This illustrates that HIV/AIDS management is a complex undertaking that requires continuous innovation both in the drugs we employ and the manner we practice care (Kato, 2024).

8.4.2. Importance of Adherence to Treatment

It truly is all about patients remaining involved in their treatment regimens in the long term. It's not merely taking medicine on time; antiretroviral therapy is complex and requires individuals to modify their day-to-day lifestyle. Research mostly indicates that the relationship between providers and patients makes a huge difference when it comes to adhering to treatment regimens. Providers' own stories, how they give care, their own style, can influence a patient's engagement in ways that don't always seem evident. When you get at these provider perceptions, you learn that it's a combination of simple, straightforward communication, some real emotional support, and even the atmosphere of the health care environment that contributes to establishing trust (Chapman et al., 2015).

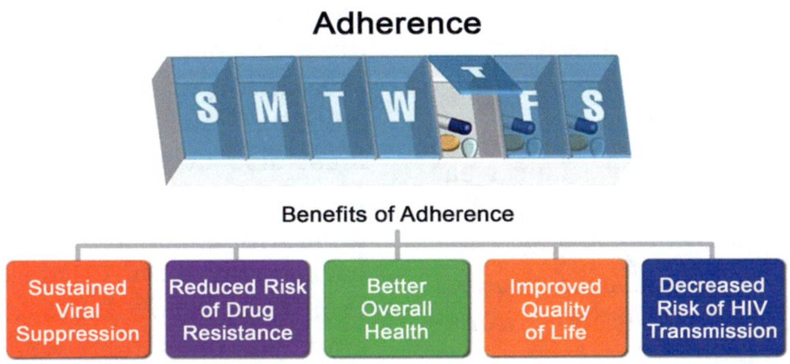

Figure 8.12. Importance of adherence to treatment.

Source: Clinicalinfo.HIV.gov. (n.d.). *Importance of Adherence to Treatment.*

Overall, if we listen to these tidbits, patients comply more with treatment, which then allows viral loads to fall and halts disease progression. Individuals undergoing HIV/AIDS treatment frequently encounter a whole set of personal and environmental barriers. At other times, it's simply unclear why the drug is such a big deal, and other times the interaction with clinicians is lacking, and to add insult to injury, experiences of stigma can get in the way. In most instances, studies conducted in Nigerian healthcare environments highlight that gender disparities and restricted access to specialist services only serve to compound things—layering additional obstacles on top of already challenging problems. Patients who are struggling with depression or other issues in their lives might not be able to maintain their antiretroviral therapy as consistently as they need to, which saps the treatment's strength. In general, best results depend on patients achieving at least 95% of their doses, but this is made challenging by both personal setbacks and larger social forces. Essentially, focused interventions that enhance patient education and increase clinical relationship trust more are central (Okuboyejo & Omogbadegun, 2013). Adherence isn't solely a matter of an individual—it severely impacts public health overall as well. When patients miss doses or fail to complete, it devastates the treatment, possibly fueling drug resistance and allowing the virus to transmit in communities. This not only increases the pressure on our healthcare systems but also erodes the hard work achieved to date against HIV/AIDS. Improved adherence is associated with reduced viral loads, reduced complications from disease, and, quite frankly, an improved quality of life for those living with HIV/AIDS. In the vast majority of situations, ramping up provider education, embracing genuinely patient-driven care, and providing adaptable treatment plans isn't merely a medical necessity, it fulfills an ethical responsibility to empower people and facilitate more equitable, more accessible care (Chapman et al., 2015; Okuboyejo & Omogbadegun, 2013). In the end, these concerted efforts stem the epidemic and advance enduring advancements in worldwide health (Figure 8.12).

8.4.3. Emerging Treatments and Research

Recent advances in HIV/AIDS medical research have really changed the way physicians treat the disease. No longer are therapies mired in the days of monotherapy – today, combination ART slows down the virus and even reduces challenging opportunistic infections. Long-acting medicines, for example, allow for patients to maintain longer intervals before needing another dosage, which particularly benefits individuals confronted with daily economic and social struggle. PrEP has also emerged as a leading approach to preventing new infections in the most vulnerable. Although these advances hold great promise, challenges such as drug resistance and unequal access continue to arise. In most instances, getting all these treatments to work effectively entails examining a combination of biological, social, and systemic factors to provide equitable healthcare (Ezeja, 2024). In the meantime, research isn't just about new drugs—it's also examining how HIV affects other conditions. Consider hearing loss, for instance; it's been seen as a significant, though not well-known, side effect in individuals with HIV/AIDS, especially those who have jobs that expose them to loud noises. The ototoxicity of certain antiretrovirals, combined with the immune burdens of HIV and even other diseases such as TB, appears to heighten the risk of hearing issues. In most instances, this translates to patients requiring more than viral suppression; they require vigilant monitoring of a variety of side effects. Rising data from high-prevalence regions like South Africa suggests the advantage of a more holistic health approach – one that considers both outcomes of treatment and quality-of-life concerns, such as sensory well-being (Khoza-Shangase, 2025). The future of HIV/AIDS treatment depends on new innovations and care that takes into account the entire individual. Scientists are working towards vaccine and immunotherapy treatments that could block infection or even produce permanent cures. Broadly, these breakthroughs rely on robust clinical trials and global collaboration. Public health programs must also overcome structural barriers, such as stigma and few resources—to allow these breakthroughs to have their full impact. There's even a new trend to add regular hearing tests to HIV treatment, indicating a more widespread emphasis on patient well-being. It's all about pouring money into research, outreach, and policy reform to translate scientific advances into daily life, hopefully leading to finally bringing the epidemic to an end (Ezeja, 2024; Khoza-Shangase, 2025).

8.5. Impact on Public Health

HIV/AIDS challenges don't just affect an individual's health; they ripple out and unsettle entire public health systems worldwide. The strain on healthcare infrastructure—especially in low-income areas hit hardest by the disease—is real and hard to ignore. Programs like the Ryan White HIV/AIDS Program (RWHAP) and AIDS Drug Assistance Programs (ADAPs) play a major role by offering essential care and support to folks without proper insurance. During crises such as the COVID-19 pandemic, these services found it tough to keep patients qualified while switching over to remote delivery. Still, innovations including telehealth platforms, home delivery of meds, and looser enrollment rules have, generally speaking, done a decent job keeping care accessible. To summarize, these shifts underscore the need for flexible, resilient public health systems that continue to back vulnerable people with HIV/AIDS, helping to avoid further health disparities (McManus et al., 2023). In regions where HIV/AIDS is especially burdensome, like sub-Saharan Africa—the impact sharpens due to a lack of resources and issues with sticking to treatments. For example, studies in Ethiopia have noted surprisingly high rates of first-line ART failure, which really complicates efforts to manage the epidemic and reduce disease and death. The fact that treatment sometimes falters so quickly highlights the urgent need for better public health measures that focus on patient adherence and early detection of complications. It turns out that factors such as age and how rigorously patients follow their treatment plans heavily sway outcomes, revealing significant gaps in patient education and follow-up care. This evidence calls for more targeted counseling and sturdier monitoring systems in public health programs to keep ART effective and improve overall health results (Wondimgezahu et al., 2023). The broader picture of HIV/AIDS also pushes us to keep rethinking ideas and updating policies as patient needs change. HIV care programs must juggle efficiency with a truly patient-centered approach, especially when social and behavioral factors constantly play a part in treatment adherence and disease progression. Digital health advances that came out during recent emergencies have taught us valuable lessons about extending access to care for marginalized groups. Interestingly, these shifts hint at a potential for wider benefits across various public health sectors, boosting both service delivery and patient retention. Addressing the mix of healthcare access, treatment adherence, and social influences is key to taming the HIV/AIDS epidemic. Future public health strategies should definitely prioritize making these innovations sustainable to ensure fair, ongoing care for populations affected by HIV/AIDS (McManus et al., 2023) (Figure 8.13).

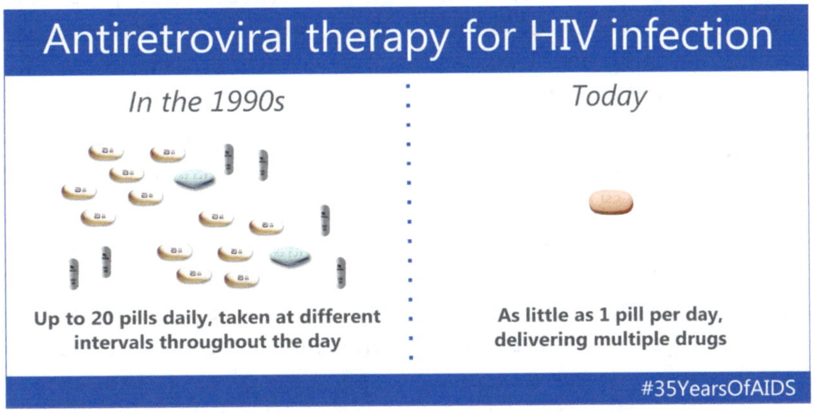

Figure 8.13. AIDS drug assistance programs.

Source: By NIAID - https://www.flickr.com/photos/niaid/27423001115/, CC BY 2.0, https://commons.wikimedia.org/w/index.php?curid=67904533

8.5.1. Global Statistics and Trends

Advances in medical science haven't stopped infectious diseases from leaving their mark on global death rates. Mortality records from 1990–2021 show noticeable shifts in why people die—

COVID-19, for example, dragged life expectancy down between 2019 and 2021. Even with the pandemic hogging the spotlight, HIV/AIDS still makes its presence known, especially in low- and middle-income areas. terms, though death from most infections has fallen to summarize, the disproportionate burden of HIV/AIDS highlights persistent health inequalities. Variations in healthcare units, availability of antiretroviral treatment—and prevention methods too—only serve to make things more difficult to overcome; deaths due to this disease cluster within certain populations, which effectively highlights the complex nature of modern-day global health issues (Naghavi et al., 2024). Taking a closer glance, the disproportionate distribution of HIV/AIDS globally becomes fairly evident—sub-Saharan Africa carries an especially great burden. That region experiences significantly higher infection and death rates; limited life-saving treatment access and late diagnosis factor heavily. A powerful example is Kaposi sarcoma, an AIDS-defining malignancy that appears much more frequently in high HIV prevalence settings, flaunting well-defined geographic disparities. And the lack of solid cancer registries and valid mortality data in most low-HDI countries confuses the picture, making it difficult to establish tailored health responses. Although some areas have experienced gains from increased HIV treatment and prevention, obstacles remain where health infrastructure is poor, and it's made painfully evident that closer monitoring—and a more equitable distribution of resources—are necessary (Carrilho & Lunet, 2023). Globally, there has been some success in reducing the number of deaths from HIV/AIDS, but the epidemic persists and refuses to end, requiring sustained public health effort. In most high-income nations, enhanced access to antiretroviral therapy combined with prevention strategies such as education and safe sex habits have typically resulted in significant reductions in HIV-related diseases and deaths. Conversely, increasing HIV-related diseases in certain European populations, in all candor, necessitate ongoing surveillance and prevention interventions targeted toward vulnerable groups. The evolving face of HIV/AIDS, and diseases such as Kaposi sarcoma that accompany it, illustriousies the urgent need for integrated health approaches that combine early diagnosis, mass treatment, and focused prevention initiatives. Knowing these evolving trends is important for policymakers so they can allocate resources effectively and create interventions that are at par with the ever-changing spread of the epidemic (Carrilho & Lunet, 2023; Naghavi et al., 2024).

8.5.2. Disparities in HIV/AIDS Prevalence

HIV/AIDS remains a stubborn health challenge and continues to persist, and its transmission isn't uniform across the board. You see how groups vary greatly since factors such as gender and age influence the figures in ways you wouldn't have anticipated. Women between 20 and 49, for instance, tend to show higher rates—not just because their bodies may be more prone to infection but also due to social and cultural hurdles that keep many from getting proper care. It's not only about individual risk either; where someone lives matters too. These regions, with their substandard healthcare infrastructure and lack of awareness in society, bear a greater burden, so the entire picture is a complicated mosaic (Dalatu, 2025). Another complication added to the mix is the way certain complications strike segments of the HIV-positive harder than others. Consider anemia, for instance—it arises more frequently in those who have HIV. Those yet to begin antiretroviral therapy (so-called ART-naïve individuals) appear to be more adversely affected by anemia compared to those already receiving the treatment. There also appears to be a discernible pattern with at-risk groups such as children and pregnant women each having their own risk factors. In most lower-middle-income settings, the issue peaks even higher relative to upper-middle-income settings, demonstrating how issues of economics combine with health factors (Shrivastav et al., 2025). Working with these unequal patterns requires that we examine the complex combination of biology, social forces, and money concerns that fuel the epidemic. Policies in most instances must provide for ensuring that health care is not only for the privileged few but extends to women in their childbearing years, children, and economically struggling individuals. It assists in monitoring shared concerns like anemia and low CD4 levels through regular screenings; these measures, grounded in extensive data, can over time chip away at moderating the risks locally and worldwide (Dalatu, 2025; Shrivastav et al., 2025) (Figure 8.14).

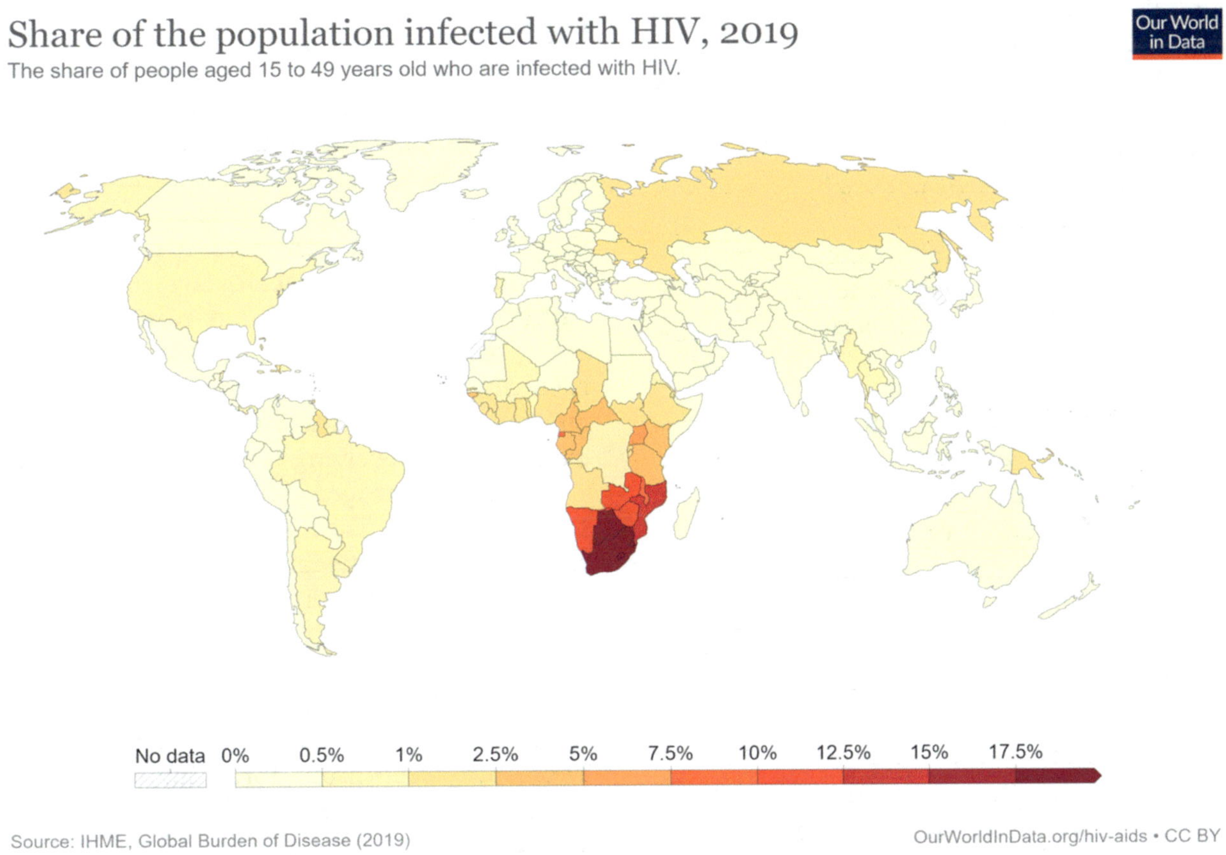

Figure 8.14. HIV/AIDS prevalence.

Source: By Our world in data - https://ourworldindata.org/hiv-aids, CC BY-SA 4.0, https://commons.wikimedia.org/w/index.php?curid=135466504

8.5.3. Public Health Initiatives and Prevention Strategies

Many years ago, the battle against HIV/AIDS shifted with a combination of public health actions that transformed infection control, the way infections are maintained under control and the quality of life for individuals living with the virus. Testing and counseling now appear immediately, flagging problems before they escalate so rapid remedies can occur. There is also a harm reduction effort, programs distributing condoms and even needle exchanges work to reduce risk for those who are most at risk. Education on HIV prevention now appears in schools and in community organizations, which serves to dispel myths and encourage individuals toward safer practices. All of these activities, in most instances, complement each other to bridge access gaps and respond to the needs of varied populations hardest hit by the epidemic. Biomedical prevention interventions have truly transformed HIV strategy, rendering public health initiatives even more potent. PrEP, a daily pill that reduces the risk of infection dramatically, is a prime example of a breakthrough; combined with ART in individuals already infected with HIV, these treatments can reduce viral loads to near zero—virtually eliminating transmission risk. Groups such as the Bill & Melinda Gates Foundation have worked hard to bring these treatments to regions where healthcare is scarce (Mugaiga, 2024).

Public education campaigns, on the whole, also emphasize adherence to treatment, maintaining regular testing, and reducing stigma, all in an effort to increase steady use. These medical breakthroughs and social efforts combined create a strong shield, one that does not just keep new cases at bay but also assists those who are already afflicted. Examining HIV/AIDS closely in conjunction with other health conditions and social ills continues to be important. Death trends, for example, indicate complications such as testicular cancer in certain HIV-positive individuals illustrating persistent disparities necessitating additional attention (Naz et al., 2025). Information largely indicates racial and ethnic minorities experiencing greater mortality rates fueled by socioeconomic and geographic challenges. Government health policies now increasingly rely on culturally relevant care and authentic community involvement to assist in closing these gaps and encourage earlier screenings. Regional variations, likewise, suggest that local, adapted interventions can genuinely make the difference. By monitoring these subtle risk factors closely, prevention strategies can remain subtle and prepared to adapt to the continually changing nature of this intricate epidemic.

8.6. Stigma and Discrimination

HIV/AIDS is not only a disease—it's part of a larger context where social inequalities combination with brutal stigma and discrimination. Most individuals, particularly those in marginalized sexual and gender groups, are shut off by outmoded ideologies that mark them as outsiders. It usually means they can't access the healthcare they require (Gibb et al., 2020). The day-to-day stress of being set aside manifests itself in their bodies, resulting in poorer health in general. Fear and misinformation about HIV prevent people from testing, receiving treatment, or enrolling in prevention programs. In a lot of healthcare settings, some discriminatory behaviors only create mistrust between patients and providers, which is critical when working with something like HIV. To summarize, stopping this cycle requires more than medical solutions—it demands culturally sensitive measures and policy reforms that prioritize dignity and inclusion. There are some groundbreaking, community-driven solutions making a difference. Consider Thailand's Key Population-led Health Services (KPLHS) program, for instance; this initiative essentially allows the very individuals impacted to take control of HIV prevention and treatment themselves (Vannakit et al., 2020). By doing this, not only do they avoid the stigma that surrounds mainstream clinics, but they also provide services that are based on actual, local needs. Lay health workers from groups like MSM, trans, and sex workers, having received training and some sort of certification, now provide care that's confidential and, quite frankly, less judgmental. This change has been associated with speedier diagnosis, quicker referrals to antiretroviral treatment, and more retention in care—definitive indications that allowing communities to take the lead can make HIV/AIDS control the game-changer it could become. At first glance, stigma and discrimination sting even worse than just excluding individuals from health access. They compound other stressors such as social isolation, violence, and economic decline, all of which deplete mental health and even make treatment more difficult for individuals to maintain (Gibb et al., 2020). All things considered, existing under that kind of persistent stress can cause actual physiological responses to stress, a self-perpetuating cycle that further increases health disparities. Conversely, social support and strong communities also at times provide a buffering effect, demonstrating how much inclusive, supportive environments matter. In most instances, addressing stigma involves delving deep into the origin of social exclusion while aligning health strategies with an improved understanding of cultural dynamics. All of this has to come together if we're to empower affected individuals and eventually see lasting progress against the HIV/AIDS epidemic (Figure 8.15).

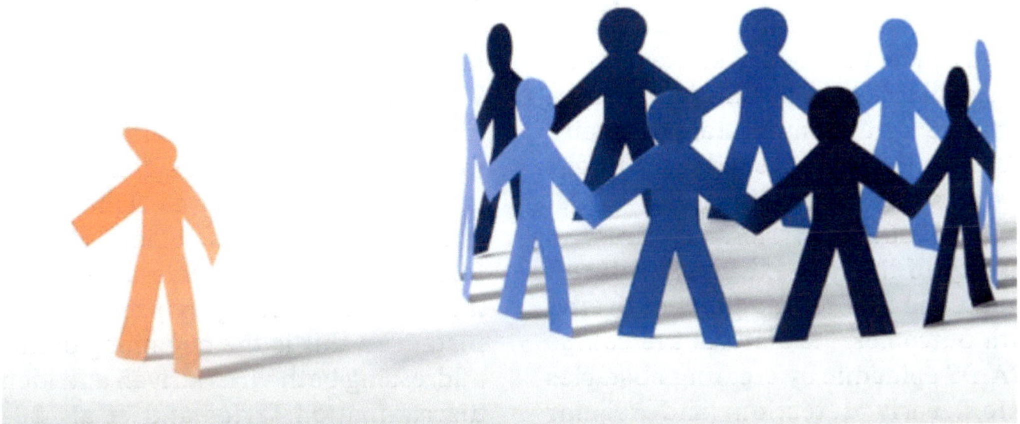

Figure 8.15. Stigma surrounding HIV/AIDS.

Source: HealthyPlace. (n.d.). *Stigma and Discrimination.*

8.6.1. Social Stigma Surrounding HIV/AIDS

The perspective of society and personal health combination in manners that profoundly impact how individuals cope with diseases such as HIV/AIDS. People living with HIV frequently cope with a stack of burdens, and stigma , that fusion of judgment and rejection , raps sharply on the mind as well as on day-to-day health habits. It appears as discrimination and exclusion, particularly in such environments as hospitals, where prejudices based on HIV status, or even sexual orientation and ethnicity, are at work. This type of exclusion leads to fear and concealment, which, in the majority of instances, prevents individuals from plunging into care that they require or continuing antiretroviral regimens. For instance, a study in the Dominican Republic tended to find that when patients feel discriminated against in clinics, they're less likely to adhere to their medication regimens (Kerr et al., 2024). In some sense, these findings make clear that stigma is not simply a latent sociocultural problem , it becomes a very concrete impediment to adequate treatment and equality in healthcare. Once you look into stigma, you immediately notice how established it is among vulnerable populations, such as men who have sex with men (MSM) and people living with HIV (PLHIV). These populations, in most instances, experience a number of overlapping stigmas that combine social prejudices surrounding ethnicity, sexual orientation, and HIV infection. The exclusion doesn't just hurt mental well-being; it also interferes with how willing people are to get tested or stick with treatment plans. Some literature notes that stigma goes way beyond one-on-one encounters, seeping into overall community behavior and coloring how everyone thinks about HIV and the possibilities for social re-entry. The way different stigmas overlap usually makes health gaps worse, trapping individuals in cycles of being pushed aside. This interlaced challenge requires strategies that address individual emotions and the larger, more structural causes of discrimination (Carneiro et al., 2022). Identifying these layers, public health programs can more effectively target interventions to reduce barriers to care and improve quality of life. It's extremely difficult to overestimate the role stigma plays in overall public health outcomes. , it distorts the course of the HIV/AIDS epidemic by creating obstacles to prevention, early detection, and regular treatment measures. Most individuals, due to fear of social condemnation, delay early testing, which subsequently prolongs diagnoses and the likelihood of further transmission. Furthermore, when individuals begin to internalize stigma, they become less confident, socially withdrawn, and challenged by adhering to long-term treatment required for viral suppression. With all this, healthcare systems evidently must invest in culturally sensitive training and policies that resist discrimination. Concurrently, tackling stigma on a broader, structural level—by establishing policies that facilitate inclusion and equity—is just as crucial. All of these mutually reinforcing strategies have, over the long term, the ability to dismantle stigma's grip and to produce improved HIV care outcomes in diverse populations (Carneiro et al., 2022; Kerr et al., 2024).

8.6.2. Impact of Stigma on Individuals and Communities

Individuals with HIV/AIDS discover that day-to-day social attitudes hugely influence their life—most times bringing about a sense of exclusion and discrimination. It is not even the health problems that are at play; the shame associated with HIV will tend to surface via stress on the mind, cases of coercion, loss of employment, and being isolated socially, which only serves to make life more difficult to manage. People in vulnerable groups, such as men who have sex with men, transgender people, sex workers, and drug users—, to be hit with additional layers of bias, compounding their challenges. This intersection of biases can prevent a person from reporting their condition and makes it more difficult to access treatment, while also dampening the effort to fight for their rights and advocate for inclusion. Metrics like the Stigma Index 2.0 provide a better, albeit dirty, image of these complex problems, and in most instances, this is the beginning of interventions addressing both virus-driven and identity-based discrimination (Friedland et al., 2018). Social arrangements and health systems combined contribute to keeping stigma going, tending to worsen conditions such as increased HIV-related mortality and wide social divisions. In most rural communities, where cultural beliefs and skewed gender roles remain the order of the day, the stigma gets internalized; individuals may end up postponing seeking help or adhering to their medication regimen. Simultaneously, problems such as alcohol use, problematic relationships with caregivers, and even dangerous cultural activities end up becoming complex with these negative attitudes, creating severe barriers to effective health care. It is not uncommon for an unstable relationship between patients and their health providers—driven by such stigmatizing practices—to shut out open communication and deter early visits. Certain community-based interventions involving participatory action research have, overall, been promising through slowly deconstructing these systemic issues, establishing a mutually reinforced sense of knowledge and ultimately developing greater trust between residents and the health system (Brooks et al., 2017). Stigma's impacts can radiate far beyond the person themselves—it can cascade through entire communities, eroding social bonds and public health initiatives in the process. When fear and stigma make it unsafe to confess one's HIV status, silence prevails and frequently perpetuates a cycle of disinformation that hampers prevention. All too frequently, this stigma serves to isolate individuals with HIV, eroding the support networks that are so important to both mental and physical health. In addition, stigma most severely affects marginalized groups, perpetuating established social inequalities and preventing them from participating fully in economic and social life. To truly transform these patterns, strategies for combating stigma must extend far beyond the single individual; they must also address the wider social habits and structures through which discrimination persists. Most times, participatory, evidence-informed approaches to empowering the affected can create a sense of mutual responsibility and settings where stigma is challenged and increasingly eroded (Brooks et al., 2017; Friedland et al., 2018).

8.6.3. Strategies to Combat Stigma

Lowering the negative communication about HIV/AIDS truly comes through in making individuals receive treatment that they so much need. Peer support programs are now employed in clinics whereby the HIV individual builds a form of community. Such individuals tend to feel less isolated. Studies indicate that when people get consistent, warm support from other people who really understand what they're experiencing, bad treatment in health facilities falls off dramatically. Support like that not only keeps patients adhering to their care regimens but even encourages them to take antiretroviral meds regularly by relieving anxieties such as fear and suspicion of physicians. By and large, integrating peer accompaniment into daily healthcare appears to enhance both mental health and appropriate use of medication, suggesting a wider place for such concepts in HIV care systems (Noveyani et al., 2024). And there's one more wrinkle in all of this that appears from the cultural and social forces impacting marginalized populations, consider, for instance, Latino men who have sex with men. When HIV stigma is combined with sexual minority and cultural stigmatization, it only makes prevention and treatment a more difficult door to open. It's evident that overcoming these intersecting stigmas requires individualized methods that are respectful of each culture. For example, ensuring and safeguarding confidentiality goes a long way in soothing fears of judgment by society. Candid, forthright education regarding HIV and prevention can also erode established myths that serve only to fuel the blaze. And when healthcare providers are warm and empathetic, it creates a sort of trust that inspires people to enter safer spaces for services. Overall, these approaches complement each other to create more equitable access to healthcare and emphasize the necessity of culturally competent stigma-reduction models (Zhu et al., 2024). As stigma is such a complex problem, it is understandable to combine both sweeping policy changes with boots-on-the-ground, individual-level support for sustained change. Efforts to train medical personnel and educate the public generally can gradually destroy established biases, more often substituting them with understanding and compassion. At a more macro level, having rights-protecting policies for individuals with HIV, together with good anti-discrimination legislation, lays the groundwork for a systemic shift. In the meantime, peer support—and services attuned to cultural realities—address the individual side of things so no one slips through the cracks. When all these strategies are combined, they help create an environment in which stigma no longer gets in the way of prevention efforts or interferes with treatment regimens. Ultimately, continued research and some adaptable alterchanges in our approaches are essential to staying ahead of shifting social environments and carrying the torch in the worldwide struggle against HIV/AIDS (Figure 8.16).

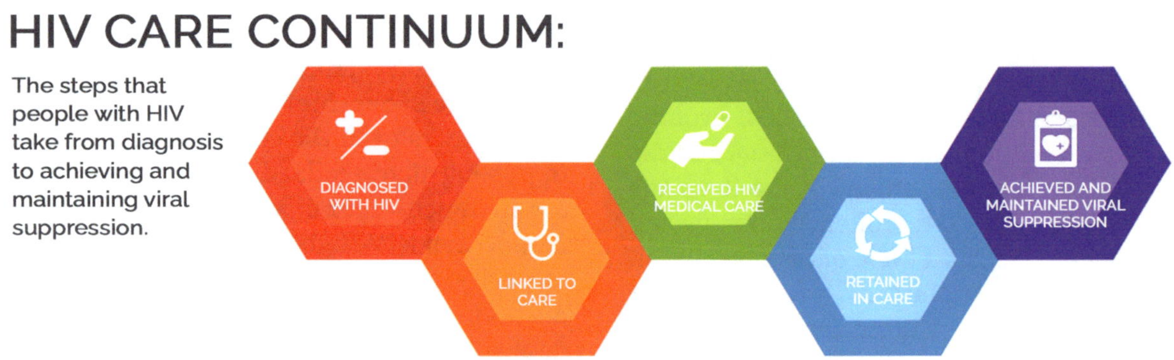

Figure 8.16. HIV care continuum.

Source: HIV.gov. (n.d.). *HIV Care Continuum.*

CLOSER LOOK

SOCIAL, CULTURAL, AND GLOBAL HEALTH IMPACTS OF HIV/AIDS

HIV/AIDS is not only a biomedical challenge but also a profound social and cultural issue with wide-reaching global health consequences. Since its emergence in the early 1980s, the epidemic has reshaped societies, health systems, and international cooperation.

Socially, HIV/AIDS has been associated with stigma and discrimination. Individuals living with HIV often face isolation, loss of employment, and denial of healthcare services. This stigma discourages testing and treatment, allowing the virus to spread further. Families and communities are also affected as caregivers shoulder emotional and financial burdens, while children orphaned by AIDS face heightened vulnerability.

Cultural factors strongly influence the dynamics of the epidemic. In many societies, discussions about sexuality, gender roles, and drug use remain taboo, limiting awareness and prevention efforts. Harmful practices such as gender inequality, transactional sex, or denial of condom use increase vulnerability, especially among women and marginalized groups. Religious beliefs sometimes promote abstinence-only approaches, which may reduce comprehensive sexual education, while cultural solidarity can also inspire strong community-based care networks.

On a global health scale, HIV/AIDS has strained healthcare systems, particularly in sub-Saharan Africa, which bears the highest burden. The epidemic has reduced life expectancy, diminished workforce productivity, and hindered economic growth. Internationally, it has spurred massive health investments, such as the Global Fund and PEPFAR, which have expanded access to antiretroviral therapy and strengthened public health infrastructure. Importantly, HIV/AIDS has highlighted the need for a rights-based approach to health, emphasizing equity, gender empowerment, and the fight against stigma.

HIV/AIDS is more than a medical condition—it is a global social phenomenon. Addressing it requires integrating medical care with education, cultural sensitivity, and international solidarity to reduce stigma, promote prevention, and ensure universal access to treatment.

Summary

HIV/AIDS is more than biology—it's enmeshed in a whole array of social issues that are all too easily forgotten. Women with HIV/AIDS, for example, often find themselves facing several types of abuse, physical, sexual, and psychological—, can arise both within their home environments and in society at large. These cruel circumstances find their way into limiting their access to consistent health care, support groups, and group activities, all this serving to increase their vulnerability even more. Rather than just adhering to a medical solution, it appears evident that addressing the problem involves methods that combine various types of expertise; nursing professionals and other health practitioners have an important role in identifying these struggles and advocating for care models that combine clinical treatment with actual social support. For the most part, more integrated forms of assistance have a way of discontinuing the vicious cycle of exposure and promoting positive health outcomes in these women (Bastos et al., 2016). The labor marketplace has the same narrative to share, particularly regarding young women caught at the confluence of HIV/AIDS and socio-economic declines. In most instances, structural imbalances are as much about healthcare as they also define work options. When policies force compulsory HIV testing as a prerequisite for work, they have the potential to drive already vulnerable groups deeper into the shadows, making it even less likely that infected individuals will seek out the assistance they require. These actions are likely to fail to address the underlying issues, contributing to stigma rather than inclusion or prevention. On the other hand, public policies must depend on protecting confidentiality, avoiding discrimination, and providing caring systems inviting voluntary testing and good treatment with opportunities in workplaces left open (Ow, 2014). To put everything in a nutshell, a struggle against HIV/AIDS requires means integrating medical, social, and economic remedies right from the onset. Understanding how problems such as gender-based violence or workplace discrimination affect health is crucial if policies and care interventions are to function effectively. Health professionals need to be prepared to back services that combine clinical care with effective social assistance, and policymakers, in the majority of instances, must construct systems that reduce stigma while protecting individuals' rights. Together, these general efforts can increase treatment compliance, strengthen the marginalized, and eventually decelerate the epidemic's spread. The fact that women suffer both from violence and workplace discrimination serves as a reminder that a compassionate, expansive, even if sometimes errored, strategy is key to controlling HIV/AIDS globally (Ow, 2014; Bastos et al., 2016).

Advances in the treatment of HIV have truly transformed the game for individuals who live with the virus. ART—, therapy, is at the center of care, fighting to suppress the virus and reduce the risk of serious disease and death. If people initiate ART at precisely the right moment and, ahem, adhere to it, their results can look an awful lot like those of people without HIV. Much of this progress hangs on a mess of guidelines that determine how to start treatment, which drug combinations to use, and even how to manage adhering to the regimen. For instance, the British HIV Association's guidelines—developed following comprehensive, hands-on evaluations of how treatments weigh effectiveness, side effects, and expense—are emphatic about getting onto treatment early, regular check-ins, and individualizing care for populations such as pregnant women and adolescents. Moreover, when patients are involved in the decision-making about how their care is provided, it can increase both engagement and health, demonstrating that an interdisciplinary team is central to the management of HIV (Waters et al., 2022). ART isn't simply about solo therapy—it impacts huge waves on the front of public health. When the virus is suppressed, the likelihood of transmission sexually plummets, a change that's transforming prevention strategies. Universal treatment is an enormous ambition; in the majority of instances, figures from high-income environments indicate almost complete viral suppression in treated patients, which reduces new infections and improves community health. As for money, although individuals previously concerned themselves with expenses, ART has proved to be fairly cost-effective. Savings have arrived courtesy of generic medications and clever shopping strategies, though juggling low cost with patient-specific options remains a challenge. And with fewer late diagnoses and improved connections to treatment, not only do patient outcomes improve, but also overall expenditure on hospital stays and associated issues falls. ART's numerous advantages extend from enhancing individual lives all the way to strengthening society's battle against HIV (Waters et al., 2022). Developing and collaborating on these treatment guidelines is extremely vital for maintaining care at an optimal level and advancing HIV treatment. Applying review templates, such as the PRISMA 2020 guidelines, tends to ensure that the evidence supporting recommendations is both strong and straightforwardly presented. This type of solid strategy assists with the meaningful assessment of treatment choices and provides clinicians that little extra boost of confidence. Having individuals who are living with HIV involved in establishing these guidelines makes the entire experience more accessible and palatable, it engenders trust and can improve adherence. Periodic revisions, supported by good research and observational data, remain salient for addressing emerging problems such as drug resistance or other complicating diseases. In our ever-changing field, open reporting and ongoing evaluations help ensure that everyday practices keep pace with the latest evidence—ultimately boosting care quality and health outcomes for everyone with HIV/AIDS worldwide.

References

1. Aboulafia, D., Ambinder, R. F., Cesarman, E., Henry, et al. (2018). Safety and preliminary efficacy of vorinostat with R-EPOCH in high-risk HIV-associated non-Hodgkin's lymphoma (AMC-075). *Clinical Lymphoma Myeloma and Leukemia, 18*(3), 180–190.e2. https://core.ac.uk/download/212865067.pdf (accessed on 7 May 2025).
2. Aisah, S. P., Tjut Adek, R., & Yunizar, Z. (2024). Web-based expert system application for early diagnosis of HIV/AIDS using the Naive Bayes method. *Journal of Advanced Computer Knowledge and Algorithms, 1(4).* https://www.semanticscholar.org/paper/0d0886134aa9d0db8ba514a4504f4dd98d8418ab (accessed on 7 May 2025).
3. Alum, E., Uti, D. E., Paul-Chima, U. O., & Alum, B. N. (2024). Toward a cure–Advancing HIV/AIDS treatment modalities beyond antiretroviral therapy: A review. *Medicine, 103*(27), e38768. https://www.semanticscholar.org/paper/47d0d95e3b9c04687d9d6c1efb1ba8aef8694ab1 (accessed on 7 May 2025).
4. Ananworanich, J., Chomchey, N., Chomont, N., de Souza, et al. (2012). Impact of multi-targeted antiretroviral treatment on gut T cell depletion and HIV reservoir seeding during acute HIV infection. *PLOS ONE, 7*(3), e33948. https://doi.org/10.1371/journal.pone.0033948 (accessed on 7 May 2025).
5. Bastos da Silva, E., Cocco da Costa, M., Janh, A., & Streck, M. T. H. (2016). Everyday's violence situations against women with HIV/AIDS: Implications for care. *Journal of Nursing Ufpe Online, 10,* 2463–2470. https://www.semanticscholar.org/paper/0a783441a41c8a7719d4f6b3d1ca33a81c34465a (accessed on 7 May 2025).
6. Bhandari, K., & Giri, S. (2025). Perception of participants towards prevention and control of HIV/AIDS: A qualitative study. *Kaladarpan , 5(1), 123–137.* https://www.semanticscholar.org/paper/33c9b0068bc441e5806b5d207d2e58a60171a914 (accessed on 7 May 2025).
7. Bloom, D. E., Humair, S., & Bärnighausen, T. (2025). A mathematical model for estimating the number of health workers required for universal antiretroviral treatment. https://core.ac.uk/download/pdf/6684677.pdf (accessed on 7 May 2025).
8. Brooks, C., D'Ambruoso, L., Kazimierczak, K. A., Ngobeni, S., Twine, R., Tollman, S., Kahn, K., et al. (2017). Introducing visual participatory methods to develop local knowledge on HIV in rural South Africa. *BMJ Global Health, 2,* e000231. https://doi.org/10.1136/bmjgh-2016-000231.
9. Cambrea, S. C., Marcu, E. A., Cucli, E., Badiu, D., Penciu, R. C., Petcu, C. L., Dumea, E., et al. (2022). Clinical and biological risk factors associated with increased mother-to-child transmission of HIV in two South-East HIV/AIDS regional centers in Romania. *Medicina, 58,* 275. https://doi.org/10.3390/medicina58020275.
10. Carneiro, A. M. F., Rodrigues, Y. C., Gomes, J. S., Lima, L. N. G. C., Lima, K. B. B., & Dolabela, M. (2022). The negative impact of stigma perceived by men who have sex with men (MSM): An integrative review. *International Journal of Current Microbiology and Applied Sciences, 11*(6), 366–378. https://www.semanticscholar.org/paper/f155462c48c18dfda55a7bd206c30043df024026 (accessed on 7 May 2025).
11. Carrilho, C., & Lunet, N. (2023). Global trends in Kaposi sarcoma incidence and mortality: The need for action to reduce inequalities. *The Lancet Global Health, 11,* e1479. https://doi.org/10.1016/s2214-109x(23)00413-8.

12. Chapman, C. A. (2015). *To A Better Understanding of Professional Practice: Provider Decision-Making When Delivering HIV Services* (Master's thesis, Loma Linda University). Loma Linda University Electronic Theses, Dissertations & Projects, 514. https://core.ac.uk/download/161855329.pdf (accessed on 7 May 2025).

13. Cumberland, W. G., Yang, O. O., & Yeghiazarian, L. (2013). A stochastic multi-scale model of HIV-1 transmission for decision-making: Application to an MSM population. *PLOS ONE, 8*(11), e70578. https://core.ac.uk/download/323076961.pdf (accessed on 7 May 2025).

14. Dalatu, P. (2025). Statistical analysis of HIV/AIDS prevalence and gender disparities at General Hospital Mubi North (2010 to 2024). *International Journal of Development Mathematics (IJDM), 2(1).* https://www.semanticscholar.org/paper/0f58439a2b77460e99823c0889d9ca89d6e4976e (accessed on 7 May 2025).

15. Das, N., Sunny, N., & Panda, P. K. (2024). A case of HIV/AIDS–Existence of four symbiotic opportunistic co-infections. *International Journal of Scientific Research, 13(10), 25–27.* https://www.semanticscholar.org/paper/20bacc27930c65ae41d3355bbda180f9cb3daeba (accessed on 7 May 2025).

16. Denu, M. K. I., Revoori, R., Buadu, M. A., Oladele, O., & Berko, K. P. (2024). Hypertension among persons living with HIV/AIDS and its association with HIV-related health factors. *AIDS Research and Therapy, 21(1), 5.* https://www.semanticscholar.org/paper/c7e7aa5012dc29f478385d01bf3dacfca3e862fb (accessed on 7 May 2025).

17. Des Jarlais, D. C. (2017). Harm reduction in the USA: The research perspective and an archive to David Purchase. *Harm Reduction Journal, 14.* https://doi.org/10.1186/s12954-017-0178-6 (accessed on 7 May 2025).

18. Ezeja, C. C. (2024). Advancements in HIV/AIDS treatment and prevention. *Newport International Journal of Public Health and Pharmacy, 5(2), 74–77.* https://www.semanticscholar.org/paper/e8f399cdf8fd11bd7d503e0b0fe8e6b332398939 (accessed on 7 May 2025).

19. Friedland, B., Sprague, L., Nyblade, L., Baral, S., Pulerwitz, J., Gottert, A., Amanyeiwe, U., et al. (2018). Measuring intersecting stigma among key populations living with HIV: Implementing the people living with HIV Stigma Index 2.0. *Journal of the International AIDS Society, 21.* https://doi.org/10.1002/jia2.25131.

20. Gibb, J. K., DuBois, L. Z., Williams, S., McKerracher, L., Juster, R. P., & Fields, J. (2020). Sexual and gender minority health vulnerabilities during the COVID-19 health crisis. *American Journal of Human Biology, 32*(5), e23499. https://doi.org/10.1002/ajhb.23499.

21. Guo, L., Fu, Y., Xie, X., Yan, W., & Long, H. (2024). Comparative efficacy and safety of ANV-based versus EFV-based ART in the management of persons living with HIV: A real-world study in Guizhou, China. *AIDS Research and Human Retroviruses, 40(8), 482–488.* https://www.semanticscholar.org/paper/09af8228e4fcab4c5a4c1120b53b71009204d7c3 (accessed on 7 May 2025).

22. Haberer, J. E., Bangsberg, D. R., Baeten, J. M., Curran, K., Koechlin, F., Amico, K. R., Anderson, P. L., et al. (2015). Defining success with HIV pre-exposure prophylaxis. *AIDS, 29*(11), 1277–1285. https://doi.org/10.1097/QAD.0000000000000647.

23. Haynes, B. F., & Mascola, J. R. (2017). The quest for an antibody-based HIV vaccine. *Immunological Reviews, 275,* 5–10. https://doi.org/10.1111/imr.12517.

24. Hlaing, M. C. S., Conway, J., & Grewal, S. (2024). Immune reconstitution-induced sarcoidosis following initiation of antiretroviral therapy in an HIV-positive patient. *Rheumatology Advances in Practice, 8*, Article P28. https://www.semanticscholar.org/paper/ad823812b0860fa43ac384cf332f9fbca9915450 (accessed on 7 May 2025).

25. James, S. L., Abate, D., Abate, K. H., Abay, S. M., Abbafati, C., Abbasi, N., Abbastabar, H., et al. (2018). Global, regional, and national incidence, prevalence, and years lived with disability for 354 diseases and injuries for 195 countries and territories, 1990–2017: A systematic analysis for the Global Burden of Disease Study 2017. *The Lancet, 392*, 1789–1858. https://doi.org/10.1016/s0140-6736(18)32279-7.

26. Jiang, H., Zhou, Y., & Tang, W. (2020). Maintaining HIV care during the COVID-19 pandemic. *The Lancet HIV, 7*(5), e308–e309. https://doi.org/10.1016/S2352-3018(20)30105-3.

27. Kato, J. K. (2024). Innovations in HIV treatment and care in Uganda: Evaluating the impact of new antiretroviral therapies and healthcare models. *IDOSR Journal of Applied Sciences, 9(2), 72–75.* https://www.semanticscholar.org/paper/603ff225b219132750565111 23c8f278ade1522e (accessed on 7 May 2025).

28. Kerr, J., Yigit, I., Long, D. M., Paulino-Ramírez, R., Waters, J., Hao, J., Nyblade, L., et al. (2024). HIV and intersectional stigma among people living with HIV and healthcare workers and antiretroviral therapy adherence in the Dominican Republic. *International Journal of STD & AIDS, 35(11), 840–849.* https://www.semanticscholar.org/paper/e07e110da6a78d15537b3578e8055f21a9d29e01 (accessed on 7 May 2025).

29. Kharsany, A. B. M., & Abdool Karim, Q. (2016). HIV infection and AIDS in Sub-Saharan Africa: Current status, challenges, and opportunities. *The Open AIDS Journal, 10*, 34–48. https://doi.org/10.2174/1874613601610010034.

30. Khoza-Shangase, K. (2025). The association between HIV/AIDS, ototoxicity of its treatments, and occupational noise-induced hearing loss: A narrative review mapping the existing literature and identifying research gaps. *International Journal of Environmental Research and Public Health, 22, 487.* https://www.semanticscholar.org/paper/a1dce79975b3bb3eae32e4cebd99b5897f4f13e7 (accessed on 7 May 2025).

31. Livingston, G., Huntley, J., Sommerlad, A., Ames, D., Ballard, C., Banerjee, S., Brayne, C., et al. (2020). Dementia prevention, intervention, and care: 2020 report of the Lancet Commission. *The Lancet, 396*(10248), 413–446. https://doi.org/10.1016/S0140-6736(20)30367-6.

32. Mami, D. M., Cuthrell, K. M., & Manteghian, M. (2024). Burden of HIV on society: Current management options and future prospective. *International STD Research & Reviews, 13*(1). https://www.semanticscholar.org/paper/22035e43dfccafec35a92b7c12ac522401e3b3ab (accessed on 7 May 2025).

33. McManus, K. A., Strumpf, A., Killelea, A., Horn, T., Steen, A., An, Z., Schurman, E., et al. (2023). Ryan White HIV/AIDS Part B and AIDS Drug Assistance Programs during COVID-19: Safety net public health programs' challenges and innovations. *Frontiers in Public Health, 11, 1172009.* https://www.semanticscholar.org/paper/707a60367c2e7a087574db1bfb14f634ca90cd0a (accessed on 7 May 2025).

34. Mugaiga, M. I. (2024). Prevention and treatment of HIV/AIDS: The Gates Foundation's role in reducing incidence and extending lives. *Research Output Journal of Public Health and*

Medicine, 4(1), 53–58. https://www.semanticscholar.org/paper/794aba5d6d5cf02255622c4080544cc34035b888 (accessed on 7 May 2025).

35. Naghavi, M., Ong, K. L., Aali, A., Ababneh, H., Abate, Y. H., Abbafati, C., Abbasgholizadeh, R., et al. (2024). Global burden of 288 causes of death and life expectancy decomposition in 204 countries and territories and 811 subnational locations, 1990–2021: A systematic analysis for the Global Burden of Disease Study 2021. *The Lancet, 403*(10435), 2100–2132. https://doi.org/10.1016/S0140-6736(24)00367-2.

36. Naz, S., Naz, H., Ali, K., Hanif, M., Jaiswal, V., & Patel, N. (2025). Regional and racial disparities in testicular cancer-related mortality among HIV/AIDS adults in the United States and Texas: A 21-year retrospective study (1999–2020). *Journal of Clinical Oncology, 43(5).* https://www.semanticscholar.org/paper/44e9fe1ce9a1e9a17aedf1bd48a30e1e43a9c2e9 (accessed on 7 May 2025).

37. Neff, V. (2009). *The NGO Sector in Community Development: Emerging Roles, Strategies and Identities.* https://core.ac.uk/download/56323318.pdf (accessed on 7 May 2025).

38. Ninson, R. (2023). Assess the knowledge pregnant women have on HIV/AIDS, mother-to-child transmission of HIV/AIDS, and how PMTCT services are utilized in a tertiary health facility in the Gambia. *Texila International Journal of Public Health, 11(2).* https://www.semanticscholar.org/paper/b50f7a989b9e0e30a8a1d21b31951ab9f855fa55 (accessed on 7 May 2025).

39. Noveyani, A. E., Cahyani, T. D., Yunita, K., Latifah, A., Maulana, M. F., & Lyan, Y. B. (2024). Group support's effect on stigma reduction and medication adherence improvement among HIV-positive individuals. *Caring: Indonesian Journal of Nursing Science, 6*(1). https://www.semanticscholar.org/paper/1f1463728d6303b7f5b6c448e47b8adbbe20f303 (accessed on 7 May 2025).

40. Okuboyejo, S., & Omogbadegun, Z. O. (2013). Investigating cognitive, behavioral, and environmental barriers to HIV/AIDS patients' adherence in Nigeria. *International Association of Providers of AIDS Care (IAPAC) Journal, 12*, 40. http://eprints.covenantuniversity.edu.ng/id/eprint/8339 (accessed on 7 May 2025).

41. Ow, T. (2014). HIV/AIDS: The labor market implications of compulsory testing. *West Indian Medical Journal, 62*, 364–367. https://www.semanticscholar.org/paper/2dee9506446d63b68b45f82f4fa3a65c697c5304 (accessed on 7 May 2025).

42. Page, M. J., Moher, D., Bossuyt, P. M., Boutron, I., Hoffmann, T., Mulrow, C. D., Shamseer, L., et al. (2021). PRISMA 2020 explanation and elaboration: Updated guidance and exemplars for reporting systematic reviews. *BMJ, 372*, n160. https://doi.org/10.1136/bmj.n160.

43. Rahmouni, M., Clerc, S., Spadoni, J., Labib, T., Tison, M., Medina-Santos, R., Bensussan, A., et al. (2025). Deep analysis of the major histocompatibility complex genetic associations using covariate analysis and haploblocks unravels new mechanisms for the molecular etiology of elite control in AIDS. *BMC Immunology, 26(1), 1.* https://www.semanticscholar.org/paper/cab344e9557bd3ddd781dc4deabc35ec4ba7bd1a (accessed on 7 May 2025).

44. Reid, S., & Dwyer, J. (2005). Insomnia in HIV infection: A systematic review of prevalence, correlates, and management. *Psychosomatic Medicine, 67*, 260–269. https://www.semanticscholar.org/paper/007bef7e8db5614228e34f8f945bece5cd93dd4b (accessed on 7 May 2025).

45. Shrivastav, V., Y. M., Ramachandran, A., Makwana, N. R., & Parmar, D. (2025). Prevalence and risk factors of anemia among people living with HIV/AIDS in Southeast Asia: A systematic review and meta-analysis. *BMC Infectious Diseases, 25(1), 550.* https://www.semanticscholar.org/paper/df44123bf3ef1627f8ae7b4db64a20bed90b2257 (accessed on 7 May 2025).

46. Silveira, A. B., Silveira, G. B., Cassol, J., Neuburger, W., Modolo, F., & Silva, H. F. (2025). The importance of dentistry on the diagnosis of HIV: A case report of oral Kaposi's sarcoma. *Revita Foco, 18*(4). https://www.semanticscholar.org/paper/4af5b9d956da7056c38550b704aa23ea24334ced (accessed on 7 May 2025).

47. Simooya, C., Silumbwe, A., Halwindi, H., Zulu, J. M., & Nzala, S. (2023). Exploring communication and implementation challenges of the HIV/AIDS policy change to test-and-treat-all in selected public health facilities in Lusaka District, Zambia. *Implementation Science Communications, 4.* https://doi.org/10.1186/s43058-023-00430-6.

48. Snowden, F. M. (2019). *Epidemics and Society: From the Black Death to the Present.* Yale University Press.

49. Terrault, N. A., Bzowej, N., Chang, K. M., Hwang, J., Jonas, M. M., & Murad, M. H. (2015). AASLD guidelines for treatment of chronic hepatitis B. *Hepatology, 63*, 261–283. https://doi.org/10.1002/hep.28156.

50. Timmons-Vendryes, R., Swendeman, D., Cisneros Asca, J., Cáceres, C., Comulada, W., Bazargan-Hejazi, S., & Silva-Santisteban, A. (2025). Sexual hygiene: Is it time for a renewed focus for HIV/STI prevention? *Advances in Global Health, 4(1), 2453630.* https://www.semanticscholar.org/paper/d090b4d2bfe38c37952ed158e31861265ba40682 (accessed on 7 May 2025).

51. Torre, L. A., Bray, F., Siegel, R. L., Ferlay, J., Lortet-Tieulent, J., & Jemal, A. (2015). Global cancer statistics, 2012. *CA: A Cancer Journal for Clinicians, 65*(2), 87–108. https://doi.org/10.3322/caac.21262.

52. Tratrat, C., Petrou, A., Fesatidou, M., Haroun, M., Chohan, M., & Geronikaki, A. (2025). Rational design, synthesis, and biological evaluation of novel thiazole/thiazolidinones multitarget anti-Human Immunodeficiency Virus molecules. *Pharmaceuticals, 18, 298.* https://www.semanticscholar.org/paper/82f657853a9cfff0971fb9ab7c7dabdc42606f85 (accessed on 7 May 2025).

53. Vannakit, R., Janyam, S., Linjongrat, D., Chanlearn, P., Sittikarn, S., Pengnonyang, S., Janamnuaysook, R., et al. (2020). Give the community the tools and they will help finish the job: Key population-led health services for ending AIDS in Thailand. *Journal of the International AIDS Society, 23.* https://doi.org/10.1002/jia2.25535.

54. Waters, L., Winston, A., Reeves, I., Boffito, M., Churchill, D., Cromarty, B., Dunn, D., et al. (2022). BHIVA guidelines on antiretroviral treatment for adults living with HIV-1 2022. *HIV Medicine, 23*(S1), 3–115. https://doi.org/10.1111/hiv.13446.

55. Wondimgezahu, S. M., & Tefera, T. (2023). Incidence and predictors of treatment failure among adults on first-line antiretroviral therapy in Gullele Sub City, Addis Ababa, Ethiopia: A retrospective study in selected public health facilities. *International Journal of Virology and AIDS, 10, 092.* https://www.semanticscholar.org/paper/78775cb7dbd4ec983afc234900bfb5f788066e99 (accessed on 7 May 2025).

56. Wulandari, S., & Utomo, B. M. (2025). The effectiveness of PMTCT education in increasing pregnant mothers' knowledge on HIV/AIDS prevention for their babies. *Professional Evidence-*

based Research and Advances in Wellness and Treatment, 2(1). https://www.semanticscholar.org/paper/846ae71727744e2c50b41a0bd3c3d466188ed7c3 (accessed on 7 May 2025).

57. Yimer, A., Kassaw, A. A. K., Surur, S., & Mussa, E. (2024). Prevalence of misconceptions about HIV/AIDS transmission and associated factors among reproductive-age women in Ethiopia: A nationwide study. *BMC Infectious Diseases, 24.* https://www.semanticscholar.org/paper/bffcab959636c3f7a84c0912a3d36aa8ba5b31f6 (accessed on 7 May 2025).

58. Zhu, H., Stadnick, N., Stockman, J., Katague, M., Moore, V., Torres, V., Cano, R., et al. (2024). Intersectional stigma among Latino MSM and HIV prevention: Barriers to HIV prevention and strategies to overcome the barriers. *AIDS Care, 37(1), 88–98*. https://www.semanticscholar.org/paper/ad7830e85418e79d56aab86401c01fd62139eef1 (accessed on 7 May 2025).

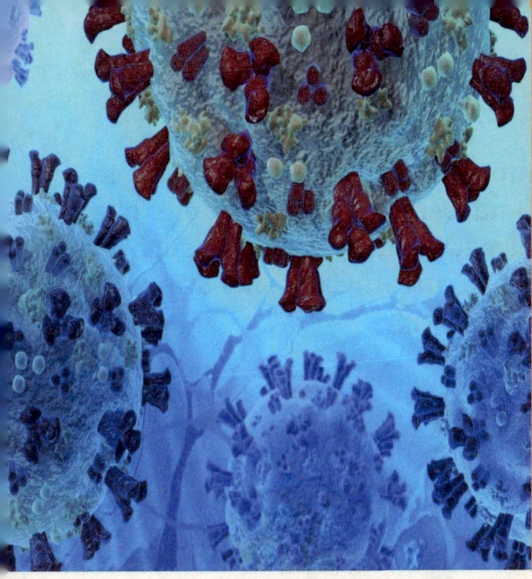

Chapter 9

SARS, MERS, AND COVID-19

Contents

Introduction

Infectious diseases have plagued us for centuries, typically creeping in from animal reservoirs and disrupting communities at random. Coronaviruses, for example, aren't limited to animals, they can cross over to humans and lead to very serious respiratory issues. Consider SARS, MERS, and the more recent COVID-19; all struck in some manner. They all tend to exhibit similar symptoms and patterns of spread, but their origins, scope, and the reactions they evoked vary significantly. Learning these subtleties isn't purely theoretical—it's what informs us about how these threats evolve over time and why we require many public health solutions. In retrospect, SARS erupted in 2002, followed by MERS in 2012, both associated, in the majority of instances, with animal contacts. These occurrences truly brought home the message that viruses are capable of jumping across species lines when we don't expect it. Next was COVID-19, SARS-CoV-2, which spread more rapidly and farther than its ancestors. Research has highlighted a tangled web of mutations and various virus lineages; for instance, in Bangladesh several strains and importation events were observed during the pandemic's course (Mahmud et al., 2025). For the most part, these evolutionary clues provide a firmer hold on viral transmission and even vaccine performance. But animal involvement adds another layer to the tale. The infected farmed mink episode demonstrated that SARS-CoV-2 is not discriminatory—transmission can ping-pong between animals and humans, further complicating control efforts. Denmark's reaction, with a huge mink cull to stop further transmission, speaks to the complicated dynamics of zoonotic spillover and reverse transmission (Rasmussen et al., 2024). It all serves to emphasize why proper genomic screening, several experience across disciplines, and an integrated One Health approach are quite essential in monitoring, and addressing, both present and future coronavirus problems.

Overview of Coronaviruses

Coronaviruses are a gigantic family of insects that can cause you anything from a common cold to pretty much horrible breathing issues. They've got these spiky bits on their surface–like tiny crowns–that allow them to cling onto our cells and initiate an infection. People used to believe they were fairly innocuous, until the SARS epidemic of 2002 further MERS in 2012 proved that these viruses pack a pretty big punch. Both of those viruses originated from animals before spreading to humans, a typical instance of zoonotic transmission that can rapidly become local problems full-blown global concerns. For the most part, observing how these infections unfold has led us to see how they're constructed, how they transmit from host to host, and why occasionally they become epic health dangers. Further came SARS-CoV-2, the COVID-19 virus, and it upended everything—making it an unprecedented crisis that opened the world's eyes, being the fifth major pandemic since the infamous 1918 flu. It all began in Wuhan, China, and before long, infections had traveled far and wide with symptoms such as a dry cough, fever, sore throat, and difficulty breathing.

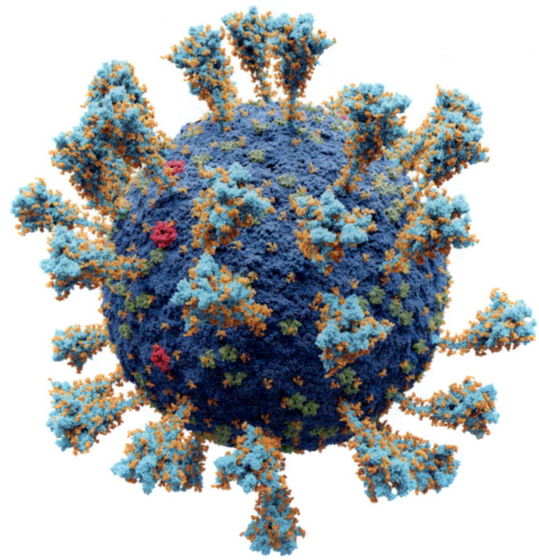

Figure 9.1. Coronavirus structure.

Source: By Alexey Solodovnikov (Idea, Producer, CG, Editor), Valeria Arkhipova (Scientific Consultant) - Own work. Scientific consultants:Nikitin N.A., Doctor of Biological Sciences, Department of Virology, Faculty of Biology, Lomonosov Moscow State University. Borisevich S.S. Candidate of Chemical Sciences, Specialist in Molecular Modeling of Viral Surface Proteins, Senior Researcher, Head of the "Quantum & Dynamics»,Laboratory of Chemical Physics, Ufa Institute of Chemistry RASArkhipova V.I., specialization in Fundamental and Applied chemistry, senior engineer, RNA Chemistry Laboratory, Institute of chemical biology and fundamental medicine SB RAS, CC BY-SA 4.0, https://commons.wikimedia.org/w/index.php?curid=104914011

This virus spun its web across communities much quicker than the previous ones, accelerating the transmission of the disease in unprecedented manners. Despite the myriad research that has been carried out, there isn't as yet one ideal antiviral—scientists have spent time reshuffling older drugs while vaccines keep getting adjusted. In general, deciphering its molecular turns—how it survives, reproduces, and communicates—is what's been informing public health interventions and treatment protocols, keeping the virus in check (Manjinder et al., 2020). It's not only the lungs that bear the brunt; there's increasingly evidence that such viruses could also play havoc with the brain. Some research suggests that after the initial respiratory symptoms, the virus can quietly make its way into the nervous system, potentially causing issues such as confused thinking and other neurological breakdowns. The hippocampus, the part that controls our memory, appears particularly vulnerable, and this has brought worry about long-term consequences, such as memory loss and even a greater likelihood of conditions such as Alzheimer's. While we're still not clear on just how common or long-lasting these brain effects are, this emerging data really stresses the need to keep an eye on both the breathing problems and the wider, more systemic fallout of coronavirus infections (Chan et al., 2020) (Figure 9.1).

Importance of Studying Severe Acute Respiratory Syndrome (SARS), Middle East Respiratory Syndrome (MERS), and Coronavirus Disease 2019 (COVID-19)

Viral epidemiology and genomics are two hands that go together when you explore diseases such as SARS, MERS, and COVID-19. Scientists now track how these pests travel—advanced sequencing technologies pick up on timing and location of the virus spread, whether persisting nearby or crossing borders. Combining genetic clues with daily demographics assists in mapping out unforeseen paths of transmission, which in turn gets health authorities to think more intelligently about how they respond to outbreaks. And sometimes it's simply observing whether the virus persists in clumps close together or suddenly appears unexpectedly distant and widespread; that slight distinction can truly alter how we approach containment. New computer models, as well, are providing us with nearly real-time photographs—a useful advantage while looking ahead. Since every disease acts differently, this type of in-depth analysis equips scientists and policymakers alike with methods to better predict and combat future pandemics (Hill et al., 2021). When it comes to the human element of pandemics such as COVID-19, things become even more complicated. Frontline healthcare workers are the ones bearing the burden of these crises—they're pushed to work in insane stress and with a perpetual risk of themselves becoming ill. Their emotional toll, echoed so many times across so many stories, indicates a severe need for greater support, even if our complete understanding of their experiences isn't entirely apparent. Considering what they've endured through SARS, MERS, and COVID-19 is not merely for their own health; it's also a critical component of keeping our medical systems buoyant in bad times. It's this jumbled combination of human and biological elements that dictates how we plan for the next big test (Billings et al., 2021). Stepping back to see how these outbreaks compare provides us with new perspective on how viruses change, cross species, and interact with us. SARS and MERS taught us that coronaviruses, capable of jumping from animals to humans, aren't merely isolated events—they have a serious effect on communities. Further there's COVID-19, whose speedy transmission reminds us that in our urbanized, interconnected world, even a new virus can mushroom into a full-fledged pandemic in a hurry. Exploring the molecular mechanisms of these events provides clues to risk factors for future spillovers and challenges us to enhance surveillance where humans interact with animals. Including demographic information further increases the visibility of those most at risk, enabling more targeted provision of public health. Ultimately, studying SARS, MERS, and COVID-19 not only grows our scientific knowledge base but also prepares society to meet current and future infectious challenges (Billings et al., 2021; Hill et al., 2021) (Figure 9.2).

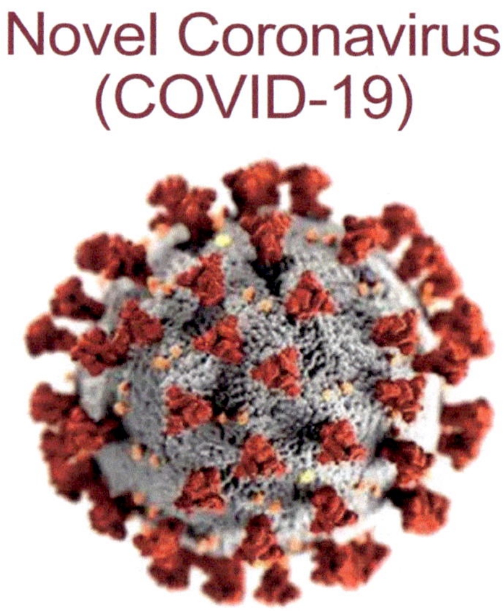

Figure 9.2. Novel coronavirus (COVID-19).

Source: Centers for Disease Control and Prevention. (n.d.). *CDC Museum COVID-19 Timeline.*

9.1. Background on Coronaviruses

Coronaviruses wear a crown of spike proteins and can infect animals and humans alike. They hop between species in ways that make it sort of difficult to keep up with them, and whereas the milder strains previously merely caused the common cold, things changed around 2003 when SARS-CoV hit the scene—overnight we had evidence that much more virulent forms were possible. Then, outbreaks like MERS-CoV followed, and most recently SARS-CoV-2 hit us with COVID-19. The scientific world, generally speaking, has been pulling together huge piles of varied data on how these viruses work, from their biology and behavior to hints for treatment. For instance, the Coronavirus Infectious Disease Ontology (CIDO) (He et al., 2022) tidily collects information regarding the virus, its interaction with hosts, and which therapies could assist, even if the arrangement isn't as neat as one would anticipate. When we examine the transmission of coronaviruses, the scene becomes even more hazy. We used to believe that transmission occurred primarily through large respiratory droplets or on surfaces, but, as the COVID-19 experience demonstrated, small aerosols can persist in the air, and travel much farther than we used to think. In most situations, this implies that strategies such as increasing ventilation, wearing masks, and maintaining a safe distance have become more crucial than ever. It's now apparent that viruses like SARS-CoV-2 may be breathing the same air as us a whole lot more than ancient models predicted, which disrupts our previous notions (Wang et al., 2021). Further there's the virus's ability to shake things up on the genetic front. a true wild card in the way outbreaks keep returning. SARS-CoV-2 specifically has mutated fairly quickly, giving rise to strains such as Delta and Omicron that have different levels of how easily contagious they are and how well they evade our immune systems. Even the CIDO system monitors such details as what amino acids they shift and how those adjustments influence protein interactions, all of which contributes to just how bad the virus could get and what treatment will be most effective. All this combined, albeit occasionally chaotic, information is gold when it comes to vaccine and antiviral drug design. More often than not, knowing these changing variables not only makes us keener diagnostically and therapeutically but also prepares us for what's to come in public health.

9.1.1. Definition and Classification of Coronaviruses

Dangerous coronaviruses have been popping up lately, making us rethink what they really are and how they slot into the viral family tree. These viruses, which belong to the Coronaviridae family, have an envelope and a single-stranded, positive-sense RNA genome, plus those crown-like spikes that you'd almost call them nature's crowns. They're not all identical, breaking down into four subgroups—Alphacoronavirus, Betacoronavirus, Gammacoronavirus, and Deltacoronavirus—but it's pretty much the alpha and beta types that infect humans. SARS-CoV-1, MERS-CoV and SARS-CoV-2 (all betacoronaviruses) are similar in evolutionary origins and molecular uniqueness, for instance. They cause respiratory diseases that range wildly in severity, and usually are tied to their genetic map and how their receptor-binding components work. Essentially, knowing these facts is important for diagnosis, monitoring, and even developing treatments during global outbreaks (Carabelli et al., 2023). Getting a bit more in-depth, the genome and protein structures determine how they act and interact with host cells. The spike (S) protein, for example, does most of the heavy lifting by binding to receptors and fusing membranes, which is how these viruses gain entry into cells. SARS-CoV-2, for instance, employs the angiotensin-converting enzyme 2 (ACE2) receptor, the same one SARS-CoV-1 employs, and that similarity in targets within tissues are quite revealing. But even with those common strategies, subtle changes such as mutations or recombination events can drastically change the ease with which they spread or evade the immune system. In the majority of instances, these genetic manipulations have been responsible for the emergence of various SARS-CoV-2 variants, each possessing a unique set of modified, inherent traits that increase its fitness and transmissibility (Carabelli et al., 2023). Simply put, these molecular refinements lead our knowledge of coronavirus classification far beyond the mere taxonomy. Further there's the fascinating question of where these viruses arise from and how they develop. Bats, for example, are usually the wildlife reservoirs of such viruses, a natural genetic melting pot where they evolve and occasionally jump to intermediate hosts before hitting humans. It's interesting to note that genetic analysis reflects approximately a 79% similarity between SARS-CoV-1 and SARS-CoV-2, yet merely some 50% if you inspect MERS-CoV (Goyal et al., 2022). Each virus appears to have its own type of host interaction and pathogenic behavior, due to these evolutionary changes. So, scientists do not only look at genetic codes in classifying them; they also take into account the way in which these viruses act in actual outbreaks, in addition to looking at different functional characteristics and epidemiological information. This more comprehensive strategy assists in creating more specific public health responses, even if sometimes the image does look a little unclear (Figure 9.3).

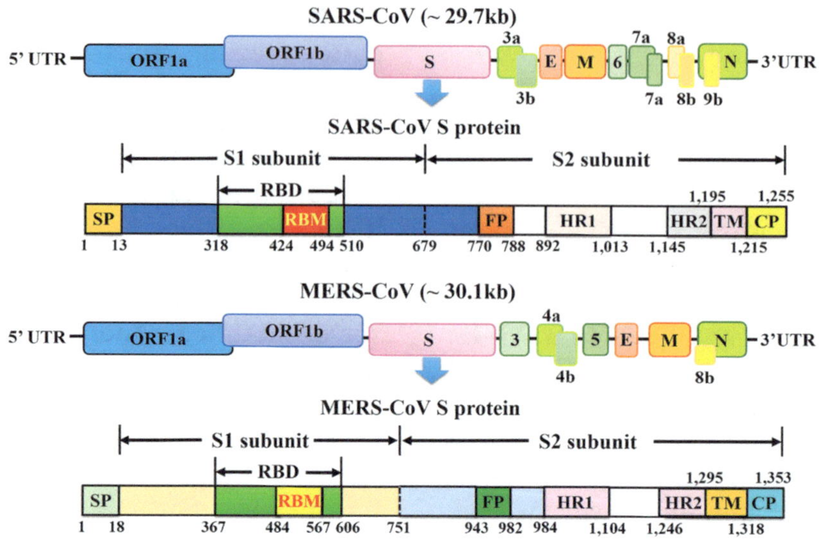

Figure 9.3. Virus variants and strains.

Source: By Zhiqi Song, Yanfeng Xu, Linlin Bao, Ling Zhang, Pin Yu, Yajin Qu, Hua Zhu, Wenjie Zhao, Yunlin Han and Chuan Qin; - https://www.mdpi.com/1999-4915/11/1/59Song, Zhiqi, Yanfeng Xu, Linlin Bao, Ling Zhang, Pin Yu, Yajin Qu, Hua Zhu, Wenjie Zhao, Yunlin Han, and Chuan Qin. 2019. "From SARS to MERS, Thrusting Coronaviruses into the Spotlight" Viruses 11, no. 1: 59. https://doi.org/10.3390/v11010059, CC BY 4.0, https://commons.wikimedia.org/w/index.php?curid=88420710

9.1.2. Historical Emergence of Coronaviruses

It was already becoming quite apparent back in the early 2000s that coronaviruses weren't the pesky microbes everyone had thought they were, suddenly they started taking a serious toll on human health. SARS surfaced in about 2002–2003, initially in China, and shortly it zoomed across national boundaries, raising alarm with its high mortality rate and merciless respiratory attacks. Before this, most coronaviruses would at best make individuals mildly ill, but SARS soon demonstrated it could spread freely from human to human with many left seriously ill and, tragically, many dead. Then, in Saudi Arabia in about 2012, MERS arrived with an even more frightening mortality rate. Both , really hammered home the fact that many of these viruses originate in animals such as bats and camels—a reminder that nature still has a lot of surprises in store. Overall, both of these early outbreaks foreshadowed just how resourceful and capricious coronaviruses could be, laying the groundwork for subsequent health crises. From SARS to MERS, we saw some disquieting trends. terms, aggressive health strategies were able to get SARS under wraps, but MERS continued to emerge sporadically—chiefly in the Middle East regions where intimate contact with camels is prevalent. Both viruses had their peculiar method of spreading; whereas SARS spread quickly, MERS, despite lesser contagion, was much more lethal. This variation in their behavior not only made containment an entirely new type of challenge but also highlighted the varied courses these viruses follow in attempting to endure in human populations. In retrospect, these outbreaks emphasized the imperative for perpetual alertness and preparedness in addressing novel, emergent coronaviruses. Further, just when it wasn't complicated enough, SARS-CoV-2 emerged in late 2019, testing our global framework by unlocking surprise complexities in the way viruses evolve, the way immunity wanes, and all the turns in their transmission dynamics (Telenti et al., 2021). History gives us a type of map for today's challenges with COVID-19. Unlike previous coronaviruses, SARS-CoV-2 was able to spin worldwide quickly, infecting humans in a continuous chain of infection that brought society to bear. Its likelihood of staying around forever is a concern , such things as declining immunity, viral mutation, and even potential animal-to-human transmission only contribute to the question mark surrounding the long term. Lessons from SARS and MERS give a rough outline of what is to come next—seasonal recurrences or possibly the emergence of new variants. The entire exercise with previous outbreaks reminds us in most instances that we need to maintain constant watchfulness, advance vaccination campaigns, and evolve public health strategies to prevent an epidemic from turning into an endemic situation. In short, controlling SARS-CoV-2 remains a tough nut to crack, making it necessary to combination lessons from history with the latest scientific breakthroughs to guide our policies and responses (Telenti et al., 2021).

9.1.3. Mechanisms of Transmission

SARS, MERS, and COVID-19 began in animals further jumped into humans, illustrating just how complex the intersection of animal hosts and human society can be. These viruses started in animal reservoirs before jumping to human beings—nominally, a textbook instance of cross-species spillover. When you're infected, droplets you breathe out can find their way into the air or settle on surfaces you may come in contact with, and if you inhale them or they hit your eyes or nose, that's when problems begin. Close contact is not the only risk; occasionally, touching an infected surface gets the job done too. The body's first line of defense, our natural immune system, works hard to shut down the infection at the start, but these viruses have become quite resourceful at evading those checkpoints, allowing them to copy rapidly and disseminate further. This covert immune evasion is a significant contributor to the way these viruses mutate and continue to pass from person to person, causing huge outbreaks (Kasuga et al., 2021). Taking a closer look, researchers have started to assemble how the shape and manner of respiratory droplets influence how these viruses spread. In essence, COVID-19, as with SARS and MERS, travels on droplets of varying shape and size. Droplets larger than say five micrometers fall rapidly, but the smaller ones—usually referred to as aerosols—may hang around for a quite remarkable time, increasing the chance of contracting it through the air. COVID-19's ability to spread even more rapidly than its predecessors is partially because it replicates well and its viral particles remain in the air and on surfaces longer. This combination of effective replication and particle stability is the reason why the virus can transmit so quickly, particularly indoors or in close areas where spacing out isn't occurring. Being aware of this has been crucial to implementing things such as wearing masks and enhanced ventilation to maintain control (Salian et al., 2021). At the molecular level, these viruses enter our cells by fitting their spike proteins onto the correct receptors on our surfaces. SARS and SARS-CoV-2 generally bind to the ACE2 receptor in most instances, whereas MERS-CoV prefers the DPP4 receptor. There is a minor but significant distinction here: for instance, SARS-CoV-2's spike binds more tightly to ACE2 than SARS's does, and that could be the reason it appears to transmit more easily. In addition, variations in how tightly these spikes bind—and where those receptors are found in our bodies—influence where the virus replicates and how much of it is shed into the environment. That, in turn, allows the virus to evade immune defenses for longer and transmit across communities. Knowledge of these viral-host interactions has been central, not only to the creation of targeted therapies but also to crafting public health measures that function to slow transmission (Kasuga et al., 2021; Salian et al., 2021) (Figure 9.4).

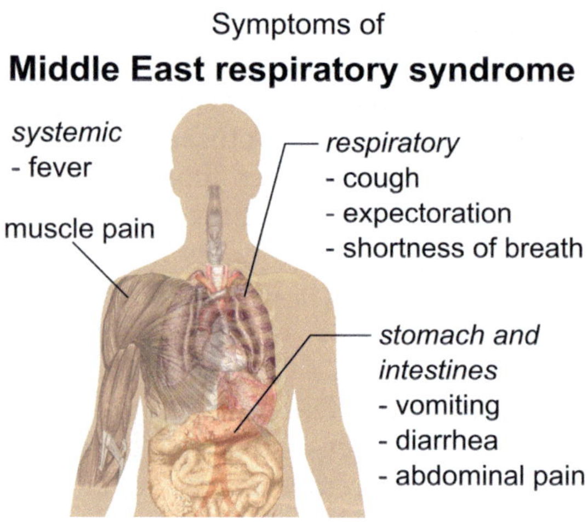

Figure 9.4. Middle East respiratory syndrome (MERS).

Source: By Mikael Häggström - Own work, CC0, https://commons.wikimedia.org/w/index.php?curid=40928291

9.2. Severe Acute Respiratory Syndrome (SARS)

In the early part of the 2000s, SARS appeared and remade our entire perception about coronavirus pandemics, highlighting how vulnerable the world could be to fresh infections. It started in Guangdong, China, and shortly, the virus jumped over borders, causing widespread sickness and an unfortunate toll in lives lost. In the majority of instances, the epidemic proved to be savage—having a mortality rate of approximately 9.5% and causing acute respiratory distress in many, which drove patients into intensive care on mechanical ventilation. Public health workers were in disarray; they followed cases, established quarantine areas, and collaborated globally, which tended to suppress the spread over a few months. However, the fact that there were no pre-existing medicines underscored our requirement for more effective monitoring systems and preventive strategies. Overall, that initial experience not only educated us on the paths and patterns of coronaviruses but also established a crucial groundwork for addressing future threats (Pustake et al., 2022). Breaking into the molecular and immunological aspect of SARS has, essentially, been a breakthrough in creating vaccines and treatments to combat subsequent coronavirus issues. Scientists saw that SARS-CoV is genetically extremely similar to SARS-CoV-2—the virus responsible for COVID-19, which allowed them to take earlier genomic and structural knowledge and use it to improve existing vaccine technology. Both viruses bind to the ACE2 receptor to infect our cells, triggering partially overlapping immune responses that, in the majority of instances, have guided the quest for the appropriate vaccine targets and antiviral medications. Evidence gathered during and after the SARS outbreak—ranging from epitope mapping to how the virus interacts within its host—paves the way for new delivery mechanisms such as lipid nanoparticles and electroporation methods. Despite these encouraging developments, hurdles remain as clinical efficacy and potential side effects still require extensive scrutiny before our being able to completely rely on our immunization initiatives against the constantly evolving viral strains (Abdolmaleki et al., 2022). From a clinical perspective, SARS appeared with a broad array of symptoms—ranging from elevated fevers and persistent coughing to worsening pneumonias that frequently broke into respiratory collapse. It was no easy task to diagnose it, with much dependence on X-ray imaging and laboratory tests such as decreased lymphocyte levels and elevated liver enzymes, which distinguished it from more common respiratory infections. Although the outbreak was ultimately brought under control, the lack of a specific antiviral therapy highlighted how important supportive care and rigorous infection control were then. The lessons that were derived from real life, having managed the patients and controlling spread, have taken a profound influence in managing subsequent epidemics like MERS and COVID-19. Early detection, prompt isolation, and effective international coordination are in most instances critical to controlling epidemics. Grasping the clinical course of SARS continues to be a pillar for enhancing how we care for patients and influence public health guidelines for upcoming coronaviruses (Pustake et al., 2022) (Figure 9.5).

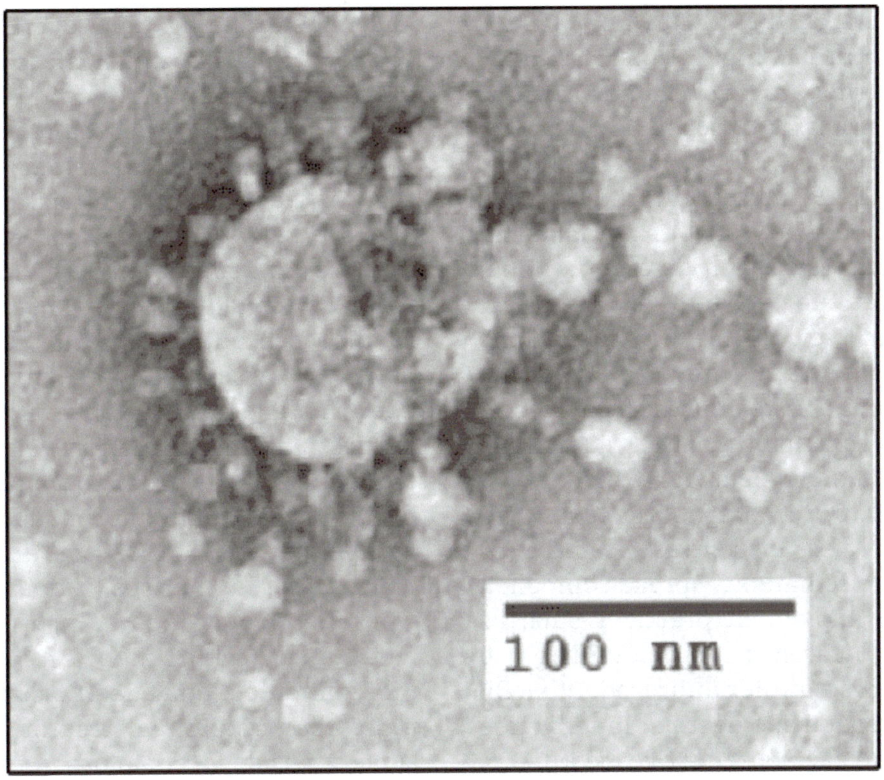

Figure 9.5. Severe acute respiratory syndrome (SARS).

Source: By Photo Credit:Content Providers(s): CDC/C.S. Goldsmith - https://www.cdc.gov/sars/lab/images.html, Public Domain, https://commons.wikimedia.org/w/index.php?curid=86419462

9.2.1. Origin and Outbreak Timeline

In the early 2000s a new coronavirus emerged and grabbed global attention with its fast spread and serious health effects. Back in 2002–2003, the SARS outbreak showed up, mainly in China, and marked our first real brush with a coronavirus seriously affecting people, leading to thousands of infections and worrisome fatality numbers. Nigh on 10 years after in 2012, another threat in the form of MERS emerged from the Arabian Peninsula, this time associated with animals—, camels—, again demonstrated that these viruses are capable of crossing species. Broadly speaking, those initial alarms set out an unbalanced template for how we now know viruses behave and guide public health action and research (Vidwans et al., 2020). By December 2019 things once again went in a strange direction in Wuhan, China, when a mysterious pneumonia started showing up. Patients presented with symptoms such as fever and respiratory issues that reminded everyone of the previous SARS and MERS outbreaks. Investigation teams quickly identified the perpetrator, a new coronavirus that would later be named SARS-CoV-2, which distinguished it from the predecessors almost from the start. Within a whirlwind, the disease swept so rapidly that the World Health Organization declared a Public Health Emergency of International Concern by the end of January 2020, and by March, it had become a global pandemic. Nicknamed COVID-19, the disease combined high transmissibility with a heavy burden, racing beyond previous outbreaks both in terms of scope and severity (Lawrenson & Buckley, 2020). Early in 2020, as news of COVID-19 filtered out, the timeline of the outbreak became a confusing amalgam of epidemiological turns and divergent global responses. What started out as a modest cluster in Wuhan grew explosively beyond the city's borders, illustrating how global travel can, candidly, be a booster for the spread of a virus. Scientists scrambled to crack its genetic code and understand its behavior, which fueled the rapid evolution of diagnostic tests and prevention strategies. In contrast to SARS or MERS, COVID-19's community spread compelled governments to implement practices such as social distancing, quarantine, and novel hygiene regulations that were rather unprecedented. By mid-2020, as infection and death numbers were rising sharply, the need for effective treatments and vaccines became too great to be ignored, triggering a concerted research effort globally (Lawrenson & Buckley, 2020; Vidwans et al., 2020).

9.2.2. Symptoms and Health Impacts

Coronaviruses such as SARS, MERS, and COVID-19 initiate a broad spectrum of breathing problems that strike individuals in varying ways based on age, underlying medical conditions, and even the virus strain itself. High temperature, cough, and difficulty in getting breath generally appear early, but quickly matters can escalate into critical distress that often equates to a stint in intensive care. It's not only the lungs taking the beating—other parts of the body, such as the kidneys, heart, and even the nervous system, can be affected too. In most instances, this set of symptoms makes it quite difficult for physicians to pinpoint one treatment regimen, and the mortality rates tend to vary per outbreak. Generally speaking, wrapping our heads around these varied signs and understanding their overall effects is key to sharpening treatment methods and helping patients better in future epidemics. Healthcare workers, on the other hand, carry a unique weight from these infections; their job puts them right in the line of risk, both physically and mentally. The physical consequences of the virus are compounded by long work shifts, increased likelihood of contracting clusters of disease, and continual contact with ill patients. Nurses and clinicians have, in all but a few instances, experienced spikes in anxiety, depression, burnout, and even post-traumatic stress disorder—problems made worse often by long shifts, sometimes inadequate protective equipment, and sheer emotional wear from working through crises. It does not help when workers are stationed in high-risk locations or without sufficient support. At any rate, solving these intersectional health concerns requires more than individual treatment—it requires some special psychological interventions and sweeping solutions to minimize risk and create a generalized workforce resilience (Çerçizaj et al., 2025). The effects of such outbreaks extend far beyond the harm to individual bodies, pervading health systems and general society. Public health crises such as COVID-19 have literally thrown a spanner into the works of providing care on a daily basis. Increased levels of absenteeism and turnover in personnel continue adding to already strained medical infrastructures, which has a tendency to bring down overall treatment capacity. The psychological and physical strain on health personnel usually ends up manifesting in a decline in quality of care and greater susceptibility to longer-term problems. Although a number of studies have highlighted these problems, much of the existing solutions tend to focus on the individual rather than taking a step back to examine larger issues, such as the necessity for improved organizational support and working conditions. Evidently, there is an urgent need for holistic strategies that maintain both individual well-being and systemic resilience in mind, so our healthcare systems can keep pace when the next crisis comes along (Fronteira et al., 2024) (Figure 9.6).

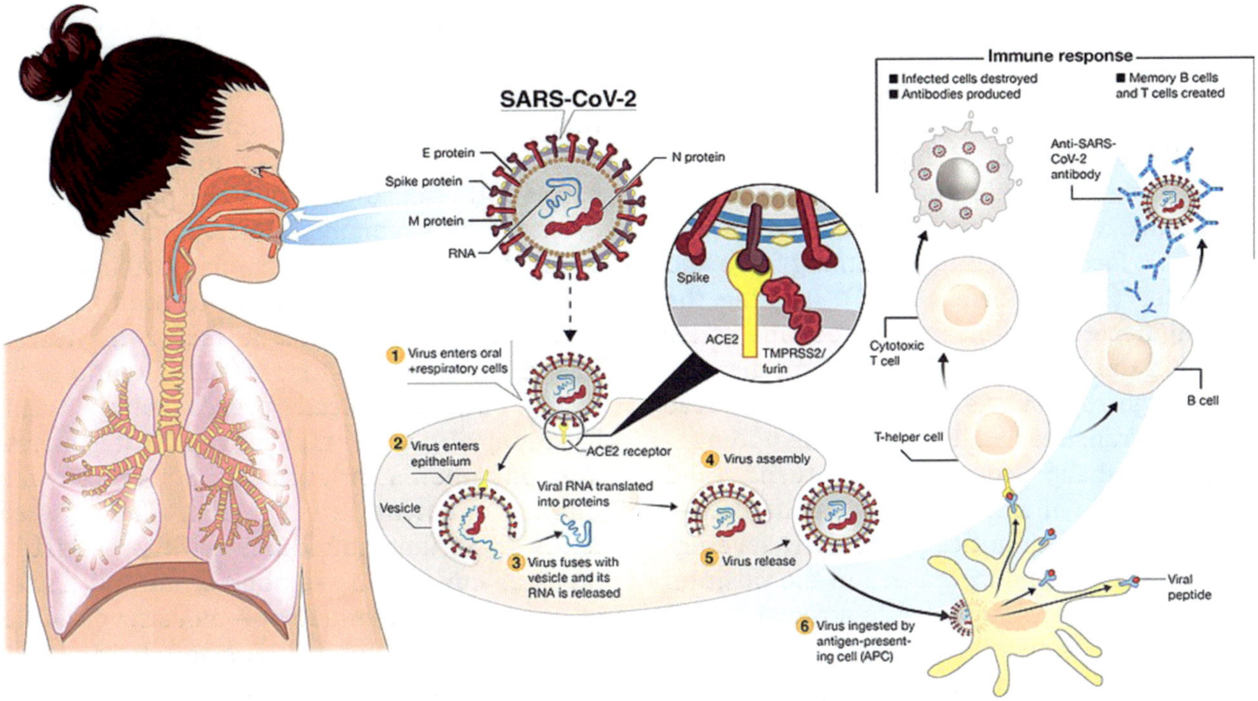

Figure 9.6. Severe acute respiratory syndrome coronavirus 2 (SARS-CoV-2).

Source: https://en.wikipedia.org/wiki/File:Fphar-11-00937-g001.jpg

9.2.3. Public Health Response and Containment Measures

New infectious diseases just don't play by any rules, so the authorities have had to get into a series of desperate maneuvers to halt the spread and prevent everyday life from disintegrating. When SARS and MERS were around, rapid actions, detection of cases, isolation, and contact tracing, were sufficient, but COVID-19 turned out to be on a whole different scale, pushing whole societies into lockdowns and rigid social distancing. How well individuals adhered to these guidelines varied considerably based on various cultural values and leadership styles; open, truthful communication proved to be a game-changer. Some countries, such as Singapore and South Korea, married learning from past epidemics to leap into mass testing and tracing, while others lagged due to delays or were simply not prepared. In brief, halting a pandemic is not merely a matter of what governments do—it is a collective action that requires the cooperation of the community, an integrated health service, and media collaboration to prevent misleading information from getting the upper hand (Peng et al., 2020). More than just attempting to bring the virus to a standstill, there's the entire other side of the equation—the emotional and social consequences of such measures. Quarantine and lockdown, while effective in slowing down the virus, tend to be packaged with additional anxiety, fear, and even social stigma for those who go through them. Communities on the front lines, such as recovering patients and health workers, can become isolated and feel separated, which further makes recovery all the more difficult. This type of stigma not only damages the affected persons but also subverts wider public health initiatives by making individuals more resistant to reporting symptoms or adhering to preventive regulations. In most instances, responding to this challenge involves employing culturally sensitive messaging that softly refutes misinformation while fostering a sense of community, with respected local leaders and media in a facilitating role in calming fears and prejudices (Peprah et al., 2020). Juggling the pressing necessity of bringing infections under control against the specter of economic disaster is a true tightrope act. As stringent controls serve to reduce transmission, they have the potential to initiate sharp economic downturns, food shortages, and increase social inequalities—striking poor communities particularly severely. This conflict puts policymakers in the position of needing to develop dynamic strategies that marry health protection with ways of reviving their economies, suited to the unique situation of each country. Global cooperation, as in the spirit of cooperation following World War II, continues to be essential to assisting low-resource countries in coping with crises and recovering from them. Being transparent about the volatility of outbreaks, and the unknowns that go along with them, tends to foster the type of trust it takes to maintain public support. Finally, learning from SARS and MERS offers useful templates for developing more sophisticated public health responses to today's and tomorrow's challenges (Peng et al., 2020).

9.3. Middle East Respiratory Syndrome (MERS)

In 2012, a virus left its stamp on the Arabian Peninsula—MERS, as it has come to be known. This zoonotic coronavirus is not your run-of-the-mill microbe; it came with a bang, appearing with a mortality rate that rounds out at nearly 35%, which is far higher than what occurred with SARS-CoV-1 and even SARS-CoV-2. It tends to begin with an uncontrolled spillover from camels (its normal animal source), followed by a limited, occasionally awkward, human spread that you predominantly observe in hospital settings. Unlike the common, community-based outbreaks of COVID-19 or previous SARS events, MERS remains limited to close-contact sites. Research, in the majority of instances, has indicated that its ability to bind to DPP4 receptors is a significant factor in how it infects lower respiratory tissues (Rando et al., 2021). Patients typically present with extreme breathing difficulties that can rapidly degenerate into pneumonia or even ARDS, necessitating intense medical intervention. The disease tends to strike individuals with pre-existing medical conditions—diabetes, kidney issues, or compromised immunity—more severely, i.e., more frequent complications and death. It's as if the virus doesn't limit its troublemaking to the lungs; it can cause widespread inflammation and disrupt other organs as well. In general, MERS transmits fairly poorly from person to person beyond very close exposure, which keeps its pandemic potential lower than SARS or COVID-19, although it remains a dominant regional threat. Scholars also observed that MERS-CoV employs similar adroit tricks as its virus relatives—manipulating interferon responses—to evade the immune system (Rando et al., 2021). MERS' spread over time truly highlights the importance of maintaining close surveillance over zoonotic sources and outbreaks within medical institutions. Despite having fewer cases worldwide than its notorious cousins, MERS consistently lays bare vulnerabilities in infection control procedures, particularly within hospitals. This has driven efforts such as more stringent screening, cautious isolation, and enhanced contact tracing—measures that, in the majority of instances, manage to stem further transmission. In the meantime, breakthroughs in deconstructing the molecular composition of MERS-CoV have fueled developments in vaccine and therapeutic research, despite the lack of an approved vaccine to date (a stark contrast to the quick deployment observed for COVID-19). Stepping back and comparing MERS to other coronaviruses not only informs us about how these viruses work but also provides us with important lessons for controlling future zoonotic threats (Rando et al., 2021) (Figure 9.7).

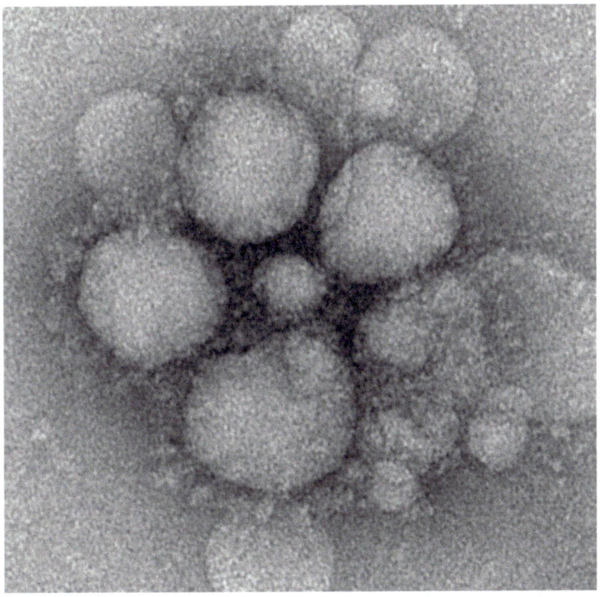

Figure 9.7. Middle East respiratory syndrome (MERS).

Source:By Cynthia Goldsmith/Maureen Metcalfe/Azaibi Tamin - https://www.cdc.gov/coronavirus/mers/photos.html, Public Domain, https://commons.wikimedia.org/w/index.php?curid=26433945

9.3.1. Origin and Outbreak Timeline

Novel coronaviruses continue to surface, fueled by the complex connection between humans and animals—a crossover that frequently allows viruses to jump from host to host. Bats, for example, appear to be playing a significant role in these incidents, with animals such as civet cats sometimes serving as a temporary bridge. Consider SARS: it's widely believed that SARS-CoV was originates in bats, transmitted through civets, further jumped to humans. This all started way back in late 2002 in China's Guangdong province and, quite quickly, accounted for more than 8,000 cases and almost 800 fatalities by early 2003. Likewise, MERS emerged in 2012 in Saudi Arabia, with dromedary camels becoming a primary reservoir. These instances, in the vast majority of instances, reveal how our intimate contact with animals can open the door for viruses to become adapted and proliferate—, out in an imperfect but revealing map of epidemic trends and zoonotic drivers. From here, these initial spark events were given fuel to build on by COVID-19. SARS-CoV-2 was initially detected in Wuhan at the end of 2019, and from the outset it showed a degree of transmissibility that greatly surpassed its forebears. Soon enough, tightly packed global cities and an interconnected world made containment a genuine headache; by March 2020, the World Health Organization had classified it as a full-blown pandemic, infecting millions and claiming numerous lives in a matter of mere months. While its origins also appear to be equally linked to bats—with some speculation regarding precisely which intermediaries assisted the leap—the virus spread so quickly that even old hands had to revise initial surveillance and detection methods (Telenti et al., 2021). Even science itself couldn't continue on its old path either. With SARS and MERS, studies filtered out through familiar, traditional publishing routes. To be contrasted was the COVID-19 pandemic that unleashed nearly panicked levels of data sharing through preprint servers like bioRxiv and medRxiv. The initial 10 months saw nearly 125,000 pandemic articles produced, numerous of which are still labeled preprints. With faster information flow came the data's influence, making it serve to inform researchers and policymakers just as quickly while hastening vaccination efforts and public health interventions at the same time as it initiating some glitches to verify information.

Overall, this rapid, and occasionally complex—shift in scientific communication has not only reshaped our approach to fighting SARS-CoV-2 but also set the stage for handling outbreaks in the future (Fraser et al., 2021).

9.3.2. Symptoms and Health Impacts

Respiratory viruses such as SARS, MERS, and COVID-19 leave us with a mess of lessons regarding how varied symptoms can be and how severe the health blow could be. Fever, cough, and respiratory difficulties tend to appear initially, suggesting a lung problem even if you don't anticipate it. For the most part, SARS and MERS appear to get right to the point quickly—off from mild symptoms to serious pneumonia and even respiratory collapse—whereas COVID-19 can turn it on its head, from hardly perceptible infections to outright acute respiratory distress (ARDS). Surprisingly, these pathogens not only play havoc with the lungs but can also set off issues in various organs. This complex image of symptoms assists public health policymakers, for the most part, in determining how to best address such constantly evolving viral threats (Mohanasundari et al., 2024).

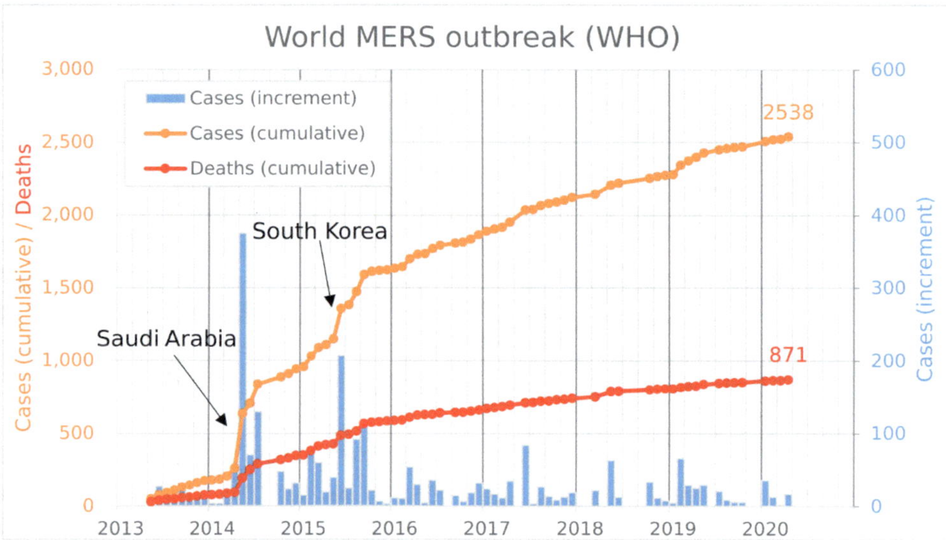

Figure 9.8. Symptoms and health impacts of respiratory viruses.

Source: By Phoenix7777 - Own workData source: MERS-CoV - Disease outbreak news. World Health Organization., CC BY-SA 4.0, https://commons.wikimedia.org/w/index.php?curid=40913864

Apart from the immediate battle with oxygen, the fallout from these viruses can persist long after the emergency would otherwise have expired. For instance, most SARS survivors found themselves coping with persistent lung conditions and even episodes of psychological distress, whereas MERS occasionally introduced an increased risk of unexpected complications such as kidney issues. Further, of course, there's COVID-19 which added its own impact with what people refer to as "long COVID"—a prolonged condition characterized by fatigue, confusion, and persistent respiratory symptoms. You could argue these conditions add layer upon layer of complication, as secondary infection and exaggerated inflammatory responses potentially cloud the issues further. Overall, these setbacks to health highlight why ongoing surveillance and individualized rehabilitation programs continue to be so important (Mohanasundari et al., 2024). Droplets containing these viruses translate into capturing the early symptoms as being instrumental in the chain of transmission being damaged . Public health campaigns—consider the COVID-19 education campaigns as an example—have pushed communities to pay more attention to symptoms and adhere to safety measures. Similar signs appear throughout SARS, MERS, and COVID-19, but the quick, at times volatile, transmission of COVID prompted everyone to act fast and unprecedentedly. In a wider, more human-focused context, combinationincorporating day-to-day issues with medical knowledge assists in the development of the appropriate type of messaging and prevention strategies, enabling it to be managed more effectively to deal with these capricious viral threats (Figure 9.8).

9.3.3. Public Health Response and Containment Measures

SARS, MERS, and COVID-19 all rattled the cage, eliciting public health responses that weren't all the same by any means—they varied quite a bit based on how easily each virus spread and the special social environments they breached. In early 2020, for instance, China surprised many by stamping out COVID-19 with a combination of rapid case finding, isolation, and relatively strict lockdowns. Their strategy was sort of two-pronged: they first plunged into halting community spread with a sweeping series of public health measures; then they pivoted to preventing any new cases, particularly those insidious imports associated with cold-chain products—from reappearing. The fact that these efforts disrupted important transmission chains made the point that, without vaccines or specific drugs, good old-fashioned public health interventions can work magic. In the majority of instances, strong action at both individual and community levels reduced reproductive numbers significantly, establishing a kind of worldwide standard for managing respiratory epidemics (Gao & Li, 2022). Conversely, the global strategy for these outbreaks appeared to be deeply embedded in the way societies and governments are programmed. Consider Singapore and South Korea, they'd already had coronavirus scares previously, and they knew how to turn that past experience into more targeted responses that minimized disruption when it came to COVID-19. Their success was due in large part to collaborative leadership, well-established health systems, and a sort of cultural milieu of compliance with health guidelines. In general, sustained, sometimes rough-around-the-edges, communication that freely identified unknowns and addressed misinformation were the hallmarks of maintaining public trust in motion. This all-around, sort-of a holistic approach—, explained in the Sociotype ecological model (where context, relations, and personal factors all co-mingle)— highlights just how diverse and culture-sensitive the public health response needs to be to mirror the communities they address (Peng et al., 2020). Although the majority of containment measures relied heavily on -non-pharmacological interventions, they were not without their challenges. The silent transmission from individuals who did not present symptoms, as well as the virus's ability to mutate quickly, threw a lot of curveballs into the equation. COVID-19, with its high percentage of asymptomatic and even pre-symptomatic infection, pushed many nations into widespread testing and mass screening regimes—efforts that did not come without concerns about social and economic consequences. Governments were in a difficult balancing act, attempting to balance these necessary interventions against the day-to-day disruptions and economic uncertainty they would create. Lessons from SARS and MERS had already foretold the need for preparedness and flexible response; in fact, these outbreaks have made explicit that continuous surveillance, rapid response times, and international coordination are absolutely essential to extinguish new threats early. Finally, histories with these coronaviruses are an important reminder that public health containment is a moving target, one that depends on scientific advances as well as sincere societal commitment to remain ahead of future epidemics (Peng et al., 2020; Gao & Li, 2022).

9.4. Coronavirus Disease 2019 (COVID-19)

SARS-CoV-2, the virus responsible for COVID-19, triggers a complex immune response that isn't as simply one might imagine. The body ramps up antibody manufacturing, mobilizes memory B and T cells, and recruits defenses within the mucosal surfaces simultaneously. Unlike most other respiratory viruses that tend to induce only a short episode of immunity, this virus has the effect of compelling the immune system to sustain systemic antibody levels long after eight months in the majority of cases. Investigations both in humans and animal models tend to highlight that antibodies targeting the spike protein receptor-binding domain are a key factor in protecting against the virus. Added to that, Fc region-driven functions enable the removal of the virus and relief from the disease. In the early days, concerns were raised about immunity being lost too rapidly, but more recent investigations show a relatively consistent level of antibodies, suggesting long-term protection similar to what is observed with SARS-CoV-1 or indeed some influenza strains. What is found to be interesting is that the severity of the infection is able to impact the strength and longevity of such antibodies (Sampson et al., 2021). The initial defense at the point of entry comes from mucosal immunity. IgA antibodies and tissue-resident T cells respond quickly at points of entry, frequently eliminating the virus before it gets a chance to replicate. Research indicates that secretory IgA may decline more rapidly than systemic IgG, although its neutralizing capacity in blocking initial infection is still remarkably strong. In the majority of instances, IgA and IgG appear to assume different functions, with one protecting the upper airways and the other guarding the deeper respiratory passages. It's intriguing that antibodies produced from common, endemic coronaviruses don't really hold up well against SARS-CoV-2, underscoring how specific your immune response needs to be. To summarize, this balance between systemic and mucosal responses appears key whether you've been infected before or received a vaccine (Sampson et al., 2021; Siggins et al., 2021).

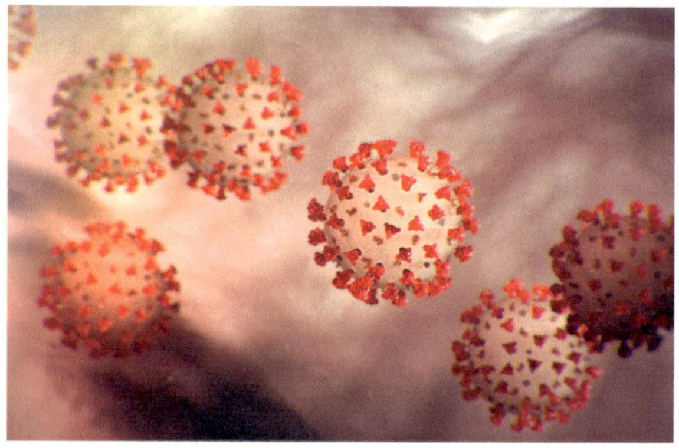

Figure 9.9. COVID-19 virus.

Source: National Foundation for Infectious Diseases. (2023). *COVID-19 Virus.*

Revisiting past data and recent research, it's evident that antibody duration is not a one-size-fits-all situation. Seasonal human coronaviruses usually cause only a partial immunity that may fade within a year, frequently resulting in milder reinfections. Pandemic viruses such as SARS-CoV-1 and SARS-CoV-2, on the other hand, tend to induce more long-lasting antibody responses. Certain experimental human challenge trials have indicated that prior immunity can typically repel a repeat viral contact, with highly high dosing of the virus being the exception. The long-term presence of neutralizing antibodies and memory immunity—up to a year or more—

indicate that the immune system maintains a functional defense, which is important for controlling spread of virus and limiting disease severity. This changing landscape is now informing public health policy and vaccine strategy to contain COVID-19, as well as other coronavirus infections (Sampson et al., 2021; Siggins et al., 2021) (Figure 9.9).

9.4.1. Origin and Outbreak Timeline

New diseases don't necessarily emerge in neat, linear fashion. In late 2019, however, there was a spike in unexplained cases of pneumonia in Wuhan, China, and scientists were racing to figure out what was going on. They took patient samples and performed some cutting-edge RNA sequencing, which isolated SARS-CoV-2, the pathogen that causes COVID-19. Oddly enough, even with this early detection, its genetic blueprint seems unlike the natural ones we're used to, leaving many to wonder if a lab misstep—accidental or even intentionally tinkered with—might have played a part. This uncertainty about that first jump from animals to humans only deepens the puzzle of tracing the virus's beginnings and makes it harder to shape strategies to avoid future global health scares (Barbari, 2024). In attempting to map how the coronavirus is transmitted, digging into its genetic past and examining infection histories tends to provide some revealing evidence. In one case, at an event in October 2021, a cohort of pilgrims coming back from Medjugorje triggered a probe that employed whole genome sequencing to map the path of the virus. Scientists observed a combination of Delta variant sub-lineages among infected individuals, suggesting that there was not merely one source behind the outbreak. Interestingly, it seems that just a single case directly traced back to the pilgrimage site, while most other infections almost certainly occurred nearer to home. For the most part, these results serve as a reminder of just how much human movement and daily activity have the potential to induce viral transmission, and they quite clearly highlight the importance of combining genomic techniques with traditional outbreak tracing (Presti et al., 2024). Layering the chronology of SARS, MERS, and COVID-19 teaches us a combination of the same and keen differences. SARS began in Guangdong, China, late in 2002, spreading largely by direct contact from person to person until finally brought under control. A decade or so later, in 2012, MERS appeared in the Middle East—, camels as a significant source, but its spread remained relatively contained. Next, COVID-19 burst onto the world stage late in 2019 and rapidly developed into a global crisis, its spread accelerating through the newer travel networks and many individuals not even recognizing they had it. The rapid detection of SARS-CoV-2 through sequencing was a great technological success; however, many unknowns regarding its actual origins continue to remain. With the virus changing all the time and various chains of transmission emerging, it is evident that we require a quicker, more coordinated international response along with strong surveillance measures (Barbari, 2024; Presti et al., 2024).

9.4.2. Symptoms and Health Impacts

SARS, MERS, and COVID-19 have an enormous difference in the way that they impact individuals. At the outset, you may experience a fever, cough, or shortness of breath, further most patients find themselves coping with symptoms months after the virus is no longer present. Most of the time, these persisting symptoms—also referred to as long COVID-19—are trouble breathing, muscle and joint pains, and even some of the mental impacts reminding us somewhat of what MERS and SARS survivors experienced. This perseverance not only complicates recovery but also adds extra workload for healthcare services that now have to monitor patients with ongoing, sometimes multidisciplinary, care requirements (Sis Aó-Almirall et al., 2021). It's not just the body that suffers; mental health tends to suffer as well, though sometimes that receives less focus. During and following outbreaks, depression and anxiety can bear heavily upon daily life and overall health. Surprisingly, some studies on traditional herbal treatments—techniques that have been attempted in Asia for centuries—indicate these may relieve the emotional burden. For the most part, this indicates that the effects of these viruses are not confined to their physical manifestations; they extend to our brains and emotions, something that necessitates rigorous attention in clinical practice as well as community support (Shahrajabian et al., 2020). If you consider the combination of symptoms in the cases of these outbreaks, it is apparent care cannot be monodimensional. It's not only about treating a cough or fever; it's also about spotting and managing long-lasting effects on both body and brain. Primary care is now leaning towards regular check-ups and follow-ups—sometimes involving several types of specialists—to help patients get back to a good quality of life. Integrating routine biomedical treatment with support for mental and social well-being has become key, even if it sometimes feels a bit complex. This dynamic strategy is slowly redefining our health systems' preparedness for any future coronaviruses (Shahrajabian et al., 2020; Sis Aó-Almirall et al., 2021) (Figure 9.10).

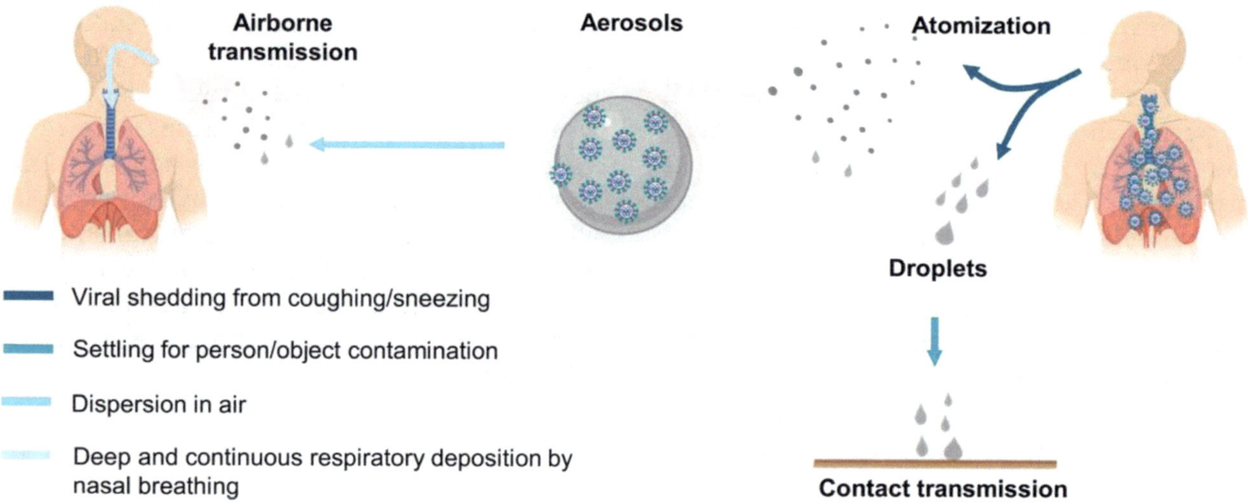

Figure 9.10. Characteristics of SARS-CoV-2 and COVID-19.

Source: By Renyi Zhang, Yixin Li, Annie L. Zhang, Yuan Wang, and Mario J. Molina - Renyi Zhang, Yixin Li, Annie L. Zhang, Yuan Wang, and Mario J. Molina; Identifying airborne transmission as the dominant route for the spread of COVID-19, PNAS June 30, 2020 117 (26) 14857-14863;https://doi.org/10.1073/pnas.2009637117, CC BY 4.0, https://commons.wikimedia.org/w/index.php?curid=99410352

9.4.3. Global Public Health Response and Vaccination Efforts

COVID-19 truly disrupted public health systems across the globe, pushing a race to implement rapid, coordinated vaccine deployments. Although researchers have overall made good headway in designing vaccines, getting them reasonably into each community is still a large pain point, particularly in middle- or low-income communities. Most African countries, for instance, have to contend with a combination of challenges: not only is the supply of vaccines low, but also maintenance of them at required temperatures and quite a lot of hesitance owing to prevalent misinformation and residual distrust. Global organizations like the COVAX facility and African Vaccine Acquisition Task Team are scrambling to procure millions of doses, but the differential delivery and political volatility make those plans difficult to execute, proving that the remedy isn't only more global cooperation but also increased local capacity to produce and deliver vaccines (Nachega et al., 2021). Short of dealing with these structural loopholes, the vision of world herd immunity is a mirage. Distribution issues aside, vaccine reluctance has also arisen as a major hurdle that works against public health efforts across the globe. In the majority of instances, vaccine reluctance has been the result of several factors: social media-encouraged disinformation, centuries-old distrust of big pharma, and continuing concerns about safety and efficacy. These hardships fall particularly hard on communities already battered by the pandemic, consider frontline workers, who frequently reside in cramped circumstances conducive to little social distancing. With structural issues such as reduced wages and limited healthcare piling on, the dangers are compounded. When you combine social class, race, and occupation-related risks, it's evident that health campaigns must address these matters more explicitly, and community outreach must be sharp to generate vaccine trust and push back against misinformation (Faghri et al., 2021). As a general rule, public health interventions must integrate social justice concepts if we intend to reach every single group. The crisis has also placed a high spotlight on how work environments influence infection risk, emphasizing that workplace safety should be a central element of any vaccination campaign. Essential workers, those trapped in on-site jobs frequently in environments in which protection is insufficient, get exposed much more to the virus, and many also fight chronic stress-related ailments that make COVID-19 worse. These underlying health concerns, combined with economic instability, such as the lack of paid sick days or job security, make it harder for individuals to adhere to quarantine protocols, thus keeping the virus in motion. To truly get vaccines to work for all, policies must address not only the short-term medical solutions; they've got to deal with the larger social and economic determinants at play. That is, increasing workplace protections, expanding access to healthcare, and providing enhanced sick leave policies (Faghri et al., 2021). Overall, a more comprehensive shift is needed to create a resilient, global response to this current health crisis.

9.5. Comparisons Among Severe Acute Respiratory Syndrome (SARS), Middle East Respiratory Syndrome (MERS), and Coronavirus Disease 2019 (COVID-19)

Looking at viral transmission and mortality rates provides us with a few important clues regarding the effects of SARS, MERS, and COVID-19 on international health. The viruses, though originating from animals and belonging to the same family—, not act identical. SARS emerged in 2002, while MERS emerged in approximately 2012, with mortality rates fluctuating at around 9.5% and 34.4%, respectively; in the majority of instances, the figures appear rather high. COVID-19, in contrast, is pegged at roughly 2.3% fatality, which is lower but comes with a much faster, almost unpredictable transmission. That quick transmission has propelled COVID-19 past the boundaries of its ancestors, triggering a global outbreak that has remade societies and stretched healthcare systems to the breaking point—even as their origins share the concept of zoonotic jumps, COVID-19 introduces its own challenges for containment and mitigation (Hafeez et al., 2021). Taking a closer look at where these viruses originate, it's apparent that the relationships between humans and animals are pivotal, particularly where live animals are bought and consumed. Live and wet markets in most low- and middle-income countries serve as busy hubs where humans, domestic animals, and wildlife intersect in ways that allow viruses to pass between species. In the vast majority of instances, research has attributed SARS and COVID-19 to these markets, suggesting that such environments facilitate the virus's transmission from animals to humans. Not only do these populated areas increase the likelihood of an initial spillover, but they also prompt the virus to make adjustments—mutating as it cycles through animal hosts.

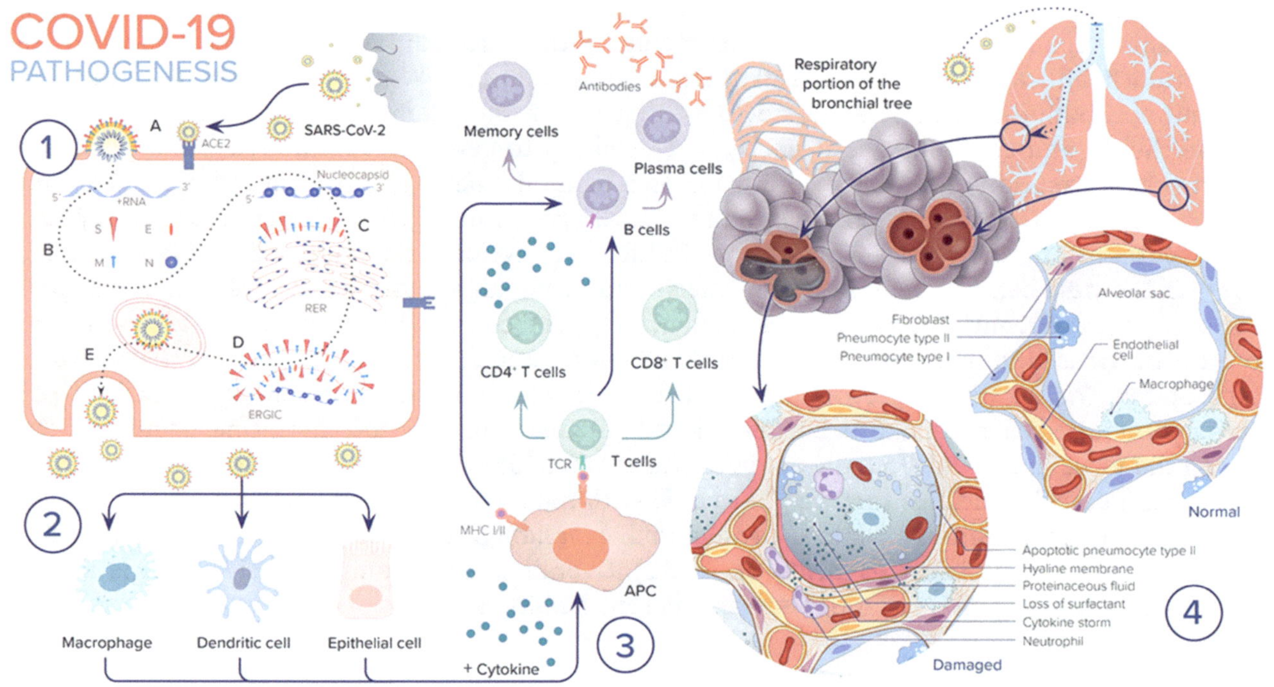

Figure 9.11. Comparisons among SARS, MERS, and COVID-19.

Source: By Nour Chams, Sana Chams, Reina Badran, Ali Shams, Abdallah Araji, Mohamad Raad, Sanjay Mukhopadhyay, Edana Stroberg, Eric J. Duval, Lisa M. Barton, and Inaya Hajj Hussein - Chams N, Chams S, Badran R, Shams A, Araji A, Raad M, Mukhopadhyay S, Stroberg E, Duval EJ, Barton LM and Hajj Hussein I (2020) COVID-19: A Multidisciplinary Review. Front. Public Health 8:383.https://doi.org/10.3389/fpubh.2020.00383, CC BY 4.0, https://commons.wikimedia.org/w/index.php?curid=99750049

Balancing their economic significance against their limitations at keeping things secure is a crucial piece in preventing future epidemics of viruses like SARS, MERS, and COVID-19 (Naguib et al., 2021). In terms of how these diseases present and spread, we find a combination of patterns that reflect different underlying mechanisms and public health challenges. Overall, SARS and MERS tended to cause serious disease—with overwhelming respiratory symptoms and greater mortalities—though their transmission was largely limited to hospitals or among people in close contact. In contrast, COVID-19 is more volatile: ranging from disease with few if any symptoms to severe disease, it makes infection within communities much easier. Its prolonged incubation time, combined with the possibility of pre-symptomatic transmission, effectively confuses the waters for containment, as opposed to the more easily trackable patterns of SARS and MERS. These differences in turn compel public health measures to adapt, relying on extensive testing, social distancing, and targeted vaccination measures to confront the novel challenges presented by COVID-19's spread and effects (Hafeez et al., 2021) (Figure 9.11).

9.5.1. Transmission Dynamics and Infection Rates

New coronavirus strains continue to cause international health concerns, at least partly because they propagate extremely rapidly and strike with big infection numbers. COVID-19, which unexpectedly emerged late in 2019, is just one dramatic case, it swept the world, overwhelming even well-planned healthcare infrastructures. This virus, as with SARS and MERS previously, began by spilling over from animals to humans (a type of spillover), then spread from person to person. In a curious twist, in most instances many of the carriers don't develop symptoms despite shedding enough virus from the upper respiratory tract to sustain outbreaks. All these factors combined cause sudden spikes in cases and complicate dealing with the outbreaks (Rohan et al., 2021). Knowing how these portions interlink is, by and large, the key to changing our response tactics as new threats emerge, even if things sometimes become complex. Where and how individuals interact truly determines how a virus gains traction. Schools, for example, tend to become small hubs where consistent close contact accelerates the transmission of viruses such as SARS-CoV-2. Frequent close interactions, particularly in classrooms, can power transmission greatly with highly contagious variants like Delta, according to some agent-based models, including those constructed from expert estimates on contact patterns. Recurring screening and the quick isolation of cases are likely to reduce infections more effectively than general quarantine procedures, which, quite honestly, so often cause unjustified absences with minimal actual effect. With reduced contacts and more prudent contact, risk declines demonstrably, highlighting the utility of individually oriented prevention measures (Woodhouse et al., 2021). These observations, strange as it seems, inform public health policy that attempts to balance infection control with keeping normal life progressing. If you look at SARS and MERS, you see each had its own uniqueness that informed their outbreak courses. SARS had a fairly high mortality rate but didn't spread very far, and its outbreaks were typically contained by strict controls and aggressive contact tracing. MERS, in contrast, spread very little among individuals, primarily remaining contained to healthcare facilities or animal contact, which resulted in only periodic outbreaks but not sustained community spread. COVID-19 turns the script around—with its capacity to transmit silently from individuals who are asymptomatic or even pre-symptomatic, it has spread worldwide with alarming rapidity. This covert transmission has translated into record-breaking infection numbers and relentless community spread. It appears that an ever-changing combination of viral evolution, unpredictable human mobility, and daily social routines is what maintains the infection levels high, requiring adaptable surveillance and intervention approaches to meet both existing and emerging outbreaks (Rohan et al., 2021).

9.5.2. Severity of Disease and Mortality Rates

New coronaviruses have emerged in recent decades, completely turning the world public health landscape around. In 2002, SARS spread rapidly from human to human with a combined 11% mortality rate that kept health officials seriously on their toes. And in 2012, MERS came onto the scene with an astonishing 37% fatality, although it didn't spread as quickly between individuals.

These viruses primarily strike the respiratory system, frequently causing serious pneumonia and even acute respiratory distress—complications that particularly plague older people and those with preexisting medical conditions. COVID-19, which emerged at the end of 2019, added further to the complication by presenting a broad range of symptoms, ranging from cases that leave you with barely a scratch to ones that verge into life-threatening disease, complicating attempts to assign an absolute death rate. Such heterogeneity emphasizes that disease severity must be taken into account in the context of each individual viral outbreak (Shah et al., 2021).

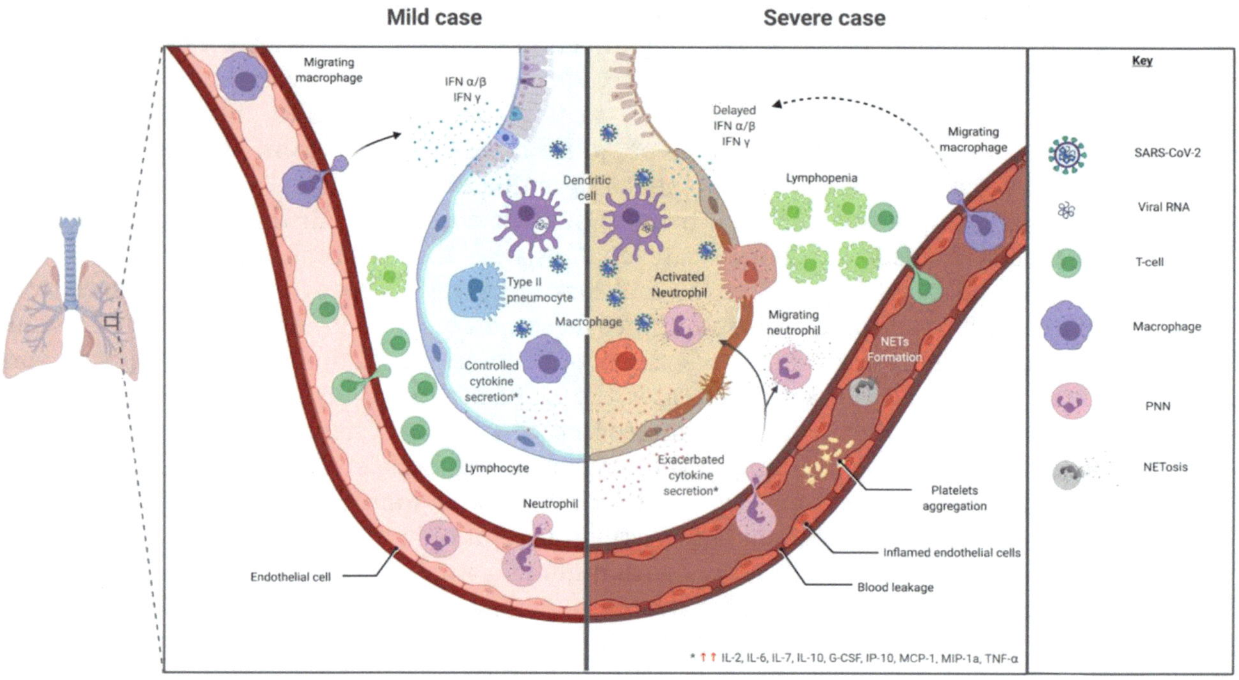

Figure 9.12. Severity of disease and mortality rates.

Source: By Grégorie Lebeau, Damien Vagner, Étienne Frumence, Xavier Guillot, Estelle Nobécourt, Loïc Raffray, and Philippe Gasque - Lebeau, G.; Vagner, D.; Frumence, É.; Ah-Pine, F.; Guillot, X.; Nobécourt, E.; Raffray, L.; Gasque, P. Deciphering SARS-CoV-2 Virologic and Immunologic Features. Int. J. Mol. Sci. 2020, 21, 5932.https://doi.org/10.3390/ijms21165932, CC BY 4.0, https://commons.wikimedia.org/w/index.php?curid=99475584

As for how lethal these viruses are, various components come into play. terms, factors like a virus's intrinsic strength, the way that our immune systems respond, and the overall infrastructure of healthcare all combine to impact outcomes. SARS-CoV-2—the virus that causes COVID-19—has proven to be more infectious than its ancestors. While SARS and MERS had a tendency to manifest as a narrower spectrum of symptoms, COVID-19 can be as mild as an upper respiratory sniffle or as severe as multi-organ failure. In most instances, older adults and individuals fighting chronic disease take the worst hit. As of early 2021, the pandemic had killed more than 2.8 million people globally—a sobering indication of its far-reaching severity. Furthermore, examination of the viruses' genetic blueprints demonstrates common enzyme targets but variation in how quickly they spread and how virulent they turn out to really determine the clinical outcomes and the fatality statistics

(Mei et al., 2021). Determining how bad and lethal these infections are isn't always black and white. Although SARS and MERS also had fairly high case-fatality ratios, their outbreaks were contained within specific regions and didn't persist long, which resulted in fewer total deaths worldwide. By contrast, COVID-19 succeeded in traveling globally—not simply because so many had few or no symptoms, but also owing to extended viral shedding—accumulating a larger total death toll even if per-case mortality was lower. Further, of course, there's "long COVID," that persistent umbrella term for post-acute manifestations still adding to the health impact well beyond the initial wave. They are combined with variations in local healthcare capacity, public reaction, and individual vulnerabilities to subtly modify the ultimate mortality landscape. Overall, ongoing surveillance and specialized medical measures are still unequivocally essential in addressing today's crisis as well as future coronavirus epidemics (Mei et al., 2021; Shah et al., 2021) (Figure 9.12).

9.5.3. Societal and Economic Impacts

SARS, MERS, and COVID-19 broke out, disrupting normal life and exposing underlying fissures in our health infrastructures and social protection. Nurses and other frontline workers were put in brutal, high-stakes conditions, with extended shifts and limited equipment—that wore them down slowly. Day by day, the sheer pressure appeared to accumulate, giving rise to anxiety, depression, burnout, and even PTSD, while the knock-on effect damaged patient care. Research, in the majority of instances, indicates that developing stronger mental health support for such workers is essential; relieving the everyday stress and making assistance more accessible can truly make a difference during crises and well beyond. Such supports not only assist the individual caregivers but also raises the general well-being of our communities (Çerçizaj et al., 2025). Economic consequences assumed many hues and dimensions as governments struggled with policies such as lockdowns, travel restrictions, and closure of workplaces. Supply chains became complex, and consumer demand plummeted, triggering a broad downturn. Interestingly, though, some experts argue that draconian policies don't necessarily translate to improved health outcomes, some nations with less stringent policies fared similarly, or even better in cases and fatalities. This suggests that policies that are too stringent could prove counterproductive, exacerbating joblessness, firm closures, and social divisions. Walking the tightrope of balancing public health imperatives against maintaining the stability of the economy is a daunting task; policymakers must then balance the social cost of controls versus their benefits in a pragmatic as well as equitable manner (Karg, 2024). Aside from matters of health and finance, such outbreaks have undermined social relations and public trust. Apprehension and stigma surrounding the virus altered the way individuals interacted—provoking, on occasion, discrimination against select groups. Extended periods of separation, anxiety, and interrupted habits negatively impacted mental health across the spectrum. At the same time, vulnerable groups, already precariously placed, were hit harder by employment insecurities and unequal access to care, exacerbating established disparities. With schools disrupted and jobs displaced, opportunities for recovery became even more uncertain, making visible a desperate need for a social safety net. An open, honest dialogue coupled with open-minded policies could perhaps heal these social cleavages. In the end, what these crises teach us is that recovering is not simply about medical solutions or economic strategy—but also about creating strong social connections and addressing embedded inequities to hold our communities together.

9.6. Lessons Learned from Past Outbreaks

Experiences with SARS and MERS in the past have paved the way for how we treat viral outbreaks today. Back then, when things went a little awry, it was clear that being able to identify an issue early on and being honest about it, whether at home or abroad, is imperative. Delaying too long to record and report cases merely allowed the virus more space to breed, which compelled most to support robust tracking mechanisms and more fluid global coordination. Our hospitals needed to adapt to unforeseen spikes in patients, while public health interventions needed to tread the fine line between working and being accepted by society. These lessons all ultimately influenced the initial COVID-19 measures, although the sheer magnitude of the outbreak ultimately revealed gaps that remain to be filled (Telenti et al., 2021).

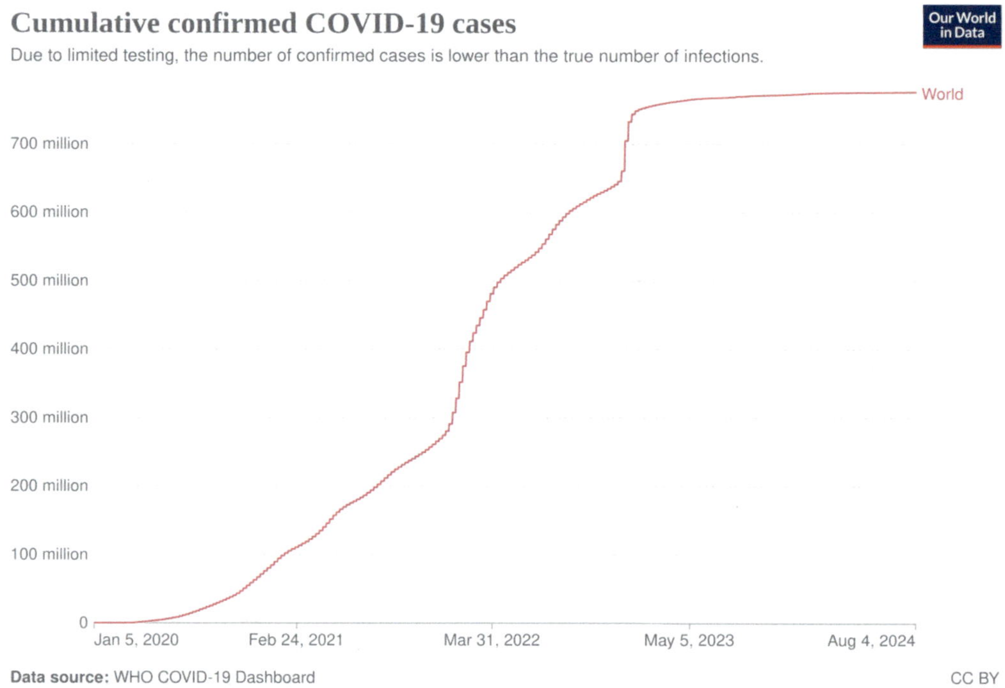

Figure 9.13. Meta-analysis and comprehensive study of coronavirus outbreaks.

Source: By Our World in Data - OWID (University of Oxford), CC BY 4.0, https://commons.wikimedia.org/w/index.php?curid=88469357

Another fundamental lesson learned from those previous scares involves vaccine development and deployment. The remarkably rapid development of COVID-19 vaccines was partly due to immunological leads acquired in previous studies of SARS-CoV and MERS-CoV. By knowing the general architecture and key targets of these viruses, researchers were able to focus on the essentials for vaccine development and accelerate the process. Of course, there were a few hiccups along the way—concerns regarding long-term immunity and fears of vaccine-related respiratory issues did arise, which compelled research aimed at creating safer, more effective choices. In the majority of instances, it also proved to be the case that getting vaccines out equitably and gaining public confidence are as crucial as the scientific advances behind them. Learning from those early experiences, many came to understand that rapid vaccine action must be accompanied by good plans for manufacture, availability, and strategies to address hesitancy (Li et al., 2020). A final key insight concerns just how flexible coronavirus transmission can be. In contrast to a few previous outbreaks that really did little more than sputter after their initial burst, SARS-CoV-2 had a disposition to continue circulating among populations, at least in part due to immunity wearing off and the virus continuing to evolve. This combination of characteristics suggests that COVID-19 could ultimately become a normal presence in our lives, requiring constant surveillance, regular vaccinations, and public health approaches that can adapt as circumstances change. Generally speaking, letting our guard down is a risky move—staying alert to new variants and changing spread patterns is key. To summarize, these experiences underscore the need to fuse insights from various fields and keep up global cooperation, so we're better prepared to handle future outbreaks and boost our overall resilience against infectious diseases (Telenti et al., 2021) (Figure 9.13)..

9.6.1. Importance of Early Detection and Response

Viruses such as SARS, MERS, and COVID-19 pushed us to respond quickly in identifying outbreaks. Early identification of a problem allows health teams to set up quickly measures that reduce transmission and prevent hospitals from becoming overwhelmed. With COVID-19, identification of people with the virus—even those who did not even become sick—was necessary because the virus transmitted quietly and even altered its shape sometimes. Testing, contact tracing, and case isolation became the day-to-day measures that laid the groundwork for slowing the spread. In the majority of instances, if not addressed promptly, circumstances would have descended into a critical international crisis with further disease and fatalities. Clearly, early diagnosis isn't simply an initial step—it's the foundation that supports initiating subsequent action such as the deployment of vaccines and technology-driven solutions (Wang, 2025). In addition to the clamor for early testing, getting onto treatment quickly makes patients do a lot better, particularly when they're very ill. COVID-19 demonstrated that quickly deploying doctors and nurses can prevent complications and hasten recovery. Physical therapists, especially those who work on breathing disorders, embraced the concept of initiating therapy as soon as severe symptoms strike, which checks the chronic problems stemming from prolonged use of a ventilator and lack of mobility. Their methods, be it through respiratory therapy, proning patients, or mobilizing them early, appear to maximize lung function, reduce ICU stays, and start rehabilitation. For the most part, it usually makes it worse to wait because it creates additional weakness and greater overall risks, so timely hospital action is especially important nowadays in coronavirus times (Alokayli et al., 2024). This isn't merely individualized care, however. Prompt detection and rapid response cascade out to inform larger public health action by merging data technology innovations with international collaboration. The entire COVID-19 ordeal demonstrated that exchanging outbreak information quickly and employing digital monitoring tools really can accelerate how we track and manage a crisis. When officials were alerted to the trends in virus transmission, they could encourage people to maintain social distancing and wear masks—actions that were fairly instrumental in slowing the spread. Furthermore, identifying emerging variants at once allowed plans to be switched around in a matter of seconds to meet the threat. Essentially, it is using together early recognition along with tech advancement and synergized global coordination as a complete system for approaching infection and hopefully avoid another emergency similar to the kind we witnessed over the COVID pandemics (Wang, 2025).

9.6.2. Role of International Cooperation in Public Health

Health emergencies have a way of stirring things up—nations find themselves depending on one another even when resources are not infinite. Cambodia, for example, demonstrated the way that decisive political resolve combined with common actions such as mask-wearing, quarantine enforcement, and pressuring vaccination programs can stem the flow of a virus. They combinationed indigenous effort with portions from international blueprints like the International Health Regulations 2005, which essentially demand sharing information freely and moving in lockstep. Despite some restrictions in laboratories and finance, their experience suggests that a common global health infrastructure helps increase measures like testing, quarantine, and deploying vaccines. It also serves as a reminder that, with unevenly distributed resources, additional international support and constant knowledge exchanges are absolutely vital (Chhim et al., 2023). Reflecting on outbreaks such as MERS you can see that trying to put together an international response is never easy. Of course, labs became a lot better at detecting disease and at coming up with tests, but delays still emerged, particularly with investigations into how viruses transmit between animals and people. This type of hiccup indicates that fighting an epidemic isn't just about human health—it requires a mix that also looks at animals and the environment. Fast data sharing and genuine trust between countries are really, really important, and to be honest, overcoming bureaucratic obstacles makes a huge difference for any global response (Ribeiro dos et al., 2022). Maintaining international collaboration strong means really drawing on past lessons while being flexible. Governments, multilateral institutions, and communities all have to get together—be it by enhancing early detection procedures, making vaccines available to everyone equitably, or merely keeping the debate regarding threats realistic. Cambodia's stepped, multi-layered response is a good case in point: combining local entrepreneurship with international coordination can seriously enhance the response effort during a health crisis. Even where there are resource gaps or quarantine arrangements aren't ideal, the future belongs to combining scientific advancements with the determination of leaders and communities, so we can have rapid, clear, and inclusive solutions to the world stage (Chhim et al., 2023; Ribeiro dos et al., 2022).

9.6.3. Need for Ongoing Research and Preparedness

Coronaviruses continue to reappear with the capacity to induce epidemics and even pandemics, which quite indicates that we need to continue exploring how they work. Ever since their discovery in the 1960s, the viruses have always managed to surprise us by way of genetic mix and match—they do not cling just to the lungs but, for example, at times strike the kidneys, like in challenging cases of SARS, MERS, and COVID-19. This type of diversity complicates it a little for treating patients, and we are left with serious questions regarding what motivates certain viruses to be fond of lining blood vessels or to cause pesky little clots. More constant research needs to be conducted, not only to have a complete picture of these microbes but to also read the signs in which they could evolve in some ways that can lead to new outbreaks. Investing in research in the areas of virology, immunology, and disease transmission assists us in identifying these dangers ahead of time while also driving advancements in treatments and vaccines that can soften the impact of what may be coming (Popov et al., 2022). Healthcare systems, for their part, have had to be prepared for these ups and downs—it's not so much a case of having one good plan. Several variables such as management decisions, the number of beds or resources a hospital possesses, and even local economic conditions all factor into how well and fast they can respond when things turn sour. Community engagement and having a clue about health have their own role here, too, making whole systems more adaptable when a virus begins its rounds. Looking back at SARS, MERS, and COVID-19, we realize that preparedness is not only a matter of doing it in hospital corridors; it's a matter of integrating local realities and considering the context. Viewing all these portions together somehow provides a stronger barrier against not only coronaviruses but also other emerging diseases (Mohammadpour et al., 2021). Lessons learned from previous outbreaks inform us that taking the initiative is our best hope for fighting off future pandemics. Preparedness must change constantly—following every new discovery of science and being responsive to how outbreaks change is essential. Spending money on improved healthcare infrastructure, educating our frontline care providers, and improving public education are all necessary to keep ahead of future threats. Additionally, when scientists, policymakers, and members of the community collaborate—despite their shortcomings—the outcome tends to be more rapid, evidence-based decision-making that saves lives. The recent pandemic has reminded us, with stark clarity, that neglecting any of these components can create severe social, economic, and health reversals. Therefore, continuing research and planning on a comprehensive, interconnected basis isn't only intelligent; it's strictly necessary to reduce the overwhelming burden of today's and tomorrow's coronavirus challenges (Mohammadpour et al., 2021; Popov et al., 2022) (Figure 9.14).

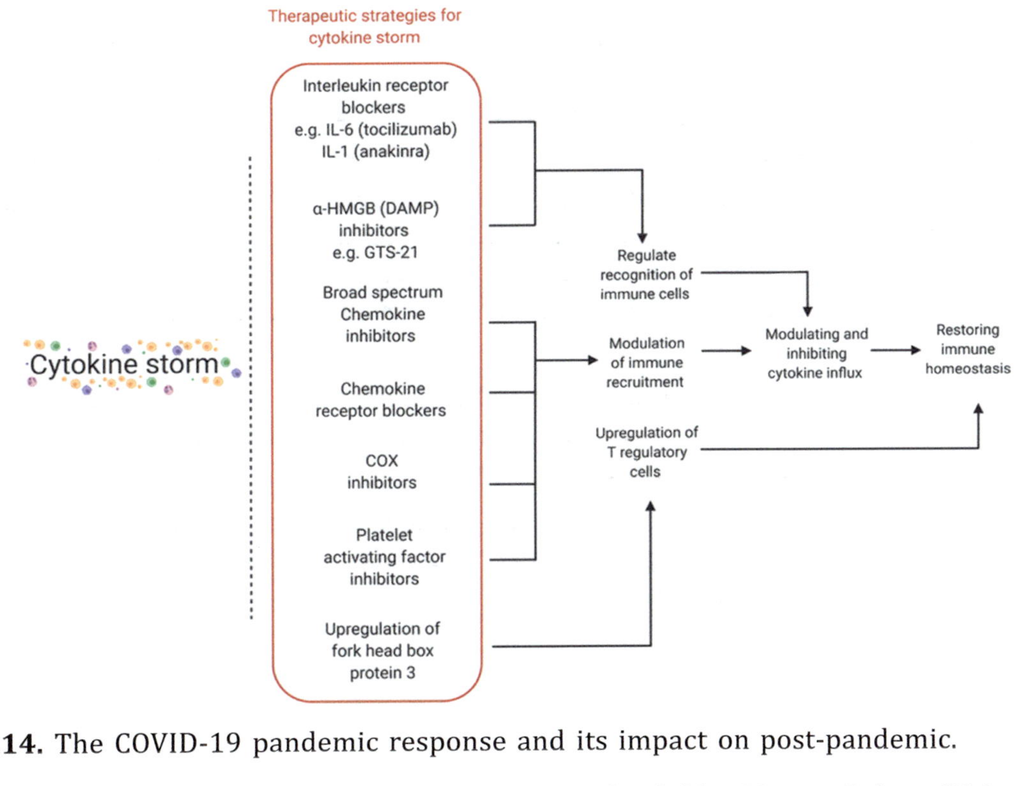

Figure 9.14. The COVID-19 pandemic response and its impact on post-pandemic.

Source: By Sonu Bhaskar, Akansha Sinha, Maciej Banach, Shikha Mittoo, Robert Weissert, Joseph S. Kass, Santhosh Rajagopal, Anupama R. Pai, and Shelby Kutty - Bhaskar S, Sinha A, Banach M, Mittoo S, Weissert R, Kass JS, Rajagopal S, Pai AR and Kutty S (2020) Cytokine Storm in COVID-19—Immunopathological Mechanisms, Clinical Considerations, and Therapeutic Approaches: The REPROGRAM Consortium Position Paper. Front. Immunol. 11:1648.https://doi.org/10.3389/fimmu.2020.01648, CC BY 4.0, https://commons.wikimedia.org/w/index.php?curid=99532048

CLOSER LOOK

VACCINE DEVELOPMENT AND FUTURE PREPAREDNESS FOR CORONAVIRUSES

The COVID-19 pandemic highlighted both the challenges and achievements of modern vaccine science. Coronaviruses, including SARS (2003), MERS (2012), and SARS-CoV-2 (2019), have demonstrated the potential for rapid global spread and severe health impacts. Developing effective vaccines against these pathogens is critical not only for outbreak control but also for long-term preparedness against future coronavirus threats.

Vaccine development for coronaviruses has benefited from advances in genomic sequencing, mRNA technology, and viral vector platforms. The unprecedented speed of COVID-19 vaccine development—delivering effective vaccines within a year—showed how global collaboration and investment can accelerate scientific innovation. These vaccines, particularly mRNA-based ones, provided strong protection and laid the foundation for adaptable platforms that can be updated quickly against new variants.

However, challenges remain. Coronaviruses mutate, leading to immune escape variants that reduce vaccine effectiveness. Achieving long-lasting immunity is difficult, as antibody levels wane and booster doses become necessary. Vaccine inequity also remains a major concern, with low-resource countries often facing delayed access, leaving populations vulnerable to outbreaks.

Future preparedness requires broad-spectrum or universal coronavirus vaccines that target conserved viral regions less prone to mutation. Research into mucosal vaccines, delivered via nasal sprays, may offer stronger protection at the site of viral entry. Beyond technology, preparedness also demands resilient global supply chains, equitable distribution mechanisms, and strong public trust to counter vaccine hesitancy.

The COVID-19 experience has underscored the importance of global cooperation, rapid surveillance, and flexible vaccine platforms. Building on these lessons, the world must invest in preparedness now—before the next pandemic emerges.

Vaccine development for coronaviruses has made extraordinary progress but must evolve further. Combining scientific innovation with global equity and preparedness will be key to preventing future coronavirus-driven health crises.

Summary

Epidemics such as SARS and MERS , and now the current COVID-19 crisis , have raised a whole host of questions when it comes to rapidly spreading viruses. Scientists worldwide have had to leap into action, attempting to understand how these viruses function, how they transmit from human to human, and how our bodies react. For the most part, vaccines have appeared as the ideal way to reduce cases to the severe, and slow transmission, but SARS-CoV-2 just continues to evolve. Since the virus remains around, moving slightly with each iteration, and our immune systems not being able to last forever, COVID-19 may very well become a normal, endemic issue. This is to say that public health plans and vaccine programs have to be rather adaptable to cope (Telenti et al., 2021). Ongoing surveillance and being ready to change course are our best bets against sudden surges or new variants. Conversely, SARS and MERS were largely controlled by robust public health actions, but when COVID-19 landed on a worldwide scale it truly pushed our health systems and coordination to the limit. A review of all three indicates that previous research and approaches now provide a boost to contemporary vaccine development and pandemic preparation. The rapid deployment of COVID-19 vaccines drew on experiences gained working with SARS and MERS earlier – an unmistakable signal of hope and the stiff challenges of initiating long-term immunity. Nevertheless, challenges such as getting vaccines to everyone, gaining public confidence, and adapting them for new strains still remain genuine concerns. Continuous research that is based on those experiences in various times is critical to adapting our immunization strategies against COVID-19 and future animal spillovers (Li et al., 2020). This integrated set of information is what we must drive us today as well as prepare for changes in the virus's behavior. Looking at the big picture, the course of SARS, MERS, and COVID-19 reminds us that the virus and our responses are locked in a kind of tug-of-war. Early expectations for a quick wipeout have given way to more realistic plans of managing COVID-19 as a seasonal issue. What this implies is that we need to monitor even small viral mutations and be prepared to update our vaccine and public health measures whenever necessary. Sustained control will not arise just from scientific advances; it relies on firm international collaboration and scaling up our health system's ability. Being vigilant for new forms or surprising animal reservoirs is essential if we ever hope to avoid another pandemic. With increased knowledge, our policies will have to adapt as well – incorporating new data with strategies that merge safety, everyday necessities, and even economic issues (Telenti et al., 2021). Overall, these interactions learn us that resilience combined with adaptive planning is what is central to protecting our future global health.

SARS, MERS, and COVID-19 suddenly highlighted how chaotic and unpredictable new coronaviruses can be for global public health. Each had its own uniqueness, but all of them transmitted quickly and got a lot of people seriously sick—and tragically, many killed. Early on, when scientists attempted to calculate how rapidly COVID-19 spread, they discovered its reproduction number was through the roof; in Wuhan, figures exceeded 3, which meant that, in the majority of instances, preventing more than half of possible transmissions was required to make any impact. Not to mention, the initial case numbers were approximate at best—, infections likely passed undetected (De Kock et al., 2021). The most important insight was that rapid, accurate tracking of the disease is absolutely essential for putting in place effective control mechanisms. Beyond the statistics, the impact on the mental health of healthcare and social care workers has become an urgent concern. COVID-19, for example, disrupted the lives of frontline staff—not just did they have serious bodily threats to contend with, but they also battled intensely with emotional pressure. Several studies have indicated that close proximity to infected patients, insufficient protective equipment, and fear of infecting loved ones all contributed to exacerbating the stress. Female nurses appeared to have a harder time, which indicates a call for more specialized mental health care in the profession. It isn't just about individual struggles either; the backing from organizations and having clear, trustworthy information play major roles in keeping the workforce standing strong. Still, research on social care workers outside hospital walls remains patchy at best, leaving us with an incomplete picture of the overall psychological impact (De Kock et al., 2021). Overall, coping with SARS, MERS, and COVID-19 has provided us with some valuable lessons regarding epidemic preparedness. Early detection of outbreaks, getting precise case numbers, and moving quickly to stem the tide are absolutely critical when dealing with these rapidly spreading viruses. Meanwhile, protecting the mental wellbeing of both healthcare and social workers is equally essential to ensure health systems don't buckle under pressure. The proof usually tends toward the necessity for combined strategies—increasing individual resilience as well as ensuring strong system-wide support—for effectively safeguarding our frontline champions. More research and innovative interventions are necessary, particularly among those groups that operate outside usual hospital environments. Ultimately, this entire experience serves to solidify that integrating sound epidemiological understanding with all-encompassing support for workers is the key to performing better at this crisis and at upcoming public health crises.

References

1. Abdolmaleki, G., Taheri, M. A., Paridehpour, S., Mohammadi, N. M., Tabatabaei, Y. A., Mousavi, T., & Amin, M. (2022). A comparison between SARS-CoV-1 and SARS-CoV-2: An update on current COVID-19 vaccines. *DARU Journal of Pharmaceutical Sciences, 30*, 379–406. https://www.semanticscholar.org/paper/bea59a1c255b36ef7fa2e8d8580efd63233e5fd1 (accessed on 7 May 2025).

2. Alokayli, W. T., & Alkhaldi, S. M. (2024). Role of ICU physiotherapy in COVID-19: A case study. *International Journal of Recent Innovations in Medicine and Clinical Research, 3(1), 44–48.* https://www.semanticscholar.org/paper/b8646884c3aa9d82e8d527178ee3c4809c924689 (accessed on 7 May 2025).

3. Barbari, A. (2024). A different perspective on the COVID-19 pandemic: Origin of the outbreak (Part 1). *Experimental and Clinical Transplantation: Official Journal of the Middle East Society for Organ Transplantation, 22*(Suppl 2), 1–14. https://www.semanticscholar.org/paper/eead5608cd43c0676f4d54f82b180297f1ac9167 (accessed on 7 May 2025).

4. Billings, J., Ching, B. C. F., Gkofa, V., Greene, T., & Bloomfield, M. (2021). Experiences of frontline healthcare workers and their views about support during COVID-19 and previous pandemics: A systematic review and qualitative meta-synthesis. *BMC Health Services Research, 21*. https://doi.org/10.1186/s12913-021-06917-z.

5. Carabelli, A. M., Peacock, T. P., Thorne, L., Harvey, W. T., Hughes, J., de Silva, T. I., Peacock, S. J., et al. (2023). SARS-CoV-2 variant biology: Immune escape, transmission, and fitness. *Nature Reviews Microbiology, 21*, 162–177. https://doi.org/10.1038/s41579-022-00841-7.

6. Çerçizaj, R., Kamberi, F., Kiçaj, E., Prifti, V., Qirko, S., & Rogozea, L. (2025). Nursing mental health issues: Prospective pathways forward from a comprehensive review of impacts before and throughout COVID-19. *Revista Romanească pentru Educație Multidimensională, 17(1), 547–587.* https://www.semanticscholar.org/paper/1a0dff004a834eea7b2c4b423e3e5a47dea88b9a (accessed on 7 May 2025).

7. Chan, D., Ritchie, K., & Watermeyer, T. (2020). The cognitive consequences of the COVID-19 epidemic: Collateral damage? *Brain Communications*. https://core.ac.uk/download/323961751.pdf (accessed on 7 May 2025).

8. Chen, R., Sun, C., Chen, J., Jen, H. J., Kang, X. L., Kao, C. C., & Chou, K. R. (2020). A large-scale survey on trauma, burnout, and posttraumatic growth among nurses during the COVID-19 pandemic. *International Journal of Mental Health Nursing, 30*, 102–116. https://doi.org/10.1111/inm.12796.

9. Chhim, S., Ku, G., Mao, S., Van Damme, W., Ir, P., Chhea, C., et al. (2023). Descriptive assessment of COVID-19 responses and lessons learnt in Cambodia, January 2020 to June 2022. *BMJ Global Health, 8*, e011922. https://www.semanticscholar.org/paper/b4647b71b2647158e1ff650be1d454ea33095317 (accessed on 7 May 2025).

10. De Kock, J. H., Latham, H. A., Leslie, S. J., Grindle, M., Munoz, S. A., Ellis, L., Polson, R., et al. (2021). A rapid review of the impact of COVID-19 on the mental health of healthcare workers: Implications for supporting psychological well-being. *BMC Public Health, 21*. https://doi.org/10.1186/s12889-020-10070-3.

11. Faghri, P. D., Dobson, M., Landsbergis, P., & Schnall, P. L. (2021). COVID-19 pandemic. *Journal of Occupational and Environmental Medicine, 63*, e245–e249. https://doi.org/10.1097/jom.0000000000002154.

12. Fraser, N., Brierley, L., Dey, G. K., Polka, J., Pálfy, M., Nanni, F., & Coates, J. A. (2021). The evolving role of preprints in the dissemination of COVID-19 research and their impact on the science communication landscape. *PLOS Biology, 19*, e3000959. https://doi.org/10.1371/journal.pbio.3000959.

13. Fronteira, I., Mathews, V. E., Bandeira Dos Santos, R. L., Matsumoto, K., Amde, W., Pereira, A., de Oliveira, A. P. C., et al. (2024). Impacts for health and care workers of COVID-19 and other public health emergencies of international concern: Living systematic review, meta-analysis, and policy recommendations. *Human Resources for Health, 22*(1), 10. https://www.semanticscholar.org/paper/4deab5766399d201f656940673d17aaea0914878 (accessed on 7 May 2025).

14. Gao, W., & Li, L. (2022). Cold-chain transmission, asymptomatic infection, mass screening, vaccine, and modelling: What we know so far for coronavirus disease 2019 control and experience in China. *Medical Review, 2*(1), 1, 2. https://www.semanticscholar.org/paper/d580203085ecef7c780ff93abf476d6477fcea3e (accessed on 7 May 2025).

15. Goyal, R., Gautam, R. K., Chopra, H., Dubey, A. K., Singla, R. K., Rayan, R. A., & Kamal, M. A. (2022). Comparative highlights on MERS-CoV, SARS-CoV-1, SARS-CoV-2, and NEO-CoV. *EXCLI Journal, 21*, 1245–1272. https://doi.org/10.17179/excli2022-5355.

16. Hafeez, S., Din, M., Zia, F., Ali, M., & Shinwari, Z. K. (2021). Emerging concerns regarding COVID-19; second wave and new variant. *Journal of Medical Virology, 93*, 4108–4110. https://doi.org/10.1002/jmv.26979.

17. He, Y., Yu, H., Huffman, A., Lin, Y., Natale, D. A., Beverley, J., Zheng, L., et al. (2022). A comprehensive update on CIDO: The community-based coronavirus infectious disease ontology. *Journal of Biomedical Semantics, 13*, 14. https://doi.org/10.1186/s13326-022-00279-z.

18. Hill, V., Ruis, C., Bajaj, S., Pybus, O. G., & Kraemer, M. U. G. (2021). Progress and challenges in virus genomic epidemiology. *Trends in Parasitology, 37*(12), 1038–1049. https://doi.org/10.1016/j.pt.2021.08.007.

19. Kamriana, K., Dewiyanti, D., Arafah, S., & Alwi, A. (2024). The effectiveness of leaflet education media on knowledge and attitudes regarding health protocol during the COVID-19 pandemic in Canrego Village, South Polongbangkeng District, Takalar District. *Journal of Midwifery and Nursing, 6(2), 564–571.* https://www.semanticscholar.org/paper/4b5b75893979ca7232405cbcbce859de3c97b3ec (accessed on 7 May 2025).

20. Kargı, B. (2024). Assessing the socioeconomic impact of stringent containment policies on COVID-19 outcomes: A comparative analysis of OECD countries in 2020–2021. *Gümüşhane Üniversitesi Sağlık Bilimleri Dergisi, 4*, 1667–1679. https://www.semanticscholar.org/paper/2faa39d52fb7b60be51be67345f4d3037977f46e (accessed on 7 May 2025).

21. Kasuga, Y., Zhu, B., Jang, K. J., & Yoo, J. S. (2021). Innate immune sensing of coronavirus and viral evasion strategies. *Experimental & Molecular Medicine, 53*, 723–736. https://doi.org/10.1038/s12276-021-00602-1.

22. Lawrenson, J., & Buckley, R. (2020). COVID-19 and the eye. *Ophthalmic & Physiological Optics,*

40, 383–388. https://www.semanticscholar.org/paper/8a44a21440801f77c7486481689145fea6b03c5b (accessed on 7 May 2025).

23. Li, Y. D., Chi, W. Y., Su, J. H., Ferrall, L., Hung, C. F., & Wu, T. C. (2020). Coronavirus vaccine development: From SARS and MERS to COVID-19. *Journal of Biomedical Science, 27*, 104. https://doi.org/10.1186/s12929-020-00695-2.
24. Lo Presti, A., Rubino, S., Ibba, G., Ambrosio, L., Di Martino, A., Ferraro, F., Rapiti, A., et al. (2024). An outbreak of COVID-19 after a pilgrimage to Medjugorje due to Delta sub-lineages. *Journal of Infection in Developing Countries, 18*(3), 332–336. https://www.semanticscholar.org/paper/fc816195aeb10b89da964a175ca2ab0df27c7ab9 (accessed on 7 May 2025).
25. Mahmud, A. S. M., Andersson, P., Bulach, D., Duchene, S., Gonçalves da Silva, A., Lin, C., Seemann, T., et al. (2025). Molecular epidemiology of SARS-CoV-2 in Bangladesh. *Viruses, 17*, 517. https://www.semanticscholar.org/paper/c26c168e7c275d5b22a00b06ea14b7d705a8eeb7 (accessed on 7 May 2025).
26. Manjinder, K., Navdeep, K., & Simranpreet, K. (2020). A review on the fifth pandemic: Coronavirus. *Asian Journal of Pharmaceutical and Clinical Research, 13*(12), 25–28. https://core.ac.uk/download/477856300.pdf (accessed on 7 May 2025).
27. Mei, M., & Tan, X. (2021). Current strategies of antiviral drug discovery for COVID-19. *Frontiers in Molecular Biosciences, 8*, 671263. https://doi.org/10.3389/fmolb.2021.671263.
28. Mohammadpour, M., Zarifinezhad, E., Ghanbarzadegan, A., Naderimanesh, K., Shaarbafchizadeh, N., & Bastani, P. (2021). Main factors affecting the readiness and responsiveness of healthcare systems during epidemic crises: A scoping review on cases of SARS, MERS, and COVID-19. *Iranian Journal of Medical Sciences, 46*, 81–92. https://www.semanticscholar.org/paper/f1b806fe518b1e61847b25dfdf530f72ea80a081 (accessed on 7 May 2025).
29. Mohanasundari, S., Kiran, K. P., Vashishtha, N., Singh, R., Rani, B., & Nagamani, N. (2024). Overview of emerging viruses, other viruses and great pandemic of the 21st century. *A and V Pub International Journal of Nursing and Medical Research, 3(1), 37–40*. https://www.semanticscholar.org/paper/0f174db412005e70365795c9c44026046063698b (accessed on 7 May 2025).
30. Nachega, J. B., Sam-Agudu, N. A., Masekela, R., van der Zalm, M. M., Nsanzimana, S., Condo, J., Ntoumi, F., et al. (2021). Addressing challenges to rolling out COVID-19 vaccines in African countries. *The Lancet Global Health, 9*, e746–e748. https://doi.org/10.1016/s2214-109x(21)00097-8.
31. Naguib, M. M., Li, R., Ling, J., Grace, D., Nguyen-Viet, H., & Lindahl, J. F. (2021). Live and wet markets: Food access versus the risk of disease emergence. *Trends in Microbiology, 29*, 573–581. https://doi.org/10.1016/j.tim.2021.02.007.
32. Peng, W., & Berry, E. (2020). Coping with the challenges of COVID-19 using the sociotype framework: A rehearsal for the next pandemic. *Rambam Maimonides Medical Journal, 12*, e0005. https://www.semanticscholar.org/paper/47516cef6ad15f39d23bb5d635587a94250473b6 (accessed on 7 May 2025).
33. Peprah, P., & Gyasi, R. M. (2020). Stigma and COVID-19 crisis: A wake-up call. *The International Journal of Health Planning and Management, 36*, 215–218. https://doi.org/10.1002/hpm.3065.
34. Popov, H., Stoyanov, G., Petkova, L., Stoyanov, D., Ivanov, M. N., & Tonchev, A. (2022). SARS,

MERS, and COVID-19-associated renal pathology. *Encyclopedia, 2,* 1710–1721. https://www.semanticscholar.org/paper/7f7ac23c40f3272aac3424b69b3eabc5bbac17e0 (accessed on 7 May 2025).

35. Pustake, M., Tambolkar, I. A., Giri, P., & Gandhi, C. (2022). SARS, MERS and COVID-19: An overview and comparison of clinical, laboratory and radiological features. *Journal of Family Medicine and Primary Care, 11,* 10–17. https://www.semanticscholar.org/paper/bf7914d2497d869c4aaa278fdafa97da1a150246 (accessed on 7 May 2025).

36. Rando, H., Maclean, A. L., Lee, A. J., Lordan, R., Ray, S., Bansal, V., Skelly, A. N., et al. (2021). Pathogenesis, symptomatology, and transmission of SARS-CoV-2 through analysis of viral genomics and structure. *mSystems, 6*(5). https://www.semanticscholar.org/paper/0435833f32fdf9b7427d8994165eefd3b6b76e83 (accessed on 7 May 2025).

37. Rasmussen, T., Qvesel, A. G., Pedersen, A. G., Olesen, A., Fonager, J., Rasmussen, M., Sieber, R., et al. (2024). Emergence and spread of SARS-CoV-2 variants from farmed mink to humans and back during the epidemic in Denmark, June–November 2020. *PLOS Pathogens, 20*(1), e1011921. https://www.semanticscholar.org/paper/11ab1c6747a76b943a22811faf834c6d622ad695 (accessed on 7 May 2025).

38. Read, J. M., Bridgen, J. R. E., Cummings, D. A. T., Ho, A., & Jewell, C. (2021). Novel coronavirus 2019-nCoV (COVID-19): Early estimation of epidemiological parameters and epidemic size estimates. *Philosophical Transactions of the Royal Society B: Biological Sciences, 376.* https://doi.org/10.1098/rstb.2020.0265.

39. Ribeiro, C. dos S., van Roode, M. Y., Farag, E., Nour, M., Moustafa, A., Ahmed, M., Haringhuizen, G., et al. (2022). A framework for measuring timeliness in the outbreak response path: Lessons learned from the Middle East respiratory syndrome (MERS) epidemic, September 2012 to January 2019. *Eurosurveillance, 27.* https://www.semanticscholar.org/paper/9f8a389862e6623e4293af542f58c55ca3af7be8 (accessed on 7 May 2025).

40. Rohan, R., Rameshwar, S., Sachin, D., Vitthal, G. K., Nilesh, M., & Vaishali, M. P. (2021). Understanding the dynamics of COVID-19 outbreak: Structure, diagnosis, prevention and treatment. *Anti-Infective Agents, 19(4), 12.* https://www.semanticscholar.org/paper/fa59c3e9452d552c4c2a068dc0355a478cfba936 (accessed on 7 May 2025).

41. Salian, V. S., Wright, J., Vedell, P. T., Nair, S., Li, C., Kandimalla, M., Tang, X., et al. (2021). COVID-19 transmission, current treatment, and future therapeutic strategies. *Molecular Pharmaceutics, 18*(3), 754–771. https://doi.org/10.1021/acs.molpharmaceut.0c00608.

42. Sampson, A., Heeney, J. L., Cantoni, D., Ferrari, M., Suau Sans, M., George, C., Di Genova, C., et al. (2021). Coronavirus pseudo types for all circulating human coronaviruses for quantification of cross-neutralizing antibody responses. *Viruses, 13,* 1579. https://doi.org/10.3390/v13081579.

43. Shah, S. Z. A., Ujjan, I. D., & Lashari, N. A. (2021). Post-acute COVID-19 syndrome. *Pakistan Journal of Medical & Health Sciences, 15*(5), 891–892. https://doi.org/10.53350/pjmhs21155891.

44. Shahrajabian, M. H., Sun, W., Soleymani, A., & Cheng, Q. (2020). Traditional herbal medicines to overcome stress, anxiety and improve mental health in outbreaks of human coronaviruses. *Phytotherapy Research, 35,* 1237–1247. https://doi.org/10.1002/ptr.6888.

45. Siggins, M. K., Thwaites, R. S., & Openshaw, P. (2021). Durability of immunity to SARS-CoV-2

and other respiratory viruses. *Trends in Microbiology, 29*, 648–662. https://doi.org/10.1016/j.tim.2021.03.016.

46. Telenti, A., Arvin, A. M., Corey, L., Corti, D., Diamond, M., García-Sastre, A., Garry, R. F., et al. (2021). After the pandemic: Perspectives on the future trajectory of COVID-19. *Nature, 596*, 495–504. https://doi.org/10.1038/s41586-021-03792-w.
47. V'kovski, P., Kratzel, A., Steiner, S., Stalder, H., & Thiel, V. (2020). Coronavirus biology and replication: Implications for SARS-CoV-2. *Nature Reviews Microbiology, 19*, 155–170. https://doi.org/10.1038/s41579-020-00468-6.
48. Vidwans, R. R., & Lankadasari, M. (2020). COVID-19: A centennial pandemic from origin to clinical trials. *Acta Biological Marshiness, 3*, 30–52. https://www.semanticscholar.org/paper/3e03092cad7f50e1d508f36dc8fe0f226a3e784c (accessed on 7 May 2025).
49. Wang, C. C., Prather, K. A., Sznitman, J., Jiménez, J. L., Lakdawala, S. S., Tüfekçi, Z., & Marr, L. C. (2021). Airborne transmission of respiratory viruses. *Science, 373*. https://doi.org/10.1126/science.abd9149.
50. Wang, K. (2025). Global strategies against COVID-19: The role of public health measures, vaccination, and technology. *Theoretical and Natural Science*. https://www.semanticscholar.org/paper/8f39ef2a5c7611c91034b5caf131ab8c1dd13f3d (accessed on 7 May 2025).
51. Woodhouse, M., Aspinall, W., Sparks, S. R. J., & COVID-19 Mapping and Mitigation in Schools. (2021). Analysis of alternative COVID-19 mitigation measures in school classrooms: An agent-based model of SARS-CoV-2 transmission. medRxiv 2021.08.30.21262826; doi: https://doi.org/10.1101/2021.08.30.21262826 (accessed on 7 May 2025).

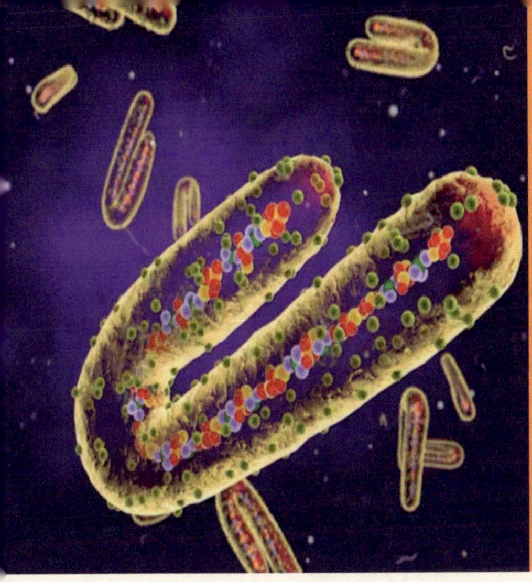

Chapter 10

EBOLA AND MARBURG VIRUSES

Contents

Introduction

Most disease hopping from animals to man continues to plague public health worldwide – they seem to emerge in the most unexpected places. Ebola and Marburg viruses, members of the Filoviridae gang, have been causing a stir because they have the potential to initiate savage, usually fatal hemorrhagic fevers. These viruses have a propensity to erupt with little notice, particularly in areas of Central and West Africa where natural circumstances and local populations intersect in ways that facilitate ease of transmission. Their epidemics strike communities forcefully, not only by inducing acute disease but by disrupting social and economic systems and overburdening public health. It's usually significant to determine where these viruses originate, how they spread, and how their symptoms present themselves so that we can devise better strategies to combat them and enhance treatments. Examining closely how Ebola and Marburg work, their natural cycles and sanctuaries still aren't completely understood, and this only makes it more difficult to stop them. Scientists tend to blame specific bat species – these organisms appear to host the viruses without appearing ill, allowing the viruses to persist in the environment. Frequently, humans become infected through direct contact with these animals or even through contaminated body fluids; then, person-to-person transmission can initiate an outbreak. Their symptoms often get mixed up with those of other local diseases, complicating early diagnosis and a prompt response. Some work on their molecular biology has noticed both overlaps and clear differences between the two, insights that help in making tests and treatments work better. All this, and those periodic flare-ups that we notice, demands increased emphasis on surveillance and study to really get a handle on such spillover occurrences (Ruiz et al., 2021; Tian et al., 2022). Large-scale outbreaks – such as that debilitating 2014–2016 Ebola outbreak in West Africa – in the last decades have pressed researchers and public health officials to really delve into understanding Ebola and Marburg. This concentration has resulted in visible achievements toward vaccines, antiviral medications, and strategies for outbreak control. However, the problem remains: the viruses mutate rapidly and appear to erupt unpredictably, which complicates vaccine efficacy and complicates treatment deployment. And the areas most affected usually lack robust healthcare and public health infrastructures, further complicating efforts toward control. In the majority of instances, integrating knowledge from virology, ecology, social sciences, and clinical medicine seems our best option for improved preparedness. A balanced strategy such as this, in the majority of instances, would be able to reduce the burden of these filovirus threats and improve overall global health security (Ruiz et al., 2021; Tian et al., 2022) (Figure 10.1).

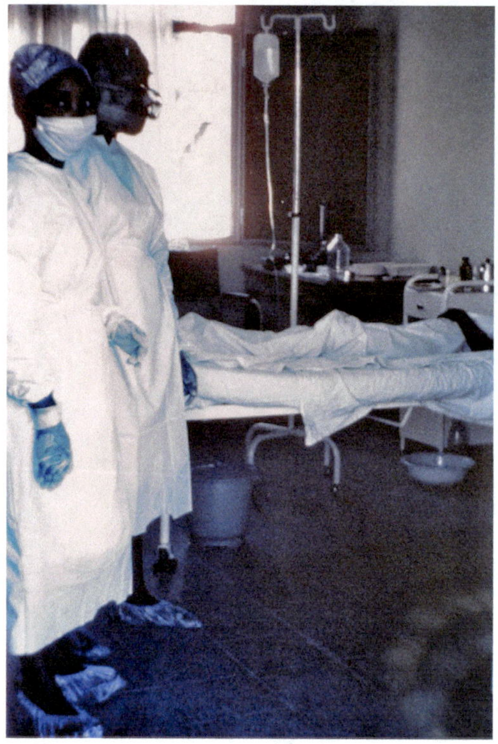

Figure 10.1. Ebola and Marburg hemorrhagic fever viruses.

Source: By Photo Credit:Content Providers(s): CDC/Dr. Lyle Conrad - This media comes from the Centers for Disease Control and Prevention's Public Health Image Library (PHIL), with identification number #7042. https://commons.wikimedia.org/w/index.php?curid=212727

Overview of Ebola and Marburg Viruses

Viral hemorrhagic fevers assault global health ruthlessly, simply because they come on so relentlessly and too many times result in tragic endings. Consider Ebola virus disease—, blazed into life back in 1976 with epidemics in Zaire and Sudan that sent the world scrambling and demonstrating only how lethal the Ebola virus truly is. The disease isn't confined to human beings alone but also to nonhuman primates. , there are five recognized forms in the Filoviridae family, such as Zaire ebolavirus and Sudan ebolavirus. The virus tends to spread when an individual gets into direct contact with fluids or blood from infected animals—usually fruit bats, chimpanzees, or monkeys—who underscore its origin from animals. Symptoms range widely, beginning with fever and body pains then progressing to fatal bleeding and even heart failure. Even though a perfect cure still eludes us, researchers are steadily working on treatments using things like monoclonal antibodies and antiviral drugs. Keeping alert and making people aware remains critical to handling outbreaks worldwide (Azad et al., 2015). Marburg virus disease is another nasty hemorrhagic fever in the same Filoviridae clan, caused by the Marburg virus. Since the last half century, almost 15 outbreaks have been documented, and a fresh outbreak in Ghana reminds us that this virus still wanders portions of Africa. Its natural host is a collection of bat species, particularly Rousettus aegyptiacus—that again indicates its zoonotic origin. In general, if the virus attacks the immune system by manipulating gene expression and suppressing interferon signals, it winds up allowing viral reproduction to go unchecked and resulting in widespread tissue destruction. Humans may begin with gastrointestinal upset that subsequently yields to bleeding complications, usually with lethal consequences. Diagnostics advances, such as RT-PCR and whole genome sequencing—have enhanced the way we identify and treat cases, and ongoing efforts are aimed at synergizing treatments such as monoclonal antibodies with antiviral drugs and even experimenting with recombinant vaccines (Alagawany et al., 2022). Although Ebola and Marburg viruses don a different name, they have many of the same deadly characteristics. Both have a propensity to cause savage hemorrhagic syndromes with extensive inflammation, multiple organ failure and, in either case, high fatality. Their emergence from animal reservoirs into humans exposes the complex interconnections between wildlife ecology and human activity. Prevention is largely a matter of strong surveillance, good public education, and rigorous infection control procedures, particularly for healthcare professionals who handle infectious fluids. There is also a glimmer of hope in the shape of promising vaccine candidates and experimental treatments that could soften the overall blow. Nevertheless, more research and an ongoing global cooperative effort are still absolutely necessary to completely crack these zoonotic threats and to formulate strategies that keep future outbreaks at bay (Alagawany et al., 2022; Azad et al., 2015).

Importance of Studying These Viruses

Ebola and Marburg viruses take their cue from a uninhibited collection of assembly strategies and propagation mechanisms that render the investigation into them a sheer necessity. These viruses are heavily dependent on a protein named VP40, which, frankly, is anything but a bystander—and it assists in the assembly of virions before their budding away from host cell membranes. If you take a closer look at VP40, you will see that its lipid-specific interactions and how it comes together through some interfaces determine how the virus assembles and ultimately leaves the cell. In most instances, untangling the specific roles of its N-terminal and C-terminal portions can lead us to a way to interfere with virus assembly without disrupting the cell's ordinary function. Considering the severe mortality rates and intermittent outbreaks of these insects, delving deep into their molecular aspects is important to designing both preventive and therapeutic measures (Amiar et al., 2021). Spillovers from animal-to-human infectious diseases have emerged as a rising concern for global public health. It's fascinating—and somewhat unnerving—that so many of the dangerous pathogens, such as Ebola and Marburg, appear to leap from animal reservoirs in unpredictable ways. This unpredictability can throw a monkey wrench into timely diagnosis and containment, particularly in areas where resources are not abundant. As a general rule, the more we know about these viruses, the better we can prepare with wiser vaccines, better diagnostics, and public health measures that really do work. And learning about the nitty-gritty details of how these spillover events occur informs us about ecological as well as molecular variables that may assist in minimizing the likelihood of even larger outbreaks in the future (Jonas et al., 2019). The socioeconomic consequences of filovirus outbreaks truly drive home the importance of ongoing investment in virus research and monitoring. Remember the 2014–2015 Ebola epidemic—a period when the epidemic not only extracted huge human misery but also put some serious strain on the economies of various West African nations (Jonas et al., 2019). By learning about how these viruses develop, transmit, and adapt to their hosts, scientists can create the path for faster diagnostic methods, more potent vaccines, and antiviral medication that could catch future crises in their infancy. In general, it is more prudent to invest funds in preventive research than to contend with the stratospheric expenses of unmanaged outbreaks. To summarize, obtaining a better handle on the uniqueness of Ebola and Marburg isn't simply about alleviating health crises—it's also an important step toward mitigating the wider social and economic shocks these viruses can impose (Amiar et al., 2021; Jonas et al., 2019) (Figure 10.2).

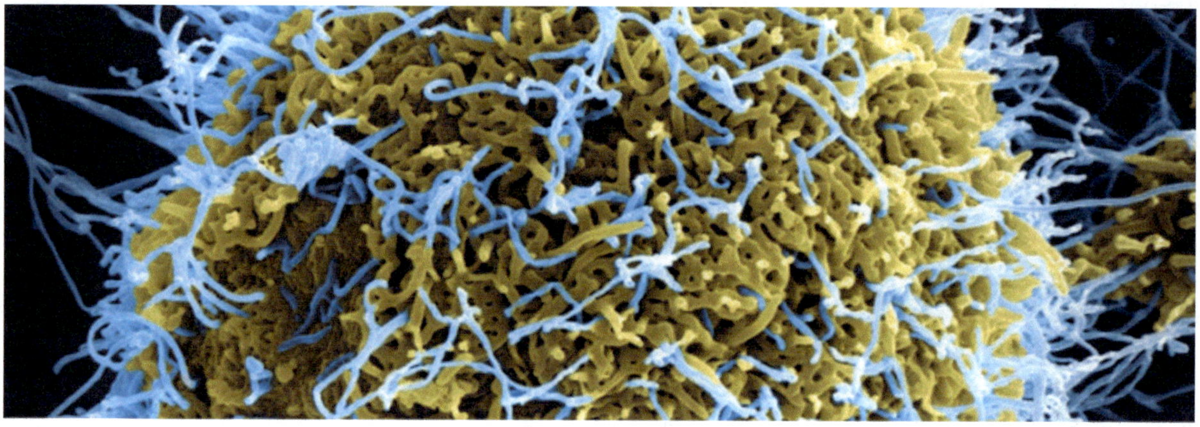

Figure 10.2. The importance of studying these viruses.

Source: J. Craig Venter Institute. (n.d.). *Genome Sequencing of Marburg and Ebola.*

10.1. History of Ebola and Marburg Viruses

Deadly viruses began making headlines toward the end of the 20th century, primarily because they appeared to be leaping from animals to humans. Ebola and Marburg—both members of the Filoviridae family—have created some genuinely catastrophic hemorrhagic fever epidemics in sub-Saharan Africa, killing dozens in their wake. In 1967, the Marburg virus first emerged when outbreaks simultaneously occurred in Marburg, Frankfurt (Germany), and Belgrade (Yugoslavia). Laboratory personnel became infected with Ugandan-imported African green monkeys with the virus, a realization that suddenly came how these viruses would erupt far from their natural settings. After that period, fatal cases, albeit occasional, have continued to remind us that it's no joke learning about their spread. For the most part, Marburg virus disease has been cataclysmic, with an average fatality rate of about 62% (Cuomo-Dannenburg et al., 2023). Ebola's story starts close to the Ebola River in the Democratic Republic of the Congo, in 1976. terms, the virus appears to have a comparable history to Marburg, as fruit bats are considered its natural host. Outbreaks soon revealed that day-to-day contact between humans and animals, particularly in far-off rural areas where bushmeat hunting is prevalent—has the potential to cause spillover events. The combination of sparse healthcare services and tight-knit communities provided additional layers of complexity to the course of the disease.

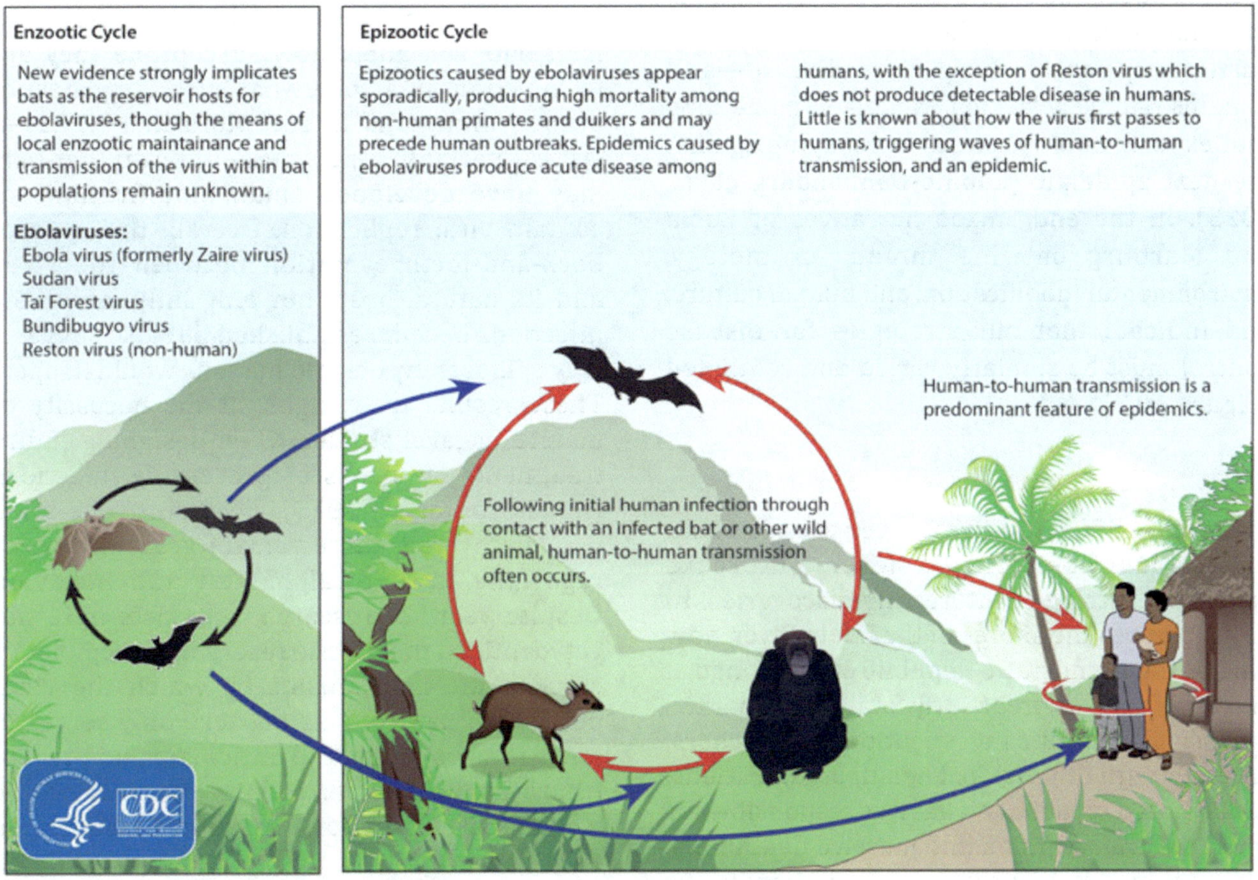

Figure 10.3. History of deadliest viruses.

Source: By Centers for Disease Control and Prevention (CDC) - https://www.cdc.gov/vhf/ebola/resources/virus-ecology.html, Public Domain, https://commons.wikimedia.org/w/index.php?curid=34451589

Ebola outbreaks became increasingly prevalent over time throughout the 1990s and 2000s, eventually peaking in the huge West African epidemic from 2013–2016. That epidemic starkly highlighted deficiencies in global preparedness and response, illustrating just how multidimensional Ebola's spread truly is (Naguib et al., 2021). Taking a closer look at both Ebola and Marburg discloses an interwoven combination of natural and man-made components. Deforestation, urbanization, and even wildlife trade pour oil on the fire by promoting the danger of these zoonotic jumps. Wet markets and live animal trading facilities commonly become surprise crossing places where viruses escape from animals into humans. Despite the fact that countless communities remain reliant upon them for income and cultural practice, their capacity to induce disease spillovers indicates that enhanced biosecurity and watchfulness through surveillance are necessary to avoid subsequent epidemics. It's also notable that mathematical modeling for such events, particularly for Marburg virus disease—still remains relatively lacking, though it's something that experts hold is central to readying against the next epidemic (Cuomo-Dannenburg et al., 2023). In the end, mixed narratives of Ebola and Marburg entwine threads of biology, environmental modification, and human culture, and indicate that our strategies for disease control must be similarly varied and combined (Figure 10.3).

10.1.1. Discovery of Ebola Virus

In the mid-1970s, a desperate need to understand mysterious hemorrhagic fever outbreaks launched a string of interesting discoveries. In 1976, close to the shores of the Ebola River, now part of the Democratic Republic of the Congo, a cluster of serious, frequently fatal cases sparked a flurry of scientific investigation. Researchers, together with other global health organizations, collaborated to identify what was responsible for the rapid transmission and massive death tolls. They ultimately identified a wholly new virus, a type of filovirus that, although bearing hints toward the Marburg virus, proved autonomous. This discovery changed the way individuals perceived viruses and epidemics in Africa, paving the way for an expanded research study of hemorrhagic fevers. In most cases, the severity of those outbreaks led to public health agendas moving toward enhanced monitoring and control measures, even venturing into apprehensions of urban and global spread (Boelaert et al., 2000). Soon enough after its perpetrator was discovered, scientists jumped headfirst into deciphering the mechanisms of its functioning and how it interacts with its hosts. It transpired that, similar to its filovirus relatives, Ebola establishes quite a complicated relationship with wild animals—primarily bats, which appear to host the virus without manifesting obvious indications of disease. For example, evidence indicated that tiny genetic variations in animals such as the African straw-colored fruit bats can affect how susceptible they are to infection. In a somewhat surprising turn of events, mutations in receptors like NPC1—a critical portal for the virus—indicate that bats may have developed small modifications to contain viral replication. Overall, this type of back-and-forth evolution between the virus and its natural hosts not only influences how infections become established but also suggests why spillover events into humans would happen. These results truly highlight the necessity of molecular-level studies when designing future treatments or means of preventing infections (Agnarsson et al., 2015). Even since the virus was discovered, there remain great mysteries regarding its natural habitat and behavior. Despite years of research, scientists have not yet identified the precise reservoir or completely cracked the mechanisms by which the virus persists in nature. This mystery only serves to make it more difficult to anticipate and prevent future epidemics, particularly considering the way the virus occasionally erupts in cities with very catastrophic consequences. Reflecting on previous Marburg and Ebola outbreaks, the following is certain: quick, concerted public health responses are essential to contain the spread and reduce deaths. These events have also demonstrated, repeatedly, how affected local communities are hit hardest and why sustained investment in surveillance, lab diagnostics, and vaccine development is so important. Finally, addressing these problems will involve marrying on-the-ground field research with laboratory research and wider epidemiological strategies to reduce the global threats of these viruses (Boelaert et al., 2000).

10.1.2. Discovery of Marburg Virus

Marburg virus initially drew attention with outbreaks dappled across African nations, with initial warnings given primarily due to its high mortality and that gruesome hemorrhagic character. Individuals in Uganda and surrounding areas paid heed when patients started developing symptoms somewhat mirroring what we eventually experienced with Ebola , a twist that had scientists working back from hints in nearly an ad hoc manner. In the majority of instances, initial field research suggested that this was not just a strange, isolated event but an indication of a virus that would lead to serious, sporadic outbreaks. Those early explorations, while a little all over the place, ultimately provided hints regarding how it transmitted and how wildlife may be involved as silent reservoirs (Amara et al., 2020). Subsequent more detailed work unraveled aspects of the Marburg mystery even further. Investigations covering quite disparate fields, from East Africa to Sierra Leone, directed fairly sharply towards some animals, and the Egyptian rousette bat (*Rousettus aegyptiacus*) kept recurring as a natural host with active infections. Approximately 2.5% of the bats were positive, and the viral strains that they harbored closely resembled those found in catastrophic human outbreaks.

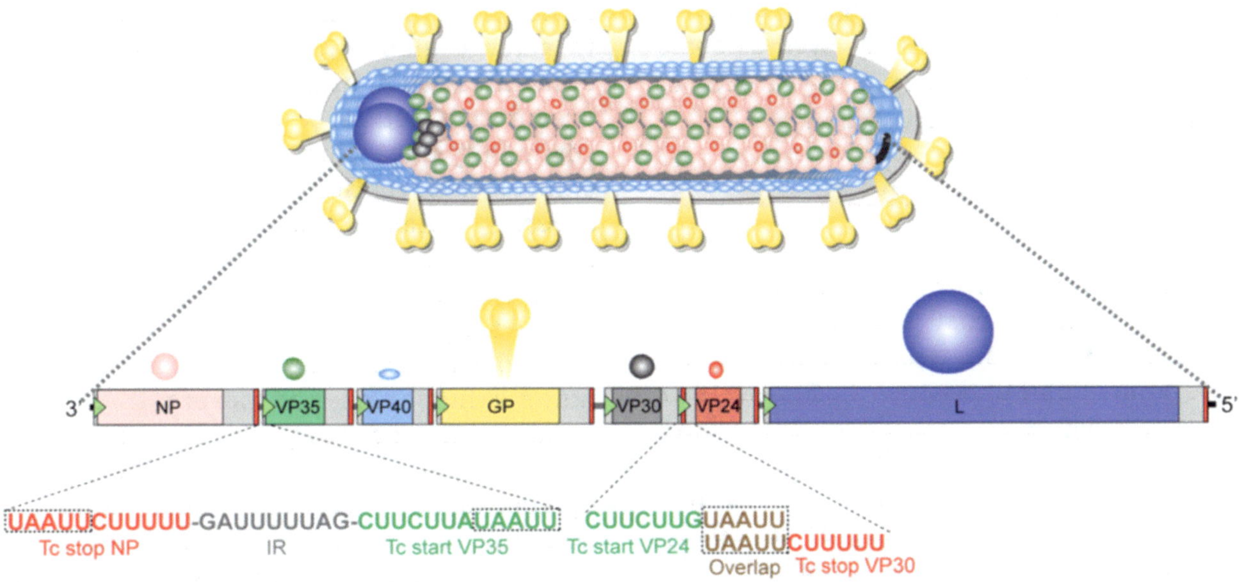

Figure 10.4. Emergence of Marburg virus.

Source: By Kristina Brauburger, Adam J. Hume, Elke Mühlberger, and Judith Olejnik - https://www.mdpi.com/1999-4915/4/10/1878/htm, CC BY 3.0, https://commons.wikimedia.org/w/index.php?curid=93995908

Overall, the results gave sound support to the hypothesis that the virus has an animal origin and highlighted why tracking new pathogens is so critical if we are going to avoid their spillover into human communities. In one sense, this research line not only completed a missing piece of the ecological jigsaw but also influenced plans to minimize zoonotic spillovers (Amara et al., 2020). Considering the broader context, understanding the emergence of Marburg virus is to position it alongside other infamous filoviruses such as Ebola, which are recognized for their unpredictable and catastrophic nature. Scientists. Placing qualifiers such as "in most cases" throughout their writing, scientists have emphasized that these viruses tend to defeat nature's own defenses—crossing species lines under the right combination of environmental and demographic pressures. It soon becomes apparent that learning about these cross-species transmission events and evolutionary uniqueness is absolutely essential. The changing story speaks to a requirement for a more concerted examination of viral evolution, animal reservoirs, and human populations—enabling us to predict and ideally cushion the impact of future epidemics. In the end, Marburg virus's tale is not merely that of one agent; it's a defining volume of our larger effort to keep infectious diseases at bay, even as some of the specifics continue to rummage around in a randomizing fashion (Figure 10.4).

10.1.3. Historical Outbreaks and Their Impact

The family of Viral hemorrhagic fevers belonging to the Filoviridae order has dislocated our healthcare system more than any other disease at one point in time or another, illustrating their outbreaks' aggressiveness. Such as Marburg virus disease; is close to Ebola, only brutal, with reports presenting fatality rates as high as 61.9% (Cuomo-Dannenburg et al., 2023). Although MVD appears less frequently than Ebola, its random appearances make immune response difficult—in the majority of instances, early identification and rapid response are the only gambles to keep the spread at bay. Unresolved questions regarding how precisely the virus transmits between individuals and holes in our general knowledge only fuel the fire, raising the risk in areas that are already at risk. Plus, the chance of infections flying under the radar, sometimes with hardly any symptoms, can let the virus stick around further resurface unexpectedly (Cuomo-Dannenburg et al., 2023). Clearly, these past challenges point toward the need for smarter, integrated monitoring and predicting methods to tackle future outbreaks head-on. Outbreaks like these do far more than just strain hospitals—they wreck communities socially and economically as well. History also teaches that crises such as Ebola and Marburn can cut through the humdrum of daily life, sweeping across healthcare infrastructure and interrupting the ordinary course of things. Routine services tend to collapse, productivity is affected, and survivors and front-line staff alike experience long-term psychological impacts. In regions where resources are already thin, such interruptions make resurgence even more difficult. As fresh zoonotic dangers continue to emerge globally, the experience of these epidemics emphasizes the imperative for preemptive action: vaccination drives, real community engagement, and rapid, concerted clinical interventions are all essential for severing transmission and damping overall mayhem. Science has benefited greatly from these outbreaks, as well—innovation holds the key to truly turning the tables. Vaccination is generally regarded as the optimal means of diminishing death and severe disease but implementing vaccines quickly once emergencies strike remains a significant challenge. Previous epidemics have frequently been tainted by delays in rolling out vaccines and treatments, demonstrating a clear lag between identifying a new pathogen and being in a position to shield individuals effectively. In turn, continuous research is working hard to test novel vaccine platforms and drive quicker development approaches. In general, examining past outbreak patterns not only refines our epidemiological models and public health responses but also refines vaccine deployment plans that are instrumental in cutting such hemorrhagic fevers off at the pass from the very beginning (Cuomo-Dannenburg et al., 2023).

10.2. Virus Structure and Classification

Viruses take all kinds of shapes, and that diversity has a lot to do with how we classify them and how they act when in a host. All viruses essentially contain their genetic material—, RNA or DNA, within a protein coat called a capsid. Occasionally, viruses such as Ebola and Marburg even acquire an additional envelope, a lipid covering borrowed from the host cell membrane, which sort of assists them in entering cells and evading the immune system. Filoviruses, for instance, are usually long and thread-like instead of the usual round or icosahedral forms. That strange structure not only throws a monkey wrench into their replication process but also alters the way they engage with immune defenses. In general, understanding these small structural nuances is central to categorizing viruses by families and designing targeted treatments and outbreak measures (Salata et al., 2019). Beyond what you can observe from the exterior, viruses are classified by what is happening in their genomes and how they replicate. Ebola and Marburg, for example, belong to the Filoviridae family, with a single-stranded, negative-sense RNA genome. Here's the catch: this RNA must be inverted into a positive-sense strand before proteins can be synthesized, and this additional step determines how quickly and aggressively these viruses can function. And slight variations in genetic sequences and how their antigens are presented splinter these viruses into smaller subfamilies. These cryptic genetic messages, duplicated here and there, enable researchers not just to distinguish them but also trace out their line of descent, which is of huge benefit in vaccinating and engineering diagnostic instruments against filoviruses (Baseler et al., 2016). Observing more carefully at Ebola and Marburg also involves paying attention to where they naturally reside and how they propagate. Both of these viruses are zoonotic—they transfer from animals to human beings—and bats are usually the ones cited as their natural reservoir. This larger ecological context is a gigantic part of their classification; it illustrates to us that these viruses form and evolve in a larger biosphere. Add to that their filamentous, elongated morphology and a strong affinity for infecting primate and human cells, and you can understand why these viruses frequently cause hemorrhagic fevers of high severity. Identifying this combination of characteristics informs public health efforts to break the chain of transmission and suppress outbreaks. In general, how a virus is constructed, its origin, and its behavior are all interconnected, furthering our general knowledge of controlling filovirus diseases (Baseler et al., 2016; Salata et al., 2019) (Figure 10.5).

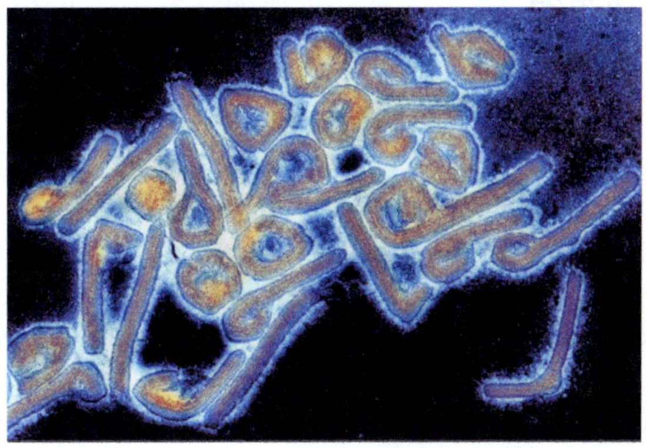

Figure 10.5. Virus structure and classification.

Source: By The University of Texas Medical Branch at Galveston. https://www.utmb.edu/newsroom/article11484.aspx - https://media.eurekalert.org/multimedia_prod/pub/web/137488_web.jpg on https://www.eurekalert.org/multimedia/pub/137488.php, CC BY-SA 4.0, https://commons.wikimedia.org/w/index.php?curid=99643704

10.2.1. Genetic Makeup of Ebola Virus

Viral infections don't simply respond to one cause – they are born from a chaotic combination of the virus's own genetic uniqueness and the characteristics of the host it encounters. Consider Ebola, say. This is explained, at least partly, by its genetic constitution, which is mostly an unpredictable sequence of around 19,000 nucleotides within a single-stranded, negative-sense RNA. It has seven structural proteins that allow it to enter cells, replicate itself, and even evade our immune systems. Small modifications in these genes can alter the way the virus behaves, so it may spread quicker or make people sicker in other populations. Scientists following these fragments of genetic information usually discover that such research not only assists in identifying mutations but also directs how interventions can be revised; they even assist in identifying stable, immunogenic areas that are the most critical in inducing protection in vaccines. Certain genetic changes in the Ebola virus have been correlated with the severity with which outbreaks struck communities. The West African outbreak, for example, showed a lot of genetic diversity between viral isolates - a indication that, most of the time, evolution can change the balance in how deadly or transmissible the virus becomes. Even the polymerase gene, the one in charge of RNA replication, has variations that could modify replication efficiency in unexpected manners. When scientists compared Ebola and its relative, the Marburg virus , both highly pathogenic filamentous viruses , they identified some conserved motifs required to ensure virus survival, but identified specific markers that perhaps account for why each one behaves differently with hosts and affects mortality rates at times. Monitoring these gene shifts, even during the midst of outbreaks, is important for detecting changes in virulence or precursors of antiviral resistance that guide public health policy. Meanwhile, the genetic configuration of those infected has a surprising influence. Host conditions, including genetic variants associated with cholesterol metabolism, appear to influence how Ebola plays out - sometimes in mannerisms that constitute the difference between life and disaster (MacDermott et al., 2021). For instance, some defensive adjustments in the PCSK9 gene could impact how the virus penetrates cells or how the immune system responds. Other genome-wide analyses have even indicated variation in genes such as Carbonic Anhydrase 5a, which seems to be associated with increased Ebola fatality rates (MacDermott et al., 2021). In a sense, the tale of Ebola's peril is not so much about its own blueprint, but also about the genetic puzzle that every individual carries. To summarize, merging viral genetics with our knowledge of host traits gives us a richer, albeit complex, picture that can ultimately steer more personalized treatment strategies.

10.2.2. Genetic Makeup of Marburg Virus

Marburg virus genetics are instrumental in determining how vile and versatile the pathogen is. Its template—a single-stranded, negative-sense RNA approximately 19 kilobases in length—comprises seven major proteins such as nucleoprotein (NP), several viral proteins (VP35, VP40, VP30, VP24), glycoprotein (GP), and the RNA-dependent RNA polymerase (L). For the most part, the configuration of these genes and the subtle variations in their sequences appear to fine-tune the virus's ability to invade host cells, evade the immune system, and replicate quickly. Recently, advances in genome sequencing joined forces with robust analysis models to enable scientists to make comparisons between various filoviruses, and this has enabled us to understand how little genetic alterations could account for why Marburg and viruses such as Ebola (Devaraj & Marianthiran, 2025) differ. These are, in a general sense, critical insights since they inform the creation of diagnostics and treatments. In recalling past outbreaks, the genetic landscape of Marburg virus is more varied than might have been anticipated. Small mutations, scattered haphazardly throughout the genome, can shift viral processes, occasionally subtly, occasionally dramatically; they even vary the virus's antigenic personality, how our immune systems perceive it. This variability matters a lot when designing vaccines or antiviral drugs, since genetic drift can shift the target sites that these interventions try to hit. In most cases, rigorous containment and research practices remind us how important it is to keep the viral genetic material secure while dodging any actual live virus contamination (Cutts et al., 2024). This balance allows genetic information to be studied safely outside of high-security laboratories, opening the door to more extensive, more detailed genetic study that is essential to keeping us ready. Exploring its molecular evolution provides further insight into where the Marburg virus may have originated. Phylogenetic studies usually point towards bats as a potential origin point, with selective forces within animal and human hosts shaping its genetic structure over time. The error-prone replication mechanism of the virus naturally results in mutations, which fuel its genetic diversity and, consequently, its adaptability. By combining genomic information with outbreak maps, scientists can follow the paths and sources of infections—a process as as it is riveting. Certain analytical techniques using deep learning have even been able to separate Marburg from similar viruses based on identifying its distinct genetic patterns (Devaraj & Marianthiran, 2025). Together, this patchwork of genetic information not only prods onward surveillance activity but also increases our ability to act decisively when new viral dangers begin to appear (Figure 10.6).

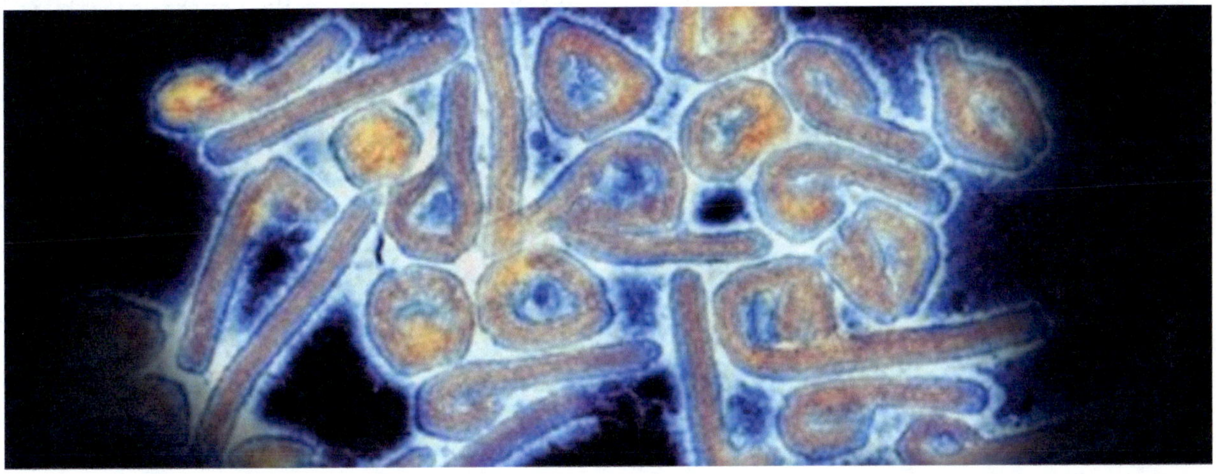

Figure 10.6. Genetic makeup of Marburg virus.

Source: Bing Images. (n.d.). *Genetic Makeup of Marburg Virus.*

10.2.3. Classification within the Filoviridae Family

Potentially highly pathogenic viruses such as Ebola and Marburg viruses compel us to depend on accurate classification techniques that aid research, diagnostics, and monitoring outbreaks. Within the negative-sense RNA viruses, the Filoviridae family truly stands out with its filamentous, elongated shape and its significant influence on human health. Categorizing such filoviruses has not been simple – their genetic diversity and the constant emergence of new variants have complicated matters for a long time. In recent times, though, advances in genome sequencing have changed the game, allowing scientists to divide species and strains with much greater precision. In essence, by aligning nucleotide sequences, scientists can separate out different genomic variants and isolates, and in the majority of instances, these improvements enhance both scientific understanding and public health interventions such as outbreak response and vaccine development (Andersen et al., 2014). One of the important portions in untangling viruses in the Filoviridae family is establishing a regular, near daily naming system. For example, the RefSeq database at the National Center for Biotechnology Information stores representative sequences that characterize major filovirus isolates, which in turn become templates for nomenclature. This nomenclature system that encompasses components like virus name, strain, host, geographic origin, sampling year, and genetic variant accommodates the steady stream of genomic data—cutting through possible uncertainty regarding variants and isolates. In general, how specialists work together here highlights that standardized taxonomy is not merely a scholarly formality, but a working instrument that cuts the comparative genomics and outbreak surveillance in evolutionary research (Andersen et al., 2014).

As more genetic data become available for Ebola and Marburg viruses, it has become evident that a stronger classification system is imperative to reflect their evolutionary relationships and public health significance. Modern molecular instruments now detect even minor genomic variations that allow for differentiation between several species and variants of the Filovirus genus. More refined classification helps identify upcoming strains, assess their pathogenic capacity, and optimize medical countermeasures in turn. On top of that, a methodical classification methodology aids ecological research by demystifying virus-host relations and transmission dynamics—even if, sometimes, the specifics get a bit muddled. As sequencing technology continues to become more affordable (and, yes, sometimes a little capricious), mixing rich genetic information into our taxonomic systems is going to fuel surveillance and assist in controlling outbreaks, ultimately enhancing public health responses globally (Andersen et al., 2014).

10.3. Transmission and Infection

Ebola and Marburg viruses are notorious for being fatal, and honestly, they become contagious to a great extent due to the way individuals interact with them. Direct contact, such as coming into contact with bodily fluids or even contaminated surfaces from an infected individual— puts these viruses ahead. Most frequently, the worst occurs late in the disease or post-mortem (when virus levels reach their zenith), leaving caregivers and those performing conventional burials in a vulnerable position. Outbreaks typically occur in areas far from medical centers; few clinical facilities make detecting and isolating cases on schedule challenging, and that only fuels fires of spread and high mortality (Sprecher et al., 2008). In most instances, knowing how local environments and common activities operate together is important in developing wiser control measures. Not all categories of contact present the same threat. How you engage with a contaminated individual—, even a corpse, counts much. It turns out that casual contact, such as eating with or talking to someone, seldom transmits the virus, particularly if the ill person isn't shedding many virus particles early on. However, when family members have direct physical contact with an ill person, the risk increases to about 32%, which indicates that actual, close contact matters. For those who are simply in proximity without contact, the risk remains relatively low. The extremely high rates of transmission observed during caregiving or funerals indicate that prolonged exposure to infected body fluids—immersed in caregiving and cultural traditions—propels the transmission (Baron et al., 2015). Obviously, an understanding of these layers is key to informing public health actions that both minimize risk and honor local customs. Despite all this knowledge, many of the details are still vague, particularly if you think about urban environments. The huge 2013–2016

West African Ebola epidemic, for instance, was an eye-opener: it indicated that transmission patterns in densely populated cities, where problems such as overcrowding and inadequate sanitation prevail, can behave in unpredictable manners relative to rural epidemics. In general, socio-political and legal obstacles can also interfere with effective surveillance and studies, subsequently making clinical prevention trials more difficult. Overcoming such obstacles is quite important if we want to reduce death rates and eliminate future epidemics with effective treatments and vaccination plans (Baron et al., 2015; Sprecher et al., 2008). More often than not, a research strategy that places local contexts at the forefront appears to be the intelligent direction to head in (Figure 10.7).

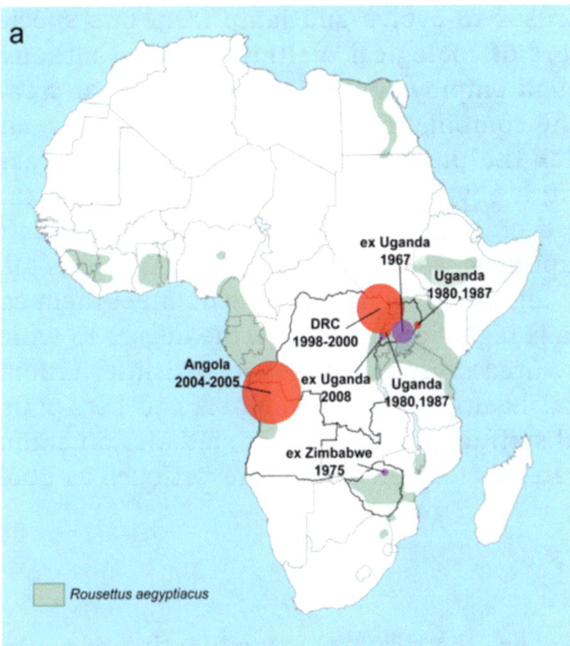

Figure 10.7. Transmission and infection of Marburg virus.

Source: By Kristina Brauburger, Adam J. Hume, Elke Mühlberger, and Judith Olejnik - https://www.mdpi.com/1999-4915/4/10/1878/htm, CC BY 3.0, https://commons.wikimedia.org/w/index.php?curid=93995910

10.3.1. Modes of Transmission In Humans

Ebola and Marburg viruses infect primarily when one is in direct contact with contaminated body fluids—not, as some may believe, through normal interaction or air. You must be in contact with fluids such as blood, saliva, sweat, vomit, feces, breast milk, urine, or sexual fluids to contract these viruses. In most resource-poor caregiving environments, where proper protective equipment is usually in short supply, this type of contact can quickly trigger an outbreak, which is why you often see clusters of family members and healthcare workers who become too intimate without proper protection. In general, knowledge of these particular routes aids in informing rapid interventions such as barrier nursing and burial practices without harm, reminding us behavior does have a direct connection to how these viruses spread (Boelaert et al., 2000). In addition to this line of contact, infections can also establish themselves by handling objects contaminated with these fluids. Common objects like clothing, bedding, and even medical devices can accumulate sufficient virus to sustain an outbreak, particularly in hospitals that do not maintain rigorous sterilization procedures. Ancient customs, such as ritual washing of the dead or shared caregiving, can introduce another variable by generating repeated contacts with contaminated fluids. In summary, public health interventions are essential in most situations to balance infection control training with a requirement to respectfully modify cultural practices, indicating how bound up the social aspect of things is in these diseases spreading (Adu-Gyamfi et al., 2019). Another striking feature of some of these viruses is that they persist even after the patient has apparently recovered. Indeed, viral RNA can be found in semen for many months, so sexual transmission can surprise everyone with a new wave of cases. This persistence makes it more difficult for those typical containment efforts that target only obviously ill individuals. Therefore, monitoring survivors and providing advice for safer sex become integral components of the overall control strategy. All of this illustrates that combat against these epidemics requires a combination of rigorous biomedical science and real community interaction, the fusion of science with daily living (Boelaert et al., 2000; Adu-Gyamfi et al., 2019).

10.3.2. Animal Reservoirs and Their Role

Sometimes it's difficult to understand how zoonotic viruses operate without taking a closer examination of where they live in nature. Ebola and Marburg, for instance, like to persist unobtrusively among fruit bats—animals that carry the viruses without falling ill themselves. These bats, congregating in huge colonies and covering large expanses of area, provide just the right conditions for the bacteria to stay around until, from time to time, they cross over onto other mammals or individuals. When people move too close—either by hunting, encroaching on bat habitats, or touching polluted surfaces—the possibility of these viruses jumping gets greater. In most instances, such natural animal hosts provide a crucial link in the chain, which is more difficult to break in epidemic-prone areas. Observe live wildlife markets. Here, in wet markets, an assortment of species ranging from bats to primates is packed into congested places where good hygiene may not always be a top consideration. In general, the cramped conditions and unsanitary environment make these markets ideal places for viruses to evolve and jump from one species to another. The animal diversity present forms a sort of biological melting pot, and although these establishments sustain local communities through employment and food, they also create agitations for viral spillovers (Naguib et al., 2021). The combination of tradition, economics, and health hazards here truly highlights just how complex the picture can be. Combatting diseases such as Ebola and Marburg is no easy accomplishment; it obviously takes a global game plan that intermeshes various types of expertise. Intersecting ecological observations with public health responses and global collaboration is usually best at capturing warning signs before outbreaks take off. Monitoring wildlife—in particular, bats—and knowing precisely how people do meet them can provide critical early warnings. But relying on the data is highly dependent on the degree to which health systems and policies integrate across nations. Greater connection between international organizations, national research institutions, and local health authorities appears to be a must. Others recommend establishing a special international staff to gather together statistics on animal reservoirs and produce more robust preparedness strategies for hemorrhagic fevers such as Ebola and Marburg (Bloom & Cadarette, 2019).

10.3.3. Factors Influencing Outbreak Spread

Infectious outbreaks do not occur out of the blue—they are the result of a combination of nature, our environment, and what we do from day to day. Ebola and Marburg, for example, primarily jump from animals to humans, with bats commonly serving as the typical carriers. When people encroach upon forested regions for agriculture, mining, or construction, they are more likely to collide with wildlife, increasing the likelihood of these spillovers. RNA viruses mutate quickly, evading our immune system and evolving to new hosts nearly sponteneously, which enhances the possibility of spreading from individual to individual. Jam-packed metropolises with uncertain healthcare only add to the problem. In general, all of this illustrates why monitoring diseases and quick action are so vital (Bloom & Cadarette, 2019; Banerjee et al., 2023). Aside from nature and the environment, how politics and money operate also determines how outbreaks get going. Flimsy health systems—those with few laboratories, insufficient medicine, and under-staffed clinics—slow down proper diagnosis and containment, allowing infections to go haywire. Political instability and wars can disrupt public health efforts, erode trust, and make people move around, and that, in turn, facilitates the virus spreading unchecked. Global travel and trade further enhance cross-border leaps, so simple containment strategies tend to fail.

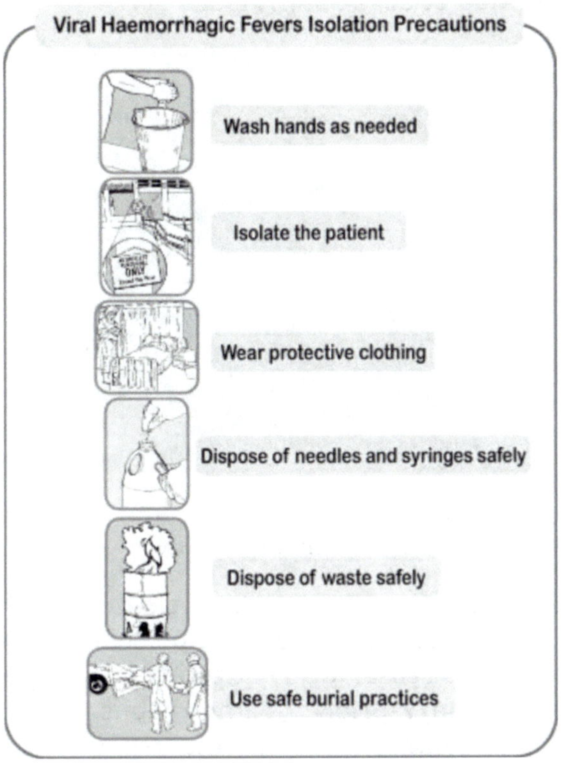

Figure 10.8. Protection

Source: By CDC - https://www.cdc.gov/vhf/abroad/pdf/african-healthcare-setting-vhf.pdf, Public Domain, https://commons.wikimedia.org/w/index.php?curid=36282107

Mixed messages, along with local tradition surrounding funerals and caregiving, add another layer of complexity to responding from communities. In most instances, halting an outbreak isn't merely a medical remedy; it's about combining effective leadership, community support, and the appropriate resources (Bloom & Cadarette, 2019; Banerjee et al., 2023). Weather patterns and changes in our environment contribute even more complexity to all this. Changes in temperature, rainfall patterns, and ecosystem changes can alter the habitat of animals that host these viruses. When forests become cleared or damaged up, the natural balance is disrupted, and humans find themselves near wild animals—ramping up the possibility of spillovers. Urban sprawl has the effect of crowding individuals into urban spaces that do not have adequate sanitation and medical care, which accelerates the rate further. All these combined, intertwined with social and economic factors, propel the way outbreaks form and develop. terms, confronting these difficulties requires scientists, community leaders, and policymakers to collaborate—with monitoring nature's changes to reframing climate policy and more intelligent urban planning (Bloom & Cadarette, 2019; Banerjee et al., 2023) (Figure 10.8).

10.4. Symptoms and Clinical Manifestations

Ebola and Marburg infections begin in a manner that resembles very much your typical fever, so they are difficult to distinguish from one another initially. Patients enter the scene with an acute onset of fever, extreme weakness, muscle aches, severe headache, and itchy sore throat. These simple flu-like symptoms, nonspecific and misleadingly easy to confuse, are often disguising the serious threat, allowing the severity of the virus to go unnoticed. As things progress, the disease tends to show its more jagged edges; for instance, disruptive gastrointestinal symptoms such as vomiting, diarrhea, and belly pain begin to manifest, which in turn cause perilous fluid depletions and jumbled-up electrolytes. The body's various systems become involved as well, as the viruses can really disrupt the blood vessel linings and trigger an extensive inflammatory response. Identification of these early hints becomes particularly critical in areas where there are no high-tech molecular tests, so physicians must rely heavily on the identification of clusters of symptoms and reconstructing any history of exposure to quickly isolate and treat infected patients, thus keeping outbreaks in check (Henrique et al., 2010). Shortly after these early warning signs, patients will present with bleeding symptoms that represent a definite turning point in the severity of the infection. You may observe small red spots (petechiae), large purple blotches (ecchymoses), mucosal bleeding, and even massive GI hemorrhage. The entire mechanism behind all of these manifestations is sort of uncontrolled: viral replication so fast, the virus evading immune system defenses, and blood clotting disturbances that in most instances veer into something akin to disseminated intravascular coagulation, usually setting the stage toward multi-organ failure. Although the word "hemorrhagic" is utilized, not all the bleeding appears the same, so the picture clinically is quite heterogeneous. Identification of these bleeding patterns serves as an indicator that the disease is progressing, and typically it suggests a poorer prognosis. Supportive treatment, particularly judicious fluid replacement and the control of clotting issues—remains a vital requirement for increasing survival in patients (Sprecher et al., 2008). Solving these diagnostic conundrums with Ebola and Marburg challenges us to refine case definitions by combining what we observe in patients with their likelihood of having been exposed. Experiments show that combining prominent symptoms, such as persistent muscle or joint pain—on top of any evidence of bleeding and exposure contact can quite effectively hone clinical diagnosis accuracy, while maintaining an acceptable level between false positives and false negatives. This approach proves to be almost indispensable in outbreak areas, especially in far-flung regions where procedures such as PCR are not always present. Improved on-the-spot reporting and real-time monitoring of symptoms may prove the key to better triaging of cases, getting those at greatest risk quarantined and treated early before the situation gets even worse. In numerous ways, these adjustments of symptom-based guidelines represent an important measure to control outbreaks and enhance the recovery prospects of areas severely affected by such lethal viruses (Henrique et al., 2010) (Figure 10.9).

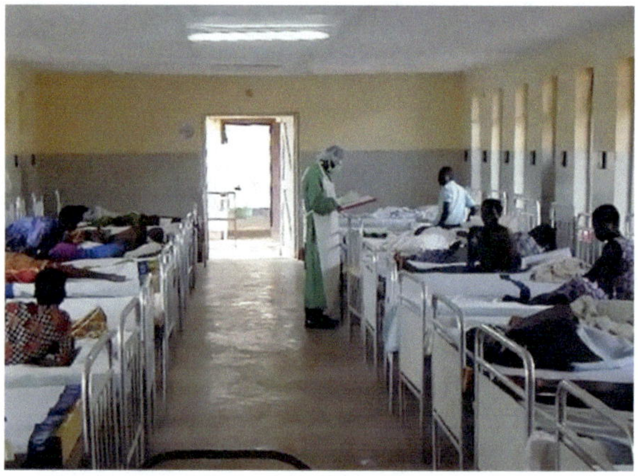

Figure 10.9. Symptoms and clinical manifestations of Marburg virus.

Source: By Daniel Bausch, Division of Viral and Rickettsial Diseases, National Center for Infectious Diseases, CDC - https://www.cdc.gov/globalidplan/7-priority_1.htm, Public Domain, https://commons.wikimedia.org/w/index.php?curid=2083669

10.4.1. Common Symptoms of Ebola Virus Disease

Ebola virus disease doesn't always come in loudly at the beginning. It can begin with a combination of symptoms that feel very much like other everyday fevers—imagine malaria or even typhoid—so it can become very difficult to identify at first. Individuals develop a sudden-onset high fever, thumping headache, painful muscles, and debilitating fatigue. These flu-like sensations persist for days, a time when the virus is actively reproducing yet hasn't yet exhibited the telltale symptoms. Subsequently, usually rather rapidly, gastrointestinal distress sets in—nausea, diarrhea, and cramps—adding to which can result in rapid dehydration and complex electrolyte imbalance. In most instances, this unforeseen spread of symptoms translates into the fact that the health workers, particularly where Ebola persists, have to be particularly vigilant so that they may be able to separate the patients and initiate supportive care in good time. Failure to pick these hints at an early stage is easily likely to lead to a delayed diagnosis and an increased possibility of spreading the infection (Sohan et al., 2022). As the disease progresses, things really only get worse. In general, advanced stages of Ebola can play havoc with the entire body, appearing as bleeding gums, nose bleeding, or even as little red dots on the skin—and sometimes, even patients experience severe internal bleeding as well. This bleeding does not occur in all cases, but if it does, it indicates that the virus is wreaking havoc , destroying the lining of blood vessels and disrupting the body's normal clotting mechanism, which can result in a severe condition called disseminated intravascular coagulation. Approximately at the same time, indicators of liver and kidney difficulties may appear; patients may develop jaundice, or a yellow color of their skin, as well as decreased urine production or abnormal lab test results, thereby complicating already complicated circumstances even further. Also possible are the instances when the patient becomes disoriented, upset, or, indeed, gets seizures—pretty obvious indications of the brain being involved. For the majority, how extreme these issues become is determined by the quantity of virus that is present and to what extent the body's immune response is off-kilter, so that if extreme support treatment isn't begun immediately, the prognosis can be extremely poor (Sohan et al., 2022). On a broader perspective, the unbelievably diverse symptoms of Ebola truly emphasize how difficult it is to treat clinically. It's not rare for patients to take a fast decline—fairly easily falling into multi-organ failure and shock, both of which are significant contributors to the high mortality rates. Recovery isn't impossible, however; early detection of the disease and initiating intensive care interventions such as meticulous fluid and electrolyte control can bring marked improvement. Early symptoms of Ebola tend to be indistinguishable from other diseases endemic in the region, and therefore physicians must rely on good diagnostic tests and improved surveillance methods. On top of that, the reality that Ebola has a zoonotic origin—entwined with other animal-borne viruses—increases the complexity, emphasizing collective action in keeping tabs on viruses and prepping for outbreaks. In the majority of instances, awareness and monitoring of these common early signs are critical to reducing mortality rates and arresting transmission in humans.

10.4.2. Common Symptoms of Marburg Virus Disease

Marburg virus disease will typically start its unobtrusive phase for anywhere from 2 to 21 days – a time when nothing feels remotely amiss. Then, almost inexplicably, patients become unwell, and those initial symptoms can truly masquerade as other relatively ordinary diseases such as malaria or typhoid. Abruptly, a fever rages on alongside throbbing headaches, chills, and sore muscles that land with a blow, as though the virus insists on announcing itself. Frequently, the disturbance isn't merely concerning fever; gastric issues like vomiting, nausea, and diarrhea enter the battleground, rapidly setting off dehydration and disrupting the equilibrium of the body. In areas where such fevers are prevalent, such erratic symptoms make it challenging for physicians to determine if they are fighting Marburg or not – a matter where special caution and quick diagnostic instincts are needed (Sohan et al., 2022). Paying attention to these initial warning signs, no matter how minor is usually essential since the disease can quickly worsen and be fatal. As the disease intensifies, it usually takes a much more ominous turn. Bleeding may start in an almost alarming fashion , from mucous membranes, pores, and even far down in the gastrointestinal tract. This bleeding, more than evident in demonstrating that the virus is ravaging the body's blood clotting and vessel integrity, is typically accompanied by a tidal wave of other issues. In most instances, organs such as the liver and kidneys begin to fail, and electrolyte disturbances, shock, and acid imbalances arise, further complicating the whole scenario. Occasionally, the infection invades the central nervous system, causing seizures, episodes of confusion, or, at worst, a coma (Sohan et al., 2022). Under these desperate circumstances, in which every second counts, quick, supportive therapy – and sometimes even experimental care – are absolutely essential. When viewing Marburg within a comparison with other hemorrhagic fevers, including Ebola, one can see many similarities of resonance. Both spread primarily through contact with contaminated body fluids and unleash disease rapidly, with usually rapid deterioration in critical cases. But Marburg has occasionally a mind of its own, as its severity and course can differ greatly depending on host-related factors and the specific strain. In the majority of outbreaks, mortality rates have varied extensively, ranging from approximately 27% to as much as 90% (Sohan et al., 2022), depending on local healthcare and topography. Generally speaking, these shared and distinct features highlight why putting together a diagnosis can be so tricky and why ongoing research into the way these viruses operate is so desperately needed. To summarize, the threat that Marburg poses pushes us to combine quick symptom recognition with rapid public health responses, even as we continue learning more about its complex nature (Figure 10.10).

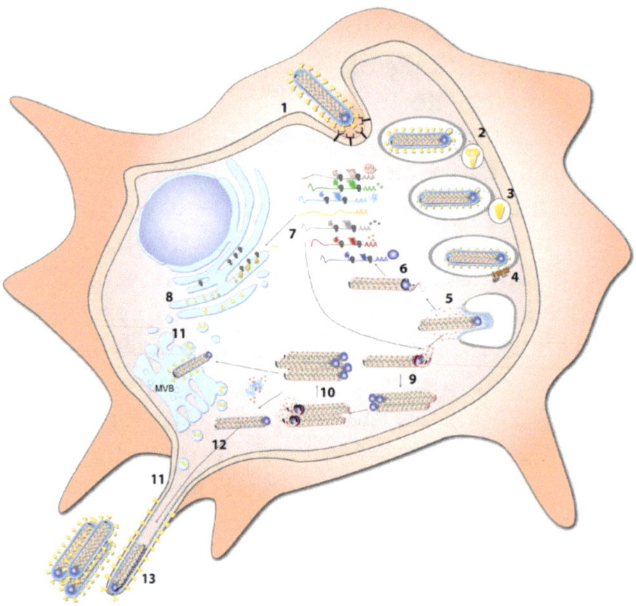

Figure 10.10. Marburg virus symptoms.

Source: By Kristina Brauburger, Adam J. Hume, Elke Mühlberger, and Judith Olejnik - https://www.mdpi.com/1999-4915/4/10/1878/htm, CC BY 3.0, https://commons.wikimedia.org/w/index.php?curid=93995911

10.4.3. Differences in Clinical Presentation

Ebola and Marburg viruses are from the same filovirus family and cause a bad hemorrhagic fever, but they don't act identically. In both instances, the diseases start with a bunch of non-specific symptoms—fever, fatigue, muscle pain, and headache—so it is difficult to distinguish between them initially. With Ebola, however, the disease has a tendency to meander into prominent gastrointestinal symptoms such as episodes of vomiting, diarrhea, and abdominal pain; these uniqueness often result in dehydration and chaos in electrolyte balance. Marburg, on the other hand, tends to play its cards with abrupt, fulminant systemic signs and signs of bleeding—i.e., petechiae or internal bleeding that is not visible—emerging more acutely. Case-fatality rates can fluctuate depending on the outbreak and viral strain, at times approaching 90% (Sprecher et al., 2008); in most cases, the nuance differences during onset mean the distinction is a minefield during early diagnosis, forcing clinicians to create outbreak responses as tailored as possible. The timing and intensity with which bleeding occurs is really what truly separates these viruses. By and large, the courses of Ebola infection go in a sort of step-by-step fashion: an early feverish phase, a stage in which the gut comes into the act, further progressing to a late hemorrhagic stage that tends to be accompanied by multi-organ complications. On the other hand, Marburg's bleeding can strike earlier and more abruptly—there tends to be severe bleeding from mucosal surfaces and from the intestines straight away, which tends to propel patients into shock sooner. Practitioners pay attention, since early bleeding in Marburg patients evidently does hasten shock and subsequently, tragically, mortality. Laboratory reports support these clinical anecdotes; Ebola survivors may have a slow convalescence with persisting symptoms, while Marburg infections sometimes terminate much more precipitously and lethally. The reasons underlying these discrepancies remain under investigation and are presumably associated with differences in how each virus infects tissues and battles the host immune response (Sprecher et al., 2008). How the infections spread also appears to be tinged with their clinical panache. Both viruses are likely to present high titers in the blood and blood-contaminated fluids when active, so these fluids become ideal vectors for infection. Interestingly, Ebola has been shown to last longer in other bodily fluids, such as semen, so that even after recovery seems complete there may exist a kind of residual risk for sexual transmission. By contrast, Marburg's history in this respect isn't so well described—data are still fairly limited. When researchers test for viral RNA by RT-PCR in a variety of fluids both during the acute disease and subsequently, it shows how complex infection control can get; importantly, a positive RT-PCR doesn't necessarily imply that the virus is still infective. This subtlety—with the understanding that not all positive results indicate transmission risk—does represent a genuine challenge to outbreak control, particularly in resource-constrained environments where such viruses tend to recur.

10.5. Diagnosis and Treatment

Ebola and Marburg disease infections need to be detected early to reduce their severe effects. Individuals may first observe symptoms such as a high fever, severe feeling of ill health, and even bleeding disorders, particularly in areas where previous outbreaks have been observed. Most of the time, physicians begin by believing such symptoms, then they resort to laboratory tests. Techniques like RT-PCR rapidly detect viral RNA when the symptoms have started, whereas tests that test for antibodies provide additional validation but are more practical later or for large-scale surveys. Unfortunately, most outbreak regions still do not have easy access to such tests due to limited infrastructure and stringent biosafety requirements. In the meantime, continued studies on how the virus exists naturally and only multiplies further reinforces the necessity to have quicker and more precise diagnosis to isolate and treat patients rapidly (Boelaert et al., 2000). As for treatment, it has been largely focused on supportive care—essentially maintaining proper fluids, electrolyte balance, and managing symptoms to prevent other complications from arising. In recent years, however, biomedical research has introduced some experimental therapies and even vaccines that have been promising, at least in the laboratory.

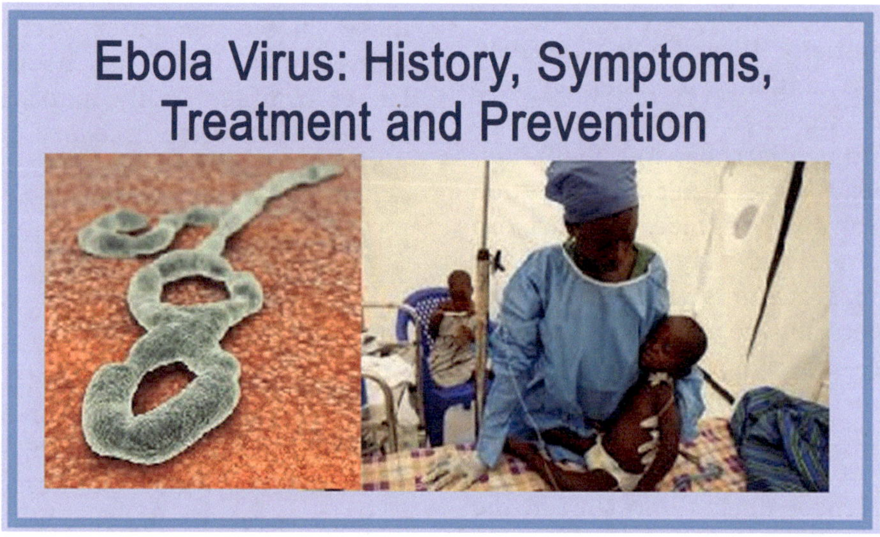

Figure 10.11. Ebola virus: History, cause, symptoms, prevention, and treatment.

Source: Jagran Josh. (n.d.). *What is Ebola Virus?.*

For example, treatments such as monoclonal antibodies and specific antivirals have proven successful in animal tests by attacking crucial viral components, which may reduce the viral load and increase chances of survival. Nevertheless, turning these research successes into therapies that work for people consistently is far from easy. Outbreaks are one-off events, and other barriers such as ethical issues and stringent regulations during epidemics make it even more challenging to conduct good-quality clinical trials (Sprecher et al., 2008). Nonetheless, scientists persist in attempting to weave these breakthroughs into outbreak responses and hoping to do better for patients. In most of Africa, socio-political and economic issues only make it harder to effectively treat and diagnose these infections. More often than not, the lack of health infrastructure, insufficient numbers of trained personnel, and distance to remote locations hinder response time. Cultural and even stigmatization-related delay also occurs in seeking care and inadvertently propels the transmission of the disease. Even promising vaccines face challenges of administration and distribution in poor-resource environments, so firm international support and astute public health planning are necessary. For future outbreak response, establishing rapid diagnostic laboratories, increasing surveillance, and engaging communities more actively are all key measures. Aligning research with these public health priorities should assist in creating more affordable diagnostic tools and scalable treatments that ultimately stem the frequently-deadly impact of Ebola and Marburg outbreaks (Boelaert et al., 2000; Sprecher et al., 2008) (Figure 10.11).

10.5.1. Diagnostic Methods for Ebola

Treating viral hemorrhagic fevers such as Ebola boils down to an early and accurate diagnosis, despite the symptoms being compounded with other diseases. Year by year, Ebola tests have moved from strict to a combination of molecular tests, which identify the RNA of the virus, and serological tests that detect the antibodies of the body. Real-time reverse transcription PCR, for instance, remains widely regarded as the gold standard for contracting the virus in its initial, active stage. However, these tests require quality facilities and experienced people, something that is not always feasible in regions that suffer from outbreaks. Serological tests—intended to indicate previous exposure through detecting antibodies—provide valuable evidence on immune response but falters in the early stage. Most often, both approaches to work together is what proves to be essential to monitoring and capping outbreaks, particularly in separating Ebola from other viruses that may be in the neighborhood. Recently, the landscape has shifted as newer diagnostic platforms rely on machine learning and genomic analyses to increase speed and accuracy. Deep learning models, for example, have been used with viral genomic data and can now differentiate Ebola from SARS-CoV-2, SARS, and MERS viruses—, one Gated Recurrent Unit-based model even achieving more than 98% accuracy in identifying Ebola sequences (Devaraj & Marianthiran, 2025). This development is overall promising, and it suggests the potential to develop portable, field-deployable tools that can analyze genomic data in real-time. By leveraging high-throughput sequencing and contemporary bioinformatics, health teams may one day be able to identify new variants in real-time and customize treatments for improved patient outcomes. There's an interesting twist even beyond human testing. Some research has focused on household animals such as dogs, sheep, and goats to determine if they could potentially be involved in the transmission of Ebola. Serological analysis in these animals has revealed low but detectable levels of antibodies to both Ebola and Marburg viruses, indicating that they may be naturally infected—, no active viral RNA being detected (Mebaley et al., 2025). Such results indicate that such animals can act as early indicators of virus circulation in regions where the disease is prevalent. It is likely that their infection results from exposure to bat guano or environments, and recognizing these routes may enable a more precise surveillance and even arrest zoonotic spillovers. Generally, the integration of molecular, serological, and even ecological information yields a wider, more resilient diagnosis and outbreak readiness strategy.

10.5.2. Diagnostic Methods for Marburg

It's not as easy to identify Marburg virus infections as one wishes. Its symptoms closely resemble those of other bleeding fevers, so rapid, accurate testing is an imperative. Rapid lab tests aid not only in the treatment of patients but also trigger public health measures to curb outbreaks. Today, technologies such as RT-PCR occupy the central place in the diagnosis of Marburg—it identifies its RNA with the appropriate sensitivity and specificity reliably. These instruments also assist in unscrambling Marburg from other related pathogens, which is rather important when symptoms overlap. Additionally, new multiplex assays—capable of testing for viruses such as both Ebola and Marburg simultaneously, increase test speed during mixed-outbreak situations (Yao et al., 2021). This approach, overall, addresses the cumbersome problem of differential diagnosis in regions where such diseases endure while equipping decision-makers with the information they require in real-time. In addition to RT-PCR, antigen detection assays are also important in the formative picture, frequently providing faster results when infections strike hard and quickly. Immunoassays targeted at viral proteins demonstrate a handy alternative in practice, particularly where sophisticated lab facilities aren't always an option. These also employ serological assays such as ELISA to detect antibodies to the Marburg virus—but such assays tend to come into their own later in infection or when collecting information for epidemiological surveys. Nonetheless, with the onset, sensitivity can plummet, so combining various approaches most of the time is best for an improved call. Incorporating these diverse test strategies into ongoing surveillance systems is a critical component of our global health security, as threats of disease become increasingly complex within our connected world (Bloom & Cadarette, 2019; Banerjee et al., 2023). Overall, having this sort of general-purpose diagnostic arsenal is the foundation of fighting and mitigating outbreak effects. Despite these advances, difficulties persist. Rolling out trustworthy Marburg diagnostics globally, particularly in resource-constrained areas where outbreaks disproportionately occur—is a challenging problem. Creating low-cost, high-throughput testing platforms that do not compromise specificity or sensitivity is essential to increasing overall capacity. Multiplex microarray technologies also present some hopeful solutions here; by testing a number of hemorrhagic fever viruses at once, they optimize resources and accelerate pathogen identification (Yao et al., 2021). Apart from that, enhancing global health networks so that testing attempts could be coordinated and important epidemiological information shared is downright imperative for timely warnings and rapid responses (Bloom & Cadarette, 2019; Banerjee et al., 2023). Ongoing research investments, improved infrastructure, and focused training will eventually enhance our preparedness to counter Marburg outbreaks—and maybe reduce both disease and mortality associated with this highly lethal virus (Figure 10.12).

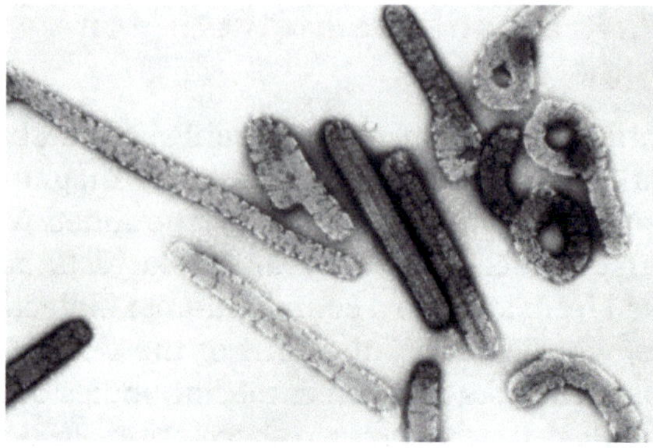

Figure 10.12. Diagnostic methods for Marburg.

Source: By Photo Credit:Content Providers(s): CDC/ Dr. Erskine Palmer, Russell Regnery, Ph.D. - This media comes from the Centers for Disease Control and Prevention's Public Health Image Library (PHIL), with identification number #275.Note: Not all PHIL images are public domain; be sure to check copyright status and credit authors and content providers. | Deutsch | English | македонски | slovenščina | +/−, Public Domain, https://commons.wikimedia.org/w/index.php?curid=157423

10.5.3. Current Treatment Options and Challenges

Keeping Ebola and Marburg virus patients alive is a serious challenge, primarily because these diseases strike severely and there is no one cure that is licensed for all. Physicians will often have to settle for mere care, fluid administration, electrolyte correction, and treatment of secondary infections—to sustain a patient. Even with much research, there isn't a single drug that people universally accept for Ebola; although some experimental drugs such as monoclonal antibodies and antivirals have had some success in initial trials and small-scale clinical environments, their availability and outcomes can greatly differ based on the outbreak and local preparedness (Adu-Gyamfi et al., 2019). Fast testing and the segregation of patients usually work in most situations, but all depends on how the local health infrastructure is. The quest for cures is made even more complex by how these viruses induce massive bleeding and systemic inflammation that usually goes horribly awry. Scientists are not only experimenting with antiviral medications, they're also exploring means of dampening down the lethal immune overresponses, colloquially referred to as a cytokine storm, that can cause vascular complications. There's still work to verify if older, established medicines slow the virus or make the immune system more responsive, and combinations of treatments, which may hit various aspects of the disease simultaneously, are getting attention. For the most part, these changing strategies emphasize the need for thoroughly planned clinical tests to double-check that any novel strategy is safe and effective (Blondiaux et al., 2015). Meanwhile, public health has significant challenges when there's an outbreak. Rapid detection and isolation of cases are crucial, but most affected areas have limited resources, delaying proper diagnosis and quarantine—, that allows the disease to spread to close contacts. This truly highlights the significance of coordinated international aid to enhance healthcare facilities, laboratories, and community interventions. Even if a region is officially declared to be Ebola-free, no guarantee exists that the threat has vanished forever, so remaining vigilant becomes imperative. In short, combined medical therapies with robust public health interventions are key to keeping these lethal infections at bay (Adu-Gyamfi et al., 2019).

10.6. Prevention and Control Measures

Halting Ebola and Marburg viruses involves combating the issue from numerous directions. It begins with early detection of cases, quarantining patients when necessary, and informing individuals what to look for. Since infection spreads primarily by direct contact with a person's body fluids, medical staff members must use the proper PPE to help reduce hospital transmissions. Separating patients and controlling materials such as needles and other sharps (which may be infected) are important aspects of this procedure. Public health outreach—advertising that reaches vulnerable populations—also aids through educating individuals about how the viruses are transmitted and what symptoms to report; this has been found to result in quicker reporting and fewer secondary infections. Because early symptoms can mimic those of far more prevalent diseases, strong surveillance combined with differential diagnosis is required to quickly detect cases and prevent them from developing into larger outbreaks. In the majority of instances, teams composed of infectious disease specialists, hospital professionals, and public health professionals collaborate to disrupt chains of transmission before things escalate into full epidemics (Sohan et al., 2022). Further there is the problem of spillover events—those instances when the virus leaps from its natural hosts in animals to humans. That problem isn't addressed by merely responding to an outbreak; it requires proactive, global action. Large initiatives like the Global Virome Project work to chart undiscovered viruses with zoonotic potential, providing early warnings that aid prevention. Now, although these massive scientific enterprises require massive investment and sometimes controversy regarding their utility, their capacity to reduce unforeseen epidemic threats simply cannot be discounted. A greater appreciation of viral ecosystems and host–virus interactions informs surveillance and vaccine programs at the human–animal interface from the very start. It is important to strengthen relations between international research centers and policymakers to implement these innovative measures that transcend national boundaries in addressing the filovirus threat (Jonas et al., 2019). In addition to being vigilant and ready, continuing with new treatments and vaccines is an important aspect of containing Ebola and Marburg outbreaks. Though no antiviral or vaccines have been officially sanctioned for the Marburg virus so far, there are clinical trials in progress using drugs such as Galidesivir and Remdesivir that have positive indications. The rapid, global coordination which helped deploy Ebola vaccines successfully presents a sort of model for accelerating access to vaccines against such viruses. In addition, inclusion of treatment regimens emphasizing supportive care, i.e., fluid replacement and symptom management, has been found to enhance chances for survival. On the community level, interventions such as quarantining contacts, implementation of safe burial practices, and limiting exposure to possible reservoir species are essential. Overall, consistent funding and research emphasis are essential to translating scientific progress into practical solutions, eventually reducing the disease and mortality due to these lethal hemorrhagic fevers (Sohan et al., 2022) (Figure 10.13).

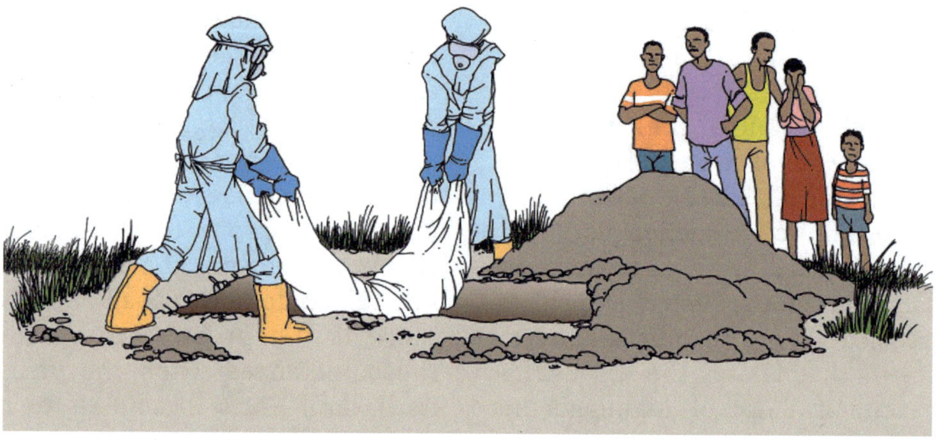

Figure 10.13. Infection prevention and control measures for Marburg virus disease.

Source: By CDC Global - Ebola illustration: safe burial, CC BY 2.0, https://commons.wikimedia.org/w/index.php?curid=66833791

10.6.1. Vaccination Efforts and Developments

Deadly viruses such as Ebola and Marburg have demonstrated, yet again, the destructive potential of hemorrhagic fevers. These deadly pathogens, infamous for their high mortality rates and rapid intensity, particularly in areas such as Sub-Saharan Africa—put our healthcare systems in some very tight spots. Recent outbreaks have placed vaccine development in overdrive, sending scientists to experiment with less orthodox techniques such as recombinant viral vectors. Specifically, research on Marburg virus vaccines has accelerated significantly, with candidates such as recombinant vesicular stomatitis virus (VSV)-based vaccines, as well as variants such as Ad26.Filo and ChAd3-MARV, being promising in initial human and preclinical trials. Although these developments are encouraging, they also highlight the complex nature of fighting such deadly diseases, requiring rigorous clinical assessments and flexible approaches in the course of outbreaks (Akhtar et al., 2024). It's not simply a matter of brilliant lab work to find a trusty vaccine. It's a complicated combination of challenges involving logistical glitches, strict regulatory guidelines, and the unpredictability of how epidemics play out. Recently, scientists have been pushing for epidemic control models that, in many instances, factor in these real-world complications by incorporating elements of risk and resilience.

It's not just the science behind the vaccines that counts; the day-to-day social and infrastructure support surrounding them counts even more. The wider, more comprehensive strategy is what is necessary to close the gap between having a vaccine on offer and seeing its actual-effectiveness in the field, particularly in areas where resources are limited and outbreaks peak hardest (Brown et al., 2017). Even with the big strides we've seen, the march toward a fully approved Marburg virus vaccine remains slow. The challenge comes from multiple fronts—a jumble of viral genetics, the unpredictable way our immune systems respond, and the sheer chaos of outbreaks, all muddling the production and distribution processes. However, groundbreaking concepts such as viral vector vaccines, DNA plasmid forms, and even virus-like particles are moving steadily through stages of clinical trials, providing a glimmer of hope. Scientists are also hard at work administering these vaccines in non-human primates and human populations, which does a great deal to shore up the argument for forthcoming approval. Agaín, combining these scientific leaps with practical outbreak control measures, albeit sometimes unevenly implemented, might reduce significantly the number of lives lost to these lethal infections, being an important step toward greater global health security (Akhtar et al., 2024).

10.6.2. Public Health Strategies for Outbreak Control

When Ebola or Marburg makes an appearance, rapid detection and isolation of the infected become the initial defense. These diseases, lethal and infectious in most instances, leave public health workers with no choice but to rely on vigilant, on-the-ground surveillance and accelerated testing. In most cases, monitoring and tracking anyone who is exposed, essentially following even the slightest indication of contact—allows us to intervene quickly when symptoms emerge. Community announcements, in which the people listen clearly to how the virus is transmitted and what practices keep it at bay, also enter the picture; even long-standing customs such as burial rites, which inadvertently assist the virus in its spread from time to time, are considered tenderly through culturally attuned guidance. These interactions create trust and push individuals towards collaboration; ultimately, combining a little surveillance, careful handling, and community outreach demonstrates that we need all these components working together to address outbreaks (Amiar et al., 2021). Employing personal protective equipment (PPE) along with precisely the type of rigorous infection prevention and control measures in hospitals is, quite simply, not negotiable. Frontline staff receive practical instruction on how to don and doff PPE correctly, and adhering to good hygiene practices reduces the likelihood of picking up something in the workplace. It's also helpful when special isolation units, rooms specially equipped to deal with highly contagious conditions, are available to treat patients in a contained environment, thus reducing the risk of spreading the rest of the facility. Add to that safe and respectful burial practices that minimize direct contact with cadavers, and you have a formula for cutting further transmission among community members. On top of that, maintaining health systems strong so they can keep daily services going even during a crisis enhances overall resilience. Overall, these combined measures are central to preventing hospital-based, or nosocomial, transmission of Ebola and Marburg (Amiar et al., 2021). Beyond the containment task at hand, long-term measures such as immunization and antiviral therapy take center stage. Vaccines against Ebola, for example, have reduced cases and saved lives, while efforts on Marburg vaccines continue to be a top priority. Meanwhile, experimental medications—whether antivirals that inhibit the virus from reproducing or immunostimulants that enhance the immune system of the body—provide encouraging assistance, albeit still requiring ample clinical evidence before they can be widely relied upon. In most instances, connecting local outbreak responses with an international network as a whole brings additional resources, exchanges practical expertise, and forms a concerted effort in monitoring the situation. Continuing investment in research ensures that new ideas continue to flow for improved diagnostics, vaccines, and treatments. Overall, this combination of prompt prevention, judicious treatment, and international cooperation is key to containing filovirus outbreaks and limiting their overall impact on public health (Amiar et al., 2021) (Figure 10.14).

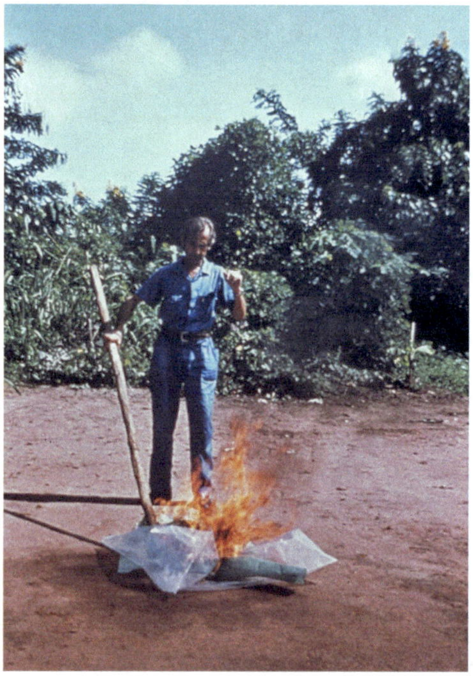

Figure 10.14. Public health strategies for outbreak control for Ebola and Marburg viruses.

Source: By CDC/ Dr. Lyle Conrad - This media comes from the Centers for Disease Control and Prevention's Public Health Image Library (PHIL), with identification number #7197.Note: Not all PHIL images are public domain; be sure to check copyright status and credit authors and content providers.| Deutsch | English | македонски | *slovenščina* | +/−, Public Domain, https://commons.wikimedia.org/w/index.php?curid=12841937

10.6.3. Role of International Organizations in Prevention

Global organizations are key movers in halting outbreaks such as Ebola and Marburg. They bring together expertise in epidemiology, virology, and public health to develop guidelines that can be readily modified when outbreaks surface. For instance, these organizations frequently establish treatment protocols and prevention measures that adhere to a similar format but remain abreast of new studies. This type of collaboration enhances a country's capacity to manage new threats as well as simplifies it to pass along information and resources, which are integral to maintaining containment. Overall, by connecting holes in local health and surveillance networks, these institutions strengthen global health security and prevent widespread spread. Simultaneously, global organizations also contribute by providing both funds and technical assistance (yes, technical assistance) to nations most affected by such diseases. These funds are vital in terms of training local healthcare professionals, establishing diagnostic laboratories, and deploying rapid response teams in outbreak areas. They even carry out public awareness campaigns which, in the majority of instances, make communities more aware of the risks of transmission and learn basic mechanisms to prevent it. Multiplication of multidisciplinary teams is possible, enabling real-time monitoring and modeling of the way transmission takes place, thus informing flexible public health interventions. Through the establishment of connections between governments, NGOs, and local actors, these institutions strengthen prevention programs and establish more robust health systems when crises occur. In the case of addressing viral hemorrhagic fevers like Ebola and Marburg, global organizations also play a significant role in research coordination and advocacy for policy. They collaborate with universities, drug companies, and governments to accelerate vaccine development and deployment of antiviral therapies. In most instances, they promote wider access to clinical trials to ensure novel treatments are adequately tested and timely integrated into clinical guidelines. In addition, these organizations advocate for the establishment of strong surveillance systems that track virus transmission and measure the effectiveness of public health interventions. Due to the dynamic nature of infectious diseases, it's usually a requirement to constantly be reassessing prevention measures – something well captured by adaptive modeling and synthesis approaches applied in other epidemics (Bhimraj et al., 2020; Tang et al., 2020). Briefly, these agencies do more than merely coordinate; they're actual innovators in the continued fight against Ebola and Marburg.

CLOSER LOOK

VIRAL STRUCTURE AND MECHANISMS OF HEMORRHAGIC FEVER

Viral hemorrhagic fevers (VHFs) are a group of severe illnesses caused by families of enveloped RNA viruses, including Arenaviridae (Lassa fever), Filoviridae (Ebola, Marburg), Bunyaviridae (Crimean-Congo hemorrhagic fever), and Flaviviridae (dengue, yellow fever). Despite their diversity, these viruses share structural and pathogenic features that lead to life-threatening disease.

Structurally, VHFs are caused by enveloped viruses with single-stranded RNA genomes. Their lipid envelopes, studded with glycoproteins, facilitate entry into host cells via receptor-mediated endocytosis. Once inside, the viral RNA is replicated and translated using host cell machinery, producing new virions that spread systemically. The simplicity of their structure, combined with rapid replication, allows these viruses to overwhelm host defenses quickly.

The mechanisms of pathogenesis in VHFs involve a combination of immune evasion, dysregulated host responses, and vascular damage. Many hemorrhagic fever viruses suppress the innate immune system by blocking interferon signaling, giving them time to replicate unchecked. As infection progresses, the immune system often responds with a cytokine storm, releasing excessive inflammatory mediators that increase vascular permeability.

This immune-mediated vascular leakage, along with direct viral damage to endothelial cells, leads to hemorrhagic symptoms such as bleeding, shock, and multi-organ failure. In dengue fever, for example, antibody-dependent enhancement can worsen secondary infections, amplifying disease severity. In Ebola, massive lymphocyte apoptosis and coagulation abnormalities further disrupt immune regulation and vascular integrity.

Transmission varies: some VHFs are spread by arthropod vectors (mosquitoes or ticks), while others involve zoonotic spillover from rodents or primates. Human-to-human transmission, especially via body fluids, is a key factor in filovirus outbreaks.

The structure of hemorrhagic fever viruses—simple yet effective—combined with their ability to hijack host immunity, explains their devastating clinical outcomes. Understanding these mechanisms is essential for developing antivirals, vaccines, and effective outbreak control strategies.

Summary

Ebola and Marburg viruses present some extremely challenging problems that remind us that we still have a long way to go in terms of new treatments and controlling outbreaks. These diseases strike hard, with extremely high mortality rates and outbreaks that appear to erupt seemingly out of nowhere, despite much effort devoted to combating them. Early studies, like the ones testing TKM-130803, brought to light both the promise and the limits of experimental treatments in such chaotic times. Researchers saw that while these drugs can climb to plasma levels way above what we'd hoped for, the moment they're given—and just how severe the infection is—can greatly change a patient's outcome. What this usually implies is that carrying a good antiviral is not sufficient; you must also get the timing right and provide added care, which is a nod to a more holistic approach to future treatment protocols (Bhimraj et al., 2020). This type of observation is, overall, important for guiding both present and future studies towards firmer, evidence-based practices. In addition to trialing new medicines, establishing quick, firm guidelines for outbreaks such as Ebola and Marburg is an important aspect of patient care. Consider, for instance, how the Infectious Diseases Society of America handled COVID-19—by soliciting opinion from experts in various fields while closely monitoring developing data. That methodology not only informed treatment decisions but also advocated more aggressively for greater patient involvement in clinical trials, so we could collect solid evidence on both safety and efficacy. That approach is a turn away from the do-nothing, use-everything policy of the past, moving toward evidence-based interventions. Because outbreaks remain a serious worldwide concern, such an adaptable, data-driven approach appears to be a wise choice for controlling viruses such as Ebola and Marburg (Bhimraj et al., 2020). Reviewing past Ebola outbreaks, it's obvious that the mixture of clinical research with trust from the community and ethical approaches is more than a wise suggestion—it's essential. Even when it got ugly with logistics or difficult ethical choices, multi-center trials were able to demonstrate that it is possible to test new treatments during an epidemic. Trust from local communities, and culturally appropriate strategies in surveillance and in patient care, were essential both in containing the virus and gathering data. And in addition, breakthroughs on how drugs travel through the body—along with siRNA therapies—are pushing us in the direction of treatments that are as individualized to the severity of the disease as humanly possible. And all of these takeaways indicate that combining scientific ingenuity with community-focused, ethical practices can increase survival rates, curtail spread, and accelerate the creation of new therapies. Finally, the future for combating Ebola and Marburg is integrating cutting-edge science with a sincere, community-focused perspective (Baseler, 2020).

Researchers have discovered new insights into how Ebola virus disease behaves using techniques such as multiplex fluorescent immunohistochemistry and *in situ* hybridization. When these are combined with whole slide imaging and some quantitative image analysis, they bring out subtleties in both the early and late stages that older, more conventional techniques may just not see. One fascinating note is that, in the majority of instances, sinusoidal macrophages within the lung are among the initial cells to react—they will secrete a proinflammatory cytokine called interleukin-6. The interferon-stimulated gene-15, however, appears in adjacent, noninfected cells instead of in those overtly invaded by the virus, suggesting a fine balance between viral replication and how the body initiates its immune response. These are observations regarding where and when the virus comes into contact with host cells that provide us with informative benchmarks for tracing the course of the disease and for informing measures to combat EBOV (Greenberg et al., 2020). While Ebola and similar viruses such as Marburg are infamous due to their very high mortality rates, completely effective treatments are yet far from finished. The new green light given for such vaccines as Merck's Ervebo is an impressive advance in prevention, but all therapeutic interventions aside from remdesivir remain on the experimental spectrum. In large measure, all of the investigation tends to reference the critical engagement of the liver—replication of viruses apparently thrives among liver macrophages, while clotting deficits related to too much production of tissue factor both among monocytes and macrophages only reinforce the sheerly systemic nature of Ebola. Nonhuman primate research, even with some discrepancies in model design, continues to be critical since they replicate human disease sufficiently well to permit extensive testing of treatments and investigation into the underlying disease mechanisms (Greenberg et al., 2020). Additionally, there's an increased interest in filoviruses' molecular world using investigations of properties such as G-quadruplexes (G4s) within their genomes. These unusual, non-canonical nucleic acid conformations, which exist in regions that assist with the regulation of the virus, are now gaining interest in Ebola and other similar pathogen research. The evidence indicates that G4s may impact essential viral operations such as replication and latency, thereby making them potentially appealing antiviral drug targets. In some instances, ligands that bind specifically to these G4s can already exhibit significant antiviral efficacy, apparently by interfering with both the genomic and transcriptomic activities of the virus. Further research into the physical and structural properties of such G4-binding molecules could be critical in refining their utility, providing a new approach to combating infections such as Ebola and Marburg.

References

1. Adu-Gyamfi, S. (2019). Ebola haemorrhagic fever in Africa: A necessary highlight. *International Journal of Public Health Science (IJPHS), 8*(1), 1–13. https://core.ac.uk/download/480549437.pdf (accessed on 7 May 2025).
2. Agnarsson, I., Allison, A. B., Almeida, G. M. F., Amman, B. R., Baker, M. L., Biesold, S. E., et al. (2015). Filovirus receptor NPC1 contributes to species-specific patterns of ebolavirus susceptibility in bats. *eLife, 4*, e11785. https://core.ac.uk/download/42368033.pdf (accessed on 7 May 2025).
3. Akhtar, A., Zaheer, A., & Hussain, D. Z. (2024). Advancements in Marburg virus vaccine development: Unravelling recent findings. A narrative review. *Student's Journal of Health Research Africa, 5*(3), 119. https://core.ac.uk/download/618348852.pdf (accessed on 7 May 2025).
4. Alagawany, M., Chakraborty, S., Chandran, D., Dhama, K., et al. (2022). Marburg virus disease: A mini-review. *Journal of Experimental Biology and Agricultural Sciences, 10*(4), 689–696. https://core.ac.uk/download/539887012.pdf (accessed on 7 May 2025).
5. Amara, E., Amman, B. R., Bairoh, F. V., Bakarr, M. Y., et al. (2020). Isolation of Angola-like Marburg virus from Egyptian rosette bats from West Africa. *Nature Communications, 11*(1), 510. https://doi.org/10.1038/s41467-020-14327-8.
6. Amiar, S., Husby, M. L., Wijesinghe, K. J., Angel, S., Bhattarai, N., Gerstman, B. S., Chapagain, P. P., et al. (2021). Lipid-specific oligomerization of the Marburg virus matrix protein VP40 is regulated by two distinct interfaces for virion assembly. *Journal of Biological Chemistry, 296*, Article 100796. https://doi.org/10.1016/j.jbc.2021.100796.
7. Andersen, K. G., Bao, Y., Bavari, S., Becker, S., et al. (2014). Filovirus RefSeq entries: Evaluation and selection of filovirus type variants, type sequences, and names. *Viruses, 6*(10), 3663–3682. https://core.ac.uk/download/42544025.pdf (accessed on 7 May 2025).
8. Azad, M., Fazeli, M., Goudarzi, M., & Seyedjavadi, S. S. (2015). Survey of clinical features, pathogenesis, and therapeutic options for Ebola hemorrhagic fever. *Journal of Paramedical Sciences (JPS), 6*(3), 114–152. https://core.ac.uk/download/483634127.pdf (accessed on 7 May 2025).
9. Ball, A. H. (2023). *Characterizing Protective Antibody Responses to Recombinant Ebola Virus Subunit Vaccines in Non-Human Primates*. https://core.ac.uk/download/590218213.pdf (accessed on 7 May 2025).
10. Banerjee, S., Sultana, Q., Mukherjee, D., Agrawal, V., Jaiswal, V., & Paudel, K. (2023). Disease-X: Accounting for the unknown. *Health Science Reports, 6*, Article e1173. https://doi.org/10.1002/hsr2.1173.
11. Baron, R. C., Bertherat, E., Blackley, D. J., Burke, R. M., Christie, A., De Roo, A., Faye, O., et al. (2015). Risk factors for transmission of Ebola or Marburg virus disease: A systematic review and meta-analysis. *International Journal of Epidemiology, 45*(1), 102–116. https://core.ac.uk/download/41991078.pdf (accessed on 7 May 2025).
12. Baseler, L., Chertow, G. M., Johnson, K. M., Feldmann, H., & Morens, D. M. (2016). The pathogenesis of Ebola virus disease. *Annual Review of Pathology: Mechanisms of Disease, 12*, 387–418. https://doi.org/10.1146/annurev-pathol-052016-100506.

13. Bhimraj, A., Morgan, R. L., Shumaker, A. H., Lavergne, V., Baden, L. R., Cheng, V. C. C., Edwards, K. M., et al. (2020). Infectious Diseases Society of America guidelines on the treatment and management of patients with COVID-19 (April 2020). *Clinical Infectious Diseases, 78*, e83–e102. https://doi.org/10.1093/cid/ciaa478.

14. Blondiaux, J., Haque, A., & Hober, D. (2015). Addressing therapeutic options for Ebola virus infection in current and future outbreaks. *Open Dartmouth: Faculty Open Access Articles*, 465. https://core.ac.uk/download/231114040.pdf (accessed on 7 May 2025).

15. Bloom, D. E., & Cadarette, D. (2019). Infectious disease threats in the twenty-first century: Strengthening the global response. *Frontiers in Immunology, 10*, Article 549. https://doi.org/10.3389/fimmu.2019.00549.

16. Boelaert, M., Borchert, M., Colebunders, R., Muyembe-Tamfum, J. J., et al. (2000). Viewpoint: Filovirus hemorrhagic fever outbreaks: Much ado about nothing? *Tropical Medicine and International Health, 5*(5), 318–324. https://core.ac.uk/download/pdf/9416886.pdf (accessed on 7 May 2025).

17. Brainard, J., Edmunds, K., Hooper, L., Hunter, P. R., et al. (2016). Presence and persistence of Ebola or Marburg virus in patients and survivors: A rapid systematic review. *PLOS Neglected Tropical Diseases, 10*(2), e0004475. https://core.ac.uk/download/41992867.pdf (accessed on 7 May 2025).

18. Brown, A. E. X., Ch'ng, Q. L., Currie, M., & Grundy, J. (2017). Some remarks about the complexity of epidemics management. *arXiv Preprint*. http://arxiv.org/abs/1705.02612 (accessed on 7 May 2025).

19. Cuomo-Dannenburg, G., McCain, K., McCabe, R., Unwin, H. J. T., Doohan, P., Nash, R. K., Hicks, J. T., et al. (2023). Marburg virus disease outbreaks, mathematical models, and disease parameters: A systematic review. *medRxiv* (Cold Spring Harbor Laboratory). https://doi.org/10.1101/2023.07.10.23292424.

20. Cutts, T., Leung, A., Banadyga, L., & Krishnan, J. (2024). Inactivation validation of Ebola, Marburg, and Lassa viruses in AVL and ethanol-treated viral cultures. *Viruses, 16*, Article 2006. https://www.semanticscholar.org/paper/d4fdce966b21559858a6a3c18db879bb47b025f6 (accessed on 7 May 2025).

21. Devaraj, A. R., & Marianthiran, V. J. (2025). Advancements in viral genomics: Gated recurrent unit modeling of SARS-CoV-2, SARS, MERS, and Ebola viruses. *Revista da Sociedade Brasileira de Medicina Tropical, 58*, e00401–2024. https://www.semanticscholar.org/paper/64d876a63a3932df83218e81918a09e280c92e35 (accessed on 7 May 2025).

22. Fan, Y., Zhao, K., Shi, Z. L., & Zhou, P. (2019). Bat coronaviruses in China. *Viruses, 11*(3), 210. https://doi.org/10.3390/v11030210.

23. Greenberg, A., Huber, B. R., Liu, D. X., Logue, J., Hischak, A. M. W., Hart, R., Abbott, M. C., et al. (2020). Quantification of viral and host biomarkers in the liver of rhesus macaques. *American Journal of Pathology, 190*, 1449–1460. https://doi.org/10.1016/j.ajpath.2020.03.003.

24. Henrique, B. M., Jeffs, B., Machado, F. P. D., Feldmann, H., Strong, J. E., Villa, L., Borchert, M., et al. (2010). Factors associated with Marburg hemorrhagic fever. *The Journal of Infectious Diseases, 201*(12), 1909–1918. https://core.ac.uk/download/pdf/9417556.pdf (accessed on 7 May 2025).

25. Jonas, O., & Seifman, R. (2019). Do we need a Global Virome Project? *The Lancet Global Health, 7*(10), e1314–e1316. https://doi.org/10.1016/s2214-109x(19)30335-3.

26. MacDermott, N. E. (2021). An investigation of genetic factors in Ebola virus disease. https://core.ac.uk/download/554492898.pdf (accessed on 7 May 2025).

27. Mebaley, T. N., Becquart, P., Fritz, M., Elguero, E., Mombo, I., Garcia, D., Bohou Kombila, L., et al. (2025). Ebola and Marburg viruses IgG detections in small ruminants and dogs from villages within outbreak areas in Gabon. *PLOS One, 20*, Article e0200000. https://www.semanticscholar.org/paper/ff9b71977b9b6e8ce89086d99948285e6b430178 (accessed on 7 May 2025).

28. Naguib, M. M., Li, R., Ling, J., Grace, D., Nguyen-Viet, H., & Lindahl, J. F. (2021). Live and wet markets: Food access versus the risk of disease emergence. *Trends in Microbiology, 29*(7), 573–581. https://doi.org/10.1016/j.tim.2021.02.007.

29. Pinzon, J. E. (2025). Filovirus research: The need for an integrated approach in time and space. https://core.ac.uk/download/pdf/10558469.pdf (accessed on 7 May 2025).

30. Ruggiero, E., & Richter, S. N. (2018). G-quadruplexes and G-quadruplex ligands: Targets and tools in antiviral therapy. *Nucleic Acids Research, 46*(6), 3270–3283. https://doi.org/10.1093/nar/gky187.

31. Ruiz-Aravena, M., McKee, C., Gamble, A., Lunn, T. J., Morris, A., Snedden, C. E., Yinda, C. K., et al. (2021). Ecology, evolution, and spillover of coronaviruses from bats. *Nature Reviews Microbiology, 20*(5), 299–314. https://doi.org/10.1038/s41579-021-00652-2.

32. Salata, C., Calistri, A., Parolin, C., & Palù, G. (2019). Coronaviruses: A paradigm of new emerging zoonotic diseases. *Pathogens and Disease, 77*. https://doi.org/10.1093/femspd/ftaa006.

33. Semancik, C. S., Cooper, C. L., Postler, T. S., Price, M., Yun, H., Zaric, M., Kuteesa, M., et al. (2024). Prevalence of human filovirus infections in sub-Saharan Africa: A systematic review and meta-analysis protocol. *Systematic Reviews, 13*. https://doi.org/10.1186/s13643-024-02626-w.

34. Sheahan, T. P., Sims, A., Leist, S. R., Schäfer, A., Won, J. J., Brown, A. J., Montgomery, S. A., et al. (2020). Comparative therapeutic efficacy of remdesivir and combination lopinavir, ritonavir, and interferon beta against MERS-CoV. *Nature Communications, 11*, Article 5390. https://doi.org/10.1038/s41467-019-13940-6.

35. Sohan, M., Shahriar, M., Bhuiyan, M. A., & Islam, M. R. (2022). Recent outbreak of Marburg virus disease: Could it be a threat for global public health? *Health Science Reports, 6*, Article e971. https://doi.org/10.1002/hsr2.971.

36. Sprecher, A. G., Anon, Baize, S., Basler, C., Bausch, D. G., et al. (2008). Treatment of Marburg and Ebola hemorrhagic fevers: A strategy for testing new drugs and vaccines under outbreak conditions. *Antiviral Research, 78*(1), 150–161. https://core.ac.uk/download/pdf/9416824.pdf (accessed on 7 May 2025).

37. Tang, B., Bragazzi, N. L., Li, Q., Tang, S., Xiao, Y., & Wu, J. (2020). An updated estimation of the risk of transmission of the novel coronavirus (2019-nCoV). *Infectious Disease Modelling, 5*, 248–255. https://doi.org/10.1016/j.idm.2020.02.001.

38. Tian, L., Pang, Z., Li, M., Lou, F., An, X., Zhu, S., Song, L., et al. (2022). Molnupiravir and its antiviral activity against COVID-19. *Frontiers in Immunology, 13*, Article 855496. https://doi.org/10.3389/fimmu.2022.855496.

39. Trovato, M., Sartorius, R., D'Apice, L., Manco, R., & De Berardinis, P. (2020). Viral emerging diseases: Challenges in developing vaccination strategies. *Frontiers in Immunology, 11*, Article 2130. https://doi.org/10.3389/fimmu.2020.02130.

40. Yao, W., Yang, Z., Lou, X., Mao, H., Yan, H., & Zhang, Y. (2021). Simultaneous detection of Ebola virus and pathogens associated with hemorrhagic fever by an oligonucleotide microarray. *Frontiers in Microbiology, 12*, Article 713372. https://doi.org/10.3389/fmicb.2021.713372.

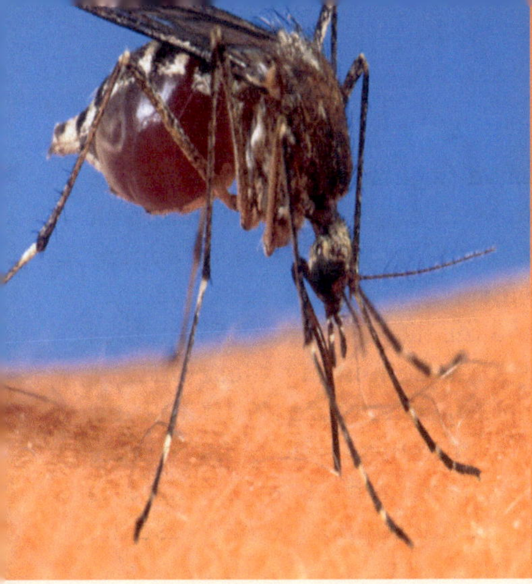

Chapter 11

ZIKA AND CHIKUNGUNYA

Contents

Introduction

Mosquito-borne diseases have proliferated recently, and it's difficult not to notice how much these viruses are destabilizing our health systems, particularly in those warm, humid regions of the world. Arboviruses, quite often, now strike communities severely, due to the ubiquitous presence of the mosquito. Zika and Chikungunya, for instance, appear where these insects are prevalent; both tend to usher in serious, even long-lasting health problems. It's worth determining not only how and why they spread but also with what frequency they recur in various regions. Weather, geography, and even the number of people who have already developed an immunity appear to have their say. And on top of it, residual antibodies and local uniqueness in the environment put another layer of complexity—so ongoing checks and surveys are still central to grasping the complete effect (Chrisafis et al., 2017). Traditional public health strategies have not always caught up with curbing Zika and Chikungunya epidemics, particularly in large diverse nations where top-down measures frequently run into logistical and social stumbling blocks.

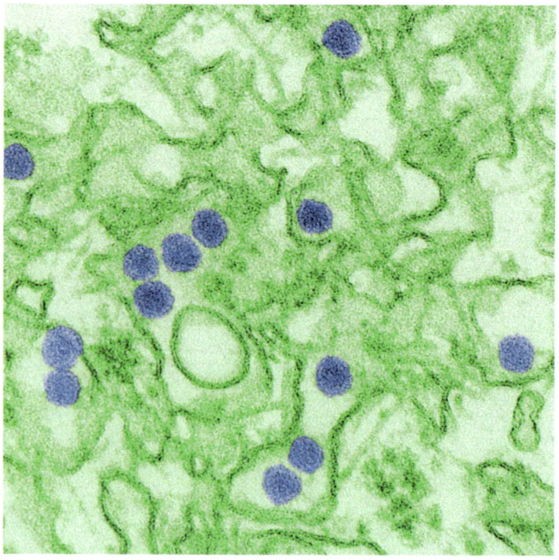

Figure 11.1. Zika, Dengue, and Chikungunya.

Source: By CDC/ Cynthia Goldsmith - http://phil.cdc.gov/phil/details.asp?pid=20541, Public Domain, https://commons.wikimedia.org/w/index.php?curid=47622558

These days, a new spin using tools such as social media metrics (ie, Twitter buzz) is filling the role as an assistive sidekick. Researchers can dig through internet talk to identify voices heard locally that amplify community-led health campaigns. These data-driven methods accomplish more than merely aiming prevention; they also provide a real-time glimpse at the way people feel and act about disease control, combining new-fangled technology with boots-on-the-ground work in a clear new package (Carlton et al., 2016). Zika and Chikungunya, however, introduce not only medical but also social and economic headache—landing hardest on the most vulnerable. Yes, they are both transmitted by mosquitoes, but they both attack in different manners. Zika, for example, receives a lot of publicity due to its connection to birth defects when transmitted from mother to baby, while Chikungunya is infamous for taking the wind out of you with crippling joint pain that could last. Outbreaks for both tend to appear when nature's just right—more rain, warmer temperatures, and the like that allow mosquitoes to thrive. In general, combating these viruses involves coming together across disciplines, monitoring environmental cues, increasing community awareness, and ensuring there is continued public health support to decrease the overall threat (Carlton et al., 2016; Chrisafis et al., 2017) (Figure 11.1).

Overview of Zika and Chikungunya Viruses

Vector-borne diseases are truly testing global health, and the problem requires that someone step in with some hands-on urgency. Viruses such as Zika and Chikungunya, for example, have been making headlines recently—not just because they crop up unexpectedly, but because they deliver a serious wallop. Aedes mosquitoes, those pest insects that make their homes in tropical and subtropical locales, are the primary vectors, allowing outbreaks to spread through populations. Not so long ago, these insects and the viruses they transmitted tended to be confined to little, far-apart urban pockets. Today, with increased travel, urban growth, and climatic changes conducive to mosquito breeding, public health experts see these diseases spread to new regions. In most instances, this trend indicates how our daily activities get complex with nature in such a manner that nature becomes a pest for health precautions. Currently, with vaccines still on the drawing board, the majority of public health measures rely on mosquito control and ongoing surveillance, even as scientists, in the majority of instances, are still preoccupied with developing vaccine concepts and treatment protocols (Trovato et al., 2020). Zika, initially believed to be a threat only to regions of Africa and Asia, proved to be much more transmissible than anticipated. Scientific studies have shown that what originated in locations such as Brazil went on to reach locations in Africa, Angola, say, in 2015–2016. Such travel touched off local epidemics that, among other problems, produced cases of congenital Zika syndrome in infants. In general, the virus doesn't merely induce a typical fever; it can also cause serious neurological issues that strike families hard. It's complicated work, too, because the presentation of Zika can appear quite similar to dengue or even Chikungunya, and doctors may find it difficult to precisely determine which virus is at fault. The situation in Angola, with its ripple effect chain of complications, emphasizes all the more how important monitoring the virus's genetic changes and human migration is (Hill et al., 2019). Chikungunya, which usually comes along with Zika courtesy of the same microbe messengers, brings its own unique type to the pot. Its most notable difference is the debilitating joint pain that appears to persist way beyond the feverish onset of the disease—something that obviously sets it apart from Zika's neurological effects. Over the past few decades, as cities grow and climates change, we've seen a steady re-emergence of these mosquito-borne viruses, a pattern that keeps both doctors and public health officials on high alert. Integrated vector management, spreading public awareness, and boosting health infrastructure are all part of the ongoing effort to reduce outbreaks. Although we have yet to pinpoint exact antiviral therapies, the impetus for vaccine production persists unabated, with increasing scientific initiative to address such health issues through preventive immunization strategies (Trovato et al., 2020) (Figure 11.2).

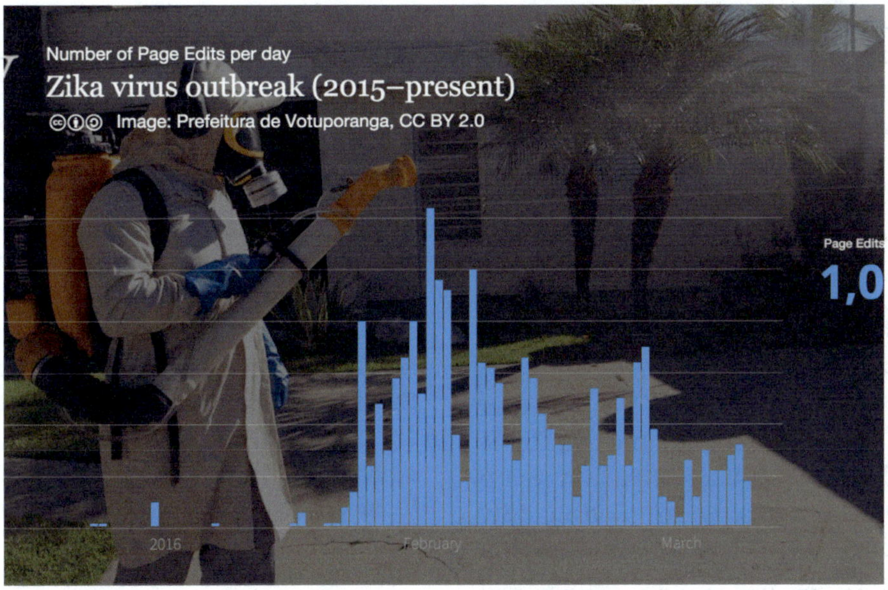

Figure 11.2. The overview of Zika and Chikungunya viruses.

Source: https://diff.wikimedia.org/2016/03/11/volunteers-zika-virus/

Importance of Studying These Diseases

Mosquito-borne diseases such as Zika and Chikungunya truly throw a spanner into public health work; they are not merely easy microbes but complex problems that require profound, thoughtful research. In the tropical and subtropical regions, these diseases can spread at neck-breaking rate, and it appears we have to consider the combination of nature, our behaviors, and even social configurations to understand why they persist and sometimes return in full force. Applying new digital techniques, such as tracking communication on Twitter, has set us into a new age of identifying outbreaks early, but these technologies tend to get it wrong when there is a change of season or the virus adjusts itself. In most instances, digging deeper through in-depth studies allows public health professionals customize their prevention strategies, utilize resources somewhat more judiciously, and alleviate the economic and health pressures on susceptible individuals (Cedrim et al., 2016). Apart from the dash to squash an outbreak, there's more at stake for studying diseases like these. Persistent mosquito populations not only weed out various pathogens at the same time but might also help new viral mutations bubble up, which could lead to unexpected epidemics. Generally speaking, getting a real feel for these tangled vector-pathogen relationships is essential if we're going to come up with smart ways to manage pests and even push vaccine development forward. Additionally, this type of work quietly tilts the scale in global health—shaping policies that ultimately protect populations who are disproportionately affected. In effect, actions to reduce mosquito populations and stem the flow of disease lay groundwork for reducing disease and deaths associated with arboviral disease, affirming why research continues to matter so much (Tidball et al., 2017). In addition to the clear public health benefits, the academic plunge into Zika and Chikungunya amps up the larger scientific capacity for facing new infectious challenges globally. Lessons surfacing from these researches, where disciplines such as virology, entomology, epidemiology, and data science unconventionally intersect, frequently inspire new partnerships and concepts. The resulting expertise not only aids in anticipating future trends and informing vaccine initiatives, it also refines our total healthcare preparedness. And consider the economic effects, piling-up healthcare costs to loss of productivity—it's a no-brainer that active disease management is the way to go. Ultimately, truly understanding these mosquitoes' diseases is central not only to managing today's outbreaks but also to creating a stronger global shield against tomorrow's health threats (Cedrim et al., 2016; Tidball et al., 2017).

11.1. Historical Background

Arbovirus threats have been on the public health radar screen for centuries, particularly in tropical, warm, and humid regions where mosquitoes breed. Zika and Chikungunya, largely transmitted by Aedes mosquitoes, had their time in the spotlight as epidemic risks. Zika was originally detected in Africa in 1947 and Chikungunya appeared in the 1950s; until the early 2000s, they sort of flew under the radar. More travel, booming cities, and dynamic environments (which provide conditions favorable to mosquito breeding) have provided these viruses with a greater platform. Nature and local economies become one in unexpected ways in most instances, making what were previously minor, localized problems into major global health concerns with far-reaching effects. It is more complicated to study these arboviruses now that there are more of them appearing in the same locales, disrupting precise diagnosis and surveillance. Tests designed to detect virus-specific antibodies—our chief instruments—tend to be misled by cross-reactions between similar viruses. Consequently, distinguishing between earlier infections of Zika, Chikungunya, and the rest becomes confused, making clinical practice and public surveillance harder. In the past, there wasn't one standard set of testing protocols or sufficient detailed information to settle how these diseases are transmitted, and the shortfall still causes trouble. Filling these testing and data gaps remains a top priority for improved virus control and for creating tests that can rapidly detect outbreaks (de Bruin et al., 2023). Politics, social atmospherics, and money have long contributed to influencing how we act regarding arbovirus outbreaks, particularly in rural or coastal areas where communities are most exposed. A glimpse at Costa Rica's battle with Zika, for example, reveals how unstable infrastructure, local traditions, and unequal political environments can stand in the way of effective mosquito eradication and disease containment. When these complications combine with environmental degradation and scarce health resources, viruses such as Zika and Chikungunya have it far too easy to spread. Studies across disciplines typically suggest that combating the outbreaks involves combating ingrained disparities and considering local realities. In most cases, it is not possible to distinguish the history of the viruses from broader issues such as governance, society, and the environment (Bomar et al., 2018).

11.1.1. Discovery of Zika Virus

Way back in the early 1900s, scientists started figuring out which bacteria could become a threat on a global level. In 1947, when they were screening for yellow fever in Uganda's Zika Forest, researchers discovered the Zika virus in a rhesus monkey. This was a milestone moment, although then Zika was largely lost in the mix behind viruses that made more readily apparent sickness. For decades, its real role in human disease remained concealed. Discovering it so far afield in the countryside brought home the notion of keeping an eye out for viruses in far-flung locations is truly critical, and it ultimately shed more light on Zika's transmission and impact on humans. Those early attempts served to place Zika into the Flaviviridae family, expanding our perception of mosquito-borne viruses and foreshadowing what was to come. Following that original discovery, Zika didn't remain in the spotlight because it only made individuals sick in a noticeable way infrequently. In general, recent developments in the fields of molecular biology and viral genomics have altered that perception by showing its genomic diversity and evolutionary history. New technologies such as metagenomics now allow researchers to identify and investigate viral genomes directly from environmental or biological samples without the need for conventional culture. This approach has not only isolated virus strains previously undetected, but it's also furthered our insight into the complex interconnection among RNA viruses, thereby enhancing work in epidemiological modeling and risk assessment (Hassan et al., 2020).

Most often, these technological advances made the world take Zika seriously, particularly after it began appearing outside of its normal niches. From a broader perspective, the Zika tale extends far beyond the realm of virology and leaks into realms such as economics and public health. Emerging diseases, after all, have a way of disturbing market patterns and disrupting civic welfare. The unexpected emergence of Zika among other epidemic viruses created both demand and supply shocks that wreaked havoc on healthcare systems as well as economic stability just like the problems we experienced in the COVID-19 pandemic (Hassan et al., 2020). Looking at the initial days of Zika's emergence reminds us how intricately interconnected scientific inquiry, public health preparedness, and economic power truly are. Just like with other newly arising viruses, putting the portions together about how Zika travels and affects society reveals why we require a balanced approach—one that intertwines virus hunting, disease management, and a candid examination of our weaknesses in an increasingly globalized world (Figure 11.3).

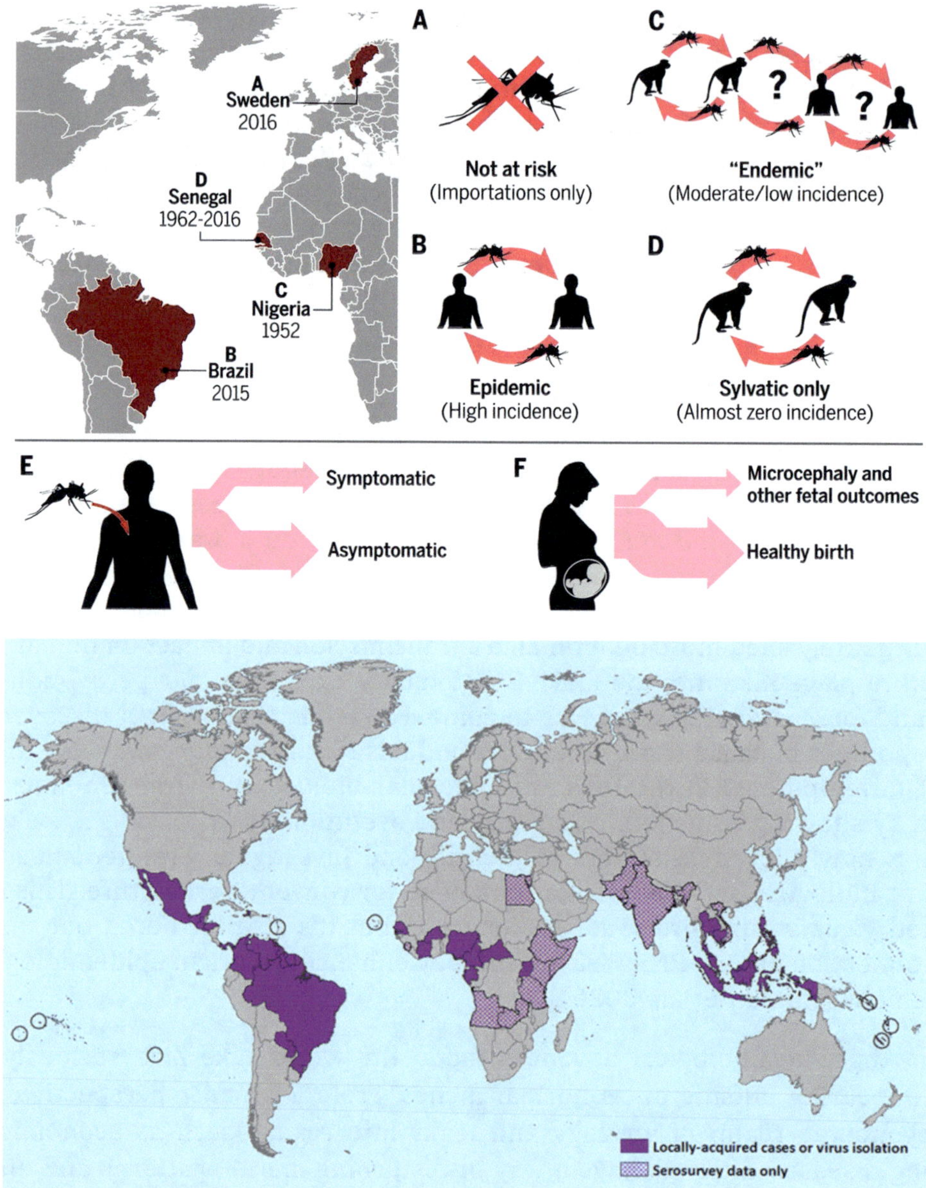

Figure 11.3. Assessing the global threat from Zika virus.

Source: By United States Centers for Disease Control and Prevention - https://www.cdc.gov/zika/images/zik-world-map_01-15-2016_web.jpg, Public Domain, https://commons.wikimedia.org/w/index.php?curid=46622992

11.1.2. Discovery of Chikungunya Virus

In the early '50s, there was a weird fever that struck suddenly, giving patients searing joint pain, rashes, and high fevers that resembled dengue quite a bit. Physicians furrowed their brows at these symptoms, which at first glance closely resembled dengue, so nothing seemed to make sense. Then, in 1952, researchers drew a sample from a patient with a fever in Tanzania and, well, that's when chikungunya first appeared. Obviously, this virus was not another pest but acted differently, flaunting peculiar biological mannerisms and clinical presentations. In the majority of instances, that involved the fact that where there were a number of mosquito-borne ailments roaming about, physicians needed to learn to distinguish between them. Researchers later discovered that determining chikungunya went hand in hand with excavating further into the mosquito universe. They ended up blaming *Aedes aegypti* and *Aedes albopictus*—two species that appeared most adept at transmitting the virus. These small pests, surprisingly resilient in human-modified environments, followed similar dynamics observed in dengue's transmission (Brady et al., 2019). By and large, their ability to thrive where people thrived resulted in outbreaks appearing more readily in hot, tropical, and even some subtropical areas. It was something of a wake-up call regarding how important it is to control these mosquito messengers when dealing with multiple viral threats. Researchers next focused on the virus's unusual replication patterns and how it damages cells. By going deep into molecular virology and screening antiviral compounds, they identified crucial stages of the virus's life cycle that could be good drug targets. In the majority of instances, such methods have been employed in research on other viruses, such as in certain flavonoid studies for infection combat (Badshah et al., 2021). The ability of chikungunya to replicate rapidly and cause intense inflammatory response practically forced researchers to experiment with various methods of treatment. Gradually, but steadily, combining knowledge from virology, entomology, and even pharmacology appeared to be the best bet to control not only chikungunya but also trio of similar infections like Zika. All this indicates that controlling emerging infections frequently requires a hybrid, sometimes complex, but always dynamic approach.

11.1.3. Evolution and Spread of Both Viruses

If you take a look at the past of arboviruses, you can notice they've been appearing in unexpected manners, changing and expanding across various areas. Most of these insects, such as Zika and Chikungunya, have appeared throughout history in several locations around the globe, suggesting that they've been coexisting with human beings for a long time. Incidences do appear to vary with weather and climate—tropical warmth and extended rain showers provide ideal areas in which to live for mosquitoes—whereas high altitudes and dry, harsh surroundings occasionally appear to suppress them. It's fascinating that antibodies, particularly in older individuals, continue to persist in the bloodstream, indicating these viruses persist longer than we would anticipate, paving the way for the outbreaks we're currently observing (Chrisafis et al., 2017). Zika is an example of just how much a virus can change throughout the years. Initially, it was initially isolated in 1947 from a rhesus monkey in Uganda and subsequently for decades it was largely confined to a narrow equatorial strip over Africa and Asia, as a general rule. Then it jumped from primates to humans, adapted quite rapidly, and by 2014 pushed its way east—to regions such as Oceania and South America. Outbreaks ensued on a huge scale, with millions infected in many countries. Its capacity to generate nerve symptoms and even propagate through sexual transmission has rendered it a public health issue of some gravitas. Its sudden, cross-species and geographical leap exhibits a form of adaptive evolution that keeps us on our toes, emphasizing enhanced surveillance and more rapid diagnostics (Ansari et al., 2016). Chikungunya, in turn, makes its own unique chapter. Long known in portions of Africa and Asia, it's returned more recently with a little more kick and a little more reach. Its dissemination is closely linked with the life of its mosquito vectors—environmental changes that enhance mosquito numbers can quickly alter cycles of transmission. In contrast to Zika, Chikungunya strikes with a sudden, severe joint pain, imparting it a distinctly perceptible clinical nuance despite following overall patterns of spread in the same way. Both viruses are reminders that subtle genetic adjustments and random ecological windows can enable them to break past established boundaries. Instances such as these truly highlight why the integration of continuous serological and entomological studies is so important in identifying and preventing future outbreaks (Ansari et al., 2016; Chrisafis et al., 2017) (Figure 11.4).

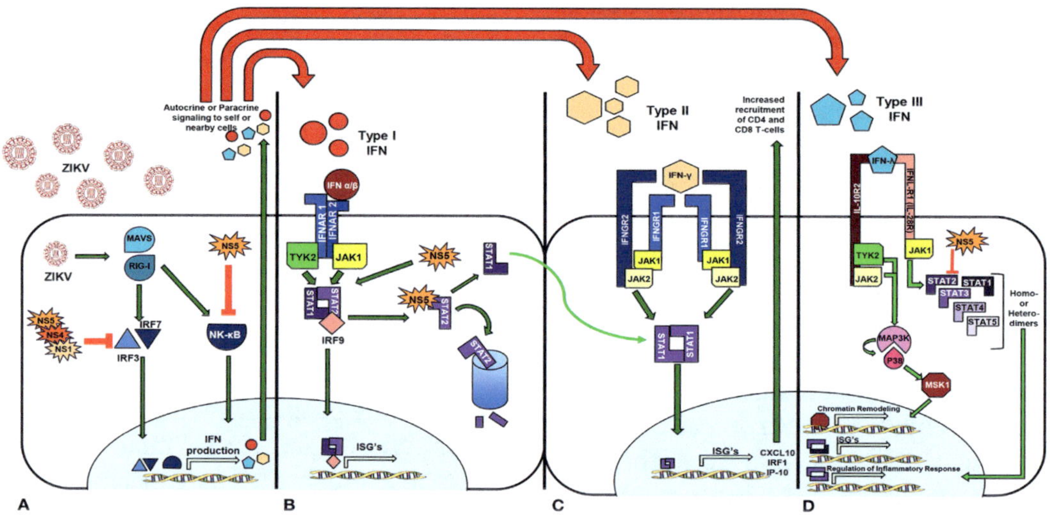

Figure 11.4. Evolution and spread of both viruses of Zika virus.

Source: Yuan, L., Huang, X. Y., Liu, Z. Y., Zhang, F., Zhu, X. L., Yu, J. Y., ... & Qin, C. F. (2018). *Evolution and Spread of Zika Virus.* Frontiers in Immunology.

11.2. Transmission Methods

Zika and Chikungunya are keeping us on our toes, in large part due to mosquitoes. Aedes mosquitoes, particularly *Aedes aegypti*, are largely responsible for spreading these viruses from person to person. This tiny mosquito has effectively made our urban centers its home, so outbreaks can sneak up on busy cities. Yes, the bite is the primary method by which these diseases are spread, but occasionally additional, secondary routes present themselves and complicate things even further. Mostly, the fact that these microbes are out and about translates into authorities advocating more massive, sweeping control efforts, and the rise and fall of mosquito populations with the seasons only serving to heighten the uncertainty. Apart from the bite, fresh evidence indicates that Zika has a few tricks in store. For instance, the virus has already been detected in semen in some studies, which leads us to suspect sexual transmission as yet another mode by which the virus can jump from person to person. In general, this added vector makes us consider beyond mosquito control itself. It particularly concerns pregnant women or intending pregnant women since conditions such as microcephaly have been associated with Zika infection. Consequently, public health professionals now integrate sexual health guidance and reproductive counseling into their efforts (Grazzini et al., 2016). And, layering it further, these viruses also raise issues regarding blood transfusions and in the healthcare sector. See, some of the people who are infected don't even have symptoms, so blood donors could inadvertently transmit Zika or Chikungunya. Blood banks are having trouble keeping it safe due to this risk, though they're attempting to boost screening protocols and modify donor deferral guidelines. National health organizations have introduced many prevention measures—albeit, admittedly, our understanding of how long the virus persists in blood isn't yet perfect. This shortcoming keeps the research into transfusion safety proceeding at a cautious, step-by-step rate (Grazzini et al., 2016) (Figure 11.5).

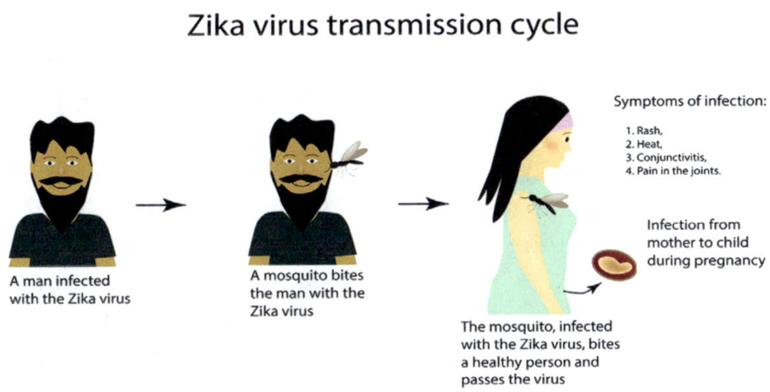

Figure 11.5. Zika-virus-transmission-cycle.

Source: VectorStock. (n.d.). *Zika Virus Transmission Cycle Infographics.*

11.2.1. Mosquito Vectors Involved

Zika and Chikungunya are more apt to spread in patterns that have to do with how their mosquito vectors live and exist. Rather than a basic human-to-human transition, these viruses spread primarily due to Aedes mosquitoes, particularly *Aedes aegypti* and its close relative, *Aedes albopictus*. Urban environments provide a definite advantage to these insects, as they usually thrive in close proximity to us and appear to favor our blood. You can observe their breeding ability even in the smallest puddles near homes, so outbreaks become more probable in hot, congested environments. In most instances, understanding outbreaks and determining control measures is all about getting what these mosquitoes do on a daily basis. In the meantime, issues compound when these mosquitoes develop resistance to our traditional insecticides. Urbanization and changing weather have compounded the challenge, so our usual control methods tend to fall behind the evolution of their behavior and increasing range. Overall, this has compelled scientists to experiment with new ideas such as employing symbiont-based methods or gene drive technologies. One interesting example is infecting the mosquitoes with Wolbachia, which appears to suppress their capacity to enable virus replication, though practical problems still exist—ecological, acceptance by the community, and real-world feasibility ironically still prevent us (Wang et al., 2022). Something different, our healthcare systems' preparedness contributes immensely when there are outbreaks. Most areas continue to experience lags in surveillance capacity, control infrastructure, and appropriate diagnostics, hindering early detection and containment. Illustratively, studies in Zanzibar reveal an evident deficit in trained personnel, standard guidelines, and laboratory tests required to address these mosquito-borne viruses. Public health education and monitoring of mosquitoes occasionally remain inadequate as well, placing communities more at risk of outbreaks. In all, increasing our surveillance, training, and outreach within communities is crucially important for maintaining Zika and Chikungunya under control (Saleh et al., 2021).

11.2.2. Other Potential Transmission Routes

Other times we think that viruses such as Zika and Chikungunya just stick with the age-old mosquito tale, but they may be doing some other moves we should investigate more. Aedes mosquitoes are the carriers of choice, no question, but it turns out that these viruses can also travel around through bodily fluids. Consider Zika – it's been detected in semen, for instance, which quite rightly raises the specter of sexual transmission.

This turn of events means that even when mosquito populations decline, the virus may persist simply through human-to-human contact. Interestingly, viral RNA residues have also been found in saliva and urine, indicating that mucosal secretions may be playing a role somehow, though we're still not entirely certain about their infective potential. Figuring out these extra routes could help us refine our predictions about virus spread and fine-tune guidelines, especially in areas where mosquito activity isn't steady. The growing complexity in transmission really calls for teamwork among virologists, epidemiologists, and experts in molecular medicine (Qin et al., 2022). Looking back, our experiences with various infectious diseases show that it's important to recognize every twist and turn in how viruses travel. Zika and Chikungunya, like most zoonotic infections, aren't always so clear about the vector-host relationship we anticipate. With increased human contact and worldwide travel, sporadic spillover events and unorthodox modes of transmission become increasingly likely. There have been cases where Zika was transmitted through blood transfusions and even from a mother to her child, which presents an entirely new set of challenges to blood safety and prenatal care practices. The same applies to Chikungunya, whose possibility of horizontal transmission from mother to child makes the monitoring of maternal infection paramount in avoiding neonatal complications. This is just to prove that our surveillance systems must expand their scope—not only on environmental determinants and mosquito abundance but also on avenues of direct human transmission (Piret & Boivin, 2021).

On another front, advances in molecular biology and vaccine technology, particularly mRNA-based therapies, are creating new avenues to address these difficult transmission modes. These rapidly advancing therapies, due to their speed and specificity, could potentially really assist us in addressing the routes that do not depend on conventional mosquito control. The rapid production cycle of mRNA vaccines allows us to possibly change course more rapidly when novel patterns develop, whether sexual or vertical transmission. If we can nail down how long the virus persists in various body fluids and tissues, we might be able to design more specific treatments to interrupt sustained spread. Overall, combining these biotechnological developments with strong epidemiological evidence appears to be the most effective strategy to tackle these arboviral threats in the long term (Qin et al., 2022) (Figure 11.6).

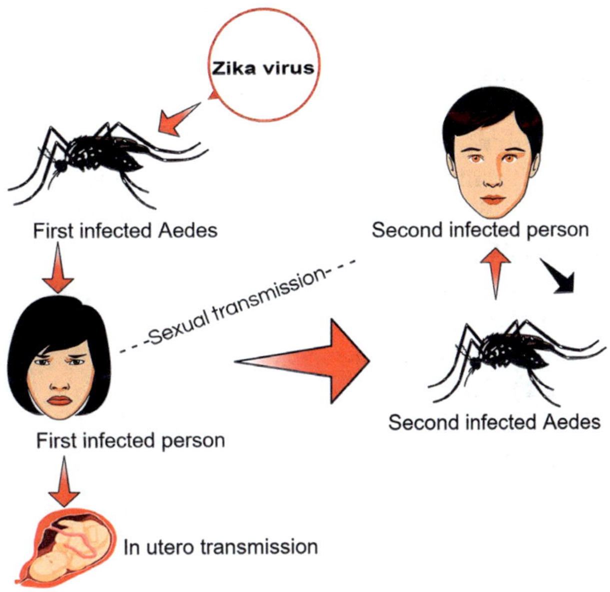

Figure 11.6. Transmission methods of Zika virus.

Source: Musso, D., & Gubler, D. J. (2016). *Transmission Methods of Zika Virus*. Frontiers in Microbiology.

11.2.3. Geographic Distribution of Transmission

Massive urban development and dense living appear to propel the transmission of Zika and chikungunya. In the tropics and subtropics, rapid expansion in the city typically creates ideal breeding grounds for mosquitoes such as *Aedes aegypti* and *Aedes albopictus*. Frequently, whenever blocks squish more than 1,000 individuals per square kilometer, there is an apparent increase in virus spread, in the majority of instances. Converting natural areas into urbanized areas leaves behind quite a lot of stagnant water—in pots or scattered rubble debris, which ultimately invites mosquitoes to reproduce. Various ecological, entomological, and epidemiological research, such as the ones discussed in (Kolimenakis et al., 2021), indicate that these high-density urban areas tend to become breeding grounds for keeping the virus alive. In general, the way we design our environment truly makes a difference in checking these diseases. Construction areas introduce a further complexity to this situation. They don't merely break ground on new buildings; they reshape the land and accumulate water-retaining containers and refuse that are wonderful egg-laying sites for vector mosquitoes. Particularly in urban areas filled with new developments, these construction areas can cause little bursts in the local mosquito population. Out-of-doors workers, who are out in these places for most of their day, are more likely to be at risk for bites, caught up in the chain of transmission. The impact of these locations is directly related to where they are located—whether on the edge of a city or urban area, right during a crowded place, which in turn determines both neighborhood and larger virus dynamics (Wilke et al., 2019). Mixing together knowledge about the behavior of mosquitoes with intelligent city planning and even safety for workers appears to be the key to addressing the transmission. City living isn't one-size-fits-all, either, and that just adds to the unpredictability. Minute variations in microhabitats—a wet stairwell, a residual barrier, or merely a random puddle—can produce mottled areas where immature and adult Aedes mosquitoes accumulate, with these patches changing season to season. Human travel, be it by building workers commuting from one site to another or householders about their daily business, facilitates the virus to jump from its point of origin. For the most part, successful public health measures rely on highly skilled surveillance and predictions taking into account these local uniqueness as well as the convoluted cocktail of mosquito activity, human movements, and urban planning (Wilke et al., 2019; Kolimenakis et al., 2021). In essence, attention to these spatial characteristics is crucial for managing outbreaks in our diverse cityscapsules.

11.3. Symptoms and Health Impacts

Chikungunya isn't a one-and-done deal; its impact appears to stick around, leaving victims with a slew of symptoms that can disrupt everyday life. In most instances, patients struck by the virus begin with a sudden episode of high fever and joint aches that can strike tough and rapid—sometimes symmetrical and almost crippling—and such severe symptoms usually persist for around 7–10 days. But that's just the start: the pain, sounding an arthritis-like sensation, may last for months and even years, a protracted journey that presents severe tests to patients as well as healthcare systems. Epidemiological research reports that approximately 75% of infected individuals have obvious signs of the infection, and approximately half report long-term problems thereafter (Rama et al., 2024). Understanding this intricate process, from the sudden flash of symptoms to the persisting discomfort, is critical to making the correct diagnosis and enacting successful care. Changing subject, Zika prefers to rollout with a lesser set of symptoms. Most only get a light rash, some fever, joint aches, or red, irritated eyes that clear in a few days. However, don't be fooled by its typically innocuous look; Zika's ability to target the nervous system means it's a whole other type of issue. Take, for example, its sinister association with fetal brain abnormalities such as microcephaly, particularly in pregnant women, casting a long shadow over its otherwise short-lived symptoms.

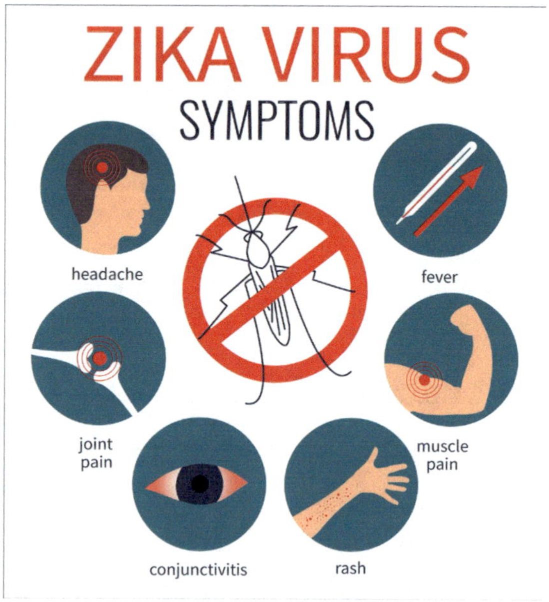

Figure 11.7. Symptoms and health impacts of Zika virus.

Source: UPMC HealthBeat. (2016). *Symptoms and Health Impacts of Zika Virus.*

The threat is not limited to infants, either—some adults will wind up fighting Guillain–Barré syndrome, an immune system assault on the nervous system. With similarities in symptoms with dengue and even Chikungunya, physicians have to depend on meticulous lab tests to prevent diagnostic missteps (Bhandari et al., 2023). If you compare both viruses side by side, they evidently throw different, albeit equally troubling, shadows. Joint pain and fever are commonalities, but whereas Chikungunya will poison its victims with long-term joint problems, Zika has an extra burden to contend with from its congenital and neurological risks. These subtleties lead to healthcare practitioners in affected areas being vigilant to note symptom particulars and adjust responses accordingly. Ultimately, an in-depth understanding of the entire gamut—from the shock of preliminary symptoms to potential long-term complications—is critical to reducing lasting effects and enhancing outcomes among populations threatened by these arboviral issues (Figure 11.7).

11.3.1. Common Symptoms of Zika Virus

Zika virus is typically transmitted through the bite of an infected Aedes mosquito, but its symptoms can easily be confused with those of dengue or even chikungunya. Picking up these signs is rather important in a case of correctly identifying the right diagnosis and determining how best to handle care in afflicted communities. Overall, individuals will often perceive a slight fever, rash, red eyes, and joint pains anywhere from a few days to about a week after they were exposed—though the symptoms are somewhat random as far as how intense they are. Strangely, they usually disappear within a week, making Zika appear less deadly than its viral relatives; but this same benign strategy can result in many cases going undetected, making it harder to contain any outbreaks. In areas where different viruses tend to combination, close monitoring through wide surveillance and employing multiple diagnostic perspectives becomes increasingly crucial (Utarini et al., 2021). Once the initial symptoms strike, most people report additional symptoms as their body begins to attack the virus. Headaches, fatigue, and muscle aches tend to accompany that initial rash and fever. Surprisingly, the rash associated with Zika tends to appear as a diffuse maculopapular type, differing from the more localized rashes so commonly witnessed in other infections. Joint pain typically involves the small joints of the feet and hands, similar to arthralgia with chikungunya, although it's typically less severe. Such overlapping syndromes can cloud the diagnostic waters, particularly in areas where these viruses are endemic, so laboratory tests are fairly indispensable to sort things out. Even where these symptoms tend to disappear by themselves, a little caution is warranted due to the possible neurological effects that sometimes accompany the virus, a worry that is very specific to pregnant women (Utarini et al., 2021). Most instances of Zika may be initially mild in nature, but familiar symptoms in some cases may end up being a prelude to something more complicated. Consider, for example, conjunctivitis—it may look mild initially but can prompt clinicians to favor a Zika diagnosis compared to other arboviral diseases. Furthermore, the constellation in which the symptoms present, typically completing within a week or less, is significantly distinct from the prolonged syndrome of chikungunya and suggests a singular clinical course for Zika. Since symptoms can be so confusing and co-infections are a real possibility, epidemiologists and vaccine scientists frequently have to balance these subtleties and imprecise diagnostic clues when strategizing public health interventions. In most situations, painstakingly disentangling these confusing clues is fundamental for providing patients with adequate treatment and for establishing intervention strategies in regions where multiple arboviruses are present.

11.3.2. Common Symptoms of Chikungunya Virus

Chikungunya may present like any other arboviral disease so that immediately renders it a tad difficult to distinguish. Within approximately 2–12 days, give or take, individuals will wake up out of the blue with a spontaneous high fever that comes out of nowhere. Immediately along with this fever, there's typically this thudding joint pain that comes on strongly, particularly within the smaller joints of the extremities; essentially, it feels like the virus's calling card. You may also experience muscle pains, a headache, or even notice a rash; though these symptoms amount to a miserable couple of days, they seldom become deadly. Physicians in regions where the virus is widespread tend to bank on the fact that the joint aches are normally both intense and bilateral, which makes them suspect Chikungunya even before all examinations are in. It's important to recognize these initial symptoms so that early intervention can stave off long-term complications. Conversely, once the initial spate of symptoms has passed, the infection may persist for weeks or even months as chronic polyarthritis—a type of chronic inflammation of the joints that is sometimes mistaken for conditions like rheumatoid arthritis (particularly if you lack that virological diagnosis to refer back to). While the fever tends to abate in a matter of days, that swelling and stiffness in the joints can truly upset regular life. Occasionally, a maculopapular rash will appear along with the fever, and although other symptoms such as fatigue, a little conjunctivitis, or even some gastrointestinal difficulties may develop, they simply aren't as indicative as the joint problems. In general, when it's put side by side with Zika virus—famous for mild joint ache but more frequent manifestations of conjunctivitis and rash—the overtly heavy joint involvement is a strong tip-off for medical professionals (Alcantara et al., 2019). Surprisingly, whereas everyone associates neurological issues such as Guillain-Barré Syndrome with Zika first, there is increasing evidence that Chikungunya sometimes plays with the nervous system as well. In exceptional instances, patients developed signs of meningoencephalitis or even neuropathy—suggesting that the virus would have some unsuspected neuroinvasive characteristics. Lab tests commonly detect a decrease in white blood cells and an increase in liver enzymes, signals that lead physicians through testing. Since both viruses tend to appear in the same locations and have some of the same symptoms, it becomes extremely difficult to distinguish between them—but also absolutely necessary for accurate patient care and monitoring. The intractable joint problems specific to Chikungunya make it even more necessary to take a close look so as not to confuse it with Zika's neurological impact. Overall, these slight yet important differences are vital to understanding the total disease burden and informing intelligent public health policies (Ansari et al., 2016; Alcantara et al., 2019) (Figure 11.8).

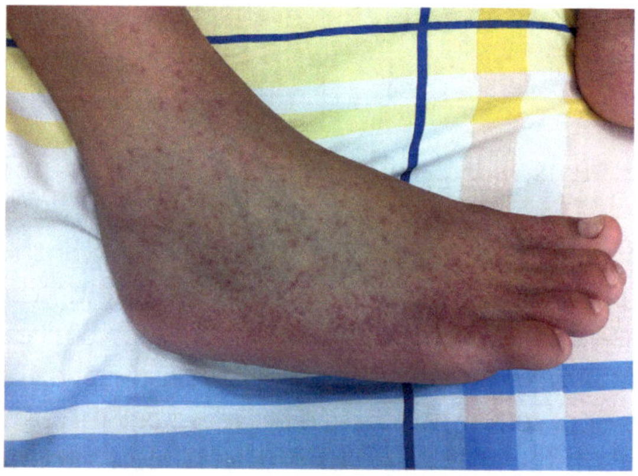

Figure 11.8. Chikungunya signs, symptoms, complications, and prevention.

Source: By Nsaa - Own work, CC BY-SA 3.0, https://commons.wikimedia.org/w/index.php?curid=23759640

11.3.3. Long-term Health Effects Associated with Both Viruses

Viral infections don't simply disappear when the fever breaks; they tend to leave a legacy of persisting problems. Zika and chikungunya, transmitted primarily by Aedes mosquitoes, have the potential to cause complications that persist long after the initial disease. Initially, Zika made headlines because of its association with birth defects such as microcephaly, but subsequently, scientists observed that adults could also experience chronic nerve problems like Guillain-Barré syndrome or even memory loss. Chikungunya, however, has the tendency to give out chronic arthritis-like joint pain that can be a mimic of rheumatoid arthritis for months or years. In most instances, these long-term problems unveil how the viruses cause chronic inflammation and play tricks with the immune system, so recovery becomes more difficult for all (Wang et al., 2022). The viruses also have a long shadow over daily lives. Congenital Zika syndrome families tend to encounter lifelong challenges such as intellectual disabilities and developmental delays that require additional hands-on care. Likewise, individuals fighting chronic chikungunya arthritis typically experience a decline in quality of life, reduced productivity, and an increase in physician visits. This array of continuing health ailments places strain on healthcare services, particularly in underserved regions. And without particular antiviral treatments or vaccines to deploy, physicians must increasingly depend on rehabilitation and pain management while attempting to construct more intelligent treatment regimens. Overall, this scenario requires an increase in research and innovation to mitigate the wider social and economic impact of these infections (Wilson et al., 2020).

Going a little deeper, the combination of residual viruses and personal immune reactions makes the picture more difficult. Certain newer research suggests that portions of viral RNA and proteins may find shelter in regions of the body such as joint tissues—those small immune refuges—that cause inflammation continually. Additionally, individual variations in immune reactions and genetic composition also appear to influence how severe or long-lasting such problems can become. These observations lead the way towards the hope of targeted drugs that modulate the immune system or clear out the portions of virus left behind. But the entire process is anarchic and unpredictable, requiring a combination of disciplines to crack it. In the majority of instances, such studies not only assure enhanced patient care; they also cast light on ways to improve vector control and prevention measures to reduce the overall burden of these diseases (Wilson et al., 2020; Wang et al., 2022).

11.4. Diagnosis and Treatment

With Zika and Chikungunya, the first major challenge is getting to a firm diagnosis. These viruses have a tangled array of early symptoms, fever, rash, and joint pain that don't lead unmistakably to one particular villain. Patients typically complain about these non-specific symptoms, so physicians are left playing possibilities rather than having a clear-cut solution. Recently, researchers have proposed some innovative solutions, such as utilizing sensor electrodes in conjunction with antibodies; the process entails an electrochemical system constructed on a combination of gold–polyaniline partnered with sulfur, nitrogen-doped graphene quantum dot nanocomposites. This combination, in a strange way, reduces cross-reaction problems and allows the system to detect signals from several of the mosquito-borne viruses, the four dengue types, Zika, and Chikungunya, simultaneously at incredibly low femtogram per milliliter. By and large, this kind of accuracy is crucial for detecting the issue early enough so that treatment may begin on time and additional transmission is contained (Nasrin et al., 2021). Shifting to treatment, there isn't any magic antiviral available that targets Zika or Chikungunya specifically, so treatment is largely supportive. Practically speaking, this involves alleviating symptoms with painkillers, fever reducers, and lots of fluids. Occasionally, when the diagnosis falters or isn't exactly on target, treatment delays or missteps can happen, an issue that can complicate a patient's recovery. That's why quick, precise tests are not just helpful; they are flat-out vital for pinning down the infection and monitoring for outbreaks. Back in the old days, organized mosquito control measures paid their dues by lowering cases, and returning to proven epidemiological and entomological strategies—addled with advances in diagnostics—can pay attention and make itself known in improved overall patient management (Wilson et al., 2020). Considering how difficult it is to diagnose and treat these infections, there appears to be no choice but a multi-layered, multifaceted strategy. Early, targeted diagnostic tools, such as those antibody-conjugated nanocomposite sensors—constitute one half of the coin, while locally adapted vector control measures, combining insecticide and non-insecticide solutions, constitute the other. These ground-level strategies serve to reduce viral transmission, thereby easing the burden that healthcare professionals have to carry. For the most part, combining sophisticated diagnostics with adaptable, community-tailored control measures not only boosts detection sensitivity but also simplifies discrimination among closely related infections, ultimately leading to more informed treatment decisions. This type of integrated, sometimes marginally imperfect, strategy has potential for maintaining control over these new arboviral threats (Nasrin et al., 2021; Wilson et al., 2020) (Figure 11.9).

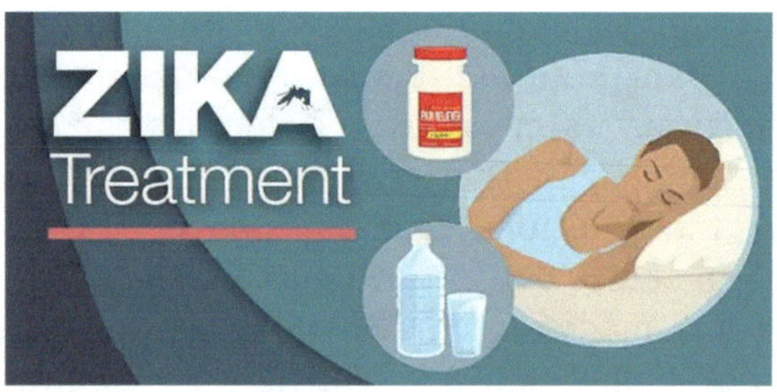

Figure 11.9. Diagnosis and treatment of Zika virus.

Source: Centers for Disease Control and Prevention. (n.d.). *Zika Diagnosis and Treatment.*

11.4.1. Diagnostic Methods for Zika Virus

Diagnosing Zika virus is not so simple as one would think. Distinguishing it from infections such as dengue and chikungunya can be downright difficult because they tend to present with similar symptoms and generally occur together in the same areas. Most of the tests available, such as the enzyme-linked immunosorbent assay (ELISA), attempt to detect Zika-specific antibodies—but unfortunately, they get confused because sometimes antibodies from other flaviviruses that are closely related cross over. Molecular tests, like reverse transcription-polymerase chain reaction (RT-PCR), are usually our first line for detecting active infections by tracking down viral RNA in urine or blood. But here's the trap: RNA detection time is relatively short, so samples must be taken quickly. Overall, new upgrades in diagnostic strategy attempt to optimize sensitivity and specificity—even where there are fewer resources—because international interest in arboviral disease and the risk of outbreaks continues to expand, a consideration commonly referenced in global health programs (Balakrishnan, 2022). Conversely, though critical laboratory testing such as RT-PCR is necessary, there has been a drive towards less complex point-of-care tests that yield quick results at the site of the issue. These quick tests (RDTs) typically detect viral antigens or immunoglobulin M antibodies. Sure, they may not always quite find the bullseye as far as sensitivity is concerned and can sometimes overcall false positives, particularly when other viruses such as chikungunya are in the mix—but they still provide a useful, field-based solution. In most cases, combining molecular methods with serological tests appears to eliminate some of the uncertainty, and continued advances are fueling the development of new assays that can identify multiple arboviruses simultaneously (Balakrishnan, 2022). Outside the laboratory bench, a good understanding of mosquito ecology and control methods genuinely assists in sharpening our overall diagnostic efforts. Having an understanding of which mosquito types are more apt to be infected and monitoring how they transmit the virus can be instrumental in predicting outbreaks and refining sample gathering. In certain instances, concepts such as genetically engineering mosquitoes to reduce virus transmission are being looked into—an endeavor that nicely complements our lab-based protocols and greater public health measures against Zika. Overall, these hybrid approaches remind us that continued progress in arboviral disease control relies on scientists, doctors, and public health professionals all coordinating together, particularly in circumstances where stealthy diagnostics would otherwise hamper efficient case detection and treatment.

11.4.2. Diagnostic Methods for Chikungunya Virus

Arboviral diseases continue to evolve and it's crucial to identify the proper tests in a hurry. Chikungunya, for instance, tends to cross-react with viruses such as Zika or Dengue so merely testing symptoms is not sufficient anymore. Laboratories now rely on techniques such as RT-PCR, which detects viral RNA during that initial, chaotic period, and it's renowned for being sensitive and specific, allowing physicians to respond rapidly and even stem outbreaks.

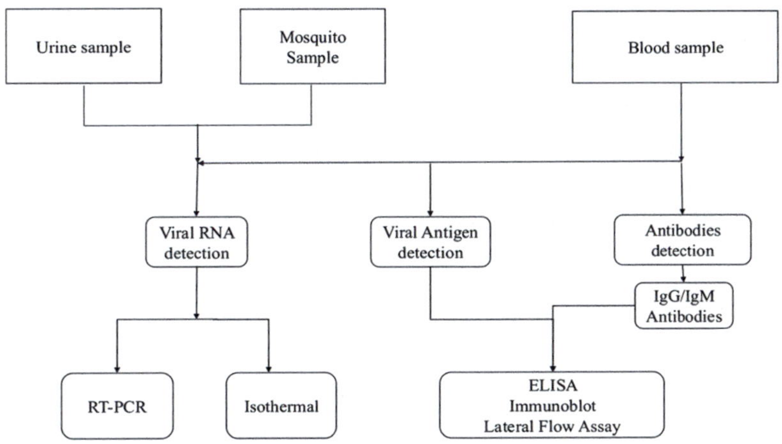

Figure 11.10. Diagnostic methods for Chikungunya virus.

Source: Nayak, K., & Mehendale, S. (2023). *Diagnostic Methods for Chikungunya Virus.* Tropical Medicine and Infectious Disease, 8(365).

There are also tests on the blood for IgM and IgG antibodies that suggest ongoing or previous infections, but these can sometimes become confused when other viruses that are similar are present. With arboviruses spreading in more complicated patterns worldwide, getting the diagnoses correct becomes an actual challenge and the lab plays a massive part, even if sometimes things become a bit confusing. Others are also experimenting with some novel test concepts, which should speed and simplify virus identification. Consider ATR-FTIR spectroscopy, for example, it's an approach that scans for subtle biochemical changes in specimens at high speeds without destroying them, and essentially relies on brilliant math tools like Principal Component Analysis and Linear Discriminant Analysis to discriminate between characteristic spectral fingerprints. It's only in its infancy within the context of viral diagnostic tests, but in many instances its low sample preparation and rapid turnaround could potentially bypass some of the technical and logistical problems associated with traditional testing, particularly in resource-limited environments. Combining this new method with old-school methods could define a useful quick screen for Chikungunya during sudden outbreaks (Lima et al., 2020). Challenges are by no means over, however. When several arboviruses, Chikungunya, Dengue, and Zika, to be precise—, co-circulating, the overlapping signals on immunoassays can really muddy the water, tending to prompt clinicians to follow up with accurate molecular tests. Further there's the reality that there are very few licensed vaccines and standardized diagnostic kits are scarce, so it's no wonder that ongoing advances in testing are essential. The World Health Organization tends to emphasize the importance of improved surveillance mechanisms, citing the importance of sensitive, specific, and simple-to-implement tests for differentiating these infections. Improved diagnostic accuracy does more than inform patient management, it also supports public health action for vector control and the management of outbreaks – particularly in regions devastated by these arboviruses (Ansari et al., 2016) (Figure 11.10).

11.4.3. Current Treatment Options and Recommendations

Treating Zika and Chikungunya is all about alleviating symptoms—there really isn't any antiviral or licensed vaccine yet. Patients are advised to rest, maintain fluids, and take over-the-counter pain relievers such as acetaminophen to alleviate fever and joint pains. Many physicians even hold off on NSAIDs until dengue is eliminated, lest they cause bleeding. Zika, specifically, receives special attention for pregnant women, as it may at times produce major problems such as microcephaly. All attempts to avoid these infections center around keeping mosquitoes in check: applying insecticides, bed nets, or repellents to avoid the Aedes species. The necessity for rapid diagnosis and public health intervention is apparent when you look at some of the nerve complications associated with Zika (Ansari et al., 2016). Climate change and international travel appear to be driving the viruses into new territory, so advice now is more in favor of more coordinated monitoring and public health response. Increasing both epidemiological and entomological surveillance can pick up outbreaks earlier and refine the mosquito control action. In most parts of the world, experts even recommend delaying pregnancy during active cases of Zika due to the severe threats to unborn infants. There are also newer guidelines for safer sex practices—because Zika is infectious that way as well. Because all treatment continues to be merely supportive care, increasing health preparedness for complications such as Guillain-Barré syndrome or prolonged joint pain is fairly important. In reality, combining environmental measures with health education can help reduce mosquito breeding sites and raise awareness, particularly among susceptible individuals (Ansari et al., 2016). At the policy level, there is increasing opinion that combating these viruses requires a combination of surveillance, control of mosquitoes, and community action. If we can standardize case definitions and methods for follow-up across borders, timely information sharing becomes much simpler. Consider the EU-wide network as an example—it facilitates cross-sector collaboration and training and could even be used as a model for other regions. Getting health and research professionals caught up on these surveillance methods certainly enhances our overall readiness. In short, current guidelines urge not only individualized treatment of patients but also long-term public health strategies that integrate monitoring, prevention, and education to address the growing threat of Zika and Chikungunya in an ever-evolving world.

11.5. Prevention Strategies

Preventing issues due to diseases such as Zika and Chikungunya largely hinges on severing the connection between infected people and the mosquito perpetrators. Urban-dwelling *Aedes aegypti*, those obnoxious primary carriers, have compelled communities to experiment with various ploys – from clearing breeding grounds around homes and neighborhoods (getting rid of stagnant water significantly reduces mosquito larvae) to word-of-mouth campaigns about maintaining the environment clean. Individuals should apply microbe spray, screen their windows, and cover up when mosquitoes are most active. Although the vaccines for these viruses are still in the planning stages, most authorities believe that effective mosquito control and community effort can reduce the rates of infection before any vaccine is widely available. New diagnostic and surveillance technology advancements now push prevention strategies into sharper focus. Equipment such as Lab On A Chip devices, CRISPR-based diagnostics, and even nano-tech have enabled instant and trustworthy results at the point of care itself – an actual game-changer when intervention speed is critical. Health authorities can now identify emerging hotspots with these improved surveillance systems, and—in general—align resources and schedules for managing the mosquito populations more strategically. Additionally, by looking at immune responses through markers such as inflammatory cytokines and markers of endothelial activation, we get a preview of how the disease progresses in the body. All these technology advancements, when coupled with conventional practices, act in concert to expedite responses and streamline prevention measures on an even larger scale (Adekola et al., 2024). Although the perfect remedy against arboviral infections may still be a robust vaccination, existing circumstances focus on the necessity of having supporting strategies such as maternal immunization and other cost-effective public health interventions. Research on vaccines for related viruses suggests that vaccinating pregnant women—transferring some passive immunity to their offspring—might prevent serious consequences in infants, our most susceptible population; fewer hospitalizations and death rates might result. Economic analyses even indicate that such maternal immunization programs tend to be cost-savers and improve quality-adjusted years of life, and hence are a wise addition to our healthcare systems. Therefore, until vaccines for Zika and Chikungunya specifically become available in the market, combining maternal immunization with sustained vector control measures and quick diagnosis tools is still an effective means of reducing the total impact of the disease (Álvarez Aldeán et al., 2024) (Figure 11.11).

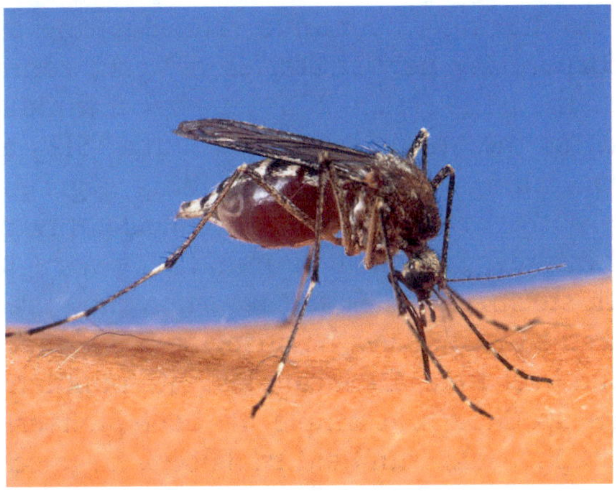

Figure 11.11. Mosquito control.

Source: By Original author: US Department of Agriculture; then denoised rescaled, enhanced with adaptive denoising filters and minimal resharpening, then unscaled to original resolution, for easier refitting at various resolutions. - Picture from the USDA website at http://www.ars.usda.gov/is/graphics/photos/aug00/k4705-9.htm, Public Domain, https://commons.wikimedia.org/w/index.php?curid=64685

11.5.1. Mosquito Control Measures

Mosquito control does have an enormous part to play in preventing outbreaks of diseases such as Zika and chikungunya , diseases that most frequently spread due to Aedes mosquitoes. Most of the time, individuals begin by eliminating the areas where those insects breed, such as puddles and other groups of stagnant water, which is particularly prevalent in congested urban areas. Further there's the application of chemicals – larvicides and adulticides – to clobber numbers, even though we fret about potential environmental harm and the microbes ultimately figuring out these solutions. Recently, scientists have even attempted biological solutions, including introducing bacterial agents like Bacillus thuringiensis israelensis (BTI) that target mosquito larvae with minimal impact on other species. However, the recalcitrant dengue and chikungunya rates in most places result in our having to continue reformulating and incorporating new strategies to gain control over the issue (Miah, 2024). newer techniques such as the sterile insect technique (SIT) are also gaining popularity, providing a greener alternative to the traditional chemical pathways. Essentially, SIT involves inundating a region with sterilized males so that when they breed with the wild females, no offspring are produced – and over time, the local mosquito population dries up. Cuba, for example, has been pioneering this approach, with field trials on a large scale promising dramatic reductions in mosquitoes. These researches, in the majority of instances, support the suggestion that SIT can complement or even replace traditional methods. The researchers continue carrying out complicated research that quantitate how severely SIT cuts disease cases, a step critical to informing public health choices as well as spending plans (Gato et al., 2024). Of course, bumps along the way include logistic and cost issues, but overall, SIT has serious potential for long-term, sustainable disease control of mosquito-borne disease. In addition to town-scale interventions, daily prevention measures also count. Applying mosquito repellents—, or purchased off the shelf—, significantly reduce those annoying bites that transmit disease, disrupting the cycle of transmission. It doesn't do any harm to install simple barriers such as window screens or bed nets that exclude moth-eaten mosquitoes from our homes. Local community actions, where neighbors exchange advice and remind one another to apply repellents and eliminate standing water, tend to enhance these efforts even further. When individual protective routines combine with environmental adjustments and biological approaches, it forms a multi-layered strategy that is more effective in dealing with the complex nature of Aedes mosquitoes and the transmission of arboviral infections (Miah, 2024). In the long term, maintaining the struggle fresh with innovative, responsive mosquito control strategies remains at the core of fighting dangers such as Zika and chikungunya globally.

11.5.2. Personal Protective Measures

Mosquito-borne diseases such as Zika and chikungunya are on the increase, which essentially means we must take care of ourselves. Although large community initiatives attempt to keep mosquitos under wraps, each individual must go the extra mile to reduce their risk. Applying a mosquito repellent is one good step, keeping those diseased little microbes at a distance. Nevertheless, eventually synthetic repellents lose their effectiveness—mosquitos develop immunity and the chemicals may damage the environment as well. In all but a few instances, opting for natural, plant-based ones appears to be an intelligent, less damaging option. These plant-based natural repellents, whose microbe-repelling properties are long established, typically have fewer environmental problems and still prove effective. Overall, utilizing them provides you with a frontline shield that beautifully complements more extensive measures to reduce the spread of these infections (Miah, 2024). Apart from repellents, the use of protective equipment and some modifications in the home contribute significantly to staying away from arboviral infections such as Zika and chikungunya. Long-sleeved shirts, trousers, or any covering garment—especially during hours when mosquitoes are flying around—can drastically reduce the likelihood of being bitten. Eliminating mosquito breeding sites around residences, like standing water in damaged containers or clogged drains, is also extremely crucial. Public health campaigns usually emphasize such remedies, but honestly, it's up to one's personal initiative.

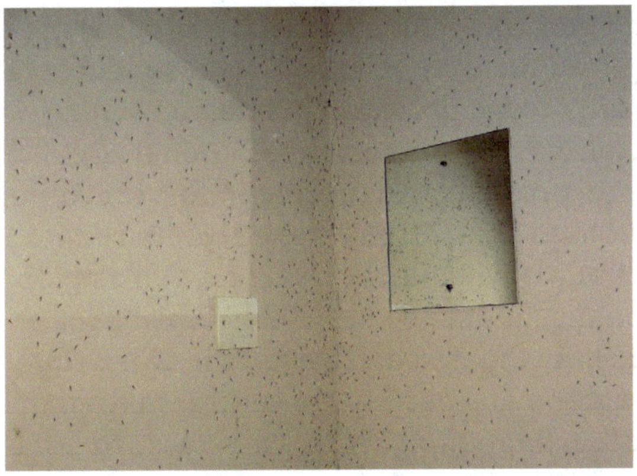

Figure 11.12. Protective tips to reduce mosquito bites and disease transmission.

Source: By Bjørn Christian Tørrissen - Own work by uploader, http://bjornfree.com/galleries.html, CC BY-SA 3.0, https://commons.wikimedia.org/w/index.php?curid=22968008

And some people even attempt DIY approaches (such as, for instance, suffocating local mosquitoes supplemented by natural deterrents), which may act synergistically to reduce the overall number of mosquitoes and biting incidence. Each of these individual steps not only makes you safer but also contributes a little to the community's war on the disease (Miah, 2024). Combining age-old botanical wisdom with modern public health strategies holds the key to a new type of personal protection against these diseases. To cite just a few examples, essential oils from certain plants such as Azadirachta, Eucalyptus, and Ocimum exhibit remarkable anti-larval and insecticidal activities, providing a convenient alternative to chemical toxins. Familiarity with how these plant substances function will allow us to adapt their use for keeping mosquitoes at bay. In general, marketing these plant-based repellents could also reduce the environmental cost associated with chemical repellents, aligning individual safety with larger ecological aims. Introducing these natural alternatives into daily practice—even imperfectly—can enhance your own protection and contribute to overall efforts to better control outbreaks (Kaushik et al., 2023) (Figure 11.12).

11.5.3. Public Health Initiatives and Education

Mosquito-borne diseases such as Zika and Chikungunya continue to cause concern to many, and fighting them involves more than responding, more than just reacting, it involves nincorporating prevention with education. Community outreach has played a crucial role in most scenarios, as it assists individuals at risk in acquiring habits that hinder virus spread. In Brazil, to cite one case, research demonstrates that when school children are taught about the *Aedes aegypti* mosquito (chief offender), they begin to see how viruses get passed along and how they can prevent it. These children, now with an improved understanding of arboviruses, help families take action in an unlikely but crucial way and continue mosquito control efforts. Interactive and culturally sensitive lessons appear to prompt people to take simple actions, such as draining standing water or adopting basic protective practices—ones that, collectively, not only raise immediate health benefits but also construct durable community resilience against epidemics (Caprara et al., 2023). Climate fluctuations, with all the uncertainty they bring, usually agitate the transmission of these diseases, so mass public health campaigns have had to come to terms with environmental changes impacting mosquito populations. Pacific Islands, for example, provide the clearest explanation of how weather and health threat combination.

Usually, scientists find that combining stable climate research and local health promotion can assist with addressing spikes of dengue, Zika, and Chikungunya. For most occasions, increasing health care systems by spreading local information works best, in particular when tight resources are on hand. When education is synchronized with these constantly changing environmental conditions, health interventions become more adaptable and effective, opening the door to a rapid response that tracks the turns and turns of disease trends (Boenecke et al., 2019). In addition, collaborating globally, such as with the World Mosquito Program, demonstrates that integrating scientific knowledge with community-based work can support public health education. These programs combine new vector control methods with practical outreach, and that in turn increases their total effect. Messaging that not only provides information but also encourages people toward improved behaviors has consistently reduced transmission rates. Making educational materials specific to a variety of different cultural contexts—and relying on local knowledge—further increases how effectively messages persist. In addition, when education institutions, households, and neighborhood health providers collaborate, a mutual sense of responsibility is created that inspires both short-term and long-term action. This collaborative environment not only assists in managing active outbreaks but also makes the public health system more resilient, preparing it better to address future occurrences with Zika and Chikungunya (Boenecke et al., 2019; Caprara et al., 2023).

11.6. Global Response and Research

Viral outbreaks have been a rising issue in recent times, with instances and severity growing by the day. Just consider how Zika and Chikungunya have emerged in every corner of the world – it's not a clear tale of microbes, but a complex one of insect-borne diseases in our world so interconnected. Early warning systems usually fell short, and public health teams were left playing catch-up to change their surveillance strategy. It now appears obvious that a worldwide response—one that combines rapid info exchange, new diagnostic concepts, and genuine community engagement—is required to stay ahead of these outbreaks. Lessons from previous pandemics, along with contemporary experiences, generally attest to the pressing requirement for coordinated responses and strengthened preparedness at both our own country levels as well as globally (Mohanasundari et al., 2024; Onyebuchi et al., 2025). At the research level, the work that has been done has been quite central to teasing out what's happening with viruses such as Zika and Chikungunya. Scientists have had to spend considerable time understanding how these viruses travel, what symptoms they introduce, and how their insect vectors act, which in turn identifies the groups at highest risk. Latest advancements in molecular diagnostics and genomic sequencing have accelerated outbreak investigations, enabling real-time tracking (even if it is imperfect) and improved prediction models. Meanwhile, scientists in epidemiology, entomology, and immunology have worked together—sometimes in surprising combinations—to craft possible vaccines and antiviral drugs by hand. Nevertheless, there are still gaps in translating these research advances into broadly applied, enduring solutions, suggesting that we still require firm investment and tighter cross-sector collaborations (Onyebuchi et al., 2025). Successfully addressing Zika and Chikungunya requires an all-hands-on-deck strategy that crosses various sectors, particularly because low-resource communities bear the impact significantly harder. It's not merely a matter of bolstering health systems; it's also ensuring communities have access to prevention measures such as effective insect management and local campaigns. Countries, as it happens, have to collaborate even once the outbreak has been contained by financing capacity-building activities that equip all to prepare for future danger. Policymakers would do well to remember recent crises to tackle longstanding healthcare disparities, while open information sharing and relatively adaptable funding mechanisms leave the utilization of resources as optimal as possible. Overall, with continuous, combined efforts in research and response, the global community has a greater chance of mitigating the effects of such viruses and strengthening defenses against emerging infectious threats (Mohanasundari et al., 2024; Onyebuchi et al., 2025) (Figure 11.13).

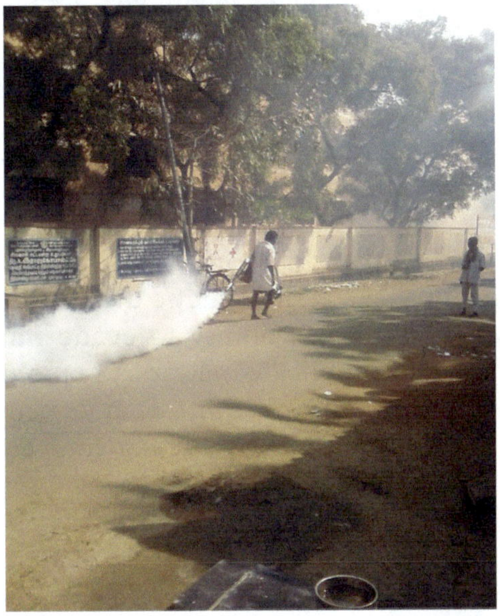

Figure 11.13. Zika virus a global health emergency.

Source: By Srithern - Own work, CC BY-SA 3.0, https://commons.wikimedia.org/w/index.php?curid=23524718

11.6.1. International Health Organizations' Roles

Diseases such as Zika and Chikungunya illustrate how crucial worldwide health teams are when outbreaks strike. These agencies serve as centers that gather snippets of epidemiological information, disseminate reliable updates, and coordinate responses that span national borders in ways you may not anticipate. Consider Zika, for example, the World Health Organization called a global health emergency that increased awareness and initiated monitoring and prevention efforts (Ansari et al., 2016). Their ability to take disconnected reports and create one comprehensive picture means that most countries receive advice sooner in most instances. They also provide technical assistance to countries that lack the appropriate infrastructure for activities such as vector control or case management. And when you think about diseases transmitted by mosquitoes—animals whose range seldom adheres to clear boundaries—it's obvious that a concerted, if at times loosely coordinated, effort is invaluable in controlling the risks to public health. And beyond data collection and raising alarms, these groups determine what the public knows and does in the face of outbreaks. They design recommendations for vulnerable populations, occasionally instructing, for instance, pregnant women to eschew travel to Zika-affected zones due to possible fetal complications (Ansari et al., 2016). Such advice doesn't only guard personal conduct. it ultimately finds its way into large-scale health policies that can impose travel restrictions or divert funds to alternative needs. They cooperate closely with governments, healthcare professionals and researchers, combining knowledge from a variety of disciplines in an entirely human, if slightly lopsided, partnership. And the integration of these ideas stirs innovation in new diagnostic tools and directs priorities toward vaccine research—a necessity, particularly with cross-reactivity with other similar viruses proving to be so challenging. To summarize, the policies and public education that follow reduce infection levels and contain the far-reaching effects of outbreaks. In addition to direct health measures, international organizations also smooth economic disruptions that outbreaks induce—especially in areas that are heavily reliant on tourism. Epidemics such as those caused by Zika and Chikungunya tend to intimidate tourists, which then devastates livelihood at the local level; after all, where fear travels, tourism declines and the economy is hit. Understanding this, the organizations collaborate with the tourism industry to combination risk communication and utilitarian travel recommendations. This combinationed approach not only prevents the spread of disease but also enhances economic confidence, sustaining travel where it is most needed. By interacting with several sectors, these groups demonstrate that fighting an outbreak is not all about medicine—, also about economics and community. Ultimately, their contribution is instrumental in developing response strategies that strike a balance between health security and the demand for economic stability.

11.6.2. Ongoing Research and Vaccine Development

Researchers have been working hard to confront the unpleasant effects of the Zika virus with new research and innovative vaccine concepts. The urgency comes from the rate at which the virus infects and its connections to serious problems such as Guillain–Barré syndrome and birth defects like microcephaly. Bands of scientists have been experimenting with combinations of vaccine platforms to design shots that will be both effective and safe while coping with the virus's unconventional pathology and uncertain spread. The initial laboratory and clinical trials already suggest vaccines capable of enhancing solid immunity. It's a delicate problem, particularly when attempting to safeguard vulnerable populations such as pregnant women and their unborn infants, which makes continuous effort a world necessity (Buitrago-Pab et al., 2024). While this is happening, other scientists are thinking outside the box by relying on new computer methods to accelerate vaccine development. Conventional vaccine development can be painstakingly slow and resource-intensive, so *in-silico* approaches are being employed to search for potential immune triggers sooner. A clever development has been employing the Immune Epitope Database web server to target small peptide motifs on the virus coat that can induce a robust immune response without inducing allergic or toxic side reactions. One peptide known as 6E, derived from the envelope protein E of the Zika virus, has appeared very encouraging, with preliminary tests indicating strong antigenicity and a favorable safety profile. However, these findings on the computer need firm *in vitro* and *in vivo* validation before they can finally support a vaccine formulation (Ansori et al., 2024). Despite learning much about how Zika functions at a molecular and immune level, translating these laboratory concepts into generally accessible vaccines is a daunting ascent. The genetic diversity of the virus and its stealth ability to evade immune systems only complicate matters. Compounding these challenges are ethical and practical concerns surrounding conducting clinical trials in vulnerable populations, such as pregnant women, which must be considered with care. Ongoing surveillance and adaptive research steps are essential to fine-tune vaccine candidates and anticipate any viral mutations that could undermine their efficacy. Global collaboration and consistent funding are essential to sustain these initiatives—not just to regulate Zika outbreaks but also to illuminate other arboviral issues like Chikungunya. Ultimately, continued investigation and a little bit of trial-and-error with vaccine development are needed to keep these mosquito-transmitted diseases at bay and minimize their public health impact (Ansori et al., 2024; Buitrago-Pab et al., 2024) (Figure 11.14).

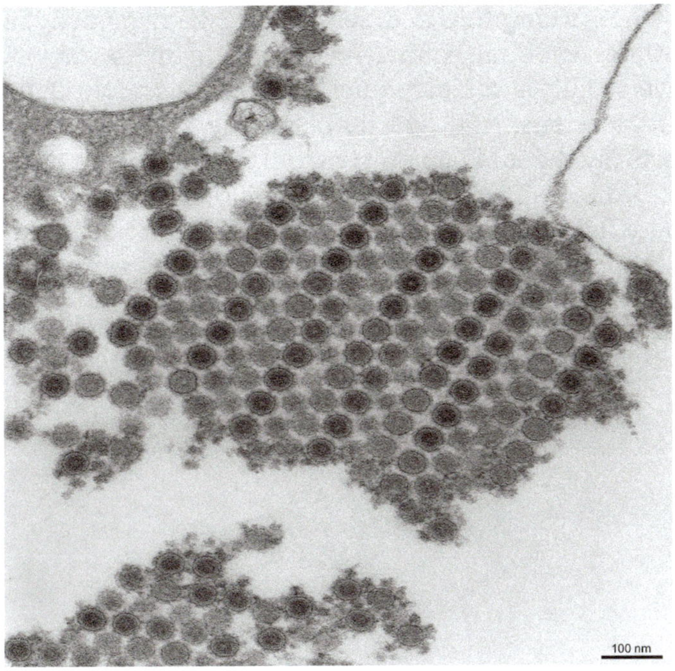

Figure 11.14. FDA grants fast track designation for a Chikungunya vaccine.

Source: By Cynthia Goldsmith - Centers for Disease Control and Prevention - http://phil.cdc.gov/PHIL_Images/17369/17369.tif, Public Domain, https://commons.wikimedia.org/w/index.php?curid=34743799

11.6.3. Challenges in Managing Outbreaks

Epidemics such as Zika and Chikungunya don't follow a clear trajectory—rather, they streak off in unpredictable directions. Zika, for instance, began in these tiny, equatorial niches further, seemingly overnight, spread from regions of Africa and Asia to the Americas. This rapid leap left public health professionals scrambling to respond, with diagnostic tools and vaccines trailing behind. It isn't merely the mosquitoes that transmit the virus; there's now talk of sexual transmission as well, and that only further complicates the issue. Further you throw in pathogens like dengue and even Chikungunya themselves—diseases that present so similarly to one another—the entire process of finding them and trying to stem outbreaks becomes all the more complicated (Ansari et al., 2016). When it comes to regulating these arboviruses, the absence of strong infrastructure truly throws a wrench in. Take Brazil: all the effort on the part of health agencies to inform and monitor groups at risk notwithstanding, the disparity between urban areas and rural areas leaves communities more vulnerable to large-scale outbreaks. In much of the rural areas, simply there are not enough health clinics and qualified personnel, so prevention and treatment programs are left with huge gaps. Grassroots programs, such as mere health education campaigns and even health workers making house calls, have proved to be effective in making people realize the danger. However, you see, while these viruses continue to mutate, sustained government support is still paramount—in general, without consistent funding and an equitable allocation of resources, the problem of controlling outbreaks just gets bigger (Tesha et al., 2016). Aside from these logistical challenges, determining stable diagnostic techniques has been the actual headache. Tests tend to get the signals confused when attempting to differentiate Zika from dengue or Chikungunya, which results in delays—sometimes even miscounts—, it is difficult to know what's happening. The reality that we don't have readily available, quick tests means early detection misses the target, postponing essential interventions. And, given that there are no licensed vaccines for Zika or Chikungunya, health efforts must double up on controlling mosquitoes and public health education. And with severe neurological complications, such as microcephaly in infants and even outbreaks of Guillain-Barré syndrome in adults, there is an obvious, urgent demand for new diagnostic and treatment technologies. In all but one instance, embracing new solutions should be a researcher's top agenda globally (Ansari et al., 2016).

CLOSER LOOK

TRANSMISSION DYNAMICS AND VECTOR CONTROL CHALLENGES

Vector-borne diseases, such as malaria, dengue, Zika, and chikungunya, are transmitted through arthropods like mosquitoes, ticks, and flies. Understanding the transmission dynamics of these diseases is essential for effective control, as it involves studying how pathogens move between vectors, hosts, and the environment. Factors such as vector density, biting behavior, host immunity, and environmental conditions influence transmission intensity and outbreak potential.

Vector ecology is closely linked to disease spread. Seasonal changes, temperature, rainfall, and humidity affect vector survival, reproduction, and feeding patterns. For example, warmer temperatures accelerate mosquito development and reduce the incubation period of pathogens like Plasmodium or dengue virus, increasing the risk of outbreaks. Urbanization, deforestation, and human mobility also create favorable conditions for vector proliferation, complicating control efforts.

Controlling vectors presents multiple challenges. Traditional methods, including insecticide spraying, bed nets, and larval habitat removal, face limitations due to insecticide resistance, behavioral adaptation of vectors, and difficulties in reaching remote or densely populated areas. Additionally, socio-economic and cultural factors, such as reluctance to use protective measures or improper water storage practices, reduce the effectiveness of control programs.

Globalization and climate change further exacerbate vector-borne disease risks. Emerging vectors are expanding their geographic ranges, introducing pathogens to populations with little immunity. Inadequate surveillance systems and limited resources in low-income regions make it difficult to detect and respond to outbreaks promptly.

Addressing these challenges requires an integrated vector management (IVM) approach, combining chemical, biological, environmental, and community-based interventions. Advances in genetic control methods, such as sterile insect techniques and gene drive mosquitoes, offer promising new strategies. Effective vector control also demands community engagement, robust urveillance, and international collaboration to prevent the spread of vector-borne diseases.

Understanding transmission dynamics and overcoming vector control challenges are critical for reducing the burden of vector-borne infections worldwide.

Summary

Mosquito-borne diseases such as Zika and Chikungunya continue to plague world health, particularly in tropical and subtropical regions. Aedes mosquitos, which breed only in the best of conditions, add an extra layer of complexity to the issue. As temperature and rain vary, they tend to create the perfect locations for breeding these mosquitoes, thereby increasing the infection rate. This is where it becomes evident that monitoring weather patterns and environmental signs is important for early detection of harmful outbreaks (Chien et al., 2019). In most instances, knowing precisely how these elements interact with each other assists in identifying high-risk areas and informs more intelligent, targeted interventions. Attempting to outsmart these diseases isn't as easy as managing mosquitos by itself. It's a good thing that the issue runs deeper. combining social, environmental, and community considerations, as well, is really important. With no antiviral medications in particular on the shelf, prevention is our best protection. Recent molecular research – for instance, investigations into how analogous viruses act in the wild – typically indicate that monitoring how such agents change, and even jump from host to host, is a necessity for keeping ahead of possible new threats (Cafiero et al., 2019). This wider view, while slightly neater, provides us with additional information on why these viruses evolve and persist, impacting the efficacy of how we ready our defenses. Overall, the increasing number of cases of Zika and Chikungunya demonstrates how climate, nature, and even our behaviors all combination together in unforeseen manners. Meteorological information has been quite valuable in informing resource mobilization and predicting outbreak patterns, but ongoing study and adaptive approaches must stay in the equation. Coupling environmental surveillance with grass-roots, community-led responses may very well close the gap in our early warning mechanisms even when faced with periodic setbacks, preventing catastrophic consequences. All of these mixed, sometimes chaotic, endeavors are important to help cut back on both disease and mortality as climate change and globalization continue to reshape the terrain (Cafiero et al., 2019; Chien et al., 2019).

Zika and Chikungunya introduce a variation of problematic issues, mostly due to their principal villain—the *Aedes aegypti* mosquito. These diseases, which constitute about what people sometimes refer to as Aedes-borne infectious diseases (ABIDs), have struck areas from Africa to the Americas and even Asia, surfacing again and again. There are international standards and lots of new ideas for controlling mosquitoes, but in the majority of instances, nations still collide with significant obstacles when implementing these ideas. Zoom in, and you notice problems on multiple levels: the large health system, close-knit community attitudes, and even people's day-to-day habits. This multi-faceted approach demonstrates that defeating these challenges requires a combination of unambiguous risk messaging, domestic cultural understanding, and behavioral modifications attuned to the setting at hand (Mulderij-Jansen et al., 2023). To put it short, it's not merely the biology of the mosquito—social and systemic concerns wedded heavily to the biology have a considerable impact. Then there's the entire aspect of things that hits our pocketbooks, like tourism, a big bucks driver that is hugely sensitive to health scares. The threat of these diseases can easily scare off travelers, with less business and putting pressure on local economies. For instance, in locations such as Guatemala, it is said through studies that by working in a collaborative effort together with media, and conveying health risk information to people in straight, straightforward fashion, tourist confidence increases, that helps to sustain the local economy in a stabilized manner (Rivera et al., 2024). Considering all of it—from media reporting to how tourists feel and even the way stakeholders react—it is evident that integrating public health initiatives with tourism management is essential to curb disease transmission and maintain economic drivers chugging along. Combined, health, social, and economic studies create a portrait in which combating Zika and Chikungunya is not a single-issue issue. Managing these diseases involves taking on mosquito control directly in addition to enlisting community engagement and candid risk interactions. More broadly, when disease outbreaks cross over with industries such as tourism, it reminds us that we require coordination between multiple disciplines—weighing health priorities against the pressure of actual commerce. Promisingly, new research is suggesting creative ideas and policy suggestions that might scale up disease prevention and community resilience. Overall, combat against Zika and Chikungunya requires an effective cocktail of scientific knowledge, public support, and intersectoral cooperation to control both health issues and the economic spillover effects (Mulderij-Jansen et al., 2023; Rivera et al., 2024).

References

1. Adekola, H., Wahab, K. A., Odunsi, O. E., Abesin, T. A., & Oyesanya, O. A. (2024). Current diagnostics and biomarkers for arboviral infections (a review on Dengue, Zika, West Nile and Chikungunya viruses). *Problems of Virology*. https://www.semanticscholar.org/paper/3dd0c580ca93e45bd4a2dc2a15ae494dba9e5309 (accessed on 7 May 2025).
2. Alcantara, L. C. J., de Siqueira, I. C., do Rosário, M. S., Ernst, T., et al. (2019). Anti-ganglioside antibodies in patients with Zika virus infection-associated Guillain-Barré syndrome in Brazil. *PLoS Neglected Tropical Diseases, 13*(9), e0007695. https://doi.org/10.1371/journal.pntd.0007695.
3. Álvarez Aldeán, J., Rivero Calle, I., Rodríguez Fernandez, R., Aceituno Mata, S., Bellmunt, A., Prades, M., Law, A., et al. (2024). Cost-effectiveness analysis of maternal immunization with RSVpreF vaccine for the prevention of respiratory syncytial virus among infants in Spain. *Infectious Diseases and Therapy, 13*(2), 1315–1331. https://www.semanticscholar.org/paper/a638b16a4ae7e4325b06d1b75f7b65d3dde07686 (accessed on 7 May 2025).
4. Ansari, A., Chang, C., Gershwin, M. E., Ortiz, B. L., et al. (2016). The Zika outbreak of the 21st century. *Journal of Autoimmunity, 68*, 1–13. https://doi.org/10.1016/j.jaut.2016.02.006.
5. Ansori, N. M., Sutriyansyah, R. A., Hilmi, M., Iman, I., Valenta, C. A., Sulung, T., Indira, N., et al. (2024). Epitope-driven vaccine development for Zika virus: A bioinformatics approach. *Journal Technology Laboratories, 98–105*. https://www.semanticscholar.org/paper/767382c759c39a7c7042956ada174adcc5a7aa18 (accessed on 7 May 2025).
6. Badshah, S., Faisal, S., Muhammad, A., Poulson, B. G., Emwas, A. H., & Jaremko, M. (2021). Antiviral activities of flavonoids. *Biomedicine & Pharmacotherapy, 140*, 111596. https://doi.org/10.1016/j.biopha.2021.111596.
7. Balakrishnan, V. S. (2022). WHO launches global initiative for arboviral diseases. *The Lancet Microbe, 3*(6), e407. https://doi.org/10.1016/s2666-5247(22)00130-6.
8. Bhandari, V., Taksande, A., & Sapkale, B. (2023). Disease transmission and diagnosis of Zika virus. *Cureus, 15*(1), Article e12345. https://www.semanticscholar.org/paper/23abc1f7df38a9639e70f3eb0e0e5e5a2d73c369 (accessed on 7 May 2025).
9. Boenecke, J., Filho, W. L., Gogoi, A., Korovou, E., et al. (2019). Climate change, health and mosquito-borne diseases: Trends and implications to the Pacific region. https://core.ac.uk/download/286710798.pdf (accessed on 7 May 2025).
10. Bomar, H. (2018). *Understanding Zika Virus in Rural Costa Rica: Integrating Medical Anthropology and Public Health*. https://core.ac.uk/download/216939681.pdf (accessed on 7 May 2025).
11. Brady, O. J., & Hay, S. I. (2019). The global expansion of dengue: How *Aedes aegypti* mosquitoes enabled the first pandemic arbovirus. *Annual Review of Entomology, 65*, 191–208. https://doi.org/10.1146/annurev-ento-011019-024918.
12. Buitrago-Pabón, A. L., Ruiz-Sáenz, S., Jiménez-Alberto, A., Aparicio-Ozores, G., Castelán-Vega, J., & Ribas-Aparicio, R. (2024). An update on Zika virus vaccine development and new research approaches. *Microbiology Research, 15*(2), 667–692. https://www.semanticscholar.org/paper/b32af7708dd50a1700093e215336d2f2446f3689 (accessed on 7 May 2025).
13. Cafiero, M. A., Carbone, A., Caruso, M., Centelleghe, C., et al. (2019). Dolphin morbillivirus in Eurasian otters, Italy. https://core.ac.uk/download/185557129.pdf (accessed on 7 May 2025).

14. Perfil dos escolares e concepções sobre as arboviroses na abordagem ecossistêmica da saúde. (2023). *Recima21, 4*(2), e422751. https://doi.org/10.47820/recima21.v4i2.2751Carlton, J., Cedrim, D., Garcia, A., McClean, P., et al. (2016). Recruiting from the network: Discovering Twitter users who can help combat Zika epidemics. http://arxiv.org/abs/1703.03928 (accessed on 7 May 2025).
15. Cedrim, D., Daniilakis, M., Garcia, A., Missier, P., et al. (2016). Tracking dengue epidemics using Twitter content classification and topic modelling. http://arxiv.org/abs/1605.00968 (accessed on 7 May 2025).
16. Chien, L. C., Perez, A., & Sy, F. (2019). Identifying high-risk areas of Zika virus infection by meteorological factors in Colombia. https://core.ac.uk/download/250588218.pdf (accessed on 7 May 2025).
17. Chrisafis, G. C. (2017). Historical patterns of arboviral seroprevalence across Africa and Asia. https://core.ac.uk/download/84397690.pdf (accessed on 7 May 2025).
18. de Bruin, E., Kasbergen, L. M. R., Koopmans, M. P. G., Nieuwenhuijse, D. F., et al. (2023). The increasing complexity of arbovirus serology: An in-depth systematic review on cross-reactivity. https://core.ac.uk/download/588754041.pdf (accessed on 7 May 2025).
19. España, G., Hogea, C., Guignard, A., ten Bosch, Q. A., Morrison, A. C., Smith, D. L., Scott, T. W., et al. (2019). Biased efficacy estimates in phase-III dengue vaccine trials due to heterogeneous exposure and differential detectability of primary infections across trial arms. *PLOS ONE, 14*(1), e0210041. https://doi.org/10.1371/journal.pone.0210041.
20. Gato, R., Menéndez, Z., Rodriguez, M., Gutiérrez-Bugallo, G., & Marquetti, M. D. C. (2024). Advancing the art of mosquito control: The journey of the sterile insect technique against *Aedes aegypti* in Cuba. *Infectious Diseases of Poverty, 13*, Article 20. https://www.semanticscholar.org/paper/3f5956bb218c5989d10d55e793e03ff133f7c720 (accessed on 7 May 2025).
21. Grazzini, G., Liumbruno, G. M., Marano, G., & Pupella, S. (2016). Zika virus and the never-ending story of emerging pathogens and transfusion medicine. *Blood Transfusion, 14*(2), 95–100. https://core.ac.uk/download/54532486.pdf (accessed on 7 May 2025).
22. Hassan, T. A., Hollander, S., van Lent, L., Schwedeler, M., & Tahoun, A. (2020). *Firm-level exposure to epidemic diseases: COVID-19, SARS, and H1N1* (NBER Working Paper No. 26971). National Bureau of Economic Research. https://doi.org/10.3386/w26971.
23. Hill, S. C., Neto de Vasconcelos, J., Neto, Z., Jandondo, D., Zé-Zé, L., Santana Aguiar, R., Xavier, J., et al. (2019). Emergence of the Asian lineage of Zika virus in Angola: An outbreak investigation. *The Lancet Infectious Diseases, 19*(10), 1138–1147. https://doi.org/10.1016/S1473-3099(19)30293-2.
24. Kaushik, M., Yadav, J., Singh, A., & Dubey, M. (2023). A systematic review of plant-based mosquito repellents and their activity. *Indian Journal of Natural Products and Resources, 14(3), 347–359.* https://www.semanticscholar.org/paper/48da6aac8eccc6b8d2a1d4863cf3460e864b2571 (accessed on 7 May 2025).
25. Kolimenakis, A., Heinz, S., Wilson, M. L., Winkler, V., Yakob, L., Michaelakis, A., Papachristos, D., et al. (2021). The role of urbanization in the spread of *Aedes* mosquitoes and the diseases they transmit: A systematic review. *PLoS Neglected Tropical Diseases, 15*, e0009631. https://doi.org/10.1371/journal.pntd.0009631.
26. Lima, K. M. G., Medeiros-De-Morais, C. D. L., & Santos, M. C. D. (2020). ATR-FTIR spectroscopy

for virus identification: A powerful alternative. https://core.ac.uk/download/326231601.pdf (accessed on 7 May 2025).

27. Luke-Currier, A., Alsamara, I., Aguilera-Cruz, J., Airapetian, K., Silaghi, L. A., & Hashim, Z. P. (2023). *On Urgently Tackling the Mosquito-Borne Diseases in the European Union*. https://core.ac.uk/download/567838799.pdf (accessed on 7 May 2025).
28. Miah, M. A. H. (2024). Dengue management through mosquito control: Asphyxiation techniques and homemade repellents for skin protection. *Ecology Journal*. https://www.semanticscholar.org/paper/b7499262688e7b258e3dbbadc0d2686f87b295ef (accessed on 7 May 2025).
29. Mohanasundari, S., Kiran, K. P., Vashishtha, N., Singh, R., Rani, B., & Nagamani, N. (2024). Overview of emerging viruses, other viruses and great pandemic of the 21st century. *A and V Pub International Journal of Nursing and Medical Research, 3(1), 37–40*. https://www.semanticscholar.org/paper/0f174db412005e70365795c9c44026046063698b (accessed on 7 May 2025).
30. Mordecai, E. A., Caldwell, J. M., Grossman, M. K., Lippi, C. A., Johnson, L. R., Neira, M., Rohr, J. R., et al. (2019). Thermal biology of mosquito-borne disease. *Ecology Letters, 22*, 1690–1708. https://doi.org/10.1111/ele.13335.
31. Mulderij-Jansen, V. (2023). *Preventing the next Aedes-borne arboviral disease epidemic*. [Thesis fully internal (DIV), University of Groningen]. University of Groningen. https://doi.org/10.33612/diss.651832082
32. Nasrin, F., Tsuruga, K., Utomo, D. I. S., Chowdhury, A. D., & Park, E. Y. (2021). Design and analysis of a single system of impedimetric biosensors for the detection of mosquito-borne viruses. *Biosensors, 11*, 376. https://doi.org/10.3390/bios11100376.
33. Onyebuchi, C., Okeke, H. N., Uzochukwu, O. H., Racheal, A. O., Kolade, E., Onyebuchi, A. O., Odekhe, E., et al. (2025). Emerging infectious diseases and global response strategies: A systematic review and meta-analysis. *International Journal of Research and Scientific Innovation*. https://www.semanticscholar.org/paper/278b7b6b2a3f4bbe997310e0677c4c9cbf456442 (accessed on 7 May 2025).
34. Piret, J., & Boivin, G. (2021). Pandemics throughout history. *Frontiers in Microbiology, 11*, Article 631736. https://doi.org/10.3389/fmicb.2020.631736.
35. Qin, S., Tang, X., Chen, Y. T., Chen, K., Fan, N., Xiao, W., Zheng, Q., & Qian, Q. (2022). mRNA-based therapeutics: Powerful and versatile tools to combat diseases. *Signal Transduction and Targeted Therapy, 7*(1), Article 1. https://doi.org/10.1038/s41392-022-01007-w.
36. Rama, K., de Roo, A. D., Louwsma, T., Hofstra, H. S., Gurgel do Amaral, G. S., Vondeling, G. T., Postma, M. J., et al. (2024). Clinical outcomes of chikungunya: A systematic literature review and meta-analysis. *PLOS Neglected Tropical Diseases, 18*(1), e0011582. https://www.semanticscholar.org/paper/865be53207b6e3aef6aaf441e8f6d7831596b60f (accessed on 7 May 2025).
37. Rivera, E. P. (2024). *Exploring the Social Dynamics of Mosquito-Borne Diseases and COVID-19 on Tourism Management* (Master's thesis, Florida International University). *Electronic Theses and Dissertations*, 4062. https://core.ac.uk/download/624161443.pdf (accessed on 7 May 2025).
38. Saleh, F., Kitau, J., Konradsen, F., Mboera, L. E. G., & Schiøler, K. L. (2021). Emerging epidemics: Is the Zanzibar healthcare system ready to detect and respond to mosquito-borne viral

diseases? *BMC Health Services Research, 21*, Article 1214. https://doi.org/10.1186/s12913-021-06867-6.

39. San Lio, R. M., Favara, G., Maugeri, A., Barchitta, M., & Agodi, A. (2023). How antimicrobial resistance is linked to climate change: An overview of two intertwined global challenges. *International Journal of Environmental Research and Public Health, 20*(3), 1681. https://doi.org/10.3390/ijerph20031681.
40. Tesha, F. (2016). *Tools and methods for Zika prevention in Cachoeira, Bahia* (Master's thesis). https://core.ac.uk/download/232738247.pdf (accessed on 7 May 2025).
41. Tidball, J. (2017). *The Buzz Behind the Bite* (Master's thesis). University of Kansas. https://core.ac.uk/download/267188350.pdf (accessed on 7 May 2025).
42. Trovato, M., Sartorius, R., D'Apice, L., Manco, R., & De Berardinis, P. (2020). Viral emerging diseases: Challenges in developing vaccination strategies. *Frontiers in Immunology, 11*, Article 2130. https://doi.org/10.3389/fimmu.2020.02130.
43. Utarini, A., Indriani, C., Ahmad, R. A., Tantowijoyo, W., Arguni, E., Ansari, M. R., Supriyati, E., et al. (2021). Efficacy of Wolbachia-infected mosquito deployments for the control of dengue. *New England Journal of Medicine, 384*, 2177–2186. https://doi.org/10.1056/nejmoa2030243.
44. Wang, G. H., Du, J., Chu, C. Y., Madhav, M., Hughes, G. L., & Champer, J. (2022). Symbionts and gene drive: Two strategies to combat vector-borne disease. *Trends in Genetics, 38*(8), 708–723. https://doi.org/10.1016/j.tig.2022.02.013.
45. Wilke, A. B. B., Cabán-Martinez, A. J., Ajelli, M., Vasquez, C., Petrie, W. D., & Beier, J. C. (2019). Mosquito adaptation to the extreme habitats of urban construction sites. *Trends in Parasitology, 35*, 607–614. https://doi.org/10.1016/j.pt.2019.05.009.
46. Wilson, A. L., Courtenay, O., Kelly-Hope, L. A., Scott, T. W., Takken, W., Torr, S. J., & Lindsay, S. W. (2020). The importance of vector control for the control and elimination of vector-borne diseases. *PLoS Neglected Tropical Diseases, 14*, e0007831. https://doi.org/10.1371/journal.pntd.0007831.
47. Zhang, Y. Z., Chen, Y., Wang, W., Qin, X. C., & Holmes, E. C. (2019). Expanding the RNA virosphere by unbiased metagenomics. *Annual Review of Virology, 6*, 119–139. https://doi.org/10.1146/annurev-virology-092818-015851.

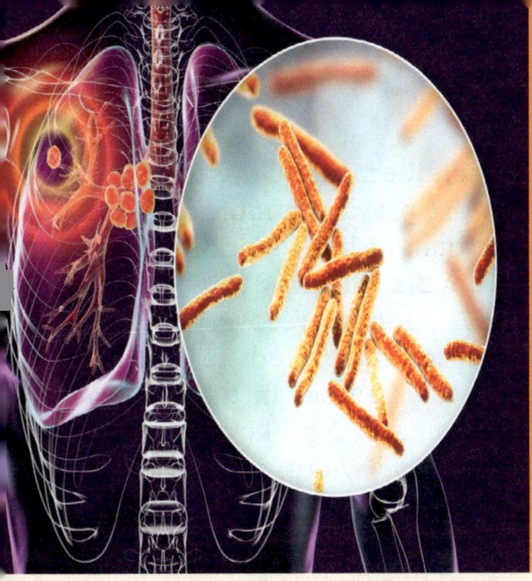

Chapter 12

TUBERCULOSIS (TB)

Contents

Introduction

In the modern changing health environment, infectious diseases become a whole lot more complicated when you add in different underlying conditions. Consider TB, for example. Caused by the bacterium *Mycobacterium tuberculosis*, it's still one of the most lethal diseases out there, particularly in areas also struggling with conditions like HIV/AIDS or diabetes. It's noteworthy that TB tends to remain hidden in its latent state, infecting about one third of the world's population, and leaving behind an ongoing, persistent threat of setting off an infectious episode. With populations shifting and disease patterns changing, there's evidently a need—broadly speaking—to get really down into the details of what's fueling infection and how to control outbreaks, a problem that's even more challenging to tackle in low-resource environments. There's been a lot of communication in recent times regarding how other diseases, specifically diabetes, fit into the TB equation. Some new research even indicates that diabetes could triple the risk of becoming infected with TB, likely because it disrupts the immune system. Sub-Saharan African research, where both TB and HIV are prevalent, indicates that metabolic problems with glucose occur far more often in TB patients than in healthy individuals, suggesting a quite complex relationship between these diseases. This double whammy truly makes treatment more difficult—patients with diabetes and TB tend to have reduced recovery, worse treatment outcomes, and increased mortality, highlighting the need for integrated healthcare strategies immediately (Faurholt-Jepsen et al., 2013). It is not only these diseases in themselves that make things so challenging; public health interventions are also hindered by large gaps in thorough data, particularly in developing nations. With little health data and widespread cultural misunderstandings, stigma, and misinformation, policymakers find it increasingly difficult to craft targeted interventions. Some researchers have even begun examining online search patterns to gauge how people think about TB and other diseases in Africa. This method—non-traditional as it is—unmasks broad concerns, suggests educational deficits, and facilitates guiding the way towards more focused health education and policy adjustments (Abebe et al., 2019). Overall, filling these info gaps is central to increasing TB awareness and engaging communities more in prevention and treatment efforts (Figure 12.1).

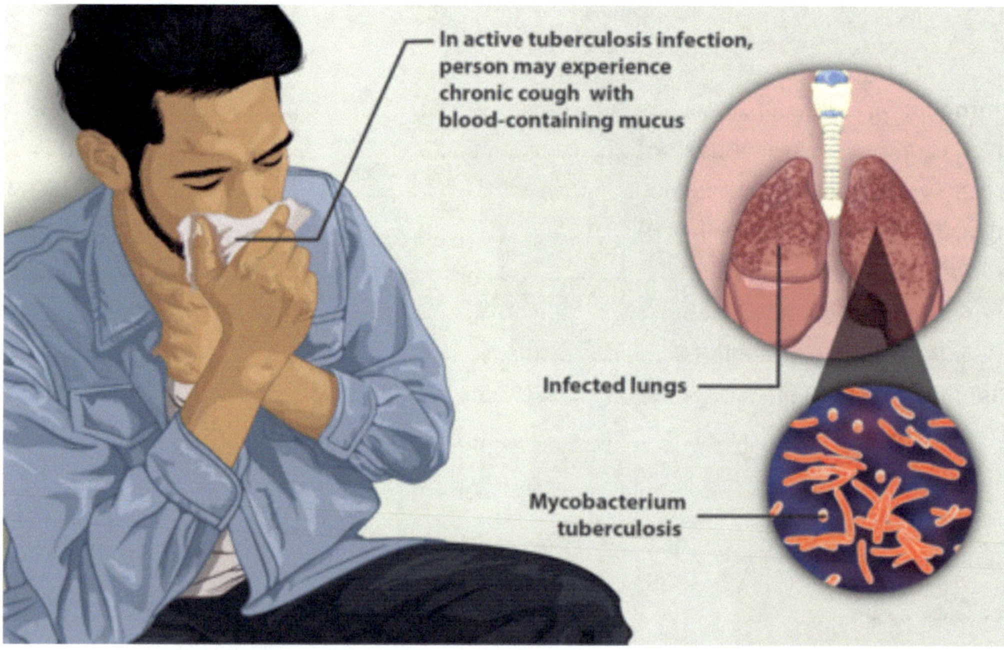

Figure 12.1. Tuberculosis (TB).

Source: By https://www.myupchar.com/ - https://www.myupchar.com/en/disease/tuberculosis-tb, CC BY-SA 4.0, https://commons.wikimedia.org/w/index.php?curid=82880185***Definition of Tuberculosis (TB)***

Infectious disease appears in two interrelated forms: one, the biology itself; and two, the significant impact they have on society globally. TB, commonly known as such by most people, is largely caused by a microbe called *Mycobacterium tuberculosis*. This bacterium likes to lodge itself in the lungs, but it will venture into other organs as well, which makes its symptoms a little here and there. When a person infected sneezes or coughs, small droplets containing the microbe hang suspended – particularly in closed, poorly aired areas. TB is a recalcitrant public health problem despite widespread control efforts. TB tends to present in two modes; one latent, silent mode without symptoms until, abruptly, it can change to an active phase characterized by prolonged cough, fever, and wasting. Evidently, knowledge of these two presentations is crucial to appropriate diagnosis and management. Taking a closer look at the molecular aspect, TB's longevity is all about *Mycobacterium tuberculosis*' clever tricks. terms, this pathogen has a pretty sophisticated cell wall and some adroit genetic modifications that enable it to evade the natural resistance of the body. More recently, scientists have been looking into its inner mechanism, discovering the enzymatic processes that, rather intriguingly, are essential to its survival and virulence. A few studies of how enzymes deal with specific molecules have even highlighted possible targets for new drugs, a vital advancement in light of the increase in drug-resistant bacteria. These studies are liable to uncover "hot-spots" in the bacterial enzymes, sites that could be used to advantage by creating molecules with precisely the correct binding affinity and eventually resulting in improved treatments. This synthesis of molecular science and clinical endeavor truly indicates how the two disciplines must collaborate in the battle against TB (Mori et al., 2021).

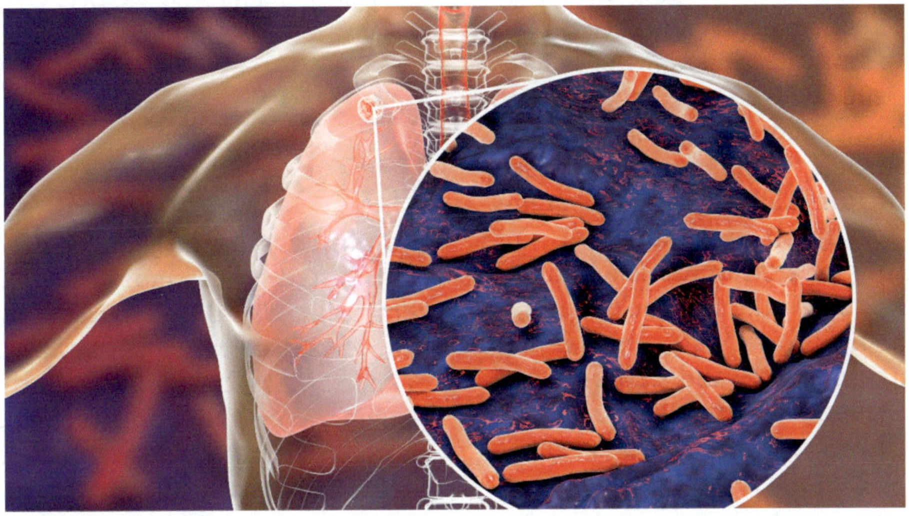

Figure 12.2. The definition of Tuberculosis (TB).

Source: Noticias en Salud. (2020). *Posibles Respuestas Inmunes a La Tuberculosis.*

On the larger end, TB is also heavily intertwined with economic and social concerns that influence how it is spread. New concepts, such as cash transfer schemes and other social protection strategies—have cropped up to combat underlying issues like poverty and restricted healthcare access. These solutions, in most instances, attempt to minimize risks and promote improved treatment by providing economic assistance to struggling families. Nevertheless, challenges persist, whether the tight conditions attached to receiving assistance, arguments regarding targeting the appropriate populations, or sustainability concerns in the long run. Observations from previous public health campaigns, particularly those that fought HIV/AIDS, indicate the potential of combining social and medical interventions to curtail the advance of TB. As a result, policy frameworks nowadays increasingly recognize that addressing social determinants is just as crucial as biomedical interventions when it comes to truly curbing TB (Boccia et al., 2016) (Figure 12.2).

Importance of Studying Tuberculosis (TB) Today

TB remains a constant threat globally, reminding us that we cannot let research slow down. Despite how far medicine has advanced, this disease still kills, striking those in low- and middle-income countries particularly hard. Boiled down, learning how *Mycobacterium tuberculosis* behaves with our immune system isn't theoretical—it leads the way to improved diagnostic techniques and treatments. Further there's drug resistance, something that only complicates the situation further and necessitates new public health strategies and new treatments. Examining the trends of the past combined with the current context also highlights problems such as established stigma, compromised access to care, and unstable healthcare systems still weighing heavily on populations (Devos & Janssens, 2017). Recent statistics indicate that TB is still a hard nut to crack when it comes to global health security, with issues like poverty, malnutrition, and cumbersome healthcare infrastructure having their say. In the majority of instances, research on TB is central to informing targeted interventions that address these very issues, which tend to spread the disease unabated. Meanwhile, probing the social and cultural aspect of TB, such as how patients adhere to treatment and how communities perceive the disease—provides valuable information for public health interventions and policy adjustments. Studies conducted in different settings, including African communities (Morgan et al., 1980), point to how context-specific, customized approaches are needed when local conditions and limited resources enter the picture. This tiered, continuous study is paramount in gradually eroding high incidence and mortality rates across the globe. Individuals traveling about so extensively today means TB control practices must do the same, therefore. Recent advances in molecular biology and genomic sequencing have unlocked unforeseen means of quick detection and even personalized treatment protocols, making ongoing research not only beneficial but downright required. Ongoing monitoring is also crucial, particularly when co-infections such as HIV/TB appear and complicate treatment strategies. The dynamic nature of TB requires us to continually re-engineer prevention strategies, enhance vaccine efficacy, and advocate for equitable healthcare provision for all. Ultimately, both scholarly investigation and practical clinical practice make up the foundation of our worldwide efforts to finally overcome this ancient issue (Morgan et al., 1980; Devos & Janssens, 2017).

12.1. Causes and Transmission

It's understanding how infections are transmitted that is most important if we want communities to be protected. TB, which is from the *Mycobacterium tuberculosis* bacterium, primarily targets the lungs but doesn't always remain there—other organs can become infected as well. When the person with active TB coughs, sneezes, or even speaks, small droplets shoot out and can persist in the air for a bit, particularly in poorly ventilated areas or where there are a lot of people. Recent research largely indicates that most cases of TB result not from the common household contacts but from the one-time, passing encounters. This new understanding of TB's journey defies old assumptions and suggests our health policies could use a re-think (McCreesh & White, 2018). Examining its migration through our social lives more closely is where some surprising information comes into view. You may believe that staying with a sick person is the greatest risk, but when solid data is combined with mathematical modeling, it becomes apparent that those fleeting contacts out in the community can have just as significant an impact. In most instances, the normal daily contacts within homes or normal social groups total less overall transmission, at least in part due to something akin to contact saturation—you just don't get much additional risk after a while—and in part due to the presence of a few superspreaders who appear to be married to generating lots of additional cases in brief periods. These findings, in the majority of instances, hint at the necessity for innovative means to identify high-risk transmitters and follow infections that extend beyond our normal day-to-day networks. In essence, public health interventions may need to move slightly toward wider, community-oriented approaches to truly capture the insidious spread of TB (McCreesh & White, 2018). At a glance at TB, the biological and social routes of its transmission merge into a larger narrative about disease burden. Globally, as mortality rates decline and populations age, the non-fatal, chronic consequences of TB are becoming more prominent. The interplay between latent and active TB with various social factors alterchanges not only who gets sick but also how easily the disease can jump from one person to another. While the direct routes of infection matter a lot, the ongoing prevalence of TB and the disabilities it can cause show that we're not only fighting new cases—we're also dealing with long-term health challenges. With increasing years now spent with TB disability, even while fewer die, health systems will need to prepare for longer care requirements. In most instances, this total burden implies that interventions must address both preventing new infections and dealing with the recalcitrant disease aftermath (Figure 12.3).

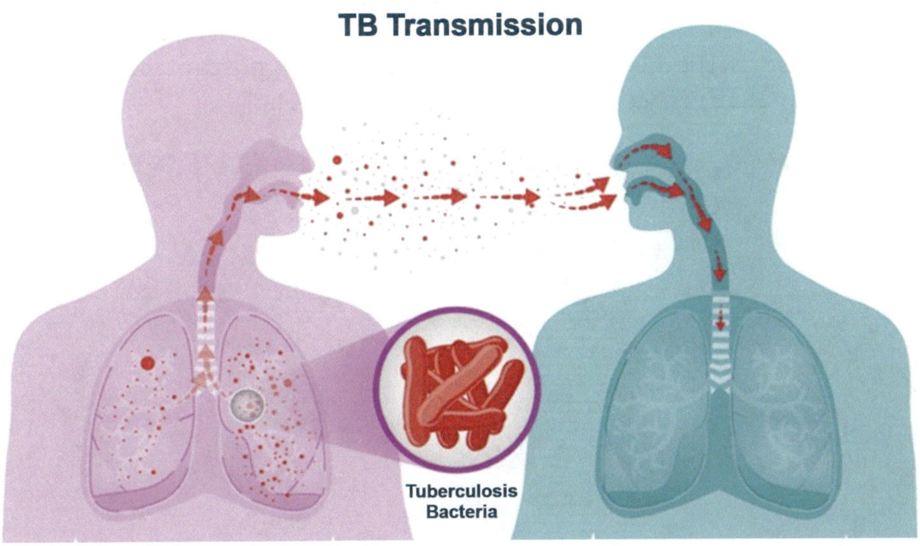

Figure 12.3. Causes and transmission for Tuberculosis (TB).

Source: Centers for Disease Control and Prevention. (n.d.). *TB Transmission.*

12.1.1. Bacterial Agent: Mycobacterium Tuberculosis

TB begins with some unique characteristics in *Mycobacterium tuberculosis* that distinguish it. This small pest has some fairly sophisticated metabolic stunts which are quite different from human cells, providing good drug targets. Scientists comparing these metabolic habits with their counterparts in Homo sapiens kept running into enzymes found only in the bacterium—there is no human equivalent. This generally holds that if we target these specific enzymes, we can restrict side effects to our cells. While drug-resistant strains increase, even when treatments may get ugly sometimes, it is a knowledge of these distinguishing metabolic factors that proves to be a vital piece to relieve the burden of global health (Arya et al., 2014). In recent research into anti-TB drugs, high-throughput screening has been well utilized to track down compounds that act in novel ways on the microbe. It appears that some of those over-the-counter non-steroidal anti-inflammatory medications—ibuprofen comes to mind and other 2-arylpropanoic acids—may stand a good chance of inhibiting *Mycobacterium tuberculosis.* These compounds appear to knock out both the drug-susceptible strains and also the multidrug-resistant strains, even targeting those resting, stationary-phase bacilli that normally evade the ordinary antibiotics. Overall, the concept is that these molecules could interfere with the bacterial protein initiation factor infB, which is a completely new target for therapy. This possible capacity to address both resistant microbes and their sneaky, latent forms is a positive indication for better results (Bhakta et al., 2013). The battle against this recalcitrant pathogen truly requires an interdisciplinary approach, summoning molecular biology, pharmacology, and bioinformatics to reveal its weaknesses. *In silico* comparisons of metabolic pathways have served to identify enzymes critical to the microbe's survival, which in turn are informing new medicinal chemistry approaches. Meanwhile, techniques such as the HT-SPOTi assay—while not ideal—provide a faster, more reproducible way of screening new compounds. When you couple empirical lab work with computational models, you get a more dynamic strategy to circumvent the limitations of existing treatments and to overcome arising drug resistance. Altogether, this multidisciplinary insight into the workings of the bacterium and how it responds to drugs is the key to eventually taking a significant bite out of the global TB pandemic (Bhakta et al., 2013; Arya et al., 2014) (Figure 12.4).

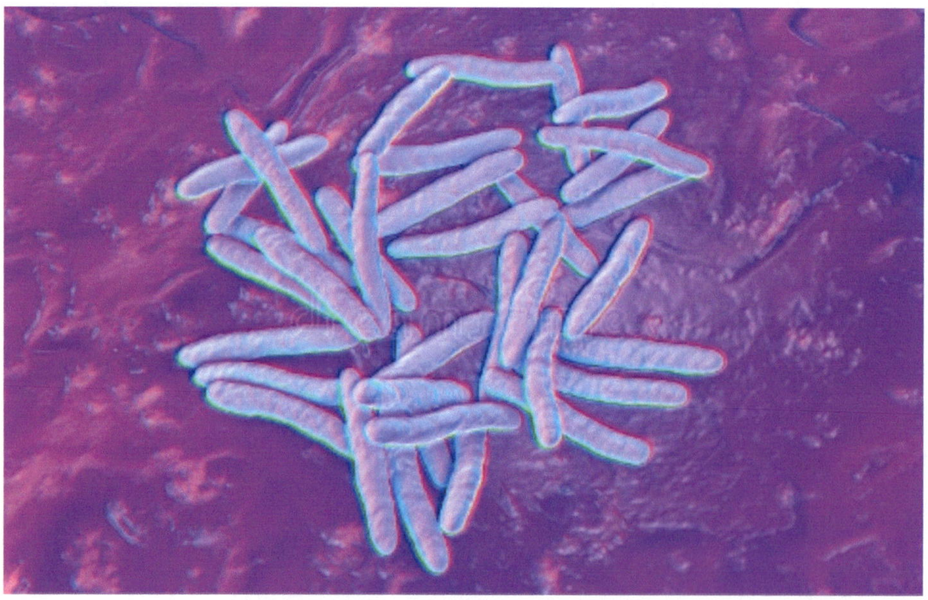

Figure 12.4. The bacterial agent: *Mycobacterium tuberculosis.*

Source: Dreamstime. (n.d.). *Bacteria Mycobacterium tuberculosis.*

12.1.2. Modes of Transmission

In retrospect, individuals used to believe that infections traveled through a mystical, near-magical atmosphere—, aspect that silently influenced the way we treat public health today. Early on, individuals used to believe that sickness drifted through these invisible miasmas, something which now seems quite naive. Then, when the germ theory caught on in the late 1800s and early 1900s, specialists began emphasizing that close proximity and droplets were the primary villains. Nevertheless, this initial model didn't give much credit to the small airborne particles we currently refer to as aerosols. Consider tuberculosis, for instance—it was largely attributed to droplets for centuries until, in 1962, evidence began to point firmly at airborne transmission, upending traditional assumptions. With an increase in interdisciplinary research, particularly during the COVID-19 period, what happens is that numerous respiratory diseases, including TB, are highly dependent on aerosols—a reality which has been left behind for too long (Jimenez et al., 2022). TB's path is not so straightforward as adhering to human-to-human transmission. In settings such as abattoirs, the risk escalates because employees are exposed to *Mycobacterium bovis*, the organism responsible for bovine TB. Experiments with abattoir workers have revealed that individuals tend not to understand fully how bTB is transmitted, how to avoid it, or why it transmits between animals and humans. Detection of tubercle lesions in cattle at slaughter suggests covert reservoirs of infection, and it is obvious that both airborne and direct contact transmission must be considered. That is, TB isn't restricted to the visible respiratory droplets—it can travel through animal sources and even surfaces, expanding the way we consider the transmission of it (Tukur, 2021). Nowadays, if one observes TB spread one can notice a fine balance between the environment, the character of the microbe, and the way humans react. Airborne transmission occurs when we inhale fine droplets containing *Mycobacterium tuberculosis*, droplets that persist and travel further than we'd anticipate. This form particularly bedevils enclosed or poorly ventilated areas, both public areas and hospitals. And yes, while being infected through contact with surfaces is less likely, it still counts in areas of less than perfect cleanliness. In general, coming to terms with these diverse modes of transmission is the first step to implementing wiser measures, such as improving ventilation, donning appropriate PPE, and educating high-risk groups like healthcare and abattoir workers about the dangers. Understanding that TB can spread via the air truly aligns with the most recent changes in infectious disease control, pushing us to tackle both droplet and aerosol routes in our prevention strategy (Tukur, 2021; Jimenez et al., 2022).

12.1.3. Risk Factors for Infection

Social and environmental settings mix together in ways that really shape who ends up at risk for TB. Being around someone infectious for long stretches, like sharing a home, seriously increases your chances because you're in constant contact with airborne *Mycobacterium tuberculosis*. In spots that are crowded and don't have good airflow, infectious droplets tend to build up, making it easier for the disease to spread. You can also look and see that where you reside is important, as some provinces register higher tuberculin skin test responses than others, suggesting local characterestics of transmission. Overall, it's not simply individual health; the day-to-day environment you inhabit lays the groundwork, so well-directed public health solutions are necessary to enhance the living environment (MacPherson et al., 2020). Immune status and age further muddy this image. Overall, children tend to be particularly susceptible for latent TB, as their defenses against infection are less effective and they have plenty of frequent close exposures to infected individuals. Curiously, household contacts of HIV-positive TB patients sometimes have lower latent infection rates than those related to HIV-negative cases—this surprising turn of events indicates that HIV co-infection may alter the infectivity of an individual or even the screening outcome, which can be a little confusing. Such revelations lead us to question the traditional concepts regarding host and pathogen interactions, illustrating that demographics and other health conditions intersect in sophisticated manners to impact TB risk (MacPherson et al., 2020).

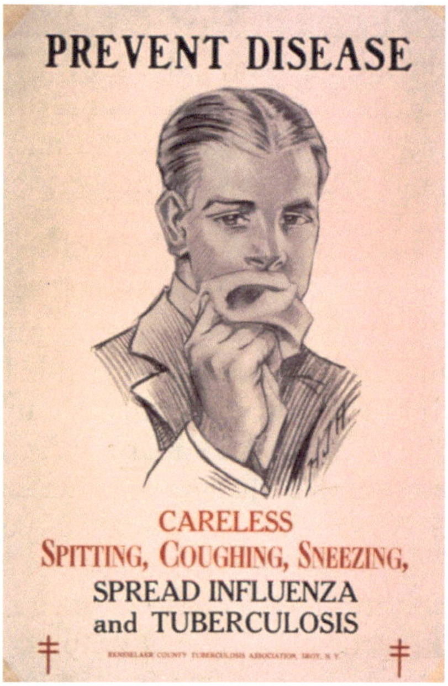
PREVENT DISEASE
CARELESS
SPITTING, COUGHING, SNEEZING,
SPREAD INFLUENZA
and TUBERCULOSIS

Figure 12.5. Tuberculosis (TB) risk factors.

Source: By Rensselaer County Tuberculosis Association. - U.S. National Library of Medicine Transferred from en.wikipedia, Public Domain, https://commons.wikimedia.org/w/index.php?curid=4352690

On a larger scale, latent TB infection is an insidious reservoir capable of igniting future outbreaks and continued health issues. Approximately one-third of the global population might be carrying latent TB bacilli, thus keeping active disease a possibility. In areas such as Africa, even though information might be lacking, it's evident that economic difficulties, increased HIV prevalence, and restricted access to healthcare all conspire together to affect rates of latent infection and the transition to active disease. In the majority of instances, examining these cross-cutting factors in greater detail is essential if we are to develop interventions that genuinely reduce TB cases in the long term. Identifying these multifaceted, interlaced risks is essential to creating public health policy that functions in high-burden environments (MacPherson et al., 2020) (Figure 12.5).

12.2. Symptoms and Diagnosis

TB doesn't always make itself known in the same manner—it can be a true chameleon depending on where it strikes. In the lungs, for instance, you tend to get a chronic cough, sometimes with blood, along with fevers, night sweats, and weight loss. But once the infection escapes the lungs, the signs get a little more subtle—perhaps stomach pains or even abnormal periods if the reproductive tract gets involved. Consider uterine TB; it can trigger intrauterine adhesions that may result in lighter-than-usual periods or difficulty conceiving, both lumped together as Ashermans syndrome. Since the lower layers of the uterine lining become damaged, patients may only experience general, subtle symptoms making TB difficult to detect on its own (Dreisler & Kjer, 2019). Overall, these differences require a thorough, complete examination, particularly in areas where TB is endemic or in people with known risk factors. Deciphering TB is a bit of a mystery, at least in part because its symptoms tend to overlap with other diseases, such as Crohn's disease, especially when the intestines are affected. Both TB and Crohn's can end up appearing very similar on initial tests, with even endoscopic observations providing a questionable image. By and large, initiating an anti-TB regimen may be of relief in either situation, but it's more often the TB patient who, after a couple of months, experiences obvious mucosal healing on follow-up scope. For a person with Crohn's, on the other hand, symptom relief may be seen without that same degree of healing, which typically requires a repeat colonoscopy to verify what's truly happening. This cautious, step-by-step manner, in which persistence of symptoms following a 3-month trial pushes the diagnosis in the direction of Crohn's, prevents errors and ensures that patients receive the correct long-term treatment (Mouli et al., 2016). In diagnosing TB in its different manifestations, physicians have the propensity to jumble up things, employing anything from varied imaging tests to invasive procedures. As an example, if TB is suspected to be attacking the uterus, doctors will begin with less invasive imaging such as contrast sonohysterography or hysterosalpingography to identify any adhesions, although these tests are more of an initial indicator than a final diagnosis. More specifically, a hysteroscopy, in which the interior of the uterus is looked at directly, allows physicians to observe and categorize any adhesions, paving the way for possible surgical measures as required. In very complicated cases, however, like when the uterine cavity almost completely disappears, an MRI could be the best choice for a complete evaluation. This combination of clinical examinations, imaging, and endoscopic methods typically increases the diagnostic accuracy and assists in personalizing treatment, particularly in patients with infertility or irregular menstrual cycles attributed to TB-induced adhesions (Dreisler & Kjer, 2019) (Figure 12.6).

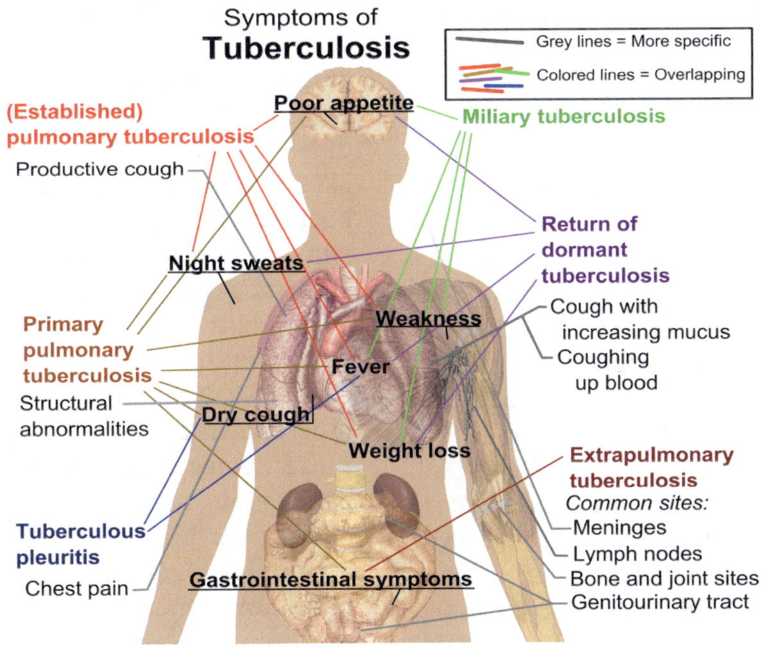

Figure 12.6. Know the symptoms of Tuberculosis (TB).

Source: By Mikael Häggström.When using this image in external works, it may be cited as:Häggström, Mikael (2014). "Medical gallery of Mikael Häggström 2014". WikiJournal of Medicine 1 (2). DOI:10.15347/wjm/2014.008. ISSN 2002-4436. Public Domain.orBy Mikael Häggström, used with permission. - All used images are in public domain., Public Domain, https://commons.wikimedia.org/w/index.php?curid=691987112.2.1. ***Common Symptoms of Tuberculosis (TB)***

TB tends to sneak up silently, so early detection is a true challenge. Most patients begin with a cough that simply refuses to let up—, three weeks and still going—, although it might appear benign at first, it gradually gets worse. That nagging cough usually produces sputum, occasionally even tinged with a hint of blood, which quite obviously indicates the damage occurring within the lungs. To these chest complaints, weight loss, night sweats, and persistent fatigue add their presence; these are indicators of the body's prolonged struggle against the *Mycobacterium tuberculosis* pathogen and indicative of a chronic state of inflammation. It is usually crucial to identify such signs early, particularly in regions where healthcare may be scarce, and delays will have more to spread and more difficult treatment results (DeHart et al., 2020). The physical aspect of TB is a root social battle, as stigma can have a tremendous impact on whether or not patients seek treatment. The overt symptoms, such as that stubborn cough and visible weight loss—can lead to social ostracism, fueling widespread fears about how infectious TB could be. This type of stigma delays diagnosis even more and interferes with regular care, effectively trapping individuals in a cycle that transmits the infection even further. Health systems truly need to broaden their perspective; they need to not only identify clinical symptoms but also address the social stigma so that people feel encouraged when they come in for treatment (Craig et al., 2018). Comprehending these social dynamics is central to more effective disease management and patient outcomes. There are more aspects to TB than the primary respiratory symptoms. At times, an annoying, low-grade fever persists in fits for weeks with accompanying nights soaking wet with sweat so that clothes and bedding become saturated—a definitive sign of the systemic extent of the infection. Numerous patients also report chest pain, which could result from pleural irritation or more generalized lung tissue damage. In later stages, the draining effect of the infection can cause generalized weakness and loss of appetite, further fueling the flames of cachexia. These secondary symptoms highlight TB's insidious, creeping nature and remind practitioners to remain vigilant, particularly in high-risk groups and in areas with limited healthcare, such as in some areas of Southeast Asia (DeHart et al., 2020). Identifying these more subtle clues early on is really almost a pillar in slowing down TB's spread and increasing survival rates.

12.2.2. Diagnostic Methods

New methods of TB diagnosis are stirring up the way the disease is detected—today doctors can now detect it sooner and with more certainty. Sputum smear microscopy, for example, continues to be utilized but frequently doesn't detect small numbers of bacteria, particularly if TB is in a location outside the lungs. Culture tests are more detailed but are often laborious, resulting in occasional undesired delays before treatment can commence. Next, molecular diagnostics intervened—consider the GeneXpert MTB/RIF test, which rapidly identifies the TB bacteria and screens for rifampicin resistance simultaneously. Such double-duty action leaves clinicians with greater latitude to determine the optimum treatment course. In fact, a study even demonstrated that the sensitivity and specificity of the assay remained robust for lung and non-lung specimens (Mechal et al., 2019). Overall, these newer approaches fill the voids created by previous techniques and ultimately enhance patient care. In addition to these commercial molecular diagnostics, CRISPR-based assays have now emerged as a genuinely promising tool for TB diagnosis. They leverage CRISPR's innate ability for high sensitivity and pinpoint precision and target the TB genetic material with a precision that sometimes borders on the astonishing. Revisiting data, the CRISPR-MTB test has turned out to be even more sensitive than culture and GeneXpert tests, additionally, it occurs quickly and requires a minimal sample to function. Notably, its capacity to identify almost single-copy levels of the pathogen in pulmonary and extra-pulmonary samples truly speaks to its potential as a game-altering diagnostic platform (Ai et al., 2019). Combining these high-level techniques into routine practice, and you may very well witness a whole turnaround in TB screening, especially where speed and precision really count. Despite all this advancement in molecular diagnostics, however, there are some potholes along the way, particularly in low-resource settings where TB is most rife. Regional variation in the prevalence of TB may cause test performance to differ significantly, such that selecting the appropriate tool requires a considered, bespoke approach. Comparative studies tend to highlight that it's a question of striking a balance between sensitivity, specificity, cost, and user-friendliness when comparing tests such as GeneXpert and CRISPR-MTB assays (Mechal et al., 2019). Further, achieving the accurate identification of rifampicin resistance is crucial in addressing multidrug-resistant TB, and molecular tests have here been seen to be in good agreement with each other in detecting resistance, resulting in more informed treatment strategies. Research continues to be crucial in optimizing these testing methods, streamlining them, and ultimately bridging the gaps in international TB control (Figure 12.7).

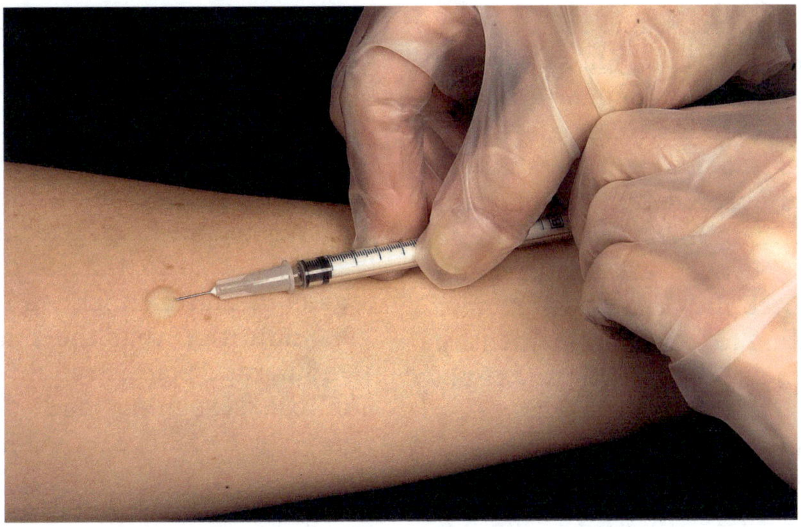

Figure 12.7. Conventional methods for diagnosis of Tuberculosis (TB).

Source: By Greg Knobloch - This media comes from the Centers for Disease Control and Prevention's Public Health Image Library (PHIL), with identification number #6806.Note: Not all PHIL images are public domain; be sure to check copyright status and credit authors and content providers. العربية | Deutsch | English | македонски | slovenščina | +/−, Public Domain, https://commons.wikimedia.org/w/index.php?curid=848106

12.2.3. Challenges in Diagnosing Tuberculosis (TB)

Diagnosis of TB is difficult since the disease appears in so many different forms and our older methods simply don't always work. Coughing and fever are easy to confuse with other lung ailments, which tends to leave physicians stumped at the beginning. X-ray tests are somewhat helpful, but they're often not detailed enough to identify TB from other such ailments. The classic sputum smear test, used for over a century, can miss the mark, especially when there aren't many bacteria around or the infection isn't in the lungs. Even the so-called gold standard, where bacteria are grown in a lab, takes weeks and delays treatment. New molecular techniques can accelerate and even test for drug resistance, but the sad truth is that such advancements are not yet available in the resource-scarce regions that are most affected (Gönül Aslan, 2024). Overall, depending on less than perfect techniques along with scarce resources really hinders rapid, precise diagnosis. Cultivating *Mycobacterium tuberculosis* from patient specimens is another significant roadblock. The pathogen behind TB is infamous for taking a long time to grow and require extremely specific environments, which further delays the entire testing process. Sputum. the primary specimen utilized for lung TB—. not contain sufficient bacteria for identification at times, particularly in children or individuals with compromised immune systems. The bacteria also tend to hide within cells, which does not help either. In general, in the absence of generally accepted, absolute criteria, it is hard to determine whether an infection is latent or about to get worse. Recent research integrating transcriptomic, proteomic, and metabolomic information is pointing toward ways to identify dependable markers of infection (Zhang et al., 2024). Nevertheless, translating these thrilling research results into routine practice is a formidable challenge. Efforts to break through these barriers are increasingly relying on new molecular technologies. GeneXpert and line probe assays are really disrupting the detection of TB by providing rapid results on both infection and drug resistance. However, these tests require specialized equipment, are expensive, and require solid infrastructure, so they can't be implemented broadly beyond richer areas (Gönül Aslan, 2024). In most instances, molecular tests may miss certain TB strains or be unable to distinguish between living and dead bacteria, distorting the diagnosis. Conversely, multiomics strategies look at the infection from a wider perspective by combining several biomarkers to create a mosaic of the infection, with the promise of earlier and more precise detection—especially in latent or initial stages (Zhang et al., 2024). While these encouraging developments exist, integrating them into existing health systems within high-burden nations remains a challenging task; evidently, there's an urgent need for rapid, low-cost, and scalable diagnostics.

12.3. Types of Tuberculosis (TB)

PTB is the form most people are aware of—it primarily affects the lungs and brings real havoc. The pathogen, *Mycobacterium tuberculosis*, targets lung tissue, resulting in a terrible, chronic cough, chest pain, and even coughing up blood at times. With every cough or sneeze, tiny droplets disseminate the bacteria, making this lung-centric phase a big contributor to spread. Nevertheless, TB is not a one-trick pony; it can stray beyond the lungs into other organs, making it all the harder to find and treat. If it seeps into organs in that manner, we refer to it as EPTB , an indication that the infection can spread to numerous places, requiring more extensive medical screening and diverse treatment regimens. EPTB occurs when the bacteria ride the bloodstream or lymphatic system into unexpected locations. It can lodge in lymph nodes, the pleura, bones, and joints, even the genitourinary tract and central nervous system. In most instances, this confusion confuses clinical diagnoses since the symptoms begin to mimic other diseases according to which organ is affected. TB meningitis and miliary TB are two rather extreme cases in point—miliary TB, for example, produces numerous small lesions all over the body, a condition which typically requires extended and more powerful treatment. Such unpredictability explains why it's so important to catch the disease early and modify therapy to the circumstances. There is another aspect to keep in mind when it comes to treating TB, and that is the problem of drug resistance and immune complications. Once the infection has developed resistance to first-line drugs such as isoniazid, treatment is much more challenging, and failure becomes a higher risk. Add to that individuals' genetic variation that influences the way they metabolize anti-TB drugs—, causing liver issues (hepatotoxicity) that restrict the extent to which the drugs can be safely employed. For instance, some polymorphisms in enzymes such as NAT2 have been associated with an increased risk of liver damage during treatment, although this is not an ideal predictor (Tostmann et al., 2014). Studies on the BCG vaccine also show it not only prevents TB but might also prevent associated conditions such as leprosy (Cunha et al., 2010). With all these turns and bends, it's obvious that an individualized strategy and continuous studies are necessary to combat TB efficiently (Figure 12.8).

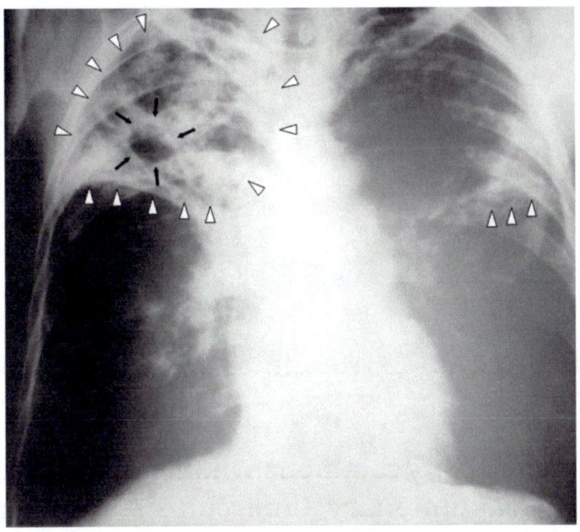

Figure 12.8. Types of Tuberculosis (TB).

Source: By Unknown author - This media comes from the Centers for Disease Control and Prevention's Public Health Image Library (PHIL), with identification number #2543.Note: Not all PHIL images are public domain; be sure to check copyright status and credit authors and content providers.العربية | Deutsch | English | македонски | slovenščina | +/−, Public Domain, https://commons.wikimedia.org/w/index.php?curid=978580

12.3.1. Pulmonary Tuberculosis (PTB)

PTB is the most frequent manner *Mycobacterium tuberculosis* presents itself in patients, primarily affecting the lungs and posing actual problems across the globe. You usually witness it when recurring symptoms such as a persistent cough, coughing up blood, and unexplained weight loss emerge—and if such signs are not treated, they can result in quite serious sickness or even death. We have made some progress with antibiotics, but mounting drug-resistant forms force treatment schemes both long and challenging. The problem strikes with additional force in developing countries, where the lags in recognizing the disease and the less-than-desirable treatments help the disease move further ahead. In most instances, addressing TB involves scaling up lab work, modifying treatment regimens, and accelerating targeted public health efforts to contain transmission and enhance patient outcomes (Christopher et al., 2022). Current management of PTB generally involves administering a combination of antibiotics for extended periods. Yes, such prolonged treatment regimens tend to be effective against drug-sensitive disease, but adherence and side effect management can be formidable challenges. Further, increased emergence of multidrug-resistant and extensively drug-resistant TB tends to make cure rates <50%. In turn, investigators are testing new concepts—even some host-directed strategies that seek to modulate the immune response of the body and reduce tissue injury—to attempt to reduce treatment durations and enhance overall recovery, particularly when co-infections or other medical issues contribute to the burden on the patient and the healthcare system (Young et al., 2019). At the global level, prevention of PTB requires improved vaccine strategies and more robust public health establishments. Consider the Bacille Calmette-Guérin (BCG) vaccine: it's used extensively but gives only partial protection to adults against lung TB, which amply indicates that we need new advances in vaccines. Socio-economic problems such as poverty and congested housing also have their role to play in transmitting TB, and the increasing specter of antimicrobial resistance (AMR) only makes things more precarious. It becomes essential, therefore, to enhance laboratory capacity, expand access to appropriate diagnostics and treatments, and enhance surveillance systems, all specific to local patterns, to reduce the overall burden of PTB (Young et al., 2019; Christopher et al., 2022).

12.3.2. Extrapulmonary Tuberculosis (EPTB)

EPTB is a puzzling component of the TB enigma, it appears in areas of the body other than the lungs, which quite literally inserts a monkey wrench into TB control. New big studies out of China indicate that this form of TB primarily affects younger people, typically those aged 15 to 34 years, and tends to infect men slightly more with an approximate male-to-female ratio of 1.51. It's an interesting aside that EPTB is very seldom an isolated entity; almost 70% of the time, you see it combined with PTB or other extrapulmonary disease. Tuberculous pleurisy, for instance, constitutes approximately half of these, with bronchial TB, lymphadenitis, and meningitis ranking in order of frequency. This diffuse pattern suggests that clinicians need to bear the potential of covert lung involvement in mind while working with TB extrapulmonary, so that they can hit diagnosis and treatment early (Kang et al., 2020). The mechanism by which EPTB operates within the body is slightly different from PTB, though both involve similar immune reactions. Both *Mycobacterium tuberculosis* and other non-tuberculous mycobacteria infect alveolar macrophages upon inhalation, initiating a type of granulomatous inflammation; however, they can move differently throughout the body and impact different patients. EPTB is typically observed more often when the immune system is weakened—consider HIV-infected patients—where the infection will disperse rather than remain confined to the lungs. These variations matter in the clinic, since they can make diagnosis more difficult. While PTB can rely on sophisticated molecular tests, EPTB usually requires a wider range of tests owing to its multiple locations and symptoms that could overlap with other diseases (Gopalaswamy et al., 2020).

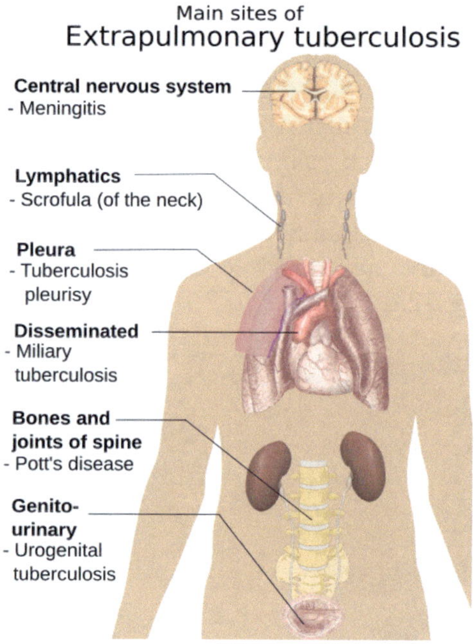

Figure 12.9. Extrapulmonary Tuberculosis (EPTB).

Source: https://commons.wikimedia.org/wiki/File:Extrapulmonary_tuberculosis_symptoms.svg

During treatment, physicians must contend with both the infection outside the lung and any potential lung complications simultaneously. Standard anti-TB regimens generally function well if the bacteria have not yet developed resistance, but delays in detecting EPTB can delay the initiation of appropriate therapy. And when pulmonary and extrapulmonary presentations appear together, additional caution is required to assess infectivity and institute appropriate isolation precautions. Evidence suggests age and gender come into play too—typically, younger patients (and especially males) are likely to have both. With such a broad presentation of EPTB, an interdisciplinary care plan—with focused imaging and microbiologic testing, among other strategies, is central to optimizing treatment, reducing outcomes, and reducing transmission. This mix of issues speaks to the continuing need for better diagnostic tools and increased awareness among health care providers (Kang et al., 2020) (Figure 12.9).

12.3.3. Multidrug-resistant Tuberculosis (MDR-TB)

TB treatment has had some unexpected turns of late, particularly with the increasing battle against multidrug-resistant TB. Ancient regimens based on first-line drugs simply do not perform as well against these resilient strains, so patients are pushed into more extended, more complex therapies. One newer 6-month, all-oral regimen—involving bedaquiline, pretomanid, linezolid, and moxifloxacin (BPaLM)—has emerged as a promising option that appears to improve compliance and reduce side effects. In general, the World Health Organization currently supports this strategy for patients with serious lung problems and even certain types of extra-PTB, moving in the direction of care that genuinely addresses the patient. Naturally, hurdles continue to exist, such as limited drug availability and complex drug interactions, particularly in scenarios involving extensive disease or when patients are unable to tolerate specific medications (Vanino et al., 2023). Despite these developments, managing MDR-TB remains a business. The challenging biology of *Mycobacterium tuberculosis* and the limitations of current treatments maintain complexity. New medicines, bedaquiline and pretomanid, for example, have expanded our options, opening the door to injection-free, shorter regimens that reduce the patient's burden. However, continued use of some drugs whose efficacy is questionable, such as high-dose isoniazid—and increasing resistance to ethambutol and pyrazinamide, strongly indicate that there is scope for change. Doctors also struggle with problems such as antimicrobial heteroresistance and cavitary lung lesions, which allow tenacious infections of bacteria to survive despite the use of multiple drugs. For the most part, these drug and biological challenges highlight the imperative for improved biomarkers to monitor for response to treatment and modulate regimens accordingly (Dookie et al., 2022). Deploying these innovative MDR-TB treatments on a worldwide level isn't as simple as might be hoped; local testing constraints and healthcare system capabilities further complicate matters. The potential of these shorter, less harsh regimens is tempered by the proviso that we can consistently identify fluoroquinolone resistance and select patients wisely in order not to produce unwanted effects. However, the developing resistance, —even to agents such as bedaquiline, overshadows these new regimens. In the meantime, continued clinical trials are in investigation of how to reduce treatment length and pill number even further, as a means of improving patients' lives and outcomes globally. In sum, overcoming these challenges will require a combination of quick diagnostics, tailored therapy, and improved patient care—a bundled solution that may ultimately prevent MDR-TB and drive us closer to the eradication of TB as a whole (Dookie et al., 2022; Vanino et al., 2023).

12.4. Treatment Options

TB therapy typically begins with prolonged regimens of combination antibiotics designed to eradicate *Mycobacterium tuberculosis* and prevent drug resistance from establishing itself. Nevertheless, when TB appears in more challenging locations, particularly within the central nervous system (CNS, the standard treatment often fails. In such instances, patients may find themselves requiring additional treatments because conventional antitubercular therapy (ATT) with corticosteroids simply is not sufficient. Certain recent analyses went so far as to explore the use of immunomodulators such as infliximab—a tumor necrosis factor-alpha blocker drug, and the initial indicators are fairly optimistic regarding enhancing disability-free survival in the really ill. This approach appears to lower both mortality rates and serious disabilities, suggesting that combining with immunotherapy may be the way forward when traditional methods fail to stimulate adequate neurological recovery (Manesh et al., 2023).

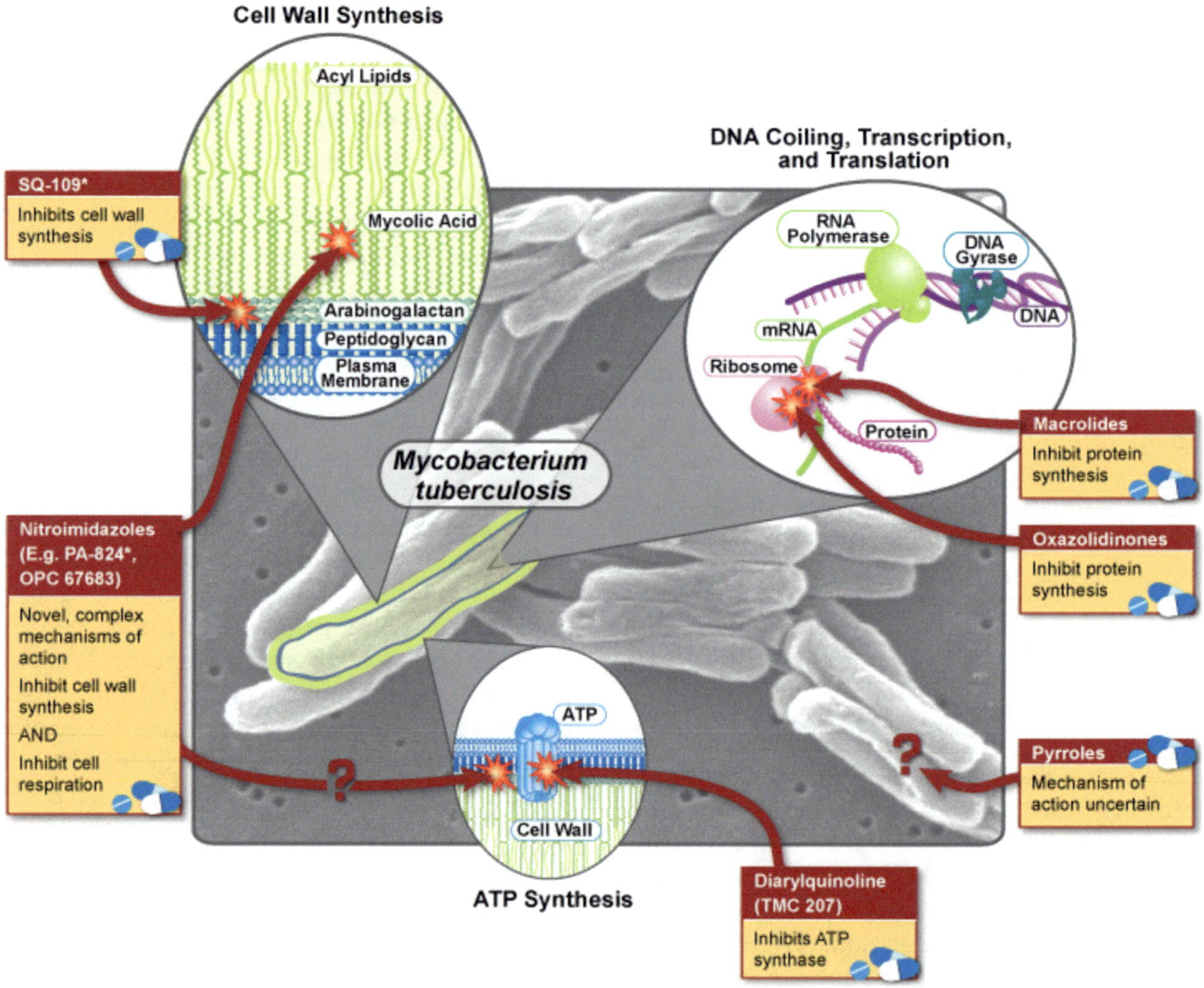

Figure 12.10. Treatment of Tuberculosis (TB).

Source: By "Photo Credit: The photo of Mycobacterium tuberculosis was obtained from the Centers for Disease Control and Prevention, CDC/ Dr. Ray Butler; Janice Carr.Illustration Credit: This illustration is in the public domain. Please credit the National Institute of Allergy and Infectious Diseases (NIAID).Illustrator: Krista Townsend" - U.S. National Institute of Allergy and Infectious Diseases (NIAID), Public Domain, https://commons.wikimedia.org/w/index.php?curid=3932505

Naturally, larger trials are usually required to establish safety and solidify treatment recommendations before this new direction can gain broad acceptance. Drug-resistant strains of TB remain a tenacious problem, challenging scientists to look beyond traditional chemotherapy. One interesting option includes plant-based compounds that could enhance what we're already doing. Ancient medicinal herbs of South Asia and Africa, for instance, have provided us with a combination of phytochemicals with potential anti-mycobacterial activity, providing a sort of safety net or even a substitute for conventional antibiotics. These plant compounds can erode bacterial burdens or even activate the body's own immune response, which can reduce the unpleasant side effects we commonly observe with chronic antibiotic therapy. Add to this the fact that employing contemporary delivery strategies such as nanoformulations assists these plant-derived agents in becoming absorbed more efficiently and functioning more effectively. Overall, the combination of natural extracts with cutting-edge technology represents a new frontier in addressing both resistance challenges and patient tolerability issues (Gautam et al., 2023). As these new concepts are unfolding, maximizing our present treatment modalities continues to be at the forefront in the battle against TB. The WHO-recommended combinations do work—but require absolute patient compliance and careful follow-up to prevent resistance and relapses. Steroids continue to play a crucial role in managing CNS cases, though, to control inflammation and its sequelae. However, the incorporation of targeted immunomodulators like infliximab could revolutions extreme TB care by enhancing neurological outcomes and preventing enduring disabilities. At the same time, combination of phytochemicals as add-ons might reduce both the duration and toxicity of standard ATT. Ultimately, a piecemeal strategy that unites antibiotics, immunotherapy, and plant-derived agents might truly revolutionize the TB treatment landscape and improve chances for recovery of patients worldwide (Gautam et al., 2023; Manesh et al., 2023) (Figure 12.10).

12.4.1. Standard Treatment Regimens

Managing TB involves adhering to a plan that is designed to eradicate *Mycobacterium tuberculosis* without allowing drug resistance and side effects to take over. Treatment usually begins with a fairly rigorous phase before subsiding into a more leisurely four-month phase, more or less six months when the TB is responsive to drugs. During those initial two months, physicians tend to prescribe a combination of isoniazid, rifampicin, pyrazinamide, and ethambutol daily to attack the bacteria from multiple directions; this combination is designed to enhance the overall impact and prevent resistance from taking hold. Yet even when this approach is effective in general, patients occasionally have difficulty with the side effects and sheer duration of the regimen, which can contribute to issues such as multidrug-resistant TB. Aside from the primary drugs, additional therapies have a significant role in keeping patients on treatment and reducing toxicity. For instance, some recent research has examined adding liver-protecting agents such as remaxol to neutralize the hepatotoxicity associated with first-line TB drugs. In one clinical trial of PTB patients, supplementing usual treatment with remaxol reduced liver complications and even enhanced cytokine profiles—this appears to have rendered patients both physically and emotionally better, enhancing their adherence to the rigorous treatment (Kolomiets et al., 2024). It's fascinating how these little changes, which combine technical medicine with good old supportive care, can make a quantifiable difference. While the straightforward plan is well suited to drug-sensitive TB, fighting drug-resistant disease requires a more tiered solution. Glancing sideways, plans for other diseases—, .g., in dog dirofilariasis, where a three-dose treatment with additional agents bested more straightforward plans—provide a nice parallel. In such challenging TB cases, the course typically takes longer, includes additional second-line medications, and requires close attention to prevent toxicity and achieve a cure (Levytska & Poliukhovych, 2024). For the most part, fine-tuning and adjusting the standard approach as more evidence becomes available is fundamental to containing TB—and its more resistant variants.

12.4.2. Challenges in Treatment Adherence

Surviving TB treatment is not as easy as it may seem. Patients must complete the course, but daily challenges make it difficult. Money problems arise in every corner—many times, patients just can't pay for the ride to the clinic, and that deficiency results in missed check-ups and worse health outcomes. More often than not, the absence of money to pay for transport halts both an individual patient's recovery and the entire community's efforts to contain TB. To this, add the fact that if doctors and patients are not communicating ideas freely, it only complicates matters further. Research tends to show that even small financial support for traveling can significantly enhance compliance, putting the spotlight on the need to overcome these financial roadblocks (Bailey et al., 2012). Apart from financial barriers, stigma is tenaciously attached to a diagnosis of TB. Being afraid of being discriminated against or excluded by friends and neighbors usually prevents individuals from getting timely help or following their medication schedule. This anxiety not only slows down diagnosis but also complicates maintaining treatment on course over the long term. In the majority of situations, that pairing of self-doubt and social isolation subverts both beginning and completing treatment. Attempts to reduce this stigma—utilizing resources such as guidance manuals to quantify and neutralize bias—can provide a more welcoming environment for those experiencing TB (Craig et al., 2018). Further there's the long grind of the regimen itself—a burden that can wear down anyone. Swallowing medication daily for months is difficult, and when symptoms subside early on, many patients are inclined to quit too early. Premature discontinuation not only jeopardizes one's own recovery but also provides an opportunity for drug-resistant strains of TB to develop. Tactics like more open-ended patient education, a more friendly give-and-take with healthcare professionals, and even hands-on techniques like directly observed therapy (DOT) have been hopeful. As a general rule, ensuring that these steps are in accord with the local culture and everyday realities is important to keeping a diverse patient population on course (Bailey et al., 2012) (Figure 12.11).

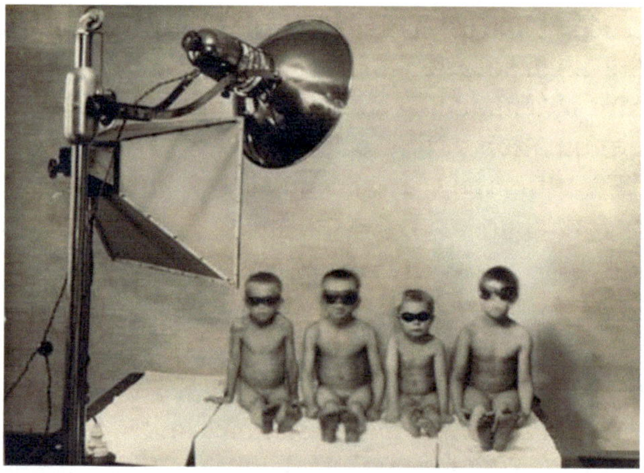

Figure 12.11. Digital adherence technologies for the management of Tuberculosis (TB).

Source: By Unknown author - http://www.pohjois-savonmuisti.fi/verkko_nayttelyt/pohjoissavonlehtikuvia/01/index-13.htm, Public Domain, https://commons.wikimedia.org/w/index.php?curid=7564674

12.4.3. Emerging Therapies and Research

Recent advances in the treatment of TB have obfuscated the traditional boundaries. Rather than remaining wedded to old-fashioned techniques that too often fall short, clinicians are beginning to investigate wiser approaches to drug delivery. Old-fashioned anti-TB drugs, for instance, sometimes fail to penetrate sufficiently into infected tissues and even may have undesirable side effects. One of the ideas that holds a lot of interest is having drug carriers that are the size of nanometers and that enhance the way the drug dissolves and remains stable, yet target the site of infection. Consider this: the very small platforms can carry the medication further release it slowly when they find the appropriate type of stimulus in the bone, which is really beneficial in conditions such as bone TB. And it doesn't stop there—combining these mini-carriers with accompaniment biomaterials or prosthetics could even combat the infection and build up damaged bone simultaneously. For to summarize, combining nanotech with medicine in this way could significantly alter the bone TB patients' game, who typically have very little effective recourse (Luo et al., 2024). Latent TB infection (LTBI) is another wildcard in this fight. Most individuals worldwide carry LTBI, unwittingly being reservoirs that can induce active disease down the line. Sure, the tuberculin skin test and interferon gamma release assays have taken us far, but they still aren't perfect when it comes to distinguishing latent TB from active TB with precision. Recently, scientists have been turning to more sophisticated techniques—molecular, immunological, and even epigenetic ones—that hold out the promise of greater precision. You may learn of novel antigen-based skin tests or metabolomic profiling, which can detect subtle micro-signals that suggest a covert infection. Along with these diagnostic advances are coming new drugs designed to combat recalcitrant strains. Even the latent bacilli are being targeted by some of these candidates, which are now making their way into clinical trials. All these new approaches might combine to make it easier to catch TB earlier and fine-tune interventions more specifically (Christian et al., 2023). Despite these promising advances, the path ahead is anything but straightforward. Nano-drug delivery systems, promising as they were in preliminary studies, have to undergo rigorous clinical tests to ensure they're safe and effective for various sets of patients. Similarly, these new diagnostic tools must surmount barriers such as prohibitively expensive price tags, specialized infrastructure requirements, and the issue of standardizing tests before they may be implemented across the board. And, it's important—to ensure that all people, particularly those in resource-poor settings where TB takes its greatest toll, can gain access to these innovations. In most cases, future research will have to juggle balancing high-tech advances with real-world practicality if we're to meet the global End TB strategy goals. As doctors and researchers continue to push boundaries, the hope is that these emerging solutions will become reliable and scalable tools, genuinely cutting down TB disease and death around the globe (Christian et al., 2023; Luo et al., 2024).

12.5. Global Impact

TB is a persistent issue across the world—made even more difficult by characterestics in the environment and social barriers that disproportionately affect the most vulnerable communities. Some recent research suggests how air quality shifts, particularly when ultra-fine particles such as PM2.5 are involved, correlate with greater numbers of TB cases in cities. When winter comes with increased PM2.5 levels, an apparent rise in TB notifications follows later; it's like toxic air saps our lung defenses, making people more susceptible to contracting TB. And when poor air drives people indoors, that added congestion can boost the rate at which the disease is transmitted. Untangling how all of these factors mesh together is fairly central to developing public health actions that avert and decelerate TB transmission (Dai et al., 2016). Overall, combining infectious disease with environmental stress yet again provides one more layer of complexity to TB's worldwide influence that really necessitates insights from a wide variety of disciplines. Stepping back to view the larger picture, interrelated health and social problems compound the TB outbreak even more challenging. Drug addiction, for instance, isn't an afterthought—fairly significantly complicates matters. Individuals with drug addiction usually have compromised health and are likely to forego treatment protocols, placing them at greater risk of TB. In most instances, drug issues contribute enormously to sickness and premature death, stealing years of productive life from people. This complex web of compromised immune systems and restricted access to care further complicates controlling TB. Worse still is the fact that the lack of solid treatment programs for drug use only fuels the cycle further, undermining global control efforts over TB and indicating the need for healthcare approaches that converge treatments for several problems.

TB's impact extends far beyond just health concerns—it disrupts economies as well, particularly in low- and middle-income regions where the disease is epidemic. Adults of working age tend to get the worst of TB, causing lost days from work and higher healthcare costs that strain fragile economies. There's also the social stigma around TB, which socially and financially disenfranchises patients, in some cases, even hindering how soon they are diagnosed and treated. When you add in variables such as environmental pollution and social issues such as drug abuse, the effect piles up, making the effort to eradicate TB all the more daunting. Global cooperation and intelligent investments in research, healthcare facilities, and public health training appear downright essential to mitigate the far-reaching consequences of TB. In short, dealing with TB by looking at its environmental and social ties is essential if we're going to finally trim down its stubborn global presence (Figure 12.12).

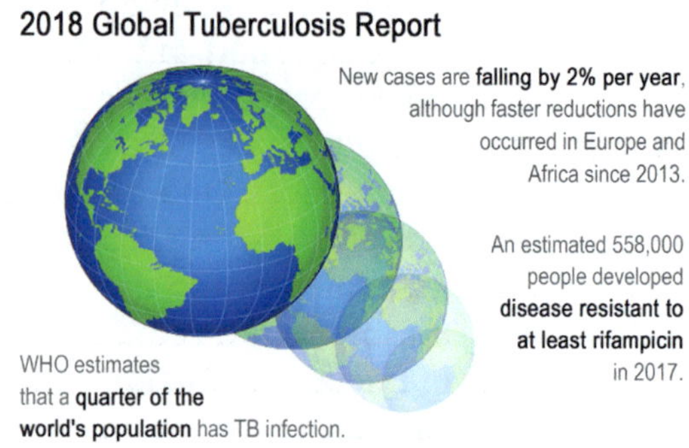

Figure 12.12. Global impact of Tuberculosis (TB).

Source: MDedge. (2018). *Global TB Statistics.*

12.5.1. Tuberculosis (TB) Prevalence Worldwide

TB remains a serious problem in much of the globe, particularly where healthcare systems are not able to keep up. Poverty, HIV co-infection, and even the finer-pointed genetic uniqueness of *Mycobacterium tuberculosis* all combine in complex and unpredictable ways. In Tanzania, for instance, research has indicated that various regions appear to have their own prevailing strains of TB, lineages such as CAS, EAI, and LAM tend to appear in specific areas. This type of local variation, by and large, suggests transmission that operates on its own small timetable and indicates that interventions may have to be individually tailored. Obtaining control of these genotype changes truly does matter if public health strategies are to find the target (Ignatova et al., 2016). Some regions of Africa and Asia continue to struggle with alarmingly high rates of TB despite improved overall control measures. The impact of HIV cannot be discounted, as individuals with weakened immunity are more likely to struggle with active TB than others. Local research has suggested that the genetic variation in the bacteria not only influences the way TB hops from one person to another but also appears to correlate with a patient's HIV status, making it a puzzle with multiple layers. For the most part, monitoring these trends, even adjusting treatment options when necessary—is essential where HIV is prevalent. New studies that combine molecular findings with clinical data are gradually unraveling this knot, giving rise to smarter and somewhat more responsive control efforts (Ignatova et al., 2016). Current statistics of TB incidence are the foundation of developing health policies and channelling funds where they are most required. Annual reports as well as larger research articles do not merely present the facts; they integrate significant findings, budgetary information, and progress reports to create a larger image of TB's hold over time. Reviews that combine molecular epidemiology with program planning facilitate easier decisions as to where additional resources can be best utilized, enhancing strategic planning. Ongoing investment, both in new research and in local healthcare strengthening—, undoubtedly, necessary if the world's TB burden is ever to be trimmed down for good.

12.5.2. Socioeconomic Factors Influencing Tuberculosis (TB) Rates

Enduring health disparities usually arrive as a package with challenging economic times - something that particularly manifests itself when you consider TB. Individuals mired in poverty or hidden away in neglected communities are likely to have a greater risk of TB, primarily due to overcrowded living areas, inadequate diet, and insufficient access to quality healthcare. In most city communities, for instance, you have densely populated surroundings that allow *Mycobacterium tuberculosis* to become cozy and spread aggressively. Joblessness and lack of proper education also have their role to play, constraining health information and making it more difficult to adopt simple preventive measures. All of this softly nudges us towards the idea that combating TB effectively entails dealing with these deeply consequential social issues. If you scratch the surface of U.S. trends, you realize that race and finances are an issue, and where you reside all combine to make TB rates different. A Chicago study, for example, indicated that U.S.-born non-Hispanic Black communities' cases of TB fell significantly in a ten-year span - despite many risk factors persisting. Overall, this suggests that whereas economic challenges enhance TB inequalities, adequately financed, focused efforts can ease those impacts. Nevertheless, the heavy burden of TB in populations with lower resources reminds us that economic status is a large, recalcitrant driver in TB control work. In the majority of instances, gaining control over these nested social and economic problems is as important as any treatment for managing TB (Armstrong et al., 2014). Digging a little further down, things become even more complicated when we consider how our bodies and the TB microbe interact. New science in areas such as microbial ecology and evolutionary biology demonstrates that TB's severity isn't all about outside pressures—it's also influenced by our environment and genes. More often than not, although tough economic times pave the way for exposure, how our body responds to infection is a fairly intricate dance between host and pathogen. This interaction pushes us towards combining policy adjustment and biomedical science to inform prevention and therapy strategies that are more effective. Understanding that TB arises from a combination of social arrangement and molecular uniqueness can, in the majority of instances, guide future public health interventions and therapy breakthroughs in a more constructive direction (Koskella et al., 2014).

12.5.3. Tuberculosis (TB) and Public Health Initiatives

Managing TB in communities largely boils down to having good, well-rounded information on hand. Health teams monitor how frequently TB arises, through what mechanisms it is spread, and among what populations risk increases. Adding context such as housing and income dynamics further illuminates why some people wind up more at risk. Yes, sure, there are speed bumps along the way, such as information arriving in patches and portions, and some concern about privacy, but when choice is guided by hard facts, resources can travel precisely where they're needed most. This process not only enhances case detection and treatment but reveals regional and demographic variations, serving to ensure fairness in the response (Thalia, 2025).

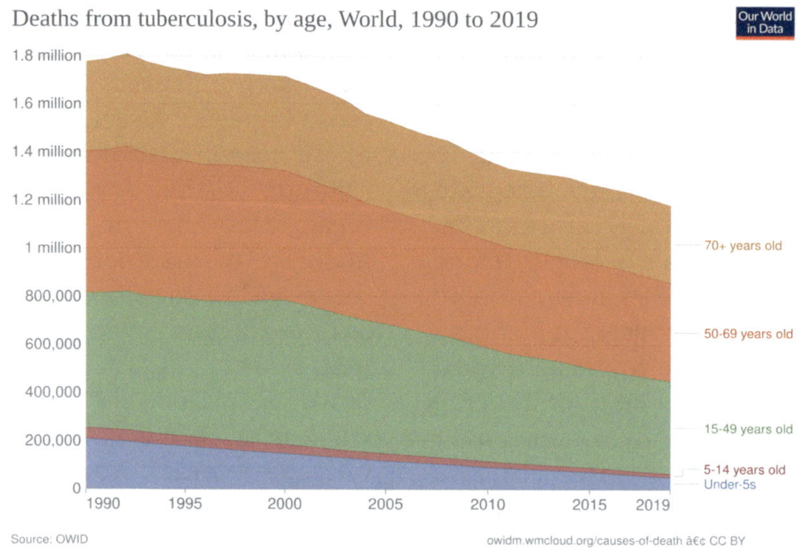

Figure 12.13. Tuberculosis (TB) and public health initiatives.

Source: By MDWiki(from Our World In Data) - https://owidm.wmcloud.org/grapher/tuberculosis-deaths-by-age, CC0, https://commons.wikimedia.org/w/index.php?curid=161670532

Incorporating insights from behavioral economics creates new opportunities for TB treatment. Classical public health is the foundation, but it can be lacking when trying to keep individuals involved in the long run. A few subtle nudges and small rewards are all that it takes to guide a patient's decision toward staying on treatment, without ever stripping away any liberty. To tailor efforts to each person's motivation – for one size does not fit all – addresses the difficult mental and social aspects of TB treatment, particularly with its lengthy regimen and the accompanying stigma. terms, newer studies highlight that if these behavioral adjustments are executed judiciously, subject to regular monitoring for ethical issues, they could enhance overall performance (Wheatley, 2024). If you mix sharp data insights with a vigilant understanding of human behavior, the entire TB management landscape begins to shift. Rather than neat numbers on one side and personal anecdotes on the other, putting these perspectives together provides policymakers with the space to create programs that address multiple needs simultaneously. Bringing communities in at the beginning fosters trust—a crucial element when attempting to break down barriers such as stigma and social exclusion. Furthermore, partnering with individuals from all sectors – from medical professionals to social workers and grassroots organizations – is seriously capable of extending the reach and life of TB control interventions. Ultimately, applying innovative data strategies in combination with behavioral concepts reduces TB cases and deaths and fosters equitability and toughness among infected groups (Wheatley, 2024; Thalia, 2025) (Figure 12.13).

12.6. Prevention Strategies

Early diagnosis, prompt treatment of latent infections, and strengthening health systems are at the center of fighting TB, particularly in areas where the disease strikes hard. Consider China, for example, it has one of the highest rates of latent TB, with about 350 million people estimated to be carrying LTBI. The nation has turned its attention to treating latent infections in high-risk groups, such as students who work with known active cases nearby. One interesting method couples a three-month course that marries rifapentine with isoniazid, typically seeking to strike a balance between treating effectively and to what extent individuals comply with the regimen. Nevertheless, there are still problems with diagnosing LTBI correctly, as older methods like the tuberculin skin test tend to yield higher counts than interferon-gamma release assays (IGRA) would indicate. In the majority of instances, pinning down precisely who is infected is crucial to preventing the leap to active disease and ending the chain of transmission (John et al., 2020). In addition to targeted treatment, an assortment of robust surveillance and harmonized public health response is essential for maintaining TB in control, particularly in areas with weak infrastructures. African countries, as a case in point, might need to consider making a priority of rebalancing investment to better detect and respond to TB, learning lessons from responding to other infectious threats, such as COVID-19. It turns out that the establishment of joint task forces, improving laboratory diagnostics and providing additional hands-on training to health staff are key measures towards increasing resilience against TB and other respiratory diseases. In most cases, these efforts take multinational cooperation and consistent political support to target the funding required for sustainable results. Modeling research, which evaluates risks of importation and regional health capacities, indicates that smart, strategic application of scarce resources can prevent outbreaks and enhance containment within epidemic-sensitive regions (Cui et al., 2020). Practical infection control measures and community engagement further provide an additional layer to TB prevention.

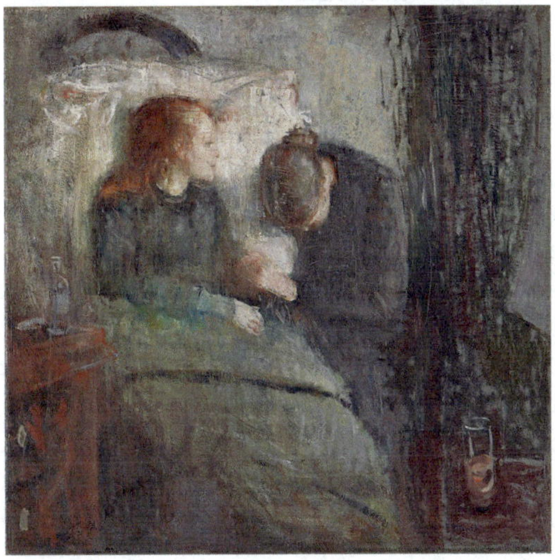

Figure 12.14. Understanding Tuberculosis (TB): Causes, risks, and prevention strategies.

Source: By Edvard Munch - http://samling.nasjonalmuseet.no/no/object/NG.M.00839 Nasjonalmuseet / Høstland, Børre, Public Domain, https://commons.wikimedia.org/w/index.php?curid=37692571

In busy or high-risk environments, strategies like keeping some social distance, enforcing sensible quarantine procedures and running health education campaigns can substantially lower transmission rates. Health workers, meanwhile, should be well-trained to implement these practices—even if that sometimes means dealing with minor logistical hiccups within healthcare settings. In addition, coupling TB control with other public health initiatives—e.g., combating co-morbidity diseases like HIV/AIDS—while augmenting supply chains for critical meds and protective equipment, truly goes a long way in cementing prevention measures. Overall, these robust strategies, alongside persistent research into new diagnostics and treatments, are crucial for achieving global TB reduction goals and ultimately eradicating the disease as a significant public health menace (Cui et al., 2020; John et al., 2020) (Figure 12.14).

12.6.1. Vaccination Efforts (Bacille Calmette-Guérin (BCG) Vaccine)

The history of the BCG vaccine is one of our greatest successes in combating TB, particularly because it has helped to reduce severe pediatric TB. In the majority of instances despite BCG being the sole licensed TB vaccine in the world, its efficacy, particularly in preventing PTB in teenagers and adults—is more likely to vary significantly. Such inconsistent performance has largely driven ongoing research and novel efforts to enhance its protective efficacy. Current debates in workshops have highlighted entire mycobacteria cell vaccines; such methods may sometimes involve genetically modified BCG strains designed to augment the immune response while reducing pathogenic threats. But hurdles remain: the absence of appropriate animal models, uncertain correlates of immune protection, and limited human challenge studies continue to impede the development towards better TB vaccines. Numerous specialists, in the majority of cases, recommend that optimizing vaccination tactics to target older age groups more effectively would be most beneficial to TB control worldwide including White et al. (2015). Beyond research breakthroughs, the effective implementation of BCG vaccination programs significantly determines TB prevention efforts. In rural or distant high-incidence locations, procrastination in the delivery of the vaccine can negate its value—especially among vulnerable children. To counteract this, some creative tactics have cropped up, such as conducting home-visit vaccination with flexible open vial strategies. For instance, research studies in places like Papua, Indonesia, show that although these tactics at times mean a little bit more wastage of vaccines, the net benefit—in terms of quality-adjusted life years as well as a decrease in cases and deaths from TB— outweighs the additional expenditure. The incremental cost-effectiveness ratios derived in these analyses suggest that such community outreach programs are fiscally responsible and provide an encouraging model for reaching populations within hard-to-reach communities (Machlaurin et al., 2023). Taking the broader perspective, scaling up BCG vaccination activities resonates with both public health returns and judicious resource allocation. Although outreach programs do have a higher initial cost than facility-based vaccinations, their potential for significantly reducing child TB incidence and death cannot be dismissed. Home vaccination strategies, especially in settings where the health infrastructure is underdeveloped, not only can ensure that vaccines are delivered on schedule but also start to reverse long-existing inequities in healthcare access that have enabled TB to take hold. terms, such measures also complement global TB control goals by working to protect the most vulnerable groups and reduce community transmission. Overall, incorporating such measures into national immunization schedules may make overall TB prevention strategies more robust and support the creation of greater equity in health outcomes (Machlaurin et al., 2023).

12.6.2. Public Health Campaigns

Controlling TB wasn't always so high-tech as it is now—it relied on a combination of medicine and community efforts to put the brakes on. At that time, early diagnosis and patient counseling were the main attractions, and campaigns even focused on habits such as public spitting on busy city streets, which helped spread the disease. Officials constructed sanatoriums and established regulations mandating that TB cases be reported, actions that accelerated awareness and initiated treatment earlier. The records indicate these measures did reduce TB mortality, but they don't account for the dramatic decline observed during the early 1900s (Anderson et al., 2019). Currently, combat against TB has assumed a more advanced taste by combining various strategies. Researchers now study TB alongside other lung infections—pneumonia, for example, using maths models to figure out which numbers (like infection and recovery rates, and campaign success) matter most. In most cases, health experts even use techniques such as Pontryagin's maximum principle to try and cut the number of infections and keep costs down simultaneously. Cost–benefit analyses suggest that even though a full-spectrum approach typically averts more cases, budget limitations tend to force officials to sometimes focus solely on TB treatment because it is the most inexpensive option (Gweryina et al., 2023). Despite these advancements of the modern era, the fight against TB is still a challenging one. Continuous public education, which at times can be a little redundant, continues to serve a vital function by motivating such factors as improved ventilation and faster trips to the doctor when symptoms develop. Public actions paired with medical treatment ensure individuals remain on their treatment regimens—a step in the direction to prevent the development of drug-resistant organisms. Evidence-driven, custom-fit approaches sensitive to realities on the ground remain essential, not to mention the fact that although initial public health actions failed to account for all the gains, their continually updated integration with novel therapies remains a cornerstone in the global battle against TB (Anderson et al., 2019; Gweryina et al., 2023).

12.6.3. Importance of Early Detection and Treatment

Infections like TB often creep up without much warning, so catching them early is a big deal—not only for the person affected but also for the community at large. Spotting TB when it's still in its early stages lets doctors jump into treatment quickly, which can ease the disease and keep it from spreading too much. If the person is diagnosed later on, the disease may have gone far enough along that treatments would be more complicated and even increase the risk of drug resistance. In short, early detection is a two-fer: it gets patients back to health quicker and prevents epidemics from running amok. A few ACF studies even indicate that it can accelerate treatment and interrupt the transmission chain—a fact that becomes extremely important in high-burden settings where delays can significantly contribute to both social and economic burdens. Prompt initiation of treatment following a diagnosis of TB is no less important. Rapid therapeutic effect can reduce bacterial load in a patient's lungs with speed, which not only tends to increase clinical outcomes but also prevents the disease from spreading further. Clinical experience generally suggests that active case finding enhances treatment success by ensuring patients present early and adhere to their treatment regimens. This, in the majority of situations, increases the likelihood of conversion of sputum—a marker that the bacteria are being cleared and that the patient is becoming less contagious. Additionally, early treatment can shorten the duration a person has TB, maintaining lung function and overall quality of life. From a program perspective, the connection of early detection with speedy treatment truly utilizes resources more effectively and reduces the long-term burden on healthcare systems (Li et al., 2024). In short, the union of rapid detection and rapid treatment appears to be key to successful TB control. Technology is now becoming part of the battle against TB in fascinating ways. New diagnostic technologies, such as those powered by AI imaging analysis, are assisting in accelerating the diagnosis of lung abnormalities just like in cases of lung cancer detection. These advances help clinicians to identify TB more rapidly and accurately from other lung conditions, which can help them design treatment that is personalized to the patient's requirements. Of course, these gadgets must undergo rigorous testing and must integrate sensibly with current clinical practices before their complete potential is reached. Nevertheless, when you combine technology advances with speedy clinical response, it appears that there is a good possibility to significantly enhance TB control programs worldwide (Li et al., 2024) (Figure 12.15).

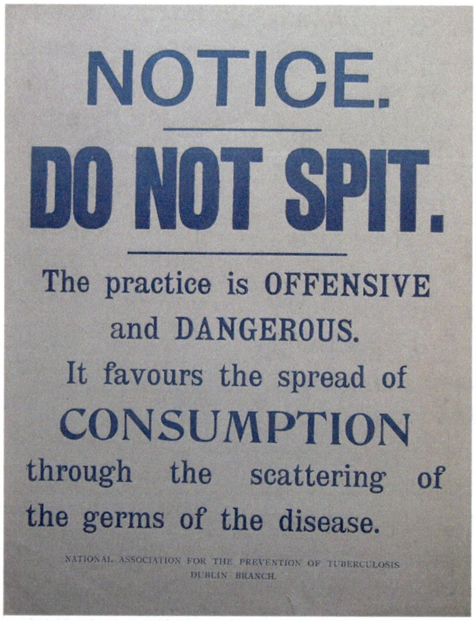

Figure 12.15. The importance of early detection and treatment.

Source: By Unknown authorNational Association for the Prevention of Tuberculosis, Dublin Branch1905 - Google Arts & Culture — notice-do-not-spit-national-association-for-the-prevention-of-tuberculosis-dublin-branch/SAFcCWlmnTtKnw, Public Domain, https://commons.wikimedia.org/w/index.php?curid=92571769

CLOSER LOOK

PATHOGENESIS AND LATENT VERSUS ACTIVE TB INFECTION

Tuberculosis (TB), caused by Mycobacterium tuberculosis, remains a leading global infectious disease, affecting millions annually. Its pathogenesis is marked by the bacterium's ability to evade the host immune system, establish infection, and persist in either latent or active forms. Understanding these mechanisms is critical for diagnosis, treatment, and prevention.

Inhalation of aerosolized droplets containing M. tuberculosis allows the bacteria to reach the alveoli, where they are phagocytosed by macrophages. However, M. tuberculosis can survive within these immune cells by inhibiting phagosome-lysosome fusion, resisting oxidative stress, and modulating host cytokine responses. This immune evasion facilitates bacterial survival and dissemination to regional lymph nodes, lungs, and sometimes extrapulmonary sites.

Following initial infection, the host immune system often contains the bacteria without eliminating them entirely, leading to latent TB infection (LTBI). In this state, individuals are asymptomatic and non-infectious, but the bacteria remain dormant within granulomas—organized aggregates of immune cells that sequester the pathogen. Latent TB can persist for years or even decades.

Active TB infection, in contrast, occurs when the host immune system fails to control bacterial replication. Reactivation may result from immunosuppression, malnutrition, or co-infection with HIV. Active TB manifests with symptoms such as chronic cough, fever, weight loss, and hemoptysis, and individuals are highly infectious. During this stage, extensive lung tissue damage occurs due to both bacterial activity and the host's inflammatory response.

Distinguishing latent from active TB is essential for treatment: latent infections require preventive therapy to reduce the risk of reactivation, while active TB necessitates multi-drug regimens to eliminate the bacteria and prevent resistance.

The pathogenesis of TB involves complex host-pathogen interactions that determine whether infection remains latent or progresses to active disease. Effective TB control relies on understanding these mechanisms to guide targeted screening, timely treatment, and public health interventions.

Summary

TB remains a difficult challenge despite advances in modern medicine and public health. Most cured patients, ironically enough, still live with lung issues, an indicator of the fact that our treatments tend to be more about eradicating the bacteria than about what happens afterward. Many individuals complete their courses of antibiotics to discover that their breathing is still problematic in the long term; this persistent problem indicates that our guidelines lack a focus on lung rehabilitation. Speaking broadly, when variables such as sex, smoking status, and blood profiles are involved, results deteriorate over time (Khosa et al., 2020). In the majority of instances, TB programs should consider beyond the mere eradication of the disease, by also providing follow-up care that enhances the quality of life. Beyond the usual lung complications, EPTB is becoming a significant percentage of cases globally. This type doesn't have the same script—the disease appears in every kind of way based on age, sex, and where individuals reside, which complicates normal diagnosis and treatment schedules. Even greater rates among women, children, and those living in specific provinces suggest that social, environmental, and biological factors all intertwine to determine the way the disease manifests and the outcome of patients (Tahseen et al., 2020). In most cases, addressing these differences means we require improved data and targeted research, so our interventions can reduce sickness and death across the board for all types of TB. When you pull all these threads together, it's apparent that the war against TB has to be multifaceted. We can't stop at infection cure; our strategy must also invest in follow-up care, such as monitoring lung function over time—to reduce chronic breathing problems and enable survivors to recover. Concurrently, increasing data on EPTB, exploring differences between regions, and identifying significant risk factors can inform smarter policies that reflect TB's complicated reality (Khosa et al., 2020; Tahseen et al., 2020). Simply put, lessening TB's impact on the world hinges on an equal combination of successful treatments, serious post-treatment rehabilitation, and subtle public health that responds to patients' and communities' diverse needs.

When addressing infectious diseases globally, knowledge of AMR is crucial—it makes TB management a headache. AMR has the tendency to increase mortality rates, prolong the duration people are ill for, and drive up healthcare costs across the globe. As far back as 2019, resistant bacteria accounted for millions of fatalities, which, in a general sense, indicates to us that having quality data is rather a priority to determine our next move. In most low-resource settings, cramped lab facilities hold back efforts to monitor and respond to outbreaks, and microbes such as *Escherichia coli* and *Staphylococcus aureus* continue to reappear as leading pathogens; multidrug-resistant TB, in particular, is particularly concerning. All of this suggests the necessity for policies that are attuned to local realities—ones that address infection control, judicious use of antibiotics, and new research on treatments and vaccines seriously. Evolving data systems in areas that lack resources, though sometimes like crawling, is vital for fully understanding AMR's impact and designing useful public health interventions (Christopher et al., 2022). Pivoting the focus to the immune aspects, regulatory T cells (Tregs) appear to have a huge influence on the course of TB and its management. These cells assist in maintaining our immune system balanced and sort of mold the way our body responds to *Mycobacterium tuberculosis*. Latest research, in the majority of instances, shows that Treg activity varies with the infection course—initially they may grow and suppress the defensive response, thus allowing the microbe to establish itself, while later, during chronic stages, they appear to relax the inflammation that, if unchecked, would cause tissue damage. This trend, so to speak, highlights just how complex the immune response is in the case of TB; it's not simply a matter of quantity of Tregs, but also quality of activity. Such findings can lead to new immunotherapies that walk a delicate tightrope between combatting the pathogen and avoiding overactive inflammation (Ahmed & Vyakarnam, 2020). Combining these epidemiologic trends and immune dynamics truly depicts the nature of the problem in combating TB. How increased AMR interacts with how Tregs modulate immune responses appears to guide both disease course and treatment outcomes. To grasp the significance of drug-resistant TB in this larger context of global AMR is to see the necessity for improved surveillance and intervention tailored to local circumstances—albeit ones that may not necessarily be simple. While simultaneously, uncovering the mechanisms of Treg function requires exploring further than merely counting cells; it necessitates qualitative understanding central to releasing more effective therapies. Looking ahead, future plans should combination enhanced data systems, cutting-edge immunological research, and well-rounded public health initiatives if we're to really cut down TB's toll. To summarize, a broadly focused strategy like this appears to be our best shot at overcoming today's challenges and eventually taking better control of this global health issue (Ahmed & Vyakarnam, 2020; Christopher et al., 2022).

References

1. Craig, G., Meershoek, A., Zwerling, A., Daftary, A., Citro, B., Smyth, C., Lewis, D., Ni Cheallaigh, D., Byrne, E., Mitchell, E. M. H., Leimane, I., Malar, J., Levy, J., van der Land, J., Macintyre, K., Johnston, L. G., Ferris France, N., Engel, N., Mumba, O., ... Nair, T. (2018). *TB STIGMA – MEASUREMENT GUIDANCE*. CHALLENGE TB. https://doi.org/10.18745/PB.20489 (accessed on 7 May 2025).

2. Abebe, R., Hill, S., Schwartz, H. A., Small, P. M., et al. (2019). *Using Search Queries to Understand Health Information Needs in Africa*. http://arxiv.org/abs/1806.05740 (accessed on 7 May 2025).

3. Ahmed, A., & Vyakarnam, A. (2020). Emerging patterns of regulatory T cell function in tuberculosis. *Clinical & Experimental Immunology, 202*(3), 273–287. https://doi.org/10.1111/cei.13488.

4. Ai, J., Zhou, X., Xu, T., Yang, M., Chen, Y., He, G., Pan, N., et al. (2019). CRISPR-based rapid and ultra-sensitive diagnostic test for *Mycobacterium tuberculosis*. *Emerging Microbes & Infections, 8*(1), 1361–1369. https://doi.org/10.1080/22221751.2019.1664939.

5. An, Y., Ni, R., Li, Z., Yang, L., Ye, Z., Li, L., Parkkila, S., et al. (2025). Tuberculosis vaccines and therapeutic drug: Challenges and future directions. *Molecular Biomedicine, 6(1), 4*. https://www.semanticscholar.org/paper/a615624943937b2573ef93b4f75890db24537a3d (accessed on 7 May 2025).

6. Anderson, D. M., Charles, K. K., Las Heras Olivares, C., & Rees, D. I. (2019). Was the first public health campaign successful? *American Economic Journal: Applied Economics, 11*(1), 143–175. https://doi.org/10.1257/app.20170411.

7. Armstrong, L., Carter, J. M., Hardison, X., & Lippold, C. (2014). Trends and disparities in TB among U.S.-born Black and White Chicago residents, 1998–2008. *Journal of Health Disparities Research and Practice, 7*(2), Article 6. https://digitalscholarship.unlv.edu/jhdrp/vol7/iss2/6 (accessed on 7 May 2025).

8. Arya, A., Amir, A., Kumar, H., Rana, K., Siddiqui, M. A., & Kapoor, N. (2014). *Mycobacterium tuberculosis* H37Rv: *In silico* drug targets identification by metabolic pathways analysis. *International Journal of Evolutionary Biology, 2014*, Article ID 284170. https://doi.org/10.1155/2014/284170.

9. Aslan, G. (2024). Diagnosing tuberculosis: Traditional and new methods against an old enemy. *Journal of Clinical Practice and Research, 5*(3), 55–62. https://www.semanticscholar.org/paper/d8ed461d2adc3126351ee07dc951a420d3a2b9b1 (accessed on 7 May 2025).

10. Bailey, A., Giorgi, A., Ashaye, A. O., Bamford, A. R., Kampmann, B., Taylor, B. R. S., Pace, C., & the TB-CHAMP Study Group. (2012). Challenges of loss to follow-up in tuberculosis research. *PLOS ONE, 7*(7), e40183. https://doi.org/10.1371/journal.pone.0040183.

11. Basera, T., Ncayiyana, J., & Engel, M. E. (2017). Prevalence and risk factors of latent tuberculosis infection in Africa: A systematic review and meta-analysis protocol. *BMJ Open, 7*, e012636. https://doi.org/10.1136/bmjopen-2016-012636.

12. Bhakta, S., Birchall, K., Evangelopoulos, D., Gibbons, S., & the TB Drug Discovery Group. (2013). Antitubercular specific activity of ibuprofen and other 2-arylpropanoic acids using the HT-SPOTi whole-cell phenotypic assay. *BMJ Open, 3*(11), e002672. https://doi.org/10.1136/bmjopen-2013-002672.

13. Boccia, D., Pedrazzoli, D., Wingfield, T., Jaramillo, E., Lönnroth, K., Lewis, J. J., Hargreaves, J., et al. (2016). Towards cash transfer interventions for tuberculosis prevention, care and control: Key operational challenges and research priorities. *BMC Infectious Diseases, 16*, Article 307. https://www.semanticscholar.org/paper/85e908c6a2322da82bd6a9fb1a2939cdeae5dcda (accessed on 7 May 2025).

14. Carnero Canales, C. S., Marquez Cazorla, J. I., Furtado Torres, A. H., Filardi, E. T. M., Delello Di Filippo, L., da Costa, P. I., Roque-Borda, C. A., et al. (2023). Advances in diagnostics and drug discovery against resistant and latent tuberculosis infection. *Pharmaceutics, 15*(10), 2409. https://doi.org/10.3390/pharmaceutics15102409.

15. Cui, X., Gao, L., & Cao, B. (2020). Management of latent tuberculosis infection in China: Exploring solutions suitable for high-burden countries. *International Journal of Infectious Diseases, 92*, S37–S40. https://doi.org/10.1016/j.ijid.2020.02.034.

16. Cunha, S. S., Merle, C. S. C., & Rodrigues, L. C. (2010). BCG vaccination and leprosy protection: Review of current evidence and status of BCG in leprosy control. *Expert Review of Vaccines, 9*(2), 209–222. https://doi.org/10.1586/erv.09.161.

17. Dai, Y., Neoh, K. G., Tong, Y. W., Wang, X., et al. (2016). On the association between outdoor PM 2.5 concentration and the seasonality of tuberculosis for Beijing and Hong Kong. *Environmental Pollution, 213*, 319–326. https://doi.org/10.1016/j.envpol.2016.02.057.

18. DeHart, C. (2020). Health concerns in Cambodia compounded by historical and rural setbacks. *Global Health Action, 13*(1), 183–191. https://doi.org/10.1080/16549716.2020.1748329.

19. Devos, I., & Janssens, A. (2017). Introduction. *European Journal of Public Health, 27*(3), 358–359. https://doi.org/10.1093/eurpub/ckx027.

20. Dookie, N., Ngema, S. L., Perumal, R., Naicker, N., Padayatchi, N., & Naidoo, K. (2022). The changing paradigm of drug-resistant tuberculosis treatment: Successes, pitfalls, and future perspectives. *Clinical Microbiology Reviews, 35*(2), e00180–19. https://doi.org/10.1128/cmr.00180-19.

21. Dreisler, E., & Kjer, J. J. (2019). Asherman's syndrome: Current perspectives on diagnosis and management. *International Journal of Women's Health, 11*, 191–198. https://doi.org/10.2147/ijwh.s165474.

22. Fang, C., He, X., Tang, F., Wang, Z., Pan, C., Zhang, Q., Wu, J., et al. (2025). Where lung cancer and tuberculosis intersect: Recent advances. *Frontiers in Immunology, 16*, 1561719. https://www.semanticscholar.org/paper/a9a7a910afbcd965e179fd4913158eb888db1f3c (accessed on 7 May 2025).

23. Faurholt-Jepsen, D. (2013). The double burden: Infectious diseases and non-communicable diseases in developing countries. *Global Health Action, 6*(1), 17222. https://doi.org/10.3402/gha.v6i0.17222.

24. Gautam, S., Qureshi, K. A., Pasha, S. B. J., Dhanasekaran, S., Aspatwar, A., Parkkila, S., Alanazi, S., et al. (2023). Medicinal plants as therapeutic alternatives to combat *Mycobacterium tuberculosis*: A comprehensive review. *Antibiotics, 12*, 541. https://doi.org/10.3390/antibiotics12030541.

25. Gweryina, R. I., Madubueze, C. E., Bajiya, V. P., & Esla, F. E. (2023). Modeling and analysis of tuberculosis and pneumonia co-infection dynamics with cost-effective strategies. *Results in Control and Optimization, 10*, 100210. https://doi.org/10.1016/j.rico.2023.100210.

26. Ignatova, A., Pawlowski, A., Shabbeer, A., Michel, A. L., Albanna, A. S., Katale, B. Z., Demay, C., & the SITVIT2 Consortium. (2016). Mapping of *Mycobacterium tuberculosis* complex genetic diversity profiles in Tanzania and other African countries. *PLOS ONE, 11*(5), e0154571. https://doi.org/10.1371/journal.pone.0154571.

27. Jimenez, J. L., Marr, L., Randall, K., Ewing, E. T., Tufekci, Z., Greenhalgh, T., Tellier, R., et al. (2022). What were the historical reasons for the resistance to recognizing airborne transmission during the COVID-19 pandemic? *Indoor Air, 32*, e13047. https://doi.org/10.1111/ina.13047.

28. Kang, W., Yu, J., Du, J., Yang, S. I., Chen, H., Liu, J., Ma, J., et al. (2020). The epidemiology of extrapulmonary tuberculosis in China: A large-scale multi-center observational study. *PLOS ONE, 15*, e0237753. https://doi.org/10.1371/journal.pone.0237753.

29. Khosa, C., Bhatt, N., Massango, I., Azam, K., Saathoff, E., Bakuli, A., Rieß, F., et al. (2020). Development of chronic lung impairment in Mozambican TB patients and associated risks. *BMC Pulmonary Medicine, 20*, Article 39. https://doi.org/10.1186/s12890-020-1167-1.

30. Koskella, B., & Lin, D. (2014). Friend and foe: Factors influencing the movement of the bacterium *Helicobacter pylori* along the parasitism-mutualism continuum. *Nature Reviews Microbiology, 12*(3), 162–173. https://core.ac.uk/download/323080778.pdf.

31. Levytska, V., & Poliukhovych, V. I. (2024). Evaluation of effectiveness and safety of therapeutic regimens for dirofilariasis in dogs. *Scientific Messenger of LNU of Veterinary Medicine and Biotechnologies, 26(116)*. https://www.semanticscholar.org/paper/b6f9635a144f6949753efc344158d0f7b5f33832 (accessed on 7 May 2025).

32. Li, Y., Wang, Y., & Qiu, Z. (2024). Artificial intelligence research advances in discrimination and diagnosis of pulmonary ground-glass nodules. *Zhonghua Jie He He Hu Xi Za Zhi = Zhonghua Jiehe He Huxi Zazhi = Chinese Journal of Tuberculosis and Respiratory Diseases, 47*(6), 566–570. https://www.semanticscholar.org/paper/000e0ccb92c2fcde50f612e53515628592d4c593 (accessed on 7 May 2025).

33. London School of Hygiene & Tropical Medicine. (2013). *Annual Report 2013*. https://core.ac.uk/download/19452766.pdf (accessed on 7 May 2025).

34. Luo, Y., Chen, H., Chen, H., Xiu, P., Zeng, J., Song, Y., Li, T., et al. (2024). Recent advances in nanotechnology-based strategies for bone tuberculosis management. *Pharmaceuticals, 17*, 170. https://doi.org/10.3390/ph17020170.

35. Machlaurin, A., Luttjeboer, J., Setiawan, D., Sytse van der Werf, T., & Postma, M. J. (2023). Non-restrictive open vial policy combined with the home visit vaccinations for improving BCG coverage in a high-incidence outreach region: A model-based cost-effectiveness analysis for Indonesia. *Journal of global health, 13*, 04049. https://doi.org/10.7189/jogh.13.04049

36. Manesh, A., Gautam, P., Kumar, S. S., Mannam, P., Jasper, A., Gunasekaran, K., Thomas, N. C., et al. (2023). Effectiveness of adjunctive high-dose infliximab therapy to improve disability-free survival among patients with severe central nervous system tuberculosis: A matched retrospective cohort study. *Clinical Infectious Diseases, 77*, 1460–1467. https://doi.org/10.1093/cid/ciad401.

37. McCreesh, N., & White, R. G. (2018). An explanation for the low proportion of tuberculosis that results from transmission between household and known social contacts. *Scientific Reports, 8*, 23797. https://doi.org/10.1038/s41598-018-23797-2.

38. Mechal, Y., Benaissa, E., Mrimar, N. E., Benlahlou, Y., Bssaibis, F., Zegmout, A., Chadli, M., et al. (2019). Evaluation of GeneXpert MTB/RIF system performances in the diagnosis of extrapulmonary tuberculosis. *BMC Infectious Diseases, 19*. https://doi.org/10.1186/s12879-019-4687-7.

39. Morgan, R. W. (1980). Basic health needs in Africa. *Health Policy and Planning, 1*(2), 121–135. https://open.bu.edu/bitstream/2144/40428/1/WP_29_Morgan_1980.pdf (accessed on 7 May 2025).

40. Mori, M., Villa, S., Ciceri, S., Colombo, D., Ferraboschi, P., & Meneghetti, F. (2021). An outline of the latest crystallographic studies on inhibitor-enzyme complexes for the design and development of new therapeutics against tuberculosis. *Molecules, 26*(6), 1712. https://doi.org/10.3390/molecules26061712.

41. Mouli, V. P., Munot, K., Ananthakrishnan, A. N., Kedia, S., Addagalla, S., Garg, S. K., Benjamin, J., et al. (2016). Endoscopic and clinical responses to anti-tubercular therapy can differentiate intestinal tuberculosis from Crohn's disease. *Alimentary Pharmacology & Therapeutics, 45*, 27–36. https://doi.org/10.1111/apt.13840.

42. Murray, C. J. L., Ikuta, K. S., Sharara, F., Swetschinski, L. R., Robles Aguilar, G., Gray, A. P., Han, C., et al. (2022). Global burden of bacterial antimicrobial resistance in 2019: A systematic analysis. *The Lancet, 399*(10325), 629–655. https://doi.org/10.1016/S0140-6736(21)02724-0.

43. Nkengasong, J. N., & Mankoula, W. (2020). Looming threat of COVID-19 infection in Africa: Act collectively, and fast. *The Lancet, 395*(10234), 841, 842. https://doi.org/10.1016/s0140-6736(20)30464-5.

44. Shah, A. P., Dave, J., Makwana, M. N., Rupani, M., & Shah, I. A. (2024). A mixed-methods study on impact of active case finding on pulmonary tuberculosis treatment outcomes in India. *Archives of Public Health, 82*. https://www.semanticscholar.org/paper/975485869d59cb075adc1869d7266a6aade54ea8 (accessed on 7 May 2025).

45. Tahseen, S., Khanzada, F. M., Baloch, A. Q., Abbas, Q., Bhutto, M. M., Alizai, A. W., Shah, Z., et al. (2020). Extrapulmonary tuberculosis in Pakistan: A nation-wide multicenter retrospective study. *PLOS ONE, 15*, e0232134. https://doi.org/10.1371/journal.pone.0232134.

46. Thalia, O. P. (2025). Data-driven decision making in public health initiatives. *Research Invention Journal of Biological and Applied Sciences, 5(1), 1–4*. https://www.semanticscholar.org/paper/a3118146cd506bca6a5661d0e2bf766c716adfa6 (accessed on 7 May 2025).

47. Tostmann, A., Wubuli, A., Roy, B., Benichou, C., Merle, C., Yee, D., & the TB-PGX Study Group. (2014). The incidence of liver injury in Uyghur patients treated for TB in Xinjiang Uyghur Autonomous Region, China, and its association with hepatic enzyme polymorphisms *NAT2, CYP2E1, GSTM1*, and *GSTT1*. *PLOS ONE, 9*(1), e85905. https://doi.org/10.1371/journal.pone.0085905.

48. Tukur, H. B. (2021). An appraisal of the knowledge, attitude, and practices of abattoir workers and butchers on bovine tuberculosis in Kaduna Central Abattoir, Kaduna State, Nigeria. *Journal of Veterinary and Biomedical Sciences, 10*(2), 56–61. https://www.semanticscholar.org/paper/cab9e253561127cf692d579bdefaf6cbeaf6992e (accessed on 7 May 2025).

49. Vanino, E., Granozzi, B., Akkerman, O. W., Muñóz-Torrico, M., Palmieri, F., Seaworth, B., Tiberi, S., et al. (2023). Update of drug-resistant tuberculosis treatment guidelines: A turning point. *International Journal of Infectious Diseases, 130*, S12–S15. https://doi.org/10.1016/j.ijid.2023.03.013.

50. Vos, T., Abajobir, A. A., Abate, K. H., Abbafati, C., Abbas, K., Abd-Allah, F., Abdulkader, R. S., et al. (2017). Global, regional, and national incidence, prevalence, and years lived with disability for 328 diseases and injuries for 195 countries, 1990–2016: A systematic analysis for the Global Burden of Disease Study 2016. *The Lancet, 390*, 1211–1259. https://doi.org/10.1016/s0140-6736(17)32154-2.

51. Wheatley, M. C. (2024). Enhancing public health strategies: The role of behavioral economics in health interventions and policy. *Premier Journal of Public Health, 14*(2), 82–89. https://www.semanticscholar.org/paper/29bd92284c03888448e07bae1efaed027081c45f (accessed on 7 May 2025).

52. Young, C., Walzl, G., & du Plessis, N. (2019). Therapeutic host-directed strategies to improve outcome in tuberculosis. *Mucosal Immunology, 13*(2), 190–204. https://doi.org/10.1038/s41385-019-0226-5.

53. Zhang, H., Shi, M., Yu, L., Ran, F., Zheng, N., Wang, X., Liu, Y., et al. (2024). Identification of a diagnostic multimers-based biomarker cluster in a mouse model of pulmonary tuberculosis. *Discovery Medicine, 36*(185), 1268–1279. https://www.semanticscholar.org/paper/c1a51cffc931515a5acbf2a2f9ca8e137d9f4909 (accessed on 7 May 2025).

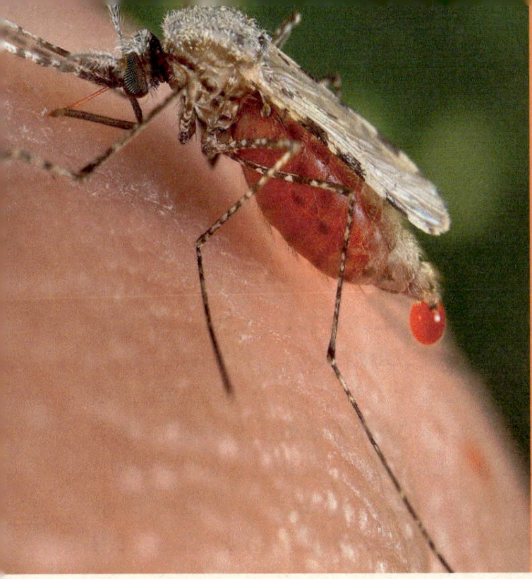

Chapter 13

MALARIA AND DENGUE

Contents

Introduction

Vectorborne diseases are a serious worldwide health problem that affect millions of lives in ways that frequently go unseen. Malaria and dengue, for example, strike tropical and subtropical areas hardest. Malaria is caused by Plasmodium parasites transmitted by Anopheles mosquitoes, and dengue is a viral disease carried by Aedes mosquitoes. These diseases, in the majority of instances, drive up healthcare expenses, reduce productivity, and put severe pressure on healthcare systems. Climate shifts, urban expansion, and even the mere existence of mosquito-friendly areas all warp the image into something complicated and complex. In the main, coming to terms with those variables is fairly crucial if we're going to develop prevention strategies that suit the local context. Education, meanwhile, is straight-up critical in controlling those diseases, particularly where they're all too prevalent. As it happens, engaging schoolchildren as health messengers can do some good; interactive presentations, group discussions, and even hands-on demonstrations about how mosquitoes reproduce and what to look for in terms of symptoms have improved knowledge among students. These initiatives don't only disseminate information regarding the insects and how to repel them (such as with nets and environmental management); they also trigger behaviors that keep families and communities safer. In most instances, this type of grassroots education snowballs, reinforcing broader public health networks (Roja et al., 2022). Retreating to take a look at the larger epidemiological landscape, infections such as dengue and malaria frequently appear in complicated patterns that are determined by their vector's biology and our own human behavior. In the US, mosquito-borne infections such as dengue continually reemerge with newer dangers such as Zika and chikungunya virus – even as tick-borne diseases appear to be on the increase. Surveillance reports occasionally indicate that although tick-related problems have been rising steadily, mosquito infection outbreaks can still strike hard in some areas. Such geographic unpredictability and the likelihood of new infections arising highlight the importance of enhanced monitoring, diagnostic work, and integrated vector management. terms, coping with these challenges requires close cooperation at both global and country levels; it's about making new tools such as vaccines and perfecting current control measures (Rosenberg et al., 2018) (Figure 13.1).

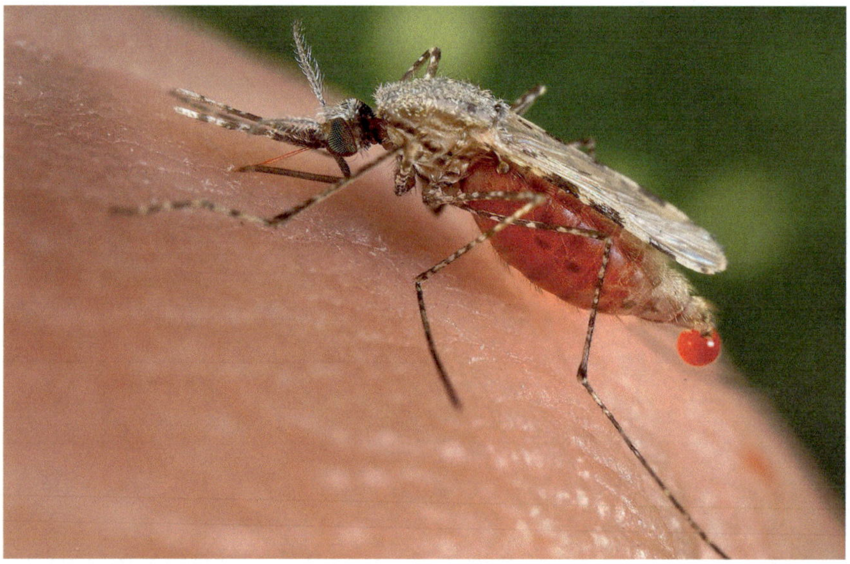

Figure 13.1. Vectorborne diseases.

Source: By Jim Gathany - This media comes from the Centers for Disease Control and Prevention's Public Health Image Library (PHIL), with identification number #5814.Note: Not all PHIL images are public domain; be sure to check copyright status and credit authors and content providers. | Deutsch | English | македонски | slovenščina | +/−, Public Domain, https://commons.wikimedia.org/w/index.php?curid=799284

Definition of Malaria

Infectious diseases are adroit. It's not only the symptoms that perplex us – it's also the mechanisms by which they take place within the body. Consider malaria, which is transmitted by those annoying Anopheles mosquitoes with Plasmodium parasites. You develop these intermittent fevers, shivering, and anemia attacks when the parasite infiltrates red blood cells, breaks them apart, and triggers the immune system of the body. By and large, the balance of power between parasite and defenses tends to swing heavily in favor of more severe sickness. In actual comparison, dengue, another mosquito-transmitted pest, has entirely different patterns of behavior when it attacks us, which makes malaria an added complexity factor. Malaria is more than a cell invasion. For example, platelets, which we tend to consider only dealing with blood clots, find themselves in the unexpected role. In most instances, these cells oscillate between keeping blood circulating smoothly and filling in as a sort of immune aid by catching onto infected red cells. Sometimes, though, the same reaction can become inflammatory in vessels or even incite trouble such as cerebral malaria by confusing clotting with vessel injury. So, while clearing the infection, platelets' zealotry may make things worse, a double-edged sword of sorts (Guo & Rondina, 2019). At a larger level, the impact of malaria is humongous, particularly in the tropical and subtropical regions where socioeconomics and the local environment enhance its spread. Described usually as a disease that extends much more than an attack by the parasite , impacting blood and vessels considerably , its significance resides both in the adversary (the parasite) and what occurs when our body responds to it. If you compare it to dengue, you observe that although they are transmitted through mosquitoes, the clinical history and causes are not identical. You may even find yourself surprised by the fact that new technologies like augmented reality are now being developed to assist in refining malaria diagnosis and education and demonstrate how slowly innovation is filtering into the fight against infectious disease (Chen et al., 2019).

Definition of Dengue

Vector-borne diseases require a consideration of both the pathogens and how they affect humans. Dengue is an acute viral disease transmitted by mosquitoes - typically *Aedes aegypti* - and it exists in four different forms, which tends to complicate immunity and increase the likelihood of a problem when a different one arrives later. The virus infiltrates the blood, further patients experience high fever, throbbing head, muscle, and joint pain, rash, and even bleeding; it's what people generally refer to as dengue fever. The condition is particularly troublesome in the tropics and subtropics where these mosquitoes are prone to thrive. Unlike some other bacterial infections which occasionally result in sepsis, dengue's complications arise primarily due to the body's immune response and bleeding blood vessels and not from bacteria intruding directly into tissues (Kristina et al., 2020). As can be readily appreciated, those distinctions imply treatment must be done in a highly differentiated manner, keeping in view both the virus and our reactions. Dengue's finicky character doesn't only derive from being a virus; it also appears with an enormous variety of symptoms. Some are almost nonexistent - perhaps only a low-grade fever - whereas others spiral into life-threatening versions such as dengue hemorrhagic fever or dengue shock syndrome, which can seriously become life-threatening. In most cases, early spotting and an accurate diagnosis are key for quick treatment and keeping outbreaks in check. Doctors often lean on several clinical signs and lab tests to sort out dengue from other fevers like malaria; after all, the symptoms can overlap more than one might expect. The World Health Organization, as a general rule, has implemented standards that emphasize supportive treatment and close monitoring for issues such as plasma leakage and bleeding (World Health Organization, 2020). These measures are meant to reduce deaths and severe disease by advocating for prompt identification and treatment—a reminder of just how critical clear definitions are in managing these diseases. In addition to the symptoms, dengue encompasses a wider picture that encompasses how it is transmitted and the contribution of mosquito behavior. Outbreaks will tend to come and go in patterns determined by weather changes, urbanization, and the general ecology of the Aedes mosquito. A detailed examination of the lifecycle of the mosquito and the small areas in which they breed informs focused control measures designed to restrict transmission. Overall, dengue has a significant global burden, infecting millions routinely and flaring in clusters due to environmental and social reasons. Because dengue has quite a few characteristics in common with malaria - consider mosquito transmission and tropical environments - a holistic approach that combines surveillance, vector control, and community engagement is crucial. This wide perspective considers dengue not only as a collection of clinical signs but as a multi-faceted public health problem that warrants concerted, global action (World Health Organization, 2020; Kristina et al., 2020) (Figure 13.2).

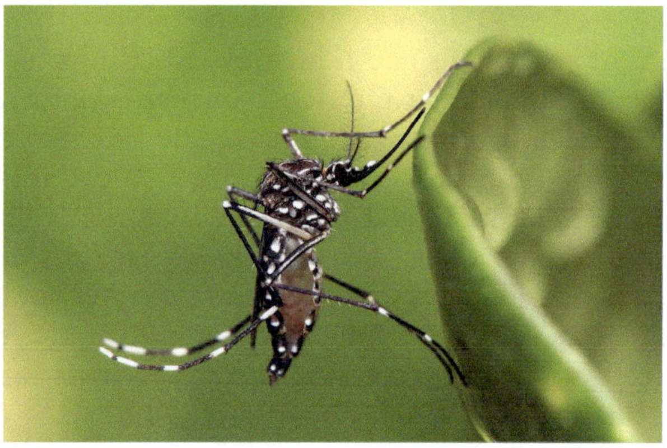

Figure 13.2. Dengue is a sudden viral disease spread by mosquitoes.

Source: By Muhammad Mahdi Karim - Own work, GFDL 1.2, https://commons.wikimedia.org/w/index.php?curid=9556152***Importance of Studying These Diseases***

Public health hinges on understanding how mosquito-borne diseases operate—a complicated web of interactions that can guide our overall health. Malaria and dengue, for instance, strike populations with a vengeance, particularly in tropical regions where mosquitoes breed like rabbits. It turns out that studying these diseases reveals how little pathogens, their mosquito vectors, and human hosts interact, and that's what scientists rely on to develop improved solutions. Occasionally, information on what mosquitoes do, our immune system, and disease transmission provides hints that lead to more targeted control concepts. Most of the time, this line of inquiry even inspires breakthroughs in vaccine research and new therapies that serve to control outbreaks; a combination of insect research, microbe exploration, and disease charting ultimately provides us with a larger perspective that is critical for public health , as is the case in many current projects (Tidball et al., 2017). Venturing into animal studies, nonhuman primates such as macaques have, in most cases, been instrumental in increasing our knowledge of these infections. Scientists have employed these primates to illuminate how diseases emerge and how our bodies combat them, ranging from diseases such as malaria to even some flavivirus-related diseases such as dengue. They closely reflect human body functions and provide a controlled environment where novel vaccines and therapies can be experimented with before reaching human testing. Their value extends beyond that of a single disease, allowing scientists to compare multiple pathogens with how hosts react, which occasionally results in insights into how we understand disease development and immunity. Overall, macaques' contribution to research demonstrates how pivotal they are in the battle against diseases such as malaria and dengue in biomedicine (Abe et al., 2008). Taking a step back, malaria and dengue affect not just the health of populations but also their economies. These diseases disproportionately affect vulnerable populations, resulting in high healthcare costs, lost productivity, and strained health services. Once research receives the investment it deserves, public health groups can drive through smarter policies, such as improved vector control, quicker diagnosis, and sound treatment regimens that reduce cases. And watching for the combination of social and environmental factors that drive disease spread can result in community-specific interventions and education initiatives. As the mosquito species and disease agents also continue to evolve, monitoring new strains and resistance is always inevitable. To summarize, exploring malaria and dengue is important not only for increasing our scientific expertise but also for developing sustainable measures that alleviate their harsh impacts worldwide (Abe et al., 2008; Tidball et al., 2017).

13.1. Historical Background

Human advancement and disease have always been complex together. Humans have developed and evolved, and concurrently, infections continued to stir things up in ways that changed entire societies. Malaria, dengue, and other vector-borne diseases have been formidable opponents—fed in part by nature's own turns and in part by human decisions. During the early 1900s, when we first began to make sense of the microbial world and learned that bacteria cause disease, there was a general assumption that we could now overcome many of these threats. Smallpox and polio, for example, dropped off the map—but it turned out pretty quickly that assuming we could eradicate malaria or dengue was a little too optimistic because these diseases continued to evolve when social and environmental contexts changed (Caminade et al., 2018). That incoherent back-and-forth between our scientific successes and the recalcitrance of these diseases indicates just how complicated controlling them truly is. Recently, things have not become any easier. Malaria and dengue have been staging unexpected returns, fueled by a combination of factors as capricious as they are diverse. Globalization, urbanization, and the relentless changes in climate have driven these diseases into new, frequently unexpected areas—areas that were previously relatively unscathed, such as cooler highlands or even more temperate climes. Weather fluctuations can be erratic as well, with temperature fluctuations, unseasonal humidity, and erratic pockets of heavy rain driving mosquito populations in unforeseen directions. Mix in human and animal migration and contrasts in public health and political stability, and you have a combination for disease persistence and re-emergence (Caminade et al., 2018). In all but a few exceptions, these trends compel us to step back and observe the intertwined combination of social and environmental elements in motion. Our biomedical advancements have done a tremendous amount of good, but they're not the magic bullet we were counting on when it comes to malaria and dengue. Those organisms responsible for these diseases, whether they're the disease-causing agents or their mosquito vectors, continue to evolve, sometimes becoming resistant to drugs and insecticides. Initial successes with diagnostics, vaccines, and therapeutics now appear to be only part of a much bigger puzzle. More often than not, we have to look beyond quick Band-Aids and consider how microbes, mosquitoes, and humans all evolve and adapt in concert; it is sort of a game of long, strategic chess. As a general rule, that requires long-term, adaptive strategies—those that integrate our biomedical advances with ideas taken from ecology and evolutionary thought (Echaubard et al., 2018). Overall, the path of fighting these diseases teaches us that contemporary health approaches need to embrace both our scientific successes and the complex, unpredictable forces of nature (Figure 13.3).

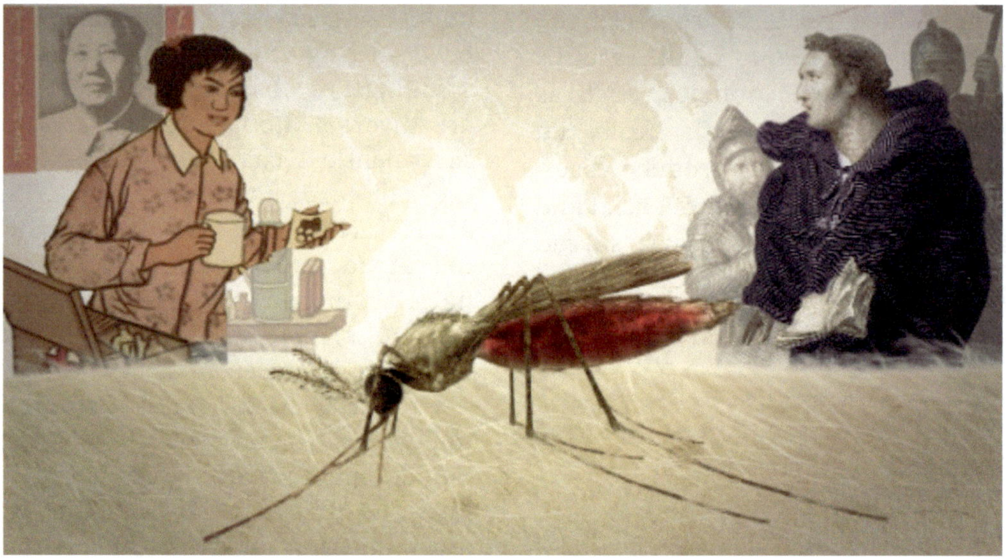

Figure 13.3. The history of Malaria drugs.

Source: NPR. (2012). *The History of Malaria Drugs.*

13.1.1. Origins of Malaria

Malaria's history stretches way back, when our primate cousins and early humans were cramped with a fluctuating environment. Millions of years ago, small Plasmodium parasites—initially partying with primates—infected humans. In tropical and subtropical areas, humans tended to stay close to pools of standing water, and those moist areas became ideal hangouts for Anopheles mosquitoes. Early on, irrigation and deforestation (which, in most instances, increased mosquito habitats) contributed to the spread of the parasite even further. With time, due to these climatic changes and human lifestyle, malaria set itself up as an ongoing health issue, even before the advent of modern medicine. Overall, the combination of our lifestyle and the natural world really set the stage for this ongoing sickness. Small, wandering Anopheles mosquitoes have played a key role in transporting malaria across continents, tying its historic origins to its worldwide presence. Various types of these mosquitoes, each flourishing under a range of climatic and environmental conditions, translate to malaria manifesting itself in various forms from region to region. As human settlements expanded and trade networks linked far-flung regions, the footprint of the disease enlarged, most apparent in Africa, Asia, and regions of the Americas. It's not solely about nature, however; urbanization and the condition of public health infrastructure also determine in what locales malaria becomes established. More often than not, contemporary science regarding vector control, even taking lessons from Aedes mosquito management strategies against dengue—tells us that nature and human systems continue to interact in complex, sometimes intractable ways (Weetman et al., 2018). More recently, climate changes and greater travel have introduced new twists to this ancient drama. Rising temperatures and altered rain patterns now drive Anopheles mosquitoes into areas where malaria used to be uncommon or under control. You can even draw parallels with the ways other vectors such as *Aedes aegypti* and *Aedes albopictus* are spreading dengue and chikungunya; it's a reminder that global environmental change impacts many diseases simultaneously. With more people on the move than ever before, parasites and their mosquito companions freely cross national boundaries, further making a control of malaria even more daunting. For the most part, comprehending the origins of malaria today involves a consideration of not only its past history thousands of years ago but also contemporary climate patterns and human migration trends that continue to reshape its future (Jan et al., 2017).

13.1.2. Origins of Dengue

Dengue fever's tale begins with the way people move and the way the environment changes, allowing its primary perpetrators, *Aedes aegypti* and *Aedes albopictus*, to spread about. Malaria, for instance, has long been associated with economic woes in disease-battered regions, but dengue's explosion—a relatively recent trend, in most instances—is gaining momentum. Urbanization and increased global travel have pushed dengue beyond its former tropical and subtropical territories. Although malaria has been around since ancient times, dengue appears to have begun in free cycles among nonhuman primates, revealing its zoonotic nature early. These early translocations remind us that chaotic ecological processes and increasing urban living tend to bring us into closer proximity with pathogens that used to remain out in the wild. Taking a closer look, comparisons between nonhuman primates , particularly macaques , have emphasized dengue's origins in zoonosis. Experiments with these animals provide a glimpse of how dengue spreads and induces disease, making some compelling comparisons to diseases such as yellow fever. The macaque model has been instrumental, both in tracking the virus's evolutionary history and in advancing work in vaccine development and treatment approaches. Generally speaking, learning about dengue's animal origins reveals just how tangled host-pathogen relationships can be, stressing the need for control measures that cover all bases. To summarize, these insights make it clear why mixing ecological studies with biomedical research is key to piecing together dengue's beginnings and planning smart public health responses (Abe et al., 2008). Different perspective, however, is that whereas dengue has just emerged onto the global scene, a long shadow by malaria extends into centuries. Research has indicated that the economic growth slowdown caused by malaria in infected regions is not merely a matter of health but also inhibits development in general.

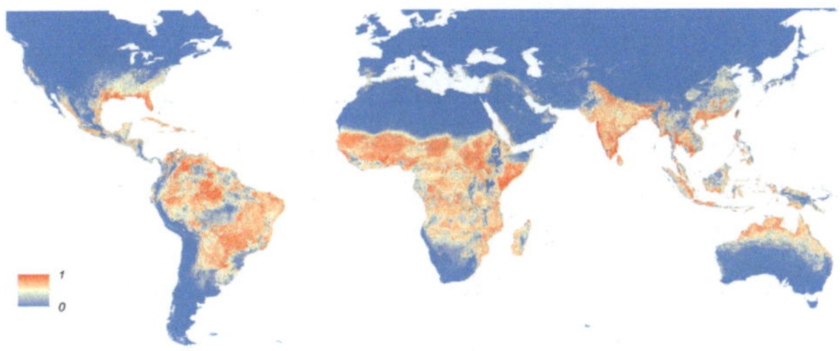

Figure 13.4. Origins of Dengue.

Source: By Moritz UG Kraemer, Marianne E Sinka, Kirsten A Duda, Adrian QN Mylne, Freya M Shearer, Christopher M Barker, Chester G Moore, Roberta G Carvalho, Giovanini E Coelho, Wim Van Bortel, Guy Hendrickx, Francis Schaffner, Iqbal RF Elyazar, Hwa-Jen Teng, Oliver J Brady, Jane P Messina, David M Pigott, Thomas W Scott, David L Smith, GR William Wint, Nick Golding, Simon I Hay - elifesciences.org/content/4/e08347, File:Global Aedes aegypti distribution.gif, CC0, https://commons.wikimedia.org/w/index.php?curid=46766801

Its historical tie and its long maintenance have been connected with gradual capital accumulation as well as a lower level of productivity, which affects arguments concerning growth and health policy. This viewpoint softly compels us to think about if dengue, with the increasing spread and rising numbers of cases, would perhaps in due course provoke corresponding economic issues at susceptible areas. Although these two diseases are dissimilar in source and mode of transmission, they both highlight the intricate relationships among health, our environment and developmental problems in the tropics. Considering dengue in conjunction with malaria provides a more complete picture, one that could assist in addressing the coinciding burdens of arboviral and parasitic diseases (Bhattacharyya, 2025) (Figure 13.4).

13.1.3. Evolution of Treatment and Prevention Methods

Treatment of vector-borne diseases such as malaria and dengue has progressed a great distance over the years. In the old days, treatment essentially involved symptom relief with fairly rudimentary drugs that frequently yielded mixed results. Over time, however, more targeted drug regimens, such as the combination therapies that are now standard in malaria treatment—have managed to stave off resistance, and patient results have tended to improve overall. While scientists probed deeper into the process of how viruses replicate and how our immune system combats invaders, new concepts like new antiviral medicines and ways to augment our immune system for fighting dengue started taking form. Such advances based on both bench molecular work and actual clinical trials have gradually transformed routine care into something more individualized and based on firm evidence. It all hints at the need for broader models that can simulate a disease's progress and the effects of various treatments, alteraltering healthcare strategies for different communities and regions (Mohareb et al., 2024). In short, we've shifted from one-size-fits-all approaches to more nuanced methods that consider the characterestics of pathogens and the unique traits of each patient. Conversely, how we avoid these diseases has also gone a large, sometimes surprising, way, partly thanks to technological advances and a greater understanding of how diseases spread. In the beginning, preventing the transmission typically involved keeping mosquitoes away with practices such as insecticide-treated bed nets and cleaning areas where they could lay eggs. These days, those tried and trusted methods are combined with new methods such as genetically modifying vector populations and creating vaccines for long-term immunity and transmission decline over time. In the majority of situations, recent research emphasizes silent carriers and varying transmission levels, genuinely making the argument for stricter surveillance and wiser, on-the-spot diagnosis. For example, employing rapid point-of-care tests in addition to more detailed PCR tests when confronted with fevers has honed our capacity to identify true pathogens, resulting in more precise measures and less unwarranted antibiotic administration (Elfving et al., 2016).

Prevention has become a multi-layered combination of technology, biology, and community-based interventions, all woven together in sometimes overlapping contexts. Since both treatment and prevention continue to advance, our models need to remain adaptive to address new challenges to malaria and dengue control. Simulation models that integrate virus behavior insights, clinical outcomes, and epidemiological information function like a crystal ball, informing public health policies and resource allocation decisions (Mohareb et al., 2024). They allow us to test how effective interventions would be in a variety of scenarios—, it's a change in the numbers of disease, shifts in community immunity, or disparate access to healthcare services. Combining these models with insights from on-the-ground research makes them more grounded in reality, allowing it to be simpler to adjust both the treatment strategies and prevention guidelines. This dance between experimentation and simulation not only sharpens our approaches but also turns the entire process of combatting these diseases into a continuously adapting, cooperative endeavor.

13.2. Transmission and Vectors

Environmental factors and disease transmission sort of combine together in a way that's difficult to overlook when we're talking about problems like malaria and dengue. Warmer by a few degrees or changes in rain—even how clouds suddenly break—, accelerate mosquito life cycles, so these insects develop faster and transmit infections faster. It's as if when the pressure is on, mosquitoes just zoom through life, and heavy rains create heaps of standing water that serves as a nursery for their eggs. Not only does this increase the absolute number of mosquitoes but gradually draws them into new regions, threatening communities that are not used to these insects. More often than not, combining nature's signals with climate information becomes just what the doctor ordered to make an educated guess about where the next outbreak will appear (Pavia et al., 2024). Scrutinizing further, the specific behaviors of various types of mosquitoes are a key indicator for how we address these ailments.

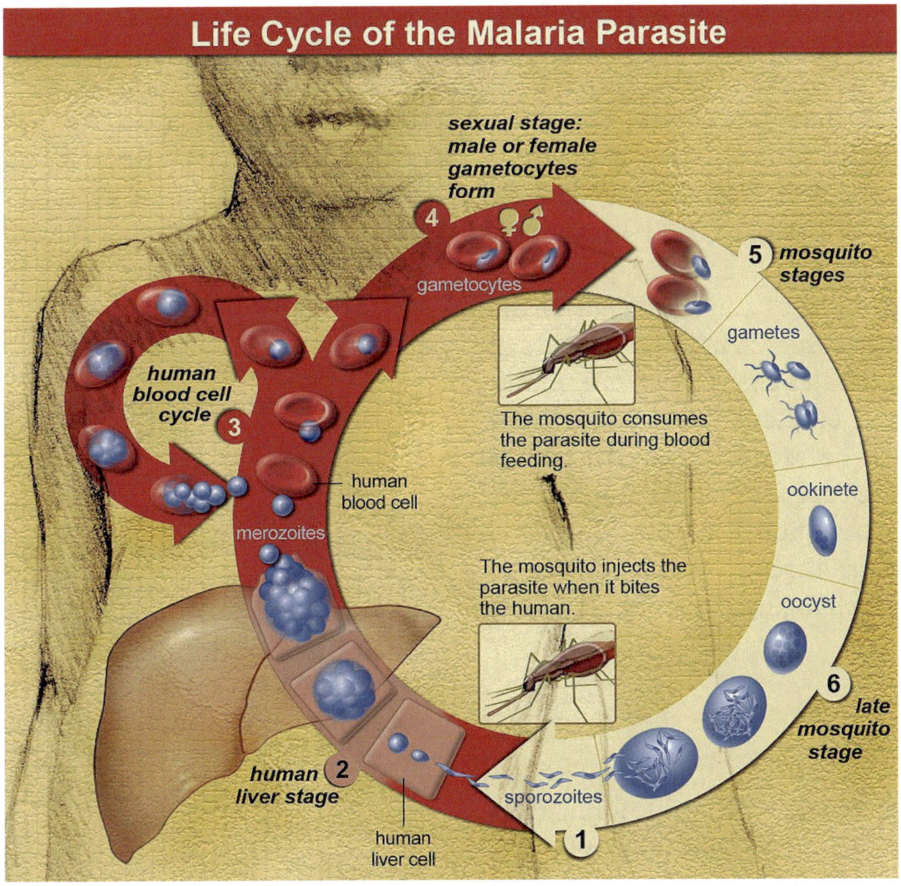

Figure 13.5. Transmission and vectors of malaria.

Source: By National Institutes of Health (NIH) - National Institutes of Health (NIH), Public Domain, https://commons.wikimedia.org/w/index.php?curid=29552307

For instance, Anopheles mosquitoes—responsible for spreading malaria by carrying Plasmodium parasites—are very different from *Aedes aegypti* and *Aedes albopictus*, responsible for dengue. Aedes mosquitoes tend to loiter in urban areas, feeding during the day, which obviously increases their likelihood of coming close to humans. Plus, a bit of extra heat can alter how quickly viruses multiply inside them, a detail that scientists call "vector competence." It turns out that understanding these little characterestics, repeated again and again through study, is really crucial if we're going to design any effective plan to lessen disease impact (Begum, 2024). Climate change isn't just a hum in the background—it actively remaps the playground for these disease vectors, keeping public health systems on their toes. Rising global temperatures and unpredictable rainfall appear to drive malaria and dengue mosquitoes into territories that weren't even considered earlier; sometimes it seems as if the ground rules keep shifting. Some of the earlier predicting models that incorporate climate trends perform reasonably well predicting these emerging patterns, at least providing some glimmer of hope of staying ahead of the issue. Concurrently, research into the genetics of pathogens demonstrates they're evolving subtly, so even our most efficient control measures occasionally must be reconsidered. All of this serves to make the case for ongoing monitoring – and, yes, a bit of global cooperation – to keep these shifting threats under control as our climate keeps changing (Pavia et al., 2024) (Figure 13.5).

13.2.1. Mosquito Species Responsible for Malaria

Mosquitoes are primarily responsible for malaria transmission due mainly to their mode of living and acting. Anopheles, for example, are the most frequently associated with being carriers of Plasmodium parasites. They tend to appear everywhere, with heat and humidity pretty much determining where they breed and bite. Overall, this combination of mosquito biology and weather ultimately determines the rate at which severe and seasonal malaria develops. Even slight changes in climate will nudge where these insects can thrive, expanding or contracting their warm homes (Jan et al., 2022). Further human behaviors and socioeconomic conditions usually modify where mosquitoes prefer to hang around, in turn increasing the threat of local epidemics. So, effective approaches to fighting malaria must reckon with both the nature of these insects and the ever-changing environment. Figuring out which Anopheles species are the main offenders is key if we're aiming for precise control. Take Anopheles gambiae, *Anopheles funestus*, and *Anopheles stephensi* – these ones are widely recognized for passing on *Plasmodium falciparum*, the parasite known to be the deadliest. Not all of them act exactly the same way; a few prefer indoor conditions to feed on people, so techniques such as indoor spraying or bed nets become quite useful. However, in most instances, promoting insecticide resistance in these mosquitoes puts a large monkey wrench into worldwide control programs. And because the prevailing mosquito forms can differ from place to place, control strategies frequently require local adjustment. The increasing resistance in addition to their ability to adapt literally points towards the necessity of new strategies, genetic or biological adjustments, perhaps, necessary to partner with conventional procedures in staying ahead of malaria (Dyck et al., 2020). Consider now Aedes mosquitoes. While they're more commonly associated with conditions such as dengue, their presence with Anopheles introduces another layer of sophistication for controlling these insects. Anopheles are typically confined to environments of clean, slow-flowing water, as opposed to the container-oriented behavior of Aedes. Even so, both species may respond to climatic fluctuations in similar ways, sometimes resulting in coincident outbreaks that strain public health infrastructures even further. There have been recent advances, including releases of sterilized insects and Wolbachia infection, aimed at limiting the populations of mosquitoes.

Though much has been expended toward controlling Aedes, scientists are now seeking similar strategies for those Anopheles with a penchant for avoiding typical indoor interventions. By and large, combining these newer strategies with old ones appears to be of major importance in reducing malaria transmission and alleviating its wider global health burden (Dyck et al., 2020).

13.2.2. Mosquito Species Responsible for Dengue

The transmission of dengue fever is closely associated with a handful of types of mosquitoes that breed in cities, primarily tropical and subtropical locations. *Aedes aegypti*, perhaps the principal offender, is a particularly effective carrier of the disease; the insect has essentially made itself at home in our cities by laying eggs in any manner of human-made water vessels around homes. Its day-biting habit, in the majority of instances, renders it even more efficient at transmitting the virus. Further there is *Aedes albopictus*, which, owing to international commerce and travel, has been spreading to new locations in unforeseen patterns. Both mosquitoes are highly resilient, thriving in high-density areas with inadequate water handling and sanitation (Allan et al., 2022).

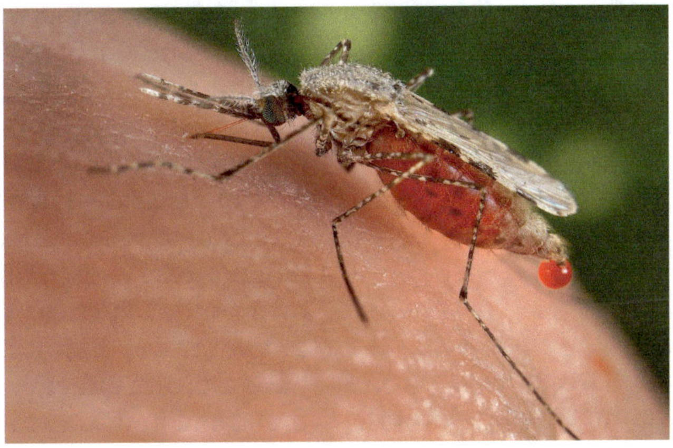

Figure 13.6. Dengue mosquito versus normal mosquito.

Source: By Jim Gathany - This media comes from the Centers for Disease Control and Prevention's Public Health Image Library (PHIL), with identification number #5814.English | македонски | slovenščina | +/−, Public Domain, https://commons.wikimedia.org/w/index.php?curid=799284

Understanding what such insects like is central to managing them and reducing disease risk. During the last few decades, the distribution of Aedes mosquitoes has expanded exponentially, presenting serious challenges for managing dengue globally. Urbanization, climate change, and rising mobility have all contributed to altering where and how concentrated such pests emerge. Indeed, these mosquitoes have invaded more than a 100 countries over roughly the past 50 years—this is partly because they can exploit manmade water containers for laying eggs, and partly due to their emerging insecticide resistance. This broad spread not only amps up the danger of dengue but also makes efforts to control them a far more tangled issue. Where Aedes species intersect with other arthropods that are hosts for other viruses, public health issues truly add up, and many advocate that measures of integrated management, addressing these uniqueness, need to be implemented urgently in our urban areas (Allan et al., 2022). With the limitations of conventional insecticide-based controls, there is a move now towards new and innovative approaches targeting these Aedes dengue carriers. Some of the most recent methods include employing symbiotic bacteria—Wolbachia, for instance—to disrupt the virus's capacity to replicate within the mosquito. Genetic engineering concepts also exist, such as gene drives, which seek to reduce or modify mosquito populations so they cannot transmit the disease with as much ease. These new interventions, when implemented, might provide scalable and more sustainable solutions to complement or even substitute chemical controls, particularly because those have the potential to encounter issues with resistance and environmental concerns. In most instances, controlling *Aedes aegypti* and *Aedes albopictus* through these biotechnological developments seems to be an important step in alleviating the worldwide dengue issue and preventing future outbreaks in susceptible urban locations (Figure 13.6).

13.2.3. Environmental Factors Influencing Transmission

Malaria and dengue, and their relatives, rely heavily on the environment where they are found—mosquitoes thrive, breed, and feed optimally under ideal circumstances. Temperature and humidity fluctuations, for instance, may alter a mosquito's functionality and even the rate at which a disease develops within it. Such changes at times fine-tune the longevity of mosquitoes or the number of bites per day, which in turn changes the rate at which diseases spread. Human activities such as urbanization and forest destruction, in the majority of instances, interfere with nature by causing additional breeding grounds and allowing mosquitoes to infest new zones. In general, understanding how nature's uniqueness and our own interact with mosquito behavior is the most important factor in developing adaptive control strategies (Bera, 2025). Rain, particularly seasonal rain, truly makes a difference in the context of dengue because it influences where Aedes mosquitoes, the prime offenders, can deposit eggs. For most areas with consistent temperature and humidity, changes in rain influence water accumulation in routine locations such as containers and natural pools, which ultimately determines the mortality of mosquito larvae. An example is a study from Sri Lanka's Colombo district, where monsoon rains are found to coincide with variations in what we refer to as vector competence—, simple capacity of mosquitoes to acquire and transmit the virus—throughout various seasons. This type of seasonal surge in mosquito ability just illustrates how dengue transmission is so sensitive to even minor alterations in the environment, and it highlights why rain data is so frequently inserted into disease predictions (Chathurangika et al., 2024). The combination of environmental conditions and mosquito biology not only adjusts to what extent mosquitoes can spread disease—it also stages the intensity and timing of when outbreaks happen. Malaria- and dengue-carrying mosquitoes thrive in their own unique niches, and slight fluctuations in temperature, humidity, or precipitation can have a direct effect on the speed at which they breed and how long they persist. Mosquitoes are experts at adjusting to new circumstances, and when you mix in human variables, it stands to reason that no one strategy will work. Rather, we need to merge climate science, mosquito research, and public health actions into a single strategy. When we gain a better understanding of these environmental drivers, we can start developing control programs that are not only a band-aid but a sustainable means of reducing the global disease burden of malaria and dengue (Chathurangika et al., 2024; Bera, 2025).

13.3. Symptoms and Diagnosis

Most patients with infectious diseases tend to present with several symptoms that overlap, making the entire diagnostic process quite complicated. Fever, body pain, tiredness, chills, nausea, and vomiting are all typical of both malaria and dengue – so much so that it is difficult to know which one is causing the problem without diagnostic tests. More often than not, when labs are not readily accessible, particularly in under-funded areas, the image becomes even more blurred. Rather than scanning one sign at a time, some doctors are now examining a complete set of signs all at once. They're typically speaking in methods that combine fuzzy criteria importance and weighted techniques in novel ways to score symptom severity and association, which can then result in a more accurate estimate about diseases such as malaria and dengue. Overall, this type of comprehensive symptom screening assists in accelerating treatments and, despite overlapping symptoms, generally enhances patient outcomes (Momena et al., 2023). Contemporary molecular diagnostics are now also a primary feature when the typical symptoms alone simply don't suffice for a diagnosis to be made. Where resources are low, rapid tests , sometimes complemented by methods such as recombinase polymerase amplification (RPA) and reverse transcription polymerase chain reaction (RT-PCR) , have been used to dismantle viruses, including the dengue virus. Even some of the studies that employ mobile labs (which sound almost like experiments) have indicated that these on-the-move assays can function almost as well as big, centralized lab tests. For example, when dengue is diagnosed in children by RT-PCR in combination with antigen capture assays, it emphasizes the fact that combining molecular testing with conventional assessments is beneficial – especially when typical fever symptoms appear to obscure the actual condition, as is also true with malaria. This type of synthesis, though maybe not always exact, makes a major contribution to identifying the suspect and guiding efficient treatment and control measures (Dieng et al., 2020). Despite all these neat new technologies, clinical judgment still has its place, particularly when diagnostic tests are delayed or altogether absent. Because both malaria and dengue tend to cause similar, non-specific fever symptoms, doctors often have to rely on a deep clinical look combined with lab checks to avoid misdiagnoses.

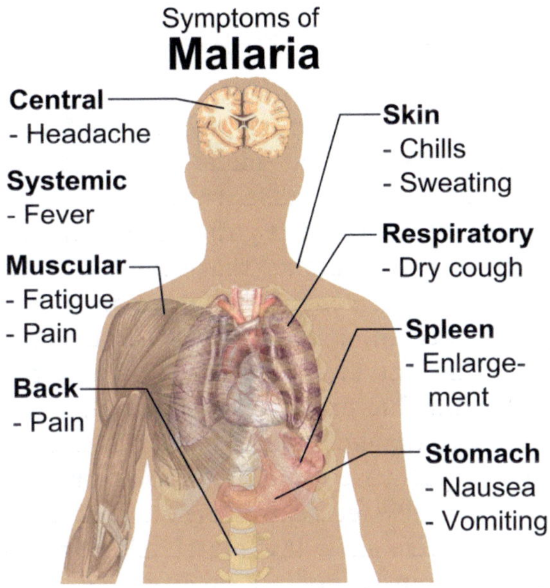

Figure 13.7. Symptoms and diagnosis of malaria.

Source: By Mikael Häggström.When using this image in external works, it may be cited as:Häggström, Mikael (2014). "Medical gallery of Mikael Häggström 2014". WikiJournal of Medicine 1 (2). DOI:10.15347/wjm/2014.008. ISSN 2002-4436. Public Domain.orBy Mikael Häggström, used with permission. - All used images are in public domain., Public Domain, https://commons.wikimedia.org/w/index.php?curid=6557991

Things like checking platelet counts (which, let's be honest, often drop in dengue), hematocrit, and liver enzymes can provide those extra clues needed to tell one disease from the other. In most cases, a multi-symptom model of assessment that combines laboratory markers with molecular testing (when available) is the best approach. A multi-layered approach – as one can imagine, a sometimes awkward-looking one – is essential in regions where both diseases are rampant because it reduces diagnostic errors, refines treatment regimens, and even reduces morbidity and mortality by averting delayed or off-target diagnoses (Dieng et al., 2020; Momena et al., 2023) (Figure 13.7).

13.3.1. Common Symptoms of Malaria

Passengers who return from tropical or subtropical areas can make it very difficult for physicians to diagnose what is behind their fever. Many times, such patients present with a mixture of symptoms that might be either malaria or even dengue. Malaria, for example, typically accompanies a set of three signs—fever, chills, and sweating—but it is how these appear and fluctuate in severity that usually directs the diagnosis. If a person has a very high temperature (usually about or above 39.5°C) and also feels extremely fatigued, the lab work may also show low platelets and anemia signs. Of course, not all cases check all the textbook boxes, but such changes in the blood typically indicate that the parasite is playing with red blood cells and the immune system, a clue which proves particularly valuable when working with patients from sub-Saharan Africa (Satarvandi et al., 2024). Besides merely having a fever and a few bizarre lab results, malaria victims occasionally complain of headaches, sore muscles, and even some gastrointestinal distress. These additional symptoms complicate things, making it difficult to distinguish malaria from other tropical diseases such as dengue. Occasionally matching up a patient's travel history with where they could have been exposed in malaria-endemic regions sorts things out somewhat. Surprisingly, dengue will present with such things as a visible rash and a fall in white blood cells, so if you don't notice those but notice anemia and low platelets, the weights generally fall in the direction of malaria. There's been some hope in employing scoring systems that combine both clinical impressions and laboratory cues to more accurately rank the probability of malaria (Satarvandi et al., 2024). Monitoring malaria's telltale characteristics isn't only about making the correct diagnosis—it also has a great deal to do with being able to treat the patient effectively, particularly in areas where many feverish diseases are prevalent. For the most part, malaria is characterized by its cyclical pattern of fever and dramatic shifts in blood counts that require immediate intervention to avoid complications. In contrast to dengue, which may carry a clearer rash and lower platelet count as well, so each presents uniquely. You find someone presenting with high temperature, chills, and diagnostic leads such as anemia and thrombocytopenia; it will serve to enable clinicians to differentiate between malaria from the other fever-like infections, e.g., typhoid or dengue. Since these overlapping signs can readily cause confusion, it's all about combining what the test reflects, what the labs indicate, and the patient's history of exposure to achieve the best result.

13.3.2. Common Symptoms of Dengue

Dengue fever comes on hard and fast, combining a combination of symptoms that can seriously disrupt your daily life. It begins with an abrupt, high fever, typically persisting for about two to seven days—often accompanied by thumping headaches and a piercing, nearly annoying pain behind the eyes. Mostly, people report the muscle and joint pain to be so severe that the disease was given the nickname "breakbone fever," a reference to the raw pain experienced throughout the body. A few days later, after the onset of the fever, you may see a rash on the skin that resembles raised red bumps or small pinpricks. This initial, feverish phase is crucial for detecting the disease and initiating care before it can deteriorate into something more severe. On the other hand, these symptoms are easily confused with other infections, making it difficult to determine whether it's dengue, particularly where diseases like malaria are also prevalent (World Health Organization, 2020). From that shaky beginning, however, dengue can turn in the wrong direction. In a majority of instances, the disease may advance to more severe stages characterized by such factors as plasma leakage, bleeding complications, and even organ damage. You may end up with patients experiencing incessant vomiting, persistent pain in the belly, nose or gum bleeding, and overall tiredness. These are indicative of the progression towards dengue hemorrhagic fever or even dengue shock syndrome. Laboratory tests may reveal low platelet counts and evidence of hemoconcentration, red alerts that the patient may be predisposed to spontaneous bleeding or shock. All of these things require physicians to be on high alert, particularly in environments where there are few medical supplies, to determine whether a patient must be hospitalized or offered additional care as expediently as possible (World Health Organization, 2020).

It's also important to know that dengue doesn't always follow the same rules. Depending on age, the environment one lives in, and an individual's background of immunity, symptoms can change quite significantly. Although most victims exhibit the typical fever and bleeding symptoms, others, particularly children or those with a previous dengue infection—may present milder or even atypical symptoms. This unpredictability makes it difficult to establish one set of blanket rules for diagnosis. And because dengue's symptoms may mimic those of other insect-borne diseases such as malaria, determining which disease is responsible usually depends on delicately balancing clinical presentation, laboratory findings, and travel history. terms, gaining a good understanding of how dengue manifests in various individuals is the key to improved public health planning and ultimately improved patient outcomes (Griffiths et al., 2018) (Figure 13.8).

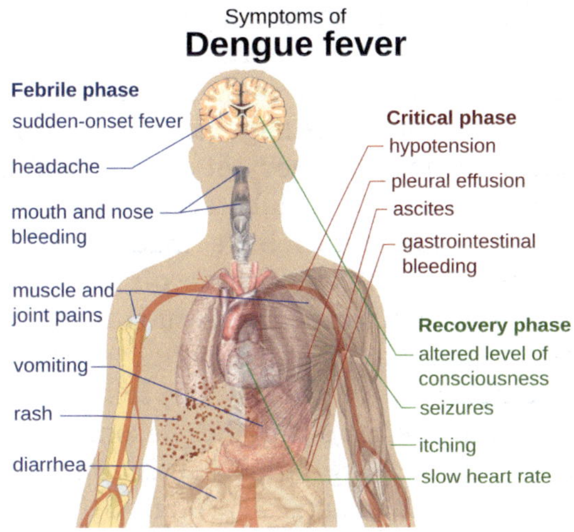

Figure 13.8. Dengue symptoms.

Source: By Mikael Häggström - All used images are in public domain; references are found in Wikipedia article at Wikipedia:Dangue fever., Public Domain, https://commons.wikimedia.org/w/index.php?curid=12712988

13.3.3. Diagnostic Methods for Both Diseases

Rapid and precise diagnosis is crucial when faced with infections like malaria and dengue-albeit they have similar symptoms most of the time, each requires its own type of treatment. Malaria diagnosis typically relies on examining blood smears under the microscope, but even that is still the superior method because it can detect and differentiate between various Plasmodium types. Rapid diagnostic tests have made inroads, partly because they're fast and easy to employ in the context of limited resources. Nevertheless, these tests do not always yield consistent results; their sensitivity and specificity vary based on changes in the parasite's genetics and even some environmental uniqueness. Dengue, however, is more challenging. Direct detection by PCR, looking for the virus's RNA, is highly sensitive but requires specialized laboratory facilities. Meanwhile, dengue-specific IgM and IgG antibody tests are widespread but fumble since their results occasionally cross-react with other flaviviruses. In general, these diagnostic challenges compel us to keep refining our methods to reduce misdiagnosis and improved patient outcomes (Gregory et al., 2018). Aside from the conventional lab techniques, recent molecular diagnostics have made available more tools for detecting these diseases early. Nucleic acid amplification tests such as PCR and loop-mediated isothermal amplification (LAMP) permit detection of pathogen-specific genetic material long before antibodies become visible. In most cases, adding antigen-detection tests to it captures non-structural protein 1 (NS1) in the very early stage of infection. Although such techniques do increase diagnostic accuracy, they have a cost: expense, technical sophistication, and dependence on properly trained staff, so they're largely limited to reference laboratories or outbreak situations where accurate epidemiological information is critical (Vos et al., 2017). In most situations, the selection of a diagnostic test is a matter of weighing accuracy, cost, and speed—all critical for informing clinical decisions and public health interventions. On the horizon, new point-of-care technologies are on the rise to simplify diagnostic challenges in countries hard-struck by malaria and dengue. New systems such as biosensors, microfluidic devices, and mobile health platforms are being engineered to combination the detection of viral proteins with parasitic antigens, assisting in distinguishing with clarity between the two infections. These handheld, user-friendly machines are set to avoid the infrastructural requirements of centralized laboratories. Even though initial pilot studies are encouraging, these methods still require rigorous testing by way of large-scale trials under diverse field settings. Of note is the importance of maintaining diagnostic accuracy; misclassification can result in incorrect treatment, thus increasing morbidity and even mortality. For the majority of situations, advancement in these new diagnostic techniques is imperative not only to enhance disease monitoring but also to refine treatment guidelines and ultimately advance patient care in regions affected by these vector-borne diseases (Vos et al., 2017; Gregory et al., 2018).

13.4. Treatment Options

Malaria and dengue introduce a whole set of challenges beyond how they're transmitted. Old malaria treatments—chloroquine and artemisinin-based combination therapies—are still at center stage, but resistant parasites have complicated the picture considerably. Dengue, by contrast, has no particular antiviral solution; treatment is generally about relieving symptoms and avoiding severe, sometimes hemorrhagic, complications. Scientists are, for the most part, experimenting with novel ideas in treatment to improve efficacy and avoid resistance. For instance, treatment for malaria nowadays frequently tries out sophisticated drug combinations and combinations therapy, while dengue treatment relies intensely on faster diagnosis and improved fluid management regimens to reduce mortality and permanent disease. Recent advances in vaccine technology, by and large, present some fairly promising avenues against these mosquito-borne pathogens. Virus-like particles (VLPs) are gaining the spotlight as a new type of subunit vaccine that functions as though it's the actual virus without any genetic ,—thus, triggering a robust immune response without the risk of infection. The VLPs, which have demonstrated remarkable immunogenicity by initiating both antibody and cell-based defenses in distinct ways from conventional vaccines, can be engineered to enhance their delivery and durability. Such adaptability makes them a future game changer in preventing malaria and dengue infections, with continuous refinements highlighting a preventive strategy that complements current therapies nicely (Nooraei et al., 2021). It is not only the drugs and vaccines that count;

managing the vector mosquito is also of vital importance. Integrated Vector Management (IVM) has taken a step forward in amalgamating innovative control strategies to reduce disease transmission. A standout strategy is the sterile insect technique (SIT), in which huge quantities of sterilized male mosquitoes are released to slowly reduce the population. This process offsets increasing insecticide resistance and the limitations of traditional control methods. Combining SIT with the incompatible insect technique (IIT), which employs Wolbachia bacteria to interfere with mosquito reproduction and restrict disease transmission, offers even greater outcomes while reducing the risk of releasing females accidentally. Early pilot trials in various countries have shown that these approaches work in urban settings, offering a sustainable and cost-effective path to reducing malaria and dengue cases. To summarize, when these vector control methods combination with medical treatments, they move us closer to a more holistic strategy that tackles both the diseases and the tiny carriers behind them (Dyck et al., 2020) (Figure 13.9).

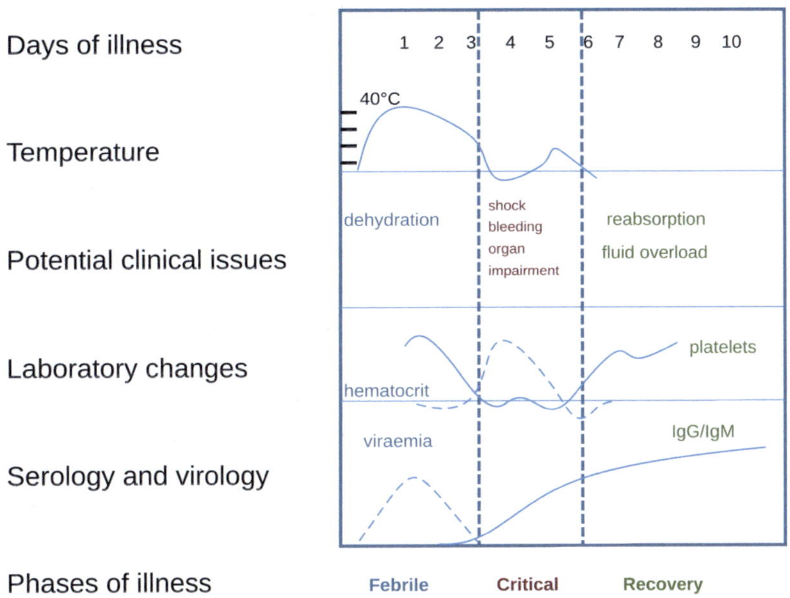

Figure 13.9. Treatment options for dengue.

Source: By Course_of_Dengue_illness.png: Dr Graham Beardsderivative work: UAwiki - This file was derived from: Course of Dengue illness.png:, CC BY-SA 3.0, https://commons.wikimedia.org/w/index.php?curid=27425148.

13.4.1. Antimalarial Medications

Medicinal chemistry has advanced a great deal and transformed the way we combat diseases such as malaria. In the good old days, medications were simple, but today we notice that ingenious drug design—combinationincorporating in heterocyclic molecules like pyridine and dihydropyridine—has significantly enhanced the efficacy of antimalarial drugs. Those nitrogen-rich ring systems appear to enable the drug to bind on to its targets within the parasite, inhibiting its growth more effectively. You also see these heterocycles appearing in a whole series of FDA-approved medications for other diseases, which only adds to their worth. Their chemical versatility provides access to entirely new medicines that may even be able to break resistance—a major barrier to malaria treatment. In most instances, as scientists keep prodding these molecular structures, there's potential for treatments that are both more powerful and less harsh on patients (Ling et al., 2021). Applying antimalarial medications in actual clinics isn't as easy as it seems. Their efficacy can vary dramatically across the different Plasmodium species, and resistance appears to emerge everywhere. Consider chloroquine, for instance—it was once the standard treatment, but widespread resistance has rendered it mostly useless, so physicians have turned to Artemisinin-based combination therapies instead. These ACTs combine quickly acting artemisinin derivatives with longer-acting partner drugs in an attempt to slow resistance development and eliminate parasites more rapidly. Nevertheless, the rising trend of ACT failure, particularly in Southeast Asia, suggests that we need new treatments and tighter pharmacovigilance urgently. And, of course, how these drugs travel and are metabolized within us (their pharmacokinetics) also has a big impact on dosing and whether or not patients remain adherent to the regimen. Continuing research into resistance processes and new drug candidates is strictly necessary to maintain therapy effectiveness in areas fighting mild as well as severe malaria (Ling et al., 2021). It's not just a matter of attempting to eradicate the microbe, though—, also developing antimalarial drugs. It's also monitoring how such medications may modulate our own immune processes. Historically, the emphasis has been on killing the organism, but new evidence indicates that certain chemicals may also change the patient's immune response, perhaps the extent to which the disease progresses or how rapidly one recovers. It's somewhat akin to what's been observed with antiviral drugs in past outbreaks, highlighting the necessity of a more multi-layered approach to treatment. Although there was much fuss about herbal immunomodulators during the COVID-19 period, solid clinical evidence of their efficacy is still wafer thin. Nevertheless, integrating immunomodulatory properties into antimalarial drug development requires extensive preclinical and clinical studies to ensure safety and efficacy. Ultimately, this strategy could enhance malaria control by not only targeting the parasite but also modulating the harmful immune responses that exacerbate the disease.

13.4.2. Treatment for Dengue Fever

Dengue fever is difficult to manage without a specific antiviral drug. Physicians typically must work by alleviating symptoms and preventing the disease from becoming risky forms such as the bleeding complications or shock experienced in some cases. Fluid balance is critical—fluids are administered cautiously to compensate for plasma leakage and maintain blood pressure levels during the critical phase of the disease. Electrolyte equilibrium and ensuring the patient remains properly hydrated are factors too, and at times blood transfusions are called for once bleeding takes off. In most low-resource settings, though, these are difficult to accomplish, which puts additional pressure on an already strained healthcare system. Generally, attempts with immune-based therapies such as convalescent plasma or monoclonal antibodies have not gone so well since the virus gets cleared quickly before shock can truly develop, and there is always that possibility of antibody-dependent enhancement - an issue raised with such therapies as Dengvaxia™ (Anthony et al., 2019). All this reinforces the imperative for affordable, effective care guidelines that can operate across various settings. In combating dengue, maintaining a leash on mosquitoes is of the utmost importance, even though it's not as easy as it's made out to be. *Aedes aegypti* likes to persist in urban jungles while *Aedes albopictus* is found persisting around temperate zones, which spoils eradication efforts. Chemical control strategies lose their oomph when mosquitoes develop resistance, and when you add in the requirement for ongoing, community-level environmental management, things get really complicated. In addition to that, vaccine development is still a pillar of dengue's control over public health. Even with some encouraging beginnings, vaccine research continues to stumble over issues such as not possessing a good animal model to test and concerns regarding causing antibody-dependent enhancement , both problems that have similarly been created with regard to Dengvaxia™ and other candidates (Anthony et al., 2019). More often than not, this puts vaccine approaches into the tricky position of trying to provoke a robust immune response without compromising safety, ideally to protect against all four types of dengue. Beyond the realm of immediate treatment, the larger impacts of dengue on society and the economy cannot be overlooked. Consider India, for instance, working every year with large dengue case numbers in addition to high healthcare costs truly places emphasis on collaborative research efforts for improved treatment and prevention. Programs like the Indo-U.S. Vaccine Action Program have been fueling innovation in vaccine development as well as in conducting clinical trials, particularly where the hardest hit by the disease are (Anthony et al., 2019). Concurrently, however, it is worthy to remember the lesser-perceived, longer-term effects of dengue; international statistics demonstrate that although mortality rates may be declining, considerable numbers of individuals remain with disabilities resulting from the disease. This trend suggests that increased support for recovery and rehabilitation services is necessary. In general, a combination of on-the-spot clinical treatment, meticulous epidemiological monitoring, and cooperation across the globe is necessary to create novel therapies and enhance healthcare facilities to conquer dengue fever.

13.4.3. Role of Supportive Care in Recovery

Recovery from diseases such as malaria and dengue relies on more than a pill and a quick fix. Antimalarial medication and conventional treatments set the stage in clinics, but sometimes it's that added layer of supportive care that truly makes a difference. When symptoms overlap or when co-infections, such as *Plasmodium falciparum* malaria and dengue—occur, the value of this care increases even further. Problems like low platelets, dehydration, or additional bacterial issues require close observation and fast response. Take providing fluids to fight plasma loss in dengue or securing blood transfusions for a bad case of anemia associated with malaria; these actions can literally halt a crisis in its path. This holistic, all-around approach not only calms immediate complaints but, in the majority of instances, stabilizes the body as a whole, reducing the bite of the disease and accelerating recovery in vulnerable populations such as children (House et al., 2025). If you look beyond the conventional clinical treatments, you soon realize that the stability and quality of care in proxy rely heavily on more general health system determinants. One large factor is training and supervision of front-line health workers - and on this front, supportive supervision schemes in areas where such diseases are prevalent have shown genuine promise. Rather than applying punishment by the back of the hand, these schemes rely on cooperative coaching—setting an atmosphere where healthcare professionals feel both incentivized and somewhat less apprehensive. In most instances, this combination of emotional boost and hands-on guidance helps pin down proper diagnoses and timely care moves that are essential when diseases become complicated. Generally speaking, the durability and effectiveness of these support measures are closely correlated with how effectively these supervision programs are established within the health system (Manzi et al., 2025). Supportive care extends far beyond what goes on within hospital walls, spilling over into how patients become informed of and take charge of their own healing. When patients and caregivers receive the inside scoop on recognizing symptoms, taking care to keep themselves hydrated, and why completing treatments is important, they become a part of the entire healing process. This partnership makes a difference, particularly in areas where resources may be limited and follow-up is not always convenient. And don't forget the worth of a good meal and a little counseling—nutritional and psychological care also enter the picture to alleviate the overall weight of the disease on body and soul. By integrating these different factors into the battle against malaria and dengue, recovery chances are significantly enhanced, reducing both the risk of complications and overall death rates associated with these diseases (House et al., 2025; Manzi et al., 2025) (Figure 13.10).

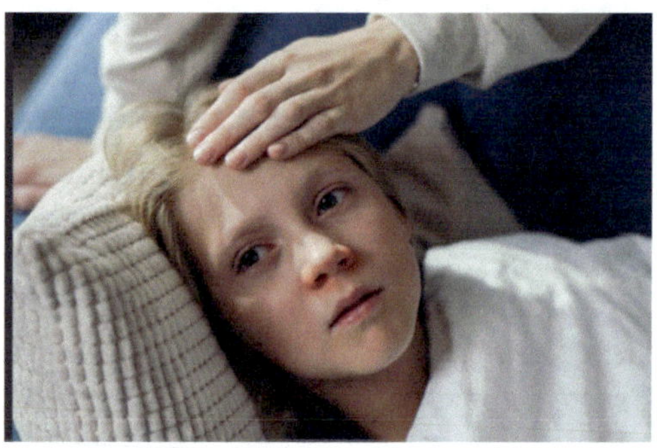

Figure 13.10. Role of supportive care in recovery.

Source: Pedi Cheshire. (2022, March). *Supportive Care.*

13.5. Prevention Strategies

Averting mosquito-borne diseases such as malaria and dengue generally involves combining a number of adaptable tactics that interfere with the transmission cycle. The concept begins with reducing human contact—sleeping under insecticide-treated bed nets each night and even wearing clothing that covers you. These individual steps reduce the likelihood of a contact with disease-carrying mosquitoes, thereby keeping disease away. Draining out stagnant water where mosquitoes breed is another easy, but effective, measure. Further there's the regulated application of insecticides to reduce mosquito numbers—but these sprays must be done with care so that they do not harm the environment or accelerate resistance. For all but the most extreme scenarios, studies have found that combining these measures with public awareness and sustained surveillance does make an impact (Butt et al., 2023). Health education and community participation also have enormous contributions. Once people know a little more, they take measures such as removing breeding sites and seeking treatment as soon as they show signs of disease. Educational programs at the community level provide useful tips that incorporate into daily life and encourage individuals to maintain preventive routines. Meanwhile, consistent government assistance, such as establishing infrastructure to monitor and respond immediately to epidemics, contributes to the overall effort. Surprisingly, when people look after themselves, that self-care tends to be the easiest and most effective route taken, with strategic application of insecticide being an important emergency measure (Butt et al., 2023). On a larger scale, intelligent utilization of healthcare means is the key. Cost-effectiveness analysis usually highlights that measures such as vector control and education are worth the investment because they yield large health returns for the expenditure incurred, which is rather significant in low- and middle-income settings. Experience with other prevention measures reveals that balancing between affordability and effectiveness counts for a great deal. Although concrete data on malaria and dengue prevention costs may be scarce in a few areas, models supporting concepts such as tax breaks for mosquito control items or insecticide-treated net subsidies can enhance public health benefits. A cautious, sometimes subtle, examination of cost versus value informs the decision to ensure that investment in preventing disease remains both wise and sustainable (Figure 13.11).

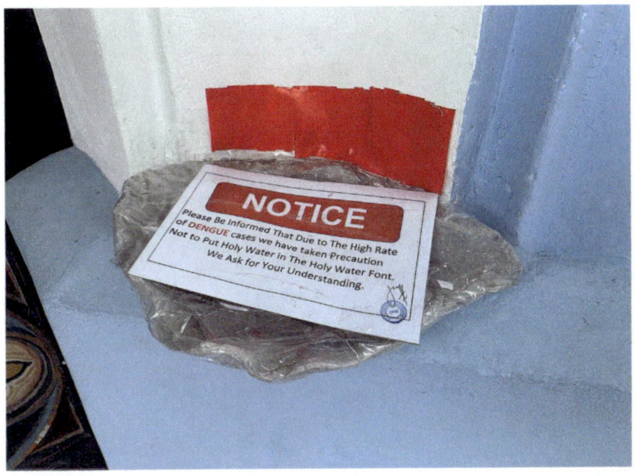

Figure 13.11. Prevent mosquito-borne diseases.

Source: By Chainwit. - Own work, CC BY 4.0, https://commons.wikimedia.org/w/index.php?curid=162168025

13.5.1. Use of Insecticide-Treated Nets for Malaria

Several have attempted various methods of reducing malaria for a long time, and one of the shining stars has been insecticide-treated nets (ITNs). These nets combine a physical barrier with a dose of insecticide to keep mosquitoes away so that individuals receive fewer bites. Not only do they protect individuals close up, but they also appear to reduce the local mosquito population, a kind of double victory. In much of sub-Saharan Africa, ITNs are the preferred means of malaria prevention. Yet, more often than not, issues such as mosquitoes adapting to the chemicals and nets being used improperly continue to arise. Lo and behold, constant adjustments and true community feedback are necessary if these nets are to continue doing their work (Zimmicrobea, 2025). Research from areas affected by malaria supports the nets' effectiveness. In Zambia's Kalumbila District, for example, when over 80% of homes had ITNs, there was an approximate 60% reduction in *Plasmodium falciparum* infection. Statistics conclusively link the use of ITNs to lower cases of malaria, indicating that although they cover individuals, they also improve health at the community level. However, interviews conducted in such regions reflect practical concerns, such as the durability of nets and whether they mesh with local traditions, which have the power to erode their effect. That is, it's not just a matter of distributing nets but also of proper, consistent use informed by social considerations (Sinzala et al., 2025). Moving forward, ITNs remain a central component of efforts to combat malaria, particularly when coupled with novel concepts like genetically altered mosquitoes. Even though the nets have lived up to their billing, maintaining their mojo involves fighting obstacles in the form of mosquito population resistance and cultural issues. In general, a policy that combinations ITNs with additional locally adapted measures—considering both health patterns and the financial scenario, appears ideal for a major impact. Science indicates that combining ITNs with innovative technological strategies can fortify malaria control, although these actions require good grassroots participation and continuous monitoring. For the time being, ITNs are not going anywhere; they are going to work alongside other interventions to continue to drive us slowly towards the eradication of malaria (Zimmicrobea, 2025).

13.5.2. Vaccination Efforts for Dengue

Dengue has quickly grown into a larger issue in recent decades. Fast-spreading Aedes mosquitoes are mostly responsible – and the tactics that used to be used to combat them, such as insecticides, aren't as effective these days because the insects are developing resistance and many breed in unmanageable containers.

This is an instance where really a better strategy is needed, one in which vaccines take center stage to play an active role. In contrast to malaria , where vaccine development has been glacial , a few dengue vaccine candidates already have reached approval, though the virus's numerous forms mean any vaccination must be effective against many different types without boomeranging on individuals. The incorporating of vaccine-induced immunity with natural infection further complicates the picture, indicating immunization campaigns must be constructed with care to enhance public health without unnecessarily increasing risks (Dyck et al., 2020).

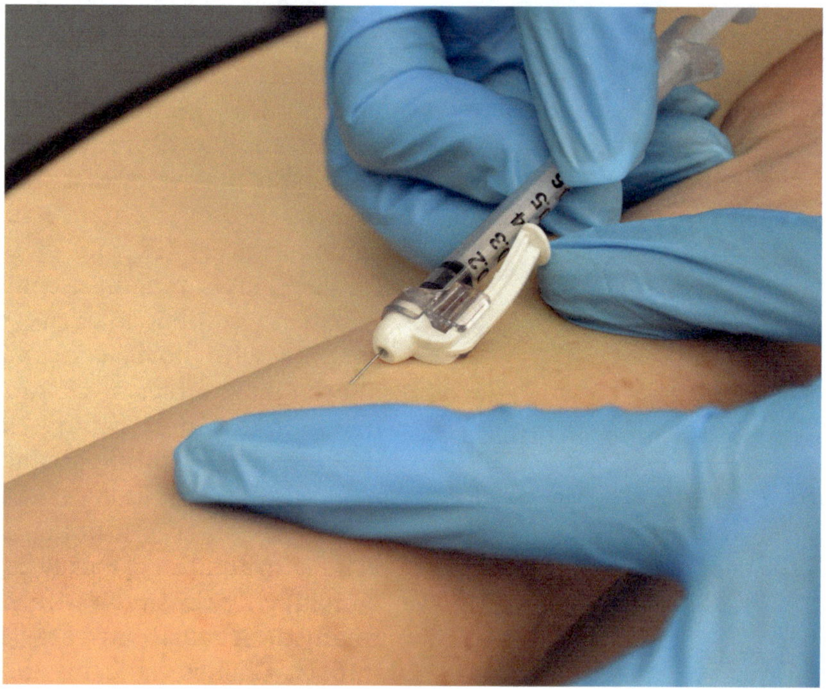

Figure 13.12. Vaccination efforts for dengue.

Source: By British Columbia Institute of Technology (BCIT). Download this book for free at http://open.bccampus.ca - https://opentextbc.ca/clinicalskills/chapter/6-7-intradermal-subcutaneous-and-intramuscular-injections/, CC BY 4.0, https://commons.wikimedia.org/w/index.php?curid=60318412

Advances in vaccines in recent years have opened numerous promising avenues for dengue prevention. New techniques, such as recombinant DNA and viral vector techniques, now allow scientists to move forward with multivalent vaccines that target all four dengue strains. Remember the frenzy during the COVID-19 pandemic, the urgency to do things quickly – but still, there is much to be said for rigorous testing. In general, the phase I to III trials are important to ensure that these vaccines are safe and highly effective in all types of individuals, particularly if there's a possibility that an inadequate immune response could even increase the severity of the disease. Combination of vaccination with other countermeasures could also give some clear, synergistic benefits that very strongly suppress dengue transmission and severe disease (Khuroo et al., 2020). Implementing dengue vaccination campaigns isn't without its own challenges. Public health systems in much of the world where dengue is prevalent have to deal with issues such as maintaining vaccines at cold temperatures, getting doses to people reliably, and persuading populations to accept them.

The virus acts differently in different places – its spread and effect can be wildly variable – so there isn't a silver bullet approach that works everywhere. Furthermore, vaccine price and equitable distribution are also important, especially as much of the stricken areas are low- and middle-income countries. To address these complex problems, international collaboration and consistent investment are truly necessary to facilitate everything from research and production to delivery. Ultimately, an effective dengue vaccination campaign would not just relieve the substantial social and economic toll of the disease but could even be a model for coordinating activity against other insect-borne diseases such as malaria, with emphasis on the merit of combining immunization with sweeping disease-control measures (Dyck et al., 2020) (Figure 13.12).

13.5.3. Community Awareness and Education Programs

Local communities engaging themselves truly makes a difference in combatting diseases caused by mosquitoes—consider malaria and dengue. Frequently, the solution is not merely medicine but individuals being educated on where these insects reproduce and how to eliminate their hideaways. If people understand that standing water can be a magnet for mosquitoes and that things as simple as nets or repellents can make a difference, then they are more likely to volunteer. In the Caribbean, for instance, Mosquito Awareness Week indicates how these unofficial school-like meetings can develop the community's capabilities. It's not merely about habit-breaking but about developing a collective feeling of responsibility, which in the majority of instances, keeps outbreaks and long-term issues at bay (Nelson et al., 2020). Education, by and large, fortifies the game plan by enabling people to identify problems earlier. If one identifies early enough the symptoms of a mosquito-borne disease, then they will seek assistance quicker—maybe lowering both the mortality and severity. Urban research typically indicates that if residents are made aware of, say, when mosquitoes are most active or where they tend to nest, they are more willing to implement simple measures to control them. This type of general know-how tends to enhance prevention and simplify the overall burden of these diseases. Therefore, always refreshing one's mind about what to do and how to think regarding these problems proves to be an important puzzle piece in regulating the influence of malaria and dengue (Nelson et al., 2020). Integrating community participation into mosquito control measures is another huge success. When locals participate too, employing their own knowledge to identify and clear mosquito breeding spots, the process feels more authentic and culturally relevant. Further there are the education sessions, which test whether people recall the tips—and give feedback in exchange—so as to really cut the health messaging to a sharper point over the long term. Open, frank communication between health workers, public health officials, and locals strengthens trust (and that's super crucial when epidemics strike). Through combining continuous education with improved surveillance and healthcare adjustments, these interventions find themselves contributing significantly to reducing transmission rates as well as the financial burden of diseases such as malaria and dengue (Nelson et al., 2020).

13.6. Global Impact

Malaria and dengue are increasing globally, and it is not one thing that causes it all. Climate changes, hotter days and more rain, couple with city populations and patchy water management to make ideal locations for the vector microbes. You have Anopheles mosquitoes moving into new locations and *Aedes aegypti* appearing where they never have before, exposing people to them unintentionally. Urban areas, too often developing haphazardly and allowing sanitation to deteriorate, contribute to the issue. Where most often rapid urban expansion comes together with changing weather, the outcome is increased disease transmission that puts a strain on healthcare, especially where resources are already scarce. terms, this complex combination requires a multidisciplinary response that harmonizes environmental management with public health strategy to control these severe infections (Zavaleta et al., 2025). The tale doesn't finish there with geography, though. New patterns indicate that dengue cases are occurring severely in older people, a bit of an anomaly given we would formerly primarily notice kids infected. This pattern reversal, and ongoing economic inequalities between countries, only compounds the problem. Low-income populations, frequently with greater exposure and less access to preventive services, carry an additional burden. Even the financial impact, lost days of work, increased cost of treatment, long-term disabilities, ripples out and struck economies with full force. In most instances, addressing all these issues entails implementing early diagnosis strategies, brighter surveillance, and more equalized health access across the board (Imlaque et al., 2025). Despite continued world efforts, malaria and dengue remain around as significant health burdens because their propagation is an unclear combination of determinants. Not only are challenges such as ambiguous diagnosis and uneven test sensitivity a problem, but effective, scaleable solutions remain elusive to nail down. We know that the solution can't be merely a biomedical solution. We must also increase community education, environmental modifications, and sturdy surveillance systems able to mobilize quickly when there are outbreaks. New technologies and enhanced global cooperation may assist as well, particularly if you keep in mind that social, economic, and environmental challenges all intertwine in complex manners. Overall, designing policies to reduce the transmission risk is no easy task, what is needed is a collaborative, multi-level global effort to confront these behemoths (Imlaque et al., 2025; Zavaleta et al., 2025) (Figure 13.13).

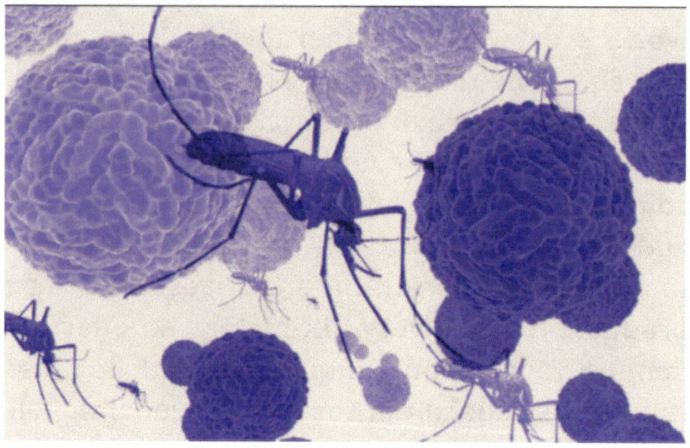

Figure 13.13. Malaria consortium: Stemming the rising tide of global dengue.

Source: Malaria Consortium. (n.d.). *Stemming the Rising Tide of Global Dengue.*

13.6.1. Malaria's Burden on Healthcare Systems

Across the world, hospitals struggle with a variety of infections—but malaria, an insect-borne disease, puts a special type of pressure that is not concerned with borders or cash. In most high-prevalence regions, caring for malaria patients means exhausting bulky resources and depending on intensive care because the disease can strike hard; this tends to overload facilities already thin from other diseases. Travelers are apt to receive good pre-trip guidance and coverage, but local people generally don't have that advantage and consequently experience more stays in the hospital and more money out of pocket. At times, when you contrast the way care is utilized overseas compared to home, it is apparent there are gaps in supportive services as well as fundamental infrastructure—a subtlety that manifests in malaria's multifaceted burden on healthcare delivery (Tozan et al., 2023). It all winds up diverting critical resources away from other health requirements and slows down the system's overall responsiveness.

Aside from the plain medical costs, malaria also adds in a great deal of insidious cost in the form of lost days of work and diminished earnings. Overall, the disease strikes working-age adults and children disproportionately, causing ripple effects throughout families that go far beyond hospital fees. Families tend to have lower incomes during episodes of sickness and convalescence, as well as additional cost in terms of travel and any additional care required. Meanwhile, health services are compelled to divert their limited resources, staff, diagnostic equipment, etc, to focus on fighting malaria rather than tackling other pressing public health problems. In low- and middle-income regions, this diversion is especially troublesome, as limited infrastructure makes each added resource strain cut more deeply, ultimately exacerbating social and economic gaps and hindering long-term development (Tozan et al., 2023). Recent global disruptions, such as those experienced during the COVID-19 pandemic, have only served to make the burden of malaria more apparent. As health systems divert attention to emerging crises, preventing and treating malaria programs can suffer, diminishing both coverage and access. This can cause delays in essential services—routine immunizations, antenatal care—that are vital to keeping malaria under control, and such delays tend to accelerate both disease and death rates. Furthermore, economic crises triggered by these disruptions only exacerbate poverty-related vulnerabilities, making it even more difficult to sustain effective malaria interventions. Finally, establishing a health system that can manage both chronic local issues such as malaria and unforeseen global risks is necessary to make sure care runs smoothly, in spite of all the bumps in the road.

13.6.2. Dengue's Economic Implications

Mosquito-borne diseases wreak havoc on more than our well-being—they empty a region's pocketbook in unforeseen ways. Dengue, for instance, has become a headache in earnest by forcing hospitals to take in more individuals, conduct additional lab tests, and incur treatment costs. This stress isn't all about the cost of medicine; it bleeds over into missed work time when people have to miss their jobs, whether they are employed in formal or more relaxed, informal environments. Population-dense tropical regions feel it even more keenly, its complexity revealed in how complex the battle against disease is with maintaining a society stable. Consider India—its runaway dengue rates, with both life-threatening diseases and deaths, end up driving up national health expenditures and dampening the economy (Naik et al., 2023). Therefore, the cost of dengue is indeed multifaceted, ranging from direct medical charges to wider effects on employee productivity and overall public health system resilience. Beneath the short-term healthcare expenditure, dengue's impact persists and disrupts community development in the long term. In areas where outbreaks recurrently occur, children are absent from school, ultimately reducing opportunities and preventing poverty from ever breaking its cycle. Expenditure on a lot of dengue control frequently translates into less expenditure on other important services such as schools or community initiatives. There's also a wave effect on industries such as tourism and commerce—when a person hears news of an outbreak, his or her travel arrangements are canceled and business operations are altered. And with increasing insecticide resistance and routine mosquito control no longer doing a fantastic job anymore, these issues only become more burdensome, necessitating a genuine need for new and permanent solutions (Wang et al., 2022). In the majority of instances, a consistent means of addressing dengue is imperative for the construction of economic resilience and reducing health disparities. Among new concepts in controlling mosquitoes is a promising avenue of escape from this economic crisis. Methods such as symbiont-based strategies or even experimental modifications of mosquito genetics promise to serve as inexpensive methods to reduce disease transmission in the long run. These new strategies could just result in reduced healthcare costs and lost workdays, and so contribute some measure of economic balance to hit areas (Wang et al., 2022). It's not that easy, though—any new policy must gain public acceptance, ride through complex ethical rapids, and fit into what local infrastructure is capable of handling. With wise and consistent investments in these technologies, public health initiatives may receive a significant shot in the arm, lowering the rate of dengue outbreaks and their economic impact. terms, managing dengue's economic toll involves merging wise scientific advancements with policymaking that can place our future on firmer ground (Naik et al., 2023) (Figure 13.14).

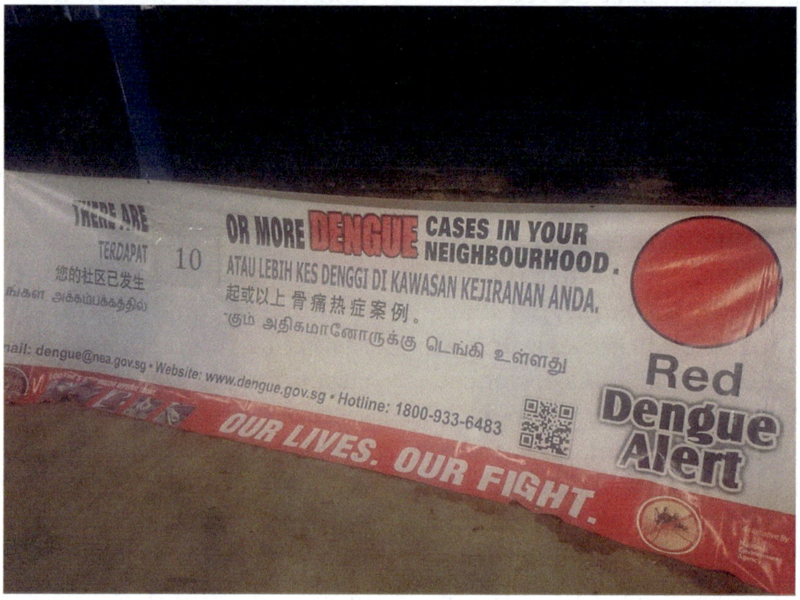
TERDAPAT
您的社区已发生
10
OR MORE DENGUE CASES IN YOUR NEIGHBOURHOOD.
ATAU LEBIH KES DENGGI DI KAWASAN KEJIRANAN ANDA.
起或以上骨痛热症案例。
அதிகமானோருக்கு டெங்கி உள்ளது
dengue@nea.gov.sg • Website: www.dengue.gov.sg • Hotline: 1800-933-6483
Red
Dengue
Alert
OUR LIVES. OUR FIGHT.

Figure 13.14. Dengue fever outbreak: Economic impact and prevention.

Source: By Skirtick - Own work, CC BY-SA 4.0, https://commons.wikimedia.org/w/index.php?curid=45030673***13.6.3. Regional Differences in Disease Prevalence***

Learning about disease patterns begins with examining the environment around us and our daily social environments. Consider malaria, for instance. Spreading isn't purely weather-related, it also appears to be related to basic things such as the number of people living in a given house. Studies generally indicate that when the average household has fewer than four members, malaria declines significantly, regardless of what the climate is like or what types of mosquitoes are present. It seems how individuals engage daily has a large role, far greater than one would anticipate. Further there's dengue, which is more likely to appear during daylight and does not at all correlate with household size. This combination of determinants highlights how disease conduct differs in ways no one could anticipate, pointing us to the complex and interconnected roles of social behavior and environment (Hulden et al., 2025). Variations in ways that diseases manifest between groups also reveal a lot about demographic and geographical factors. Consider travelers as opposed to immigrants: travelers typically contract vector-borne diseases like malaria and dengue fever, while immigrants appear to suffer more from chronic or established infection like TB and helminthiasis. In general, where you are from and how much you are already exposed already determines the types of disease you encounter within healthcare. For example, travelers returning from high-risk areas will often have more vector-borne conditions, which reinforces the notion that location plays a very big role in risk. And when you throw in some of the different transmission modes—each of which is associated with specific local social and environmental indicators—it is obvious that variables such as mosquito behavior and the public health infrastructure of an area can significantly alter the landscape (Brown et al., 2008). Meanwhile, economic and infrastructural differences form another thread of the tapestry. Malaria's relationship with poverty is fairly well established; poorer areas, tending to have larger families and reduced access to mosquito control, still battle its proliferation. The movement of the parasite, primarily through nocturnal mosquitoes, becomes amplified by how humans tend to cluster and socialize, frequently in patterns that vary quite significantly from place to place. Conversely, dengue's daytime behavior and its more relaxed association with family size direct us toward risks associated with daily outdoor labor and other urban customs you usually have in densely populated city centers. These different conditions clarify why some locations manage to drive malaria back and others do not, and why dengue will burst into view at times but be a persistent issue in some cities. In general, tailoring health approaches to such local specifics is the key to reducing the total burden of disease (Brown et al., 2008; Hulden et al., 2025).

CLOSER LOOK

LIFE CYCLE OF PLASMODIUM AND VECTOR DYNAMICS IN MALARIA

Malaria is a life-threatening disease caused by Plasmodium parasites, primarily P. falciparum, P. vivax, P. ovale, and P. malariae, transmitted through the bite of infected female Anopheles mosquitoes. Understanding the parasite's life cycle and vector dynamics is crucial for effective prevention and control.

The Plasmodium life cycle has two hosts: the mosquito vector and the human host. In humans, infection begins when sporozoites enter the bloodstream during a mosquito bite and rapidly migrate to the liver. There, they infect hepatocytes and undergo exoerythrocytic schizogony, producing thousands of merozoites. These merozoites are released into the bloodstream, infect red blood cells, and undergo erythrocytic schizogony, causing cyclical hemolysis and the characteristic fever and chills of malaria. Some merozoites differentiate into sexual forms called gametocytes, which are taken up by mosquitoes during blood meals.

Inside the mosquito, gametocytes develop into male and female gametes, fuse to form a zygote, and eventually produce sporozoites in the mosquito's salivary glands, ready to infect the next human host. This mosquito stage, called sporogony, is influenced by temperature, humidity, and mosquito lifespan, directly affecting transmission dynamics.

Vector dynamics play a pivotal role in malaria epidemiology. Anopheles mosquitoes thrive in stagnant water for breeding, and their feeding behavior, density, and longevity determine the intensity of transmission. Environmental factors such as rainfall, temperature, and land use changes can expand mosquito habitats, while insecticide resistance and human mobility further complicate control efforts.

Malaria control strategies target both parasite and vector, including insecticide-treated nets, indoor residual spraying, larval source management, and antimalarial drugs. Understanding the interplay between Plasmodium biology and vector ecology is essential for interrupting transmission and achieving malaria elimination goals.

Summary

Dengue and malaria illustrate how problematic it can be to combat disease transmitted by insects. More recent studies on these diseases discover they behave differently across time and also differ from area to area – with variables such as weather, local environment, and even financial conditions having a factor. Understand precisely where and when outbreaks would likely break out is essential in informing strategies to suit local demands and in channeling resources appropriately. Certain research even identifies seasonally high activity and local hot spots that demand ongoing monitoring and adaptive action to hold outbreaks at bay. Such a strategy not only increases preparedness but also adapts control strategies to reduce disease and mortality. Overall, these findings point to why it is so crucial to combine deep data analysis into planning for health, to remain proactive against disease outbreaks in susceptible populations, particularly where these infections are endemic (Simegn et al., 2024). On the second front, newer tech in mosquito identification is redefining how we combat these diseases. Scientists have launched sophisticated classification systems that rely on techniques such as transfer learning and ensemble methods, creating new opportunities to monitor such pests. By distinctly separating the mosquito species that are responsible for malaria and dengue, these tools help to refine the target of control measures—ie, interventions such as targeted use of insecticides and habitat manipulation can be employed more precisely. Due to such enhanced targeting, unwanted environmental effects decline and the potential for resistance is maintained low. The phenomenal precision and robust performance of these digital techniques suggest a genuine game-changer in public health, demonstrating how cutting-edge technology can make an enormous difference against vector-borne diseases (Devi, 2024). Ultimately, managing malaria and dengue requires combining robust disease understanding with contemporary technology. Health measures must rely on strong time-and-place information to rapidly identify and attack high-risk areas, and innovative mosquito identification techniques enhance our capacity to interrupt transmission cycles more efficiently. Combined, these measures create a fairly wide disease prevention and control framework—one that emphasizes precision, adaptability, and long-term outcomes. Continued investment in research, improved surveillance systems, and inventive tools remains a must if we're to ease the global burden of these diseases. Efforts like these eventually lead to better health outcomes and help build resilience against future challenges from vector-borne diseases (Devi, 2024; Simegn et al., 2024).

Vector-borne diseases continue to raise global health issues in ways that many do not even anticipate. Malaria and dengue are two heavyweights—diseases that not only accumulate high rates of disease and mortality in tropical areas but also weigh down national economies. Malaria derives its energy from Plasmodium parasites leaping between individuals through Anopheles mosquitoes, whereas dengue is spread through Aedes mosquito bites. In the majority of scenarios, this combination strains healthcare systems and hinders economic development. You may be told that monitoring outbreaks, combatting mosquito populations, and treating cases remains another best option. Recent global research suggests that local uniqueness count when addressing any of these matters (Christopher, 2022). When you combine environmental, biological, and social elements into an amalgam, it becomes obvious why adaptable, open-minded health programs are the key. Climate change is a new game changer in the equation, altering where and when malaria and dengue emerge. Increased temperatures and irregular rain patterns provide mosquitoes with comfortable niches, which can then spread the affected areas with these diseases. Overall, these changes threaten to reverse many of the gains made in keeping the diseases under control. Attempts to maintain global warming at 1.5°C do appear to have definite human health benefits by reversing some of these risks. Low- and middle-income nations, where health systems are usually strapped, are especially hit hard by these climate changes. It becomes almost unavoidable to weave climate data into public health planning if we're to build strong, resilient strategies against these ever-changing threats (Hoegh et al., 2019). Combating malaria and dengue isn't a one-trick pony—it's a combination of many approaches. Some strategies lean on solid disease tracking and environmental cleanup, while others depend on community involvement and fresh advances in medical care. Rapid diagnosis and early treatment reduce the most fatal results, and traditional strategies such as insecticide-treated bed nets, indoor spraying, and better sanitation struggle to keep mosquitoes under control. Although vaccines for dengue are still behind and only available in a handful of locations, they suggest what the future may bring. Addressing more profound problems such as poverty, urbanization, and illiteracy also creates a stronger defense in the long run. In the future, increasing research and refining data gathering—from national levels all the way down to local hotspots—will be important for developing policies that address new challenges in a really focused manner (Christopher, 2022).

References

1. Abe, A., Adams, A., Ahmed, A., Ajariyakhajorn, A., Albrecht, A., Allen, A., Apetrei, C., et al. (2008). Macaque models of human infectious disease. *ILAR Journal*, *49*(2), 220–255. https://doi.org/10.1093/ilar.49.2.220.

2. Allan, R., Budge, S., & Sauskojus, H. (2022). What sounds like Aedes, acts like Aedes, but is not Aedes? Lessons from dengue virus control for the management of invasive Anopheles. *The Lancet Global Health, 11*, e165–e169. https://doi.org/10.1016/s2214-109x(22)00454-5.

3. Begum, A. (2024). Climate change and emerging infectious diseases: Investigating the influence on transmission dynamics of vector-borne diseases. *Saudi Journal of Medical and Pharmaceutical Sciences, 10*(10), 766–775. https://www.semanticscholar.org/paper/580dc21349e537602537cfb59e0f9d363aa2efdb (accessed on 7 May 2025).

4. Bera, B. (2025). Mosquito ecology and disease transmission: Implications for global health and vector control. *Uttar Pradesh Journal of Zoology, 46*(8). https://www.semanticscholar.org/paper/bdafa99baf27722b6b43143130ad318c4e4270e0 (accessed on 7 May 2025).

5. Bhattacharyya, S. (2025). Root causes of African underdevelopment. https://core.ac.uk/download/pdf/9317792.pdf (accessed on 7 May 2025).

6. Brown, G. V., Leder, K., Matchett, E., O'Brien, et al. (2008). Disease in returned travelers and immigrants/refugees: The 6-year experience of two Australian infectious diseases units. *Journal of Travel Medicine, 13*(3), 145–152. https://core.ac.uk/download/pdf/9416725.pdf (accessed on 7 May 2025).

7. Butt, A., Imran, M., McKinney, B., Batool, S., & Aftab, H. (2023). Mathematical and stability analysis of dengue–malaria co-infection with disease control strategies. *Mathematics, 11*(22), 4600. https://www.semanticscholar.org/paper/3f71781620a3cf1d389cd3e3ce3cca6b157cb5b6 (accessed on 7 May 2025).

8. Caminade, C., McIntyre, K. M., & Jones, A. (2018). Impact of recent and future climate change on vector-borne diseases. *Annals of the New York Academy of Sciences, 1436*, 157–173. https://doi.org/10.1111/nyas.13950.

9. Chathurangika, P., Premadasa, L. S., Perera, S. S. N., & De Silva, K. (2024). Determining dengue infection risk in the Colombo district of Sri Lanka by inferencing the genetic parameters of Aedes mosquitoes. *BMC Infectious Diseases, 24(1), 944.* https://www.semanticscholar.org/paper/74c94fa95e413795cb42bf38dad8a44474b21657 (accessed on 7 May 2025).

10. Cheenammadath House, A., Hammadi, M. M., & Shafi Chicken, S. (2025). Co-infection of falciparum malaria and dengue fever: A case report. *International Journal of Advanced Research.* https://www.semanticscholar.org/paper/d96cc2ace3962e876517e1259419b755d75400b7 (accessed on 7 May 2025).

11. Chen, Y., Wang, Q., Chen, H., Song, X., Tang, H., & Tian, M. (2019). An overview of augmented reality technology. *Journal of Physics Conference Series, 1237*, 022082–022082. https://doi.org/10.1088/1742-6596/1237/2/022082.

12. Devi, B. R. (2024). Morphological analysis and classification of vector mosquitoes using novel deep learning model. *Advances in Nonlinear Variational Inequalities, 28*(1s). https://www.semanticscholar.org/paper/394003131bdd83e70d994aef0c85a08a44f8e6fa (accessed on 7 May 2025).

13. Dieng, I., Hedible, G. B., Diagne, M. M., El Wahed, A. A., Diagne, C. T., Fall, C., Richard, V., et al. (2020). Mobile laboratory reveals the circulation of dengue virus serotype I of Asian origin in Medina Gounass (Guediawaye), Senegal. *Diagnostics, 10*, 408. https://doi.org/10.3390/diagnostics10060408.

14. Dyck, V. A., Hendrichs, J., & Robinson, A. S. (2020). *Sterile Insect Technique*. CRC Press eBooks. https://doi.org/10.1201/9781003035572.

15. Echaubard, P., Rudge, J. W., & Léfèvre, T. (2018). Evolutionary perspectives on human infectious diseases: Challenges, advances, and promises. *Evolutionary Applications, 11*(3), 383–393. https://doi.org/10.1111/eva.12586.

16. Ellwanger, J. H., Kulmann-Leal, B., Kaminski, V. L., Valverde-Villegas, J. M., Gorini da Veiga, A. B., Spilki, F. R., Fearnside, P. M., et al. (2020). Beyond diversity loss and climate change: Impacts of Amazon deforestation on infectious diseases and public health. *Anais da Academia Brasileira de Ciências, 92*. https://doi.org/10.1590/0001-3765202020191375.

17. Fauci, A. S., Erbelding, E. J., Whitehead, S. S., Cassetti, M. C., Handley, F. G., & Gupta, R. (2019). Dengue vaccine clinical trials in India–An opportunity to inform the global response to a re-emerging disease challenge. *International Journal of Infectious Diseases, 84*, S4–S6. https://doi.org/10.1016/j.ijid.2019.03.016.

18. Griffiths, K., Savini, H., Brouqui, P., Simon, F., Parola, P., & Gautret, P. (2018). Surveillance of travel-associated diseases at two referral centres in Marseille, France: A 12-year survey. *Journal of Travel Medicine, 25*. https://doi.org/10.1093/jtm/tay007.

19. Guo, L., & Rondina, M. T. (2019). The era of thromboinflammation: Platelets are dynamic sensors and effector cells during infectious diseases. *Frontiers in Immunology, 10*. https://doi.org/10.3389/fimmu.2019.02204.

20. Hoegh-Guldberg, O., Jacob, D., Taylor, M. A., Bolaños, T. G., Bindi, M., Brown, S., Camilloni, I., et al. (2019). The human imperative of stabilizing global climate change at 1.5°C. *Science, 365*. https://doi.org/10.1126/science.aaw6974.

21. Hulden, L., Hulden, L., & McKitrick, R. (2025). Average household size and the eradication of malaria. *CORE*. https://core.ac.uk/download/pdf/6440939.pdf

22. Imlaque, M., Husain, S., Shewrwani, A. M. K., & Bibi, C. (2025). A review of Humma Danj (dengue fever) in Unani and conventional medicine. *International Journal of Research in Medical Sciences, 13(3)*. https://www.semanticscholar.org/paper/c324127ef11cfd0ebcfe58bfc72c8ad6821eb07c (accessed on 7 May 2025).

23. Khuroo, M. S., Khuroo, M. S., Khuroo, M. S., Sofi, A., & Khuroo, M. S. (2020). COVID-19 vaccines: A race against time in the middle of death and devastation! *Journal of Clinical and Experimental Hepatology, 10*, 610–621. https://doi.org/10.1016/j.jceh.2020.06.003.

24. Kumar, A., Kockaya, G., Kaczmarek, K., Nguyen, T. P. L., Rokhman, M., Stiensma, I., Sukma, R., et al. (2023). Cost-effectiveness of non-communicable disease prevention in Southeast Asia: A scoping review. *Frontiers in Public Health, 11,* 1206213. https://www.semanticscholar.org/paper/895cc1f36995967a9cc5ef7ee09df0971b178c84 (accessed on 7 May 2025).

25. Ling, Y., Hao, Z. Y., Liang, D., Zhang, C. L., Liu, Y., & Wang, Y. (2021). The expanding role of pyridine and dihydropyridine scaffolds in drug design. *Drug Design Development and Therapy, 15*, 4289–4338. https://doi.org/10.2147/dddt.s329547.

26. Manzi, F., Hamon, J. K., Agbodjavou, M. K., Hoyt, J., Kuwawenaruwa, A., Kionga, Y., Agossou, C., et al. (2025). How, why, and under what circumstances can supportive supervision programs improve malaria case management? A realist program theory. *Health Policy and Planning, czaf020*. https://www.semanticscholar.org/paper/75aaf3c260720a5262629e12565c51d16f3690c4 (accessed on 7 May 2025).

27. Mohareb, A., Kim, A. Y., Boyd, A., Noubary, F., Kouamé, M., Anglaret, X., Coffie, P., et al. (2024). Virological, serological and clinical outcomes in chronic hepatitis B virus infection: Development and validation of the HEPA-B simulation model. *BMJ Open, 14*. https://www.semanticscholar.org/paper/80c18070c63c3683b618530ad3f608a736960145 (accessed on 7 May 2025).

28. Momena, A. F., Mandal, S., Gazi, K. H., Giri, B. C., & Mondal, S. P. (2023). Prediagnosis of disease based on symptoms by generalized dual hesitant hexagonal fuzzy multi-criteria decision-making techniques. *Systems, 11*(231). https://doi.org/10.3390/systems11050231.

29. Murray, C. J. L. (2022). The global burden of disease study at 30 years. *Nature Medicine, 28*, 2019–2026. https://doi.org/10.1038/s41591-022-01990-1.

30. Naik, B. R., Tyagi, B. K., & Xue, R. D. (2023). Mosquito-borne diseases in India over the past 50 years and their global public health implications: A systematic review. *Journal of the American Mosquito Control Association, 39*, 258–277. https://doi.org/10.2987/23-7131.

31. Nelson, M. (2020). Public health recommendations for the control of arboviral diseases in the Caribbean. *CORE*. https://core.ac.uk/download/328827256.pdf (accessed on 7 May 2025).

32. Nooraei, S., Bahrulolum, H., Hoseini, Z. S., Katalani, C., Hajizade, A., Easton, A. J., & Ahmadian, G. (2021). Virus-like particles: Preparation, immunogenicity, and their roles as nano vaccines and drug nanocarriers. *Journal of Nanobiotechnology, 19*. https://doi.org/10.1186/s12951-021-00806-7.

33. Nugraha, R. V., Ridwansyah, H., Ghozali, M., Khairani, A. F., & Atik, N. (2020). Traditional herbal medicine candidates as complementary treatments for COVID-19: A review of their mechanisms, pros, and cons. *Evidence-based Complementary and Alternative Medicine*. https://doi.org/10.1155/2020/2560645.

34. Nurhayati. (2024). Comparison of clinical symptoms and laboratory findings in typhoid fever and dengue fever patients. *International Journal for Research in Applied Science and Engineering Technology, 12, 2381–2384*. https://www.semanticscholar.org/paper/7fd7b7deab22c367cc135f1e848b8f717481ff08 (accessed on 7 May 2025).

35. Pavia, G., Branda, F., Ciccozzi, A., Romano, C., Locci, C., Azzena, I., Pascale, N., et al. (2024). The issue of climate change and the spread of tropical diseases in Europe and Italy: Vector biology, disease transmission, genome-based monitoring, and public health implications. *Infectious Diseases, 57(2), 121–136*. https://www.semanticscholar.org/paper/8db2bec1b4609afedf77a3db10f406c77958f40b (accessed on 7 May 2025).

36. Roja, C., Lakshmi, A. S., Rani, M. A., & Eapen, A. (2022). Effect of school-based educational interventions on the knowledge of malaria and dengue among higher secondary school children in Chennai, India: A pre- and post-intervention study. *Cureus*. https://doi.org/10.7759/cureus.26536.

37. Rosenberg, R., Lindsey, N. P., Fischer, M., Gregory, C. J., Hinckley, A. F., Mead, P. S., Paz-Bailey, G., et al. (2018). Vital signs: Trends in reported vector borne disease cases–United States and territories, 2004–2016. *MMWR Morbidity and Mortality Weekly Report, 67*, 496–501. https://doi.org/10.15585/mmwr.mm6717e1.

38. Roth, G. A., Abate, D., Abate, K. H., Abay, S. M., Abbafati, C., Abbasi, N., Abbastabar, H., et al. (2018). Global, regional, and national age-sex-specific mortality for 282 causes of death in 195 countries and territories, 1980–2017: A systematic analysis for the Global Burden of Disease Study 2017. *The Lancet, 392*, 1736–1788. https://doi.org/10.1016/s0140-6736(18)32203-7.

39. Rudd, K. E., Johnson, S. C., Agesa, K. M., Shackelford, K. A., Tsoi, D., Kievlan, D., Colombara, D. V., et al. (2020). Global, regional, and national sepsis incidence and mortality, 1990–2017: Analysis for the Global Burden of Disease Study. *The Lancet, 395*, 200–211. https://doi.org/10.1016/s0140-6736(19)32989-7.

40. Satarvandi, D., van der Werff, S. D., Nauclér, P., Hildenwall, H., & Sondén, K. (2024). Scoring systems for prediction of malaria and dengue fever in non-endemic areas among travelers arriving from tropical and subtropical areas. *Emergency Medicine Journal: EMJ, 41*, 242–248. https://www.semanticscholar.org/paper/ef5f834f287fcc064f0f65675dcd595282250361 (accessed on 7 May 2025).

41. Semenza, J. C., & Suk, J. E. (2017). Vector-borne diseases and climate change: A European perspective. *FEMS Microbiology Letters, 365*. https://doi.org/10.1093/femsle/fnx244.

42. Semenza, J. C., Rocklöv, J., & Ebi, K. L. (2022). Climate change and cascading risks from infectious disease. *Infectious Diseases and Therapy, 11*, 1371–1390. https://doi.org/10.1007/s40121-022-00647-3.

43. Simegn, G., Degu, M. Z., Gebeyehu, W., Senay, A., Krishnamoorthy, J., & Tegenaw, G. S. (2024). Spatiotemporal distribution of climate-sensitive disease incidences in Ethiopia: A longitudinal retrospective analysis of malaria, meningitis, cholera, dysentery, leishmaniasis, and dengue fever between 2010 and 2022/2023. *BMC Public Health, 24(1), 697*. https://www.semanticscholar.org/paper/fbe0e0d7cda92059652896c148125a394e01226e (accessed on 7 May 2025).

44. Sinzala, C., Mulenga, D., & Kumari, N. (2025). The effects of insecticide-treated nets (ITNs) on *Plasmodium falciparum* infections in Kalumbila District, Zambia. *International Journal on Science and Technology, 16*(1). https://www.semanticscholar.org/paper/3348a9f05c254d5db7396c13feca8ba183924b56 (accessed on 7 May 2025).

45. Tidball, J. (2017). The buzz behind the bite. *Seek, 7*(1). https://core.ac.uk/download/267188350.pdf (accessed on 7 May 2025).

46. Tozan, Y., Headley, T. Y., Javelle, É., Gautret, P., Grobusch, M. P., de Pijper, C., Ásgeirsson, H., et al. (2023). Impact, healthcare utilization and costs of travel-associated mosquito-borne diseases in international travelers: A prospective study. *Journal of Travel Medicine, 30*. https://doi.org/10.1093/jtm/taad060.

47. Vaishnav, A., R., Akhiljith, K., Sreerag, K., Keshannavar, M. G., et al. (2023). Assessment of knowledge, attitude, practice towards vector-borne diseases in the urban area of Bagalkote, Karnataka, India. *International Journal of Research in Medical Sciences, 12*(1), 133–139. https://core.ac.uk/download/596246921.pdf (accessed on 7 May 2025).

48. Vos, T., Abajobir, A. A., Abate, K. H., Abbafati, C., Abbas, K., Abd-Allah, F., Abdulkader, R. S., et

al. (2017). Global, regional, and national incidence, prevalence, and years lived with disability for 328 diseases and injuries for 195 countries, 1990–2016: A systematic analysis for the Global Burden of Disease Study 2016. *The Lancet, 390*(1211–1259). https://doi.org/10.1016/s0140-6736(17)32154-2.

49. Wang, G. H., Du, J., Chu, C. Y., Madhav, M., Hughes, G. L., & Champer, J. (2022). Symbionts and gene drive: Two strategies to combat vector-borne disease. *Trends in Genetics, 38*, 708–723. https://doi.org/10.1016/j.tig.2022.02.013.

50. Weetman, D., Kamgang, B., Badolo, A., Moyes, C. L., Shearer, F. M., Coulibaly, M. B., Pinto, J., et al. (2018). Aedes mosquitoes and Aedes-borne arboviruses in Africa: Current and future threats. *International Journal of Environmental Research and Public Health, 15*, 220. https://doi.org/10.3390/ijerph15020220.

51. World Health Organization. (2020). Clinical management of severe acute respiratory infection (SARI) when COVID-19 disease is suspected: Interim guidance. *Pediatric I Medicine Rodina, 16*, 9–26. https://doi.org/10.15557/pimr.2020.0003.

52. Yoshikawa, H., Wuermli, A. J., Britto, P. R., Dreyer, B. P., Leckman, J. F., Lye, S. J., Ponguta, L. A., et al. (2020). Effects of the Global Coronavirus Disease-2019 Pandemic on Early Childhood Development: Short- and long-term risks and mitigating program and policy actions. *The Journal of Pediatrics, 223*, 188–193. https://doi.org/10.1016/j.jpeds.2020.05.020.

53. Zavaleta-Monestel, E., Rojas-Chinchilla, C., Molina-Sojo, P., Murillo-Castro, M. F., Rojas-Molina, J. P., & Martínez-Vargas, E. (2025). Impact of climate change on the global dynamics of vector-borne infectious diseases: A narrative review. *Cureus, 17*(1), e77972. https://www.semanticscholar.org/paper/36d78f4c4d2f8bc57e91de3c6bd9ad46413c2841 (accessed on 7 May 2025).

54. Zhao, T., Cai, Y., Jiang, Y., He, X., Wei, Y., Yu, Y., & Tian, X. (2023). Vaccine adjuvants: Mechanisms and platforms. *Signal Transduction and Targeted Therapy, 8*. https://doi.org/10.1038/s41392-023-01557-7.

55. Zimbuga, K. M. (2025). Efficacy of genetically modified mosquitoes vs. insecticide-treated bed nets in reducing malaria transmission in endemic regions. *NEWPORT INTERNATIONAL JOURNAL OF PUBLIC HEALTH AND PHARMACY, 6(1), 60–64*. https://www.semanticscholar.org/paper/e490f85a3f2744cbcc54ea0858def1a34b44c7e6 (accessed on 7 May 2025).

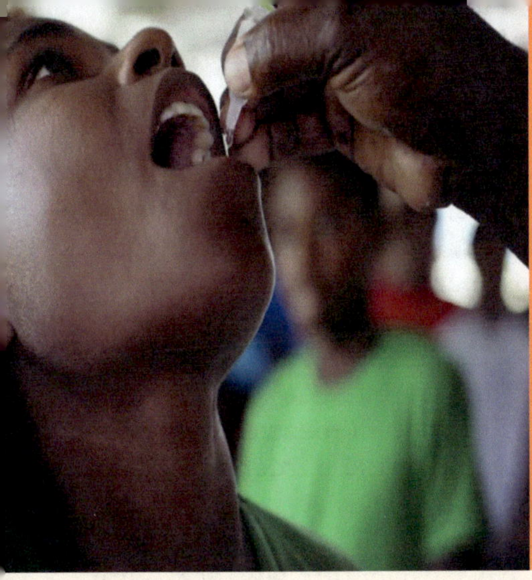

Chapter 14

MEASLES AND POLIO

Contents

Introduction

Diseases throughout history have thrown a monkey wrench into public health and altered the way communities deal with disease. Measles and polio, for instance, have long been targeted for their broad sweep and occasionally devastating aftermath, particularly for children. In the past, outbreaks occurred so frequently that these diseases accounted for high rates of disease and loss. Vaccines came nearly as a lifeline; their development and implementation serve as a living testament that immunization not only can control but sometimes even eradicate debilitating diseases. Reflecting on these trends and their aftermaths serves to demonstrate just why adhering to vaccination continues to be so crucial in preventing outbreaks. The viruses causing measles and polio are of differing family stock, but both have a wildfire potential to spread. The measles virus, a paramyxovirus, typically travels through respiratory droplets, causing fever, rash, and a compromised immune status that makes individuals more susceptible to additional infections. Polio, which comes from an enterovirus, is primarily transmitted through the fecal-oral route and can, in some instances, even result in paralysis. These unique patterns of transmission, and their different symptoms, guided vaccine strategies and shaped public health actions throughout the years. For the most part, the experiences gained from fighting these ancient enemies provide valuable tips for dealing with today's viral threats. Recent advances in vaccine work, described during the worldwide scramble against novel viruses, truly highlight how effective immunization programs not only stem disease but also hamstring its propagation (Nikolaos et al., 2021; Stanley et al., 2021). Campaigns to contain measles and polio have demonstrated just how powerful a decent vaccine can be in alleviating the burden of disease and strengthening population health. Large-scale immunization programs spurred steep declines in rates of infection – and for polio, all but eradicated it globally. Consider, for example, the oral polio vaccine and measles-mumps-rubella vaccine; both combine clever scientific advances with durable public health policy to reduce infectious risk. But challenges such as vaccine hesitancy, complicated logistics, and even viral mutations mean that continued caution is essential. A continued, broad-based vaccination campaign is still crucial to preserving these gains and preventing any resurgence. In addition, the record of these diseases warns us that forward thinking in vaccine development and early implementation are crucial to keeping the public on board and creating a strong, healthier world (Nikolaos et al., 2021; Stanley et al., 2021) (Figure 14.1).

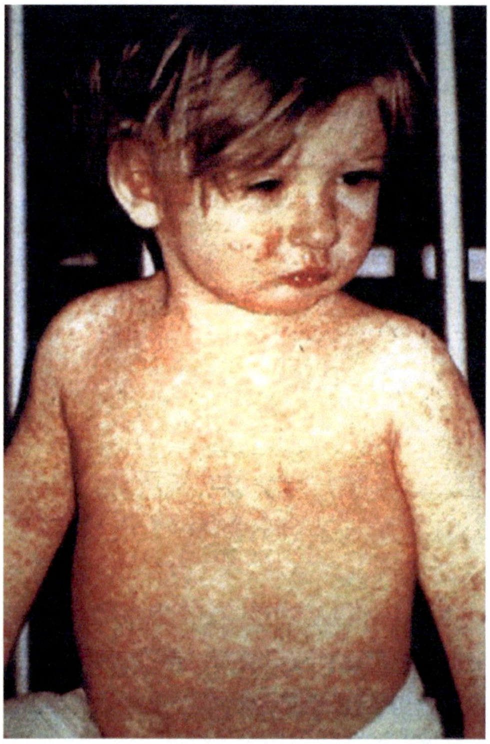

Figure 14.1. Measles cases.

Source: By CDC/NIP/Barbara Rice - http://phil.cdc.gov/phil/ (ID#: 132), Public Domain, https://commons.wikimedia.org/w/index.php?curid=210382

Definition of Measles

Infectious diseases have defined the way we perceive public health for centuries – they compelled us to develop vaccines and initiate programs to eradicate them. Measles, for example, is a viral infection that particularly affects children and teenagers. It is caused by a virus belonging to the Paramyxoviridae family, and you can contract it when a person around you coughs or sneezes. Typically, the disease begins with a fever, cough, sneezing runny nose, and watery eyes, and later a rash creeps across the skin. Even if we can stop it with a vaccine, measles still rears its ugly head, usually because not everyone gets vaccinated. In general, knowing how the virus is transmitted and functions makes us appreciate its connections with other contagious diseases such as polio, which in turn provides some useful analogies for public health. Beyond the telling signs, measles also tampers with your immune system in ways that count. The virus has a tendency to create a type of immunity lag , i.e., it makes you more vulnerable to other diseases, sometimes for weeks or even months following the initial outbreak. This residual effect is one of the main reasons that measles is still a worry despite the existence of vaccines. In the course of periods when health services do not work – such as during the COVID-19 pandemic – fewer individuals were vaccinated, and cases increased among the unvaccinated. Such failures remind us, in a concrete manner, how stretched health systems are, and reveal how important regular vaccinations are in keeping diseases like measles and polio at bay (Zohra et al., 2021). Measles is more than a viral microbe – it's intertwined with social and economic factors that define disease on a global level. It tends to strike hardest in countries with poor healthcare and low rates of vaccination, creating a hard-to-break cycle of disease and even death within vulnerable populations. Unlike polio – which tends to knock out motor neurons and lead to paralysis , measles most often induces respiratory woes and neurological complications such as pneumonia or encephalitis. Ironically, both diseases have the same problems: people dawdling over vaccinations and logistical issues that make it difficult to reach remote regions. Conquering these diseases is more than medical solutions; it also entails establishing public confidence in vaccines, untangling social health determinants, and making resources equitably shareable (Dhochak et al., 2020). In short, only through understanding these several layers can we truly hope to overcome measles—a disease far more complex than it appears on the surface.

Definition of Polio

Infectious diseases continue to challenge our global health systems, and thus it becomes essential to delve into what exactly each one has to offer. Polio—commonly referred to as poliomyelitis—is a virus that is transmitted quickly and usually disrupts the nervous system. It may cause sudden weakness in muscles that, in severe instances, results in permanent disability or even death. The virus primarily lies dormant in settings with poor sanitation and individuals are closely interacting, transmitted through the fecal-oral route. Curiously enough, it begins replicating in the intestines first before it may enter the central nervous system. Due to its infectious nature and possible catastrophic effects, polio has long been the focus of vaccination worldwide. Overall, gaining control over how the virus works and how it spreads highlights why adhering to full immunization is paramount—because dose skipping can induce outbreaks that could undo decades of gains (Biguioh et al., 2015). Simply put, what polio is all about is observing far beyond the symptoms to understand its wider impact on communities. Despite our considerable progress toward vaccine implementation, polio still appears on the radar of those areas that remain with immunity gaps and diverse societal issues deterring the access of vaccines. The World Health Organization generally brings forth the argument that vaccination constitutes the strongest protective armor we currently have against the virus. Despite this, there are challenges, particularly among individuals who have limited healthcare access or who are always in motion—refugees and migrants being good examples. National immunization plans typically must change sponteneously, tailoring programs to ensure these populations are reached and that vaccine delivery and tracking persist even when borders are diffuse. In the majority of situations, realizing these challenges—and the complex complexity of vaccine compliance—enables us to look at polio not merely as a singular disease but as an evolving public health concern intricately intertwined with social, political, and economic strands. Considered immunization plans that rely on community participation and cross-border collaboration are central to ending polio once and for all (Declich et al., 2017).

Beneath its surface, polio isn't simply a matter of its short-term symptoms; it also carries a whole range of long-term consequences that weigh on individuals and healthcare systems as much as on it. Frequently, infections pass by unremarked or bring only temporary discomfort, but sometimes in a handful of cases, the virus induces an asymmetric paralysis that affects limbs or muscles involved in respiration. This type of paralysis is often irreversible, which means it can significantly affect quality of life and necessitate long-term dependence on medical treatment and rehabilitation. And, just to make matters worse, survivors may subsequently struggle with post-polio syndrome—a syndrome characterized by recurred muscle weakness and persistent fatigue years following recovery. These clinical facts, in the majority of instances, serve to highlight precisely why promoting large-scale vaccination programs is not negotiable. By bundling the virus's biological uniqueness, its irregular pattern of spread, and the excessive burden that it inflicts upon health, experts and policymakers can design more effective prevention and control programs that are designed to reduce the global disease burden overall (Figure 14.2).

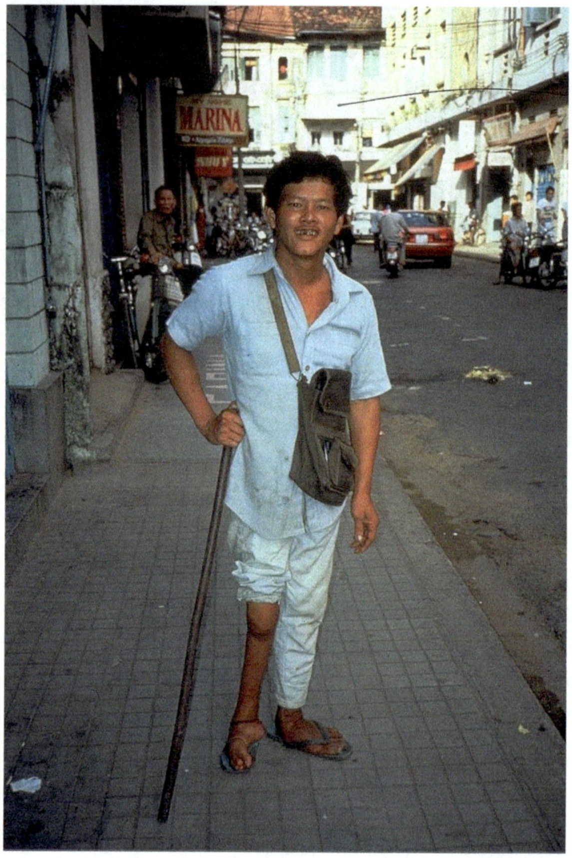

Figure 14.2. Polio—often called poliomyelitis—is a virus that spreads fast and typically messes with the nervous system.

Source: By Photo Credit:Content Providers(s): CDC/NIP/ Barbara Rice - This media comes from the Centers for Disease Control and Prevention's Public Health Image Library (PHIL), with identification number #134.Note: +/–http://www.vaccineinformation.org/polio/photos.asphttp://www.vaccineinformation.org/photos/poliiac003.jpghttp://www.vaccineinformation.org/photos/poliiac003a.jpghttp://www.vaccineinformation.org/photos/poliiac003b.jpg, Public Domain, https://commons.wikimedia.org/w/index.php?curid=1650090

Importance of Studying These Diseases

Public health begins by addressing great problems such as measles and polio. Bouncing into the fundamentals of how our genetics help us fight off infection teaches us just how our bodies and those annoying pathogens get around each other. Twins provide a clue, for the most part, that characteristics intended to be inherited in the family can play a significant role in how diseases occur, how vaccinations benefit us, and even how symptoms manifest. You begin to understand why certain people or groups may be more vulnerable, which pushes us toward creating vaccines and drugs that suit each person a little better. Ultimately, putting these genetic portions together sets the stage for more targeted intervention strategies that can improve our overall health plans (Smatti et al., 2025). Consideration of vaccination practices, therefore, provides us with an additional perspective on this entire problem. Wide sweeps that verify who's been vaccinated can alert where the system is breaking down—locales such as children receiving no shots or sporadically taking a few doses. This part of the puzzle is particularly important in economically struggling communities, where immunization holes allow these diseases to persist and even compromise herd immunity. Through examination of these immunization trends, national leaders and health people can make effective steps to close these gaps, raising overall coverage and reducing measles and polio cases (Dhalaria et al., 2025). Research on these diseases goes even further by moving global health objectives ahead. Knowing how measles and polio are spread, how vaccines work, and what hinders immunization frame solutions that resonate with communities in the location. Most of the time, incorporating knowledge from biology with day-to-day realities, such as socioeconomic barriers and healthcare access—is responsible for reaching global vaccination targets in global plans. Highlighting the mixture of genetic, economic, and health factors paints a more comprehensive picture of disease prevention. Overall, this type of work represents a genuine dedication to equitable improvements in health and the final push to eradicate measles and polio forever (Dhalaria et al., 2025; Smatti et al., 2025).

14.1. Historical Context

Measles and polio have been sparking public health controversy for many years, their control entwined with an inextricable history that is far from simple. From the beginning, witnessing communities devastated by disease and piling death rates compelled countries across the globe to understand how such diseases spread and what might halt them. In the great majority of cases, the onset of vaccines during the 20th century rendered the entire picture a new one, bringing crashing down case totals and saving lives in ways people really didn't think were possible initially. Those advances didn't materialize randomly—they were products of global cooperation and the advent of mass immunization campaigns set to eradicate those diseases. Naturally, political, social, and economic stresses, particularly in areas experiencing instability or mass-scale population migration—also clouded the issue of how vaccines made it to where they were needed. During the later decades of the 20th century and well into the early 2000s, the intricacies of vaccination plans really came to the forefront. With waves of refugees, asylum seekers and other migrants flowing across borders, many conventional healthcare infrastructures started to seem outdated. Consider, for instance, non-EU countries along the Mediterranean and Black Sea; while some of these nations wound up having complete coverage with vaccines (measles, polio, etc.), others concentrated on specific populations or restricted vaccines to children alone. Such disparate strategies usually reflect a perpetual dance between stringent resource constraints and the constantly changing public health agendas (Declich et al., 2017). The patchy history of vaccine strategies and spotty record-keeping only accentuates the historic gaps that persist in influencing the way we keep these diseases at bay today. Despite all the strides taken to develop vaccines and implement organized systems of immunization, old issues remain. Concerns such as getting access to vaccines, haphazard record-keeping and the battle to achieve smooth global coordination still make appearances. Most nations have immunization registers, yet people's frequent mobility leaves those records frequently incomplete—spurring demands for newer solutions such as online registers and improved cross-border collaboration to accurately monitor vaccination status (Declich et al., 2017). The narrative of measles and polio immunization shows, in a way, that public health strategies never stay static; they keep evolving with demographic shifts and new technologies, even as some age-old problems persist. In general, getting a grasp on this mixed historical backdrop is pretty crucial if we're ever going to design policies smart enough to finally eradicate these preventable diseases (Figure 14.3).

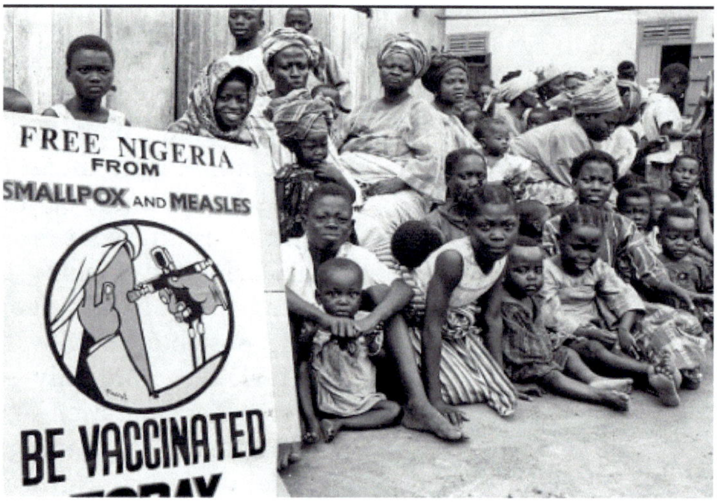

Figure 14.3. Historical context of measles and polio.

Source: The New York Times. (2011). *27DOCS-Jumbo.*

14.1.1. Origin and Early Outbreaks of Measles

Closely packed, busy human communities appear to have initiated measles as a disease to be reckoned with. At the time when cities were beginning to emerge, everyone tended to believe that the disease must have leaped from animals—most commonly believed to be cattle affected by a virus such as rinderpest, into humans. Although scientists continue to argue about when it emerged, this jump seems to have occurred millennia ago when humans transitioned from wandering around as nomads and became farmers and settled. Early instances were likely not adequately documented or became confused with other diseases, but ancient writings in countries such as the Middle East and China describe a febrile disease characterized by a characteristic rash that we currently attribute to measles. In many respects, the limited early epidemics created the pathos that was not anticipated for a disease later shown to be intractable and worldwide, primarily due to its infectiousness and grave sequelae. Reflecting on those early outbreaks, it's obvious that measles had an easy target in low-immunity communities—a scenario common in newly constructed urban settings with overcrowding and unsanitary conditions. Before the advent of vaccines, measles tore through neighborhoods with little resistance, and historical accounts commonly refer to repeating epidemics that sadly increased child mortality rates globally. In contrast to polio, which attacked more erratically and infected the nervous system, measles typically came on in abrupt, explosive surges. Parts of the world like sub-Saharan Africa and parts of Asia were repeatedly hit by this unstoppable chain of infections; decimated health systems just couldn't cope. In environments such as these, the ramifications extended far beyond mere disease—it shook social and economic equilibrium, emphasizing the unadulterated necessity for improved public health practices (Malande et al., 2019). Containment measures for measles tended to face some rather formidable challenges, particularly as the disease frequently departed before distinct symptoms could be identified. Before the advent of the modern vaccine, natural infection was absent from being the sole method of people acquiring immunity, with populations suffering outbreaks on a cyclical basis. These initial episodes, in the majority of instances, highlighted the disease's capability to cripple healthcare systems—most notably within regions that were deficient in resources or even in having standard vaccination programs. Those ancient struggles not only caused terrible loss but also helped inform broader disease-fighting strategies for combatting other diseases, such as polio, by shaping vaccination drives and responses to outbreaks. Yesterday's rapid research and rollout of vaccines, observable in the reaction to newly erupting infectious hazards, validate just how important it is to be rapid and vaccine widely to quell epidemics at their source (Trovato et al., 2020). Overall, the extensive history of measles has marked the world's public health, continuously informing current initiatives to manage infectious diseases (Figure 14.4).

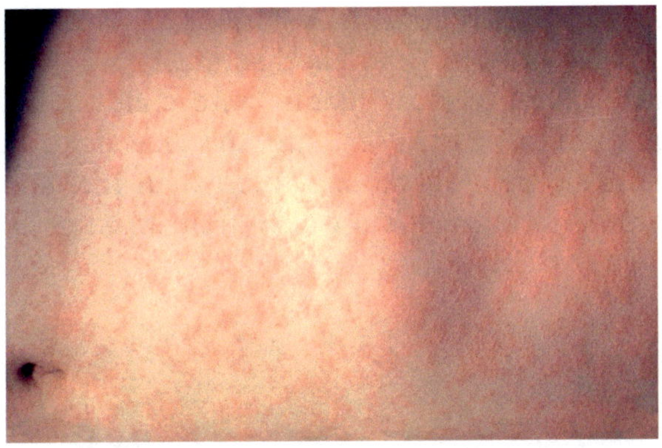

Figure 14.4. The origin and early outbreaks of measles.

Source: By Photo Credit:Content Providers(s): CDC/Dr. Heinz F. Eichenwald - This media comes from the Centers for Disease Control and Prevention's Public Health Image Library (PHIL), with identification number #3168. Note: https://commons.wikimedia.org/w/index.php?curid=4393873

14.1.2. Origin and Early Outbreaks of Polio

Poliovirus existed as far back as ancient times—its remains even appear in Egyptian mummies' bones. No one much said anything about it then, though, until somewhat strangely, the late 1800s and early 1900s when unexpected, paralyzing epidemics among children made the risk impossible to dismiss. Early accounts of the disease were sort of everywhere and everywhere in between, interspersed with portions of meandering description, until someone finally pulled it all together and laid the blame on that very virus. The outbreaks would erupt suddenly in small, localized pockets, usually during the peak summer heat when the virus seemed to rage out of control. These early, unpredictable episodes, in most cases, ended up setting the stage for later insights into how the virus spreads and why its cycles repeat—insights that later fed into efforts to stop it and even create vaccines. During the first decades of the 20th century, polio outbreaks began to emerge all over the world, with developed nations experiencing an unusual twist: improved sanitation delayed the virus encounter further into childhood or adolescence, usually making the disease strike harder. Cities, dense and filled with life, soon became viral hotspots where transmission had an easy ride.

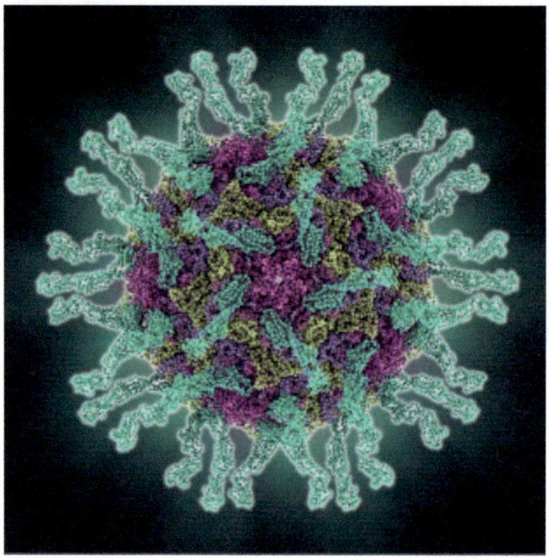

Figure 14.5. The origin and early outbreaks of polio.

Source: Science Photo Library. (n.d.). *Human Poliovirus Molecular Model.*

The fact that the virus generally traveled by the fecal-oral route didn't prevent it from taking advantage of these city spaces, and its effect on children soon captured both popular and scientific notice. For the most part, this change in who became ill and when served to uncover how social conditions combine with the disease's own characteristics to keep polio in the game, a lesson still influencing efforts to interrupt the cycle of disease. Those initial epidemics weren't merely an eye-opener regarding polio itself—they also cast a spotlight on greater challenges in managing infectious diseases that ultimately spurred vaccine research along lines akin to achievements with diseases such as measles. The brutal cost of the epidemics during the first half-century galvanized scientists and policymakers globally, prompting them to seek compulsively effective techniques in vaccination. In the majority of instances, these efforts also complemented rapid advances in virology and immunology, disciplines that started married to new concepts to fight viral dangers (Trovato et al., 2020). If you consider global health, the entire polio narrative illustrates that detecting a virus early can spur innovation in preventive technology. Vaccines revolutionized polio, but those early, disorganized outbreaks remain an essential page in the ongoing story of trying to control and understand other infectious diseases, such as measles (Sallam et al., 2023) (Figure 14.5).

14.1.3. Historical Impact on Public Health

In the 1900s, outbreaks of measles and polio rocked public health systems globally. At that time, before vaccines, these diseases struck children particularly severely, overwhelminging hospitals and leaving families in terror. With time, however, the measles vaccine emerged in the 1960s, and not long afterward, global polio vaccination campaigns gained steam. Instantly, infection rates plummeted, which was evidence that concerted immunization drives could make all the difference. Health systems had to switch gears in a hurry by ramping up surveillance, education, and mass vaccination campaigns—a shift that ultimately paved the way for contemporary methods in preventive medicine and highlighted just how crucial vaccines are when it comes to safeguarding community well-being and securing equitable access for all. The victories from such vaccination campaigns also show how tenuous our health arrangements can get when major adversities hit us. When COVID-19 burst in, usual immunization programs got disrupted; diseases we had previously managed began making unwanted comebacks. One systematic review even noted that in some polio-endemic spots cases nearly quadrupled due to halted immunization programs—fueled by movement restrictions, reduced numbers of healthcare workers, and widespread fears of virus exposure (Zohra et al., 2021). These incidents remind us, in most cases, of the thin line between crisis response and the steady upkeep of everyday health services. It's a clear warning that immunization systems must be sturdy yet subtle enough to respond to emergencies without allowing regular care to slide. In retrospect, the complex past between infectious disease and public health policy holds the main clues for addressing both old and new threats. The experiences with polio and measles demonstrate that consistent vaccination coverage is the key—and when those efforts collapse, the consequences can be terrible. The current concerns regarding viruses mutating and immunity fading, discussed recently in the context of SARS-CoV-2 (Telenti et al., 2021), resemble those earlier lessons on disease persistence and control. These turning points in history inform the design of flexible vaccine strategies that respond to shifts in virus behavior and fill gaps in immunity. Maintaining rigorous surveillance and a quick-response system are crucial. Finally, the lasting gains observed through measles and polio campaigns are a reminder that vigilance, innovation, and international cooperation are essential tools to prevent the recurrence of infectious diseases.

14.2. Symptoms and Transmission

Infectious diseases may begin on the sly, in ways that make them difficult to identify at first—they sometimes appear as nothing more than an ordinary cold. Measles, for instance, is initiated by a fever, accompanied by a cough, runny nose, and red, watery eyes; then, quite suddenly, a rash appears, signaling the disease is underway. The virus is transmitted primarily by small airborne droplets from sneezing or coughing, and, as it happens, an infected individual can usually transmit it four days before the rash even shows up and a few days afterward. These symptoms aren't skin-deep; they are indicative of a more profound viral takeover that, if not controlled, can cause serious problems such as pneumonia, particularly in areas with less-than-stellar healthcare. All this latent infectious time and concurrent symptoms usually makes measles outbreak control in susceptible populations a true headache (Uwishema et al., 2021). Things only become more complicated when regular vaccination activities get damaged—global emergencies such as COVID-19 have thrown a wrench into usual immunization activities, facilitating measles transmission even further in weaker healthcare systems. The Democratic Republic of Congo, for example, has witnessed a dramatic spike in cases because of interruptions in vaccination coverage and surveillance. A gap in such aspects as cold chain logistics has caused the detection of outbreaks to slow down, and environmental and social considerations, civil unrest being one of these—tend to cloud the water even more. Children, particularly those below five years of age, pay the ultimate price as levels of disease and even mortality increase when vaccine immunity dwindles. Given how freely the measles can travel in the air and how long carriers remain infectious, it's very obvious that consistent vaccination drives and keen health surveillance are simply indispensable (Mohan et al., 2021). Polio is yet another vaccine-preventable virus that, despite having some characteristics similar to those of measles, has a different set of rules. This virus typically spreads by the fecal-oral route, usually by contaminated food or water, which illustrates just how important good sanitation is. In the majority of instances, polio is either asymptomatic or only causes a slight, flu-like sensation, so it is not easy to catch it in the early stages. Still, on the odd occasion, it infiltrates the nervous system bringing with it sudden paralysis that can be permanent—something nobody would wish on themselves. Its insidious spread, with individuals unknowingly harboring the virus, places yet another obstacle in the path of being able to halt it. Overall, knowing these fine points of how polio travels and conceals itself is key to developing intelligent vaccination strategies and public health measures that interrupt the chain of transmission before any paralytic effects set in (Mohan et al., 2021; Uwishema et al., 2021) (Figure 14.6).

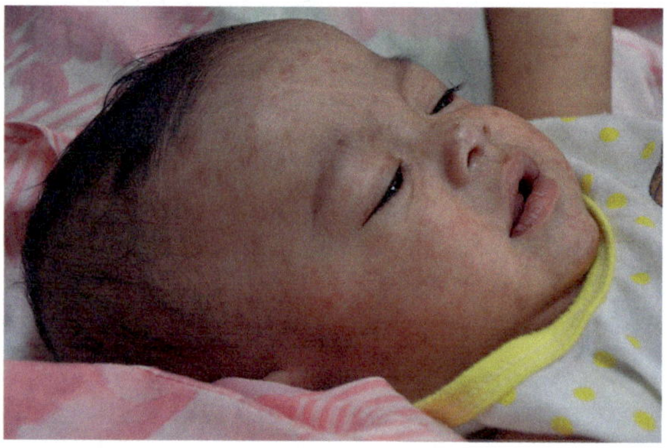

Figure 14.6. Measles: Causes, symptoms, treatment, and prevention.

Source: By CDC Global, Jim Goodson, M.P.H. - Measles is no joke, https://phil.cdc.gov/Details.aspx?pid=17980, Public Domain, https://commons.wikimedia.org/w/index.php?curid=76594880

14.2.1. Common Symptoms of Measles

Measles initially begins with several symptoms that most would mistake for another virus. A high fever appears quite rapidly, followed by a persistent cough, runny nostrils, and red, watery eyes. All of these symptoms result from the virus attacking the breathing passages along with the eye membranes, which facilitates passing on the infection and confuses early diagnosis. Two or three days before the characteristic rash shows up, minute white spots, familiarly referred to as Koplik spots, may suddenly materialize on the inner cheeks. Identification of these premonitory signs is extremely crucial for detecting the disease in time. Being aware of these hints is not only helpful to medical people; it also aids in informing public health actions such as vaccinations, which have played a pivotal role in combating measles and other such dangers such as polio (Breman et al., 2011). Soon after this initial stage, the typical rash comes onto the scene. It erupts fairly quickly across the face, neck, trunk, and limbs, serving both as a marker of the immune system's battle against the virus and as an indicator of maximum contagion. In the majority of instances, this rash is accompanied by a persistent fever and a crushing feeling of malaise—indications that the body is fighting off widespread inflammation. Physicians tend to use these , confusing symptoms to differentiate between measles and other rashes-causing diseases. And while the rash symptoms take center stage, there may be other problems such as ear infections or pneumonia that exacerbate the overall disease. These issues have prompted experts to emphasize rapid diagnosis and consistent vaccination campaigns, which in the past have served to reduce measles and keep other such diseases such as poliomyelitis at bay (Breman et al., 2011). Conversely, measles is not merely about the rash or fever—it also disrupts the body's defense mechanisms. terms, following the first attack, the virus temporarily reduces immunity, making individuals more susceptible to other diseases and respiratory difficulties that may take weeks to subside even when the rash disappears. Occasionally, though infrequently, the nervous system is attacked, manifested by irritability, an aversion to bright light, or even, in severe attacks, encephalitis. Such complications introduce a further level of risk to the infection. Scientists have been using animal models, such as macaques, for decades to solve these mysteries. These studies not only dissect how the disease functions, but they also contribute to developing improved vaccines and treatments—a reminder of why continued, hands-on research is so vital in fighting not only measles but other viral threats as well.

14.2.2. Common Symptoms of Polio

Polio tends to initiate in a bit of a covert manner. You may begin to feel a low-grade fever, a general lethargy, a headache and maybe even sore throat or strange tummy troubles. These preliminary symptoms don't strongly suggest polio because they can arise in the presence of numerous other pests, particularly in areas where the virus still pervades. In many instances, nothing overt appears at all, which quietly allows the virus to pass undetected. Identifying these clues is important because catching them early sets the stage for rapid isolation and treatment, reducing the likelihood of a worse, paralyzing attack (Jeyanathan et al., 2020). Over time, however, the virus can choose to play havoc with your nervous system. Some patients begin to experience muscle weakness and a type of uneven paralysis that usually strikes the legs more than the arms, leaving damage that may remain permanent. Occasionally even the muscles used to breathe get affected, necessitating mechanical ventilation in an emergency. Evidently, these neurological problems make it a serious issue—polio here doesn't mess around in comparison to something like measles, in which a visible rash and respiratory difficulties tend to be obvious. Due to how unpredictable the paralysis can be, early vaccination really does matter in preventing these serious consequences (Evan et al., 2020). Even after the worst of it is over, many people develop what's called post-polio syndrome years later. Eventually, muscles will start to weaken gradually, and fatigue and pain will become a constant issue. Occasionally, during this initial period, a stiff neck, some back pain, or difficulty swallowing also appear, which could suggest that the virus is affecting more than merely your motor functions. When you pit these against the rash and rampant respiratory symptoms of measles, it's a simple matter to understand how complex polio is. This quilt-like pattern of signs highlights the challenging nature of the disease control and the genuine requirement for careful public health interventions in controlling both viruses (Evan et al., 2020; Jeyanathan et al., 2020) (Figure 14.7).

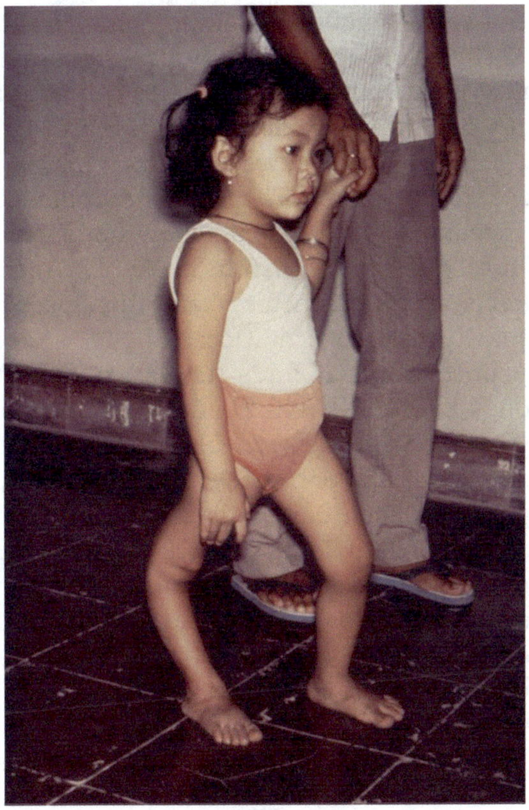

Figure 14.7. Symptoms of polio.

Source: By Photo Credit:Content Providers(s): CDC - This media comes from the Centers for Disease Control and Prevention's Public Health Image Library (PHIL), with identification number #5578.Note: Not all PHIL images are public domain; be sure to check copyright status and credit authors and content providers.العربيّة | Deutsch | English | македонски | slovenščina | +/−, Public Domain, https://commons.wikimedia.org/w/index.php?curid=211474

14.2.3. Modes of Transmission for Both Diseases

Infectious diseases transmit in a whole variety of unpredictable manners. Take measles—it's all about airborne, baby. A sneeze or a cough propels tiny droplets full of viral particles into the air that can persist for hours after the infected have departed. Densely populated, poorly ventilated areas tend to provide the perfect storm, and even a small amount of contact with throat or nasal secretions is enough. Typically, this aerial quality makes an end to measles a nightmare even with extensive vaccination (Melissa et al., 2017). With polio, however, things play a bit of a different script. The virus predominantly disappears in stool and somehow finds a route to food or water that is not hygienic, which in contexts of unsatisfactory sanitation presents a significant concern. Occasionally, and it's very uncommon, it finds its way transmitted through saliva as well. Fundamentally, polio's association with the fecal-oral pathway ties it firmly with issues of hygiene, rendering it highly responsive to environmental factors (Jeyanathan et al., 2020). Both diseases teach us how diverse modes of transmission truly determine public health action. Measles hops rapidly from one host to the next through the air, so rapid, broad-scale immunization is paramount in developing a community barrier. At the same time, combating polio isn't all about vaccines—it's about increasing hygiene and sanitation as well. Unlike measles, which essentially never hangs around, polio has the potential to persist in the environment, potentially spreading throughout a community by way of polluted water. In most instances, appreciating these distinctions assists in developing improved, more specific approaches for combating each disease (Melissa et al., 2017; Jeyanathan et al., 2020).

14.3. Vaccination and Prevention

If you consider fighting infections, it generally just boils down to biology and behavior and environment combining in unpredictable ways. Look at polio , things get complicated when not everybody gets the full vaccination and the natural environment still has carriers that can spread the virus. Math models, in most cases, help us figure out when the virus can be held in check; keeping that reproduction number below one turns out to be a must. Of course, vaccines are critical, but relying solely on them without boosting sanitation and public health systems just doesn't cut it, so a broader, more coordinated plan ends up being essential (Rahmi et al., 2025). Measles has its own challenges as well. Universal high vaccine coverage is still the target, but regional gaps create tiny weak spots where outbreaks could fire up. Long-term research consistently demonstrates a direct correlation: when vaccination levels fall, measles cases spike. In some areas, there's even less consistency – fewer communities reaching those required vaccination levels – which indicates some underlying challenges in local outreach and health engagement. A little more word on the ground and education can work wonders, particularly for making sure that vulnerable populations such as children aged under five get fully vaccinated (Gon Pçalves et al., 2024). For an effective defense against both polio and measles, having merely an active vaccine campaign is not sufficient. In most instances, combining immunization efforts with effective public health measures, improved sanitation, enhanced surveillance, and continuous health education provides a sort of safety net against a disease resurgence. Continuous monitoring, combined with rapid review of data, facilitates responsive action and wise resource reallocation. Policy-makers and health managers, in most cases, gain significantly from information that allows them to focus on specific groups or areas, and such broad-based approach not only consolidates current control measures but also lays the ground for a future where these diseases might be eradicated, reducing the overall burden of outbreak (Gon Pçalves et al., 2024; Rahmi et al., 2025) (Figure 14.8).

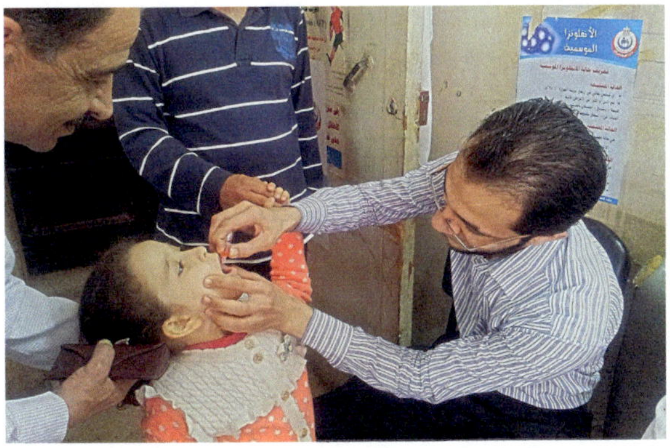

Figure 14.8. Vaccination and prevention.

Source: By CDC Global - Polio Vaccination | Egypt, CC BY 2.0, https://commons.wikimedia.org/w/index.php?curid=64849468

14.3.1. Development of the Measles Vaccine

Way back in the early to mid-20th century, all this changed dramatically as the battle against infectious diseases intensified, vaccination campaigns were established to reduce deaths among the most vulnerable. Measles, this highly contagious viral pest, particularly bothered children everywhere, and soon there was a frantic effort to halt outbreaks that were spreading a lot of disease and unfortunately, a lot of deaths in communities with patchy healthcare. During the 1950s, researchers began experimenting with isolating and attenuating measles virus strains; these initial attempts, in the majority of instances, established foundations for vaccine concepts that could be implemented to induce immunity safely.

It emerged from these experiences that not everyone received a fair chance at immunization, and this really underlined the need for wider immunization campaigns embedded in public health systems to maintain vaccine access level (Rodrigues & Plotkin, 2020). Subsequently, when the measles vaccine was developed, it was a tremendous scientific achievement due to revolutions in how we knew viruses and the immune system—scientists were able to transform live viruses into a controlled, harmless agent against the disease. The introduction of the first licensed measles vaccines in the 1960s reversed the tide, reducing cases sharply in locations that were able to implement mass immunizations. However, maintaining those high vaccination rates wasn't easy; issues such as keeping the vaccines cold and gaining public trust continued to arise. And, notably, fitting the measles shots in with the other standard vaccines only increased overall health gains, even facilitating efforts such as the campaign against polio. This combination of interventions truly exemplified just how intertwined global health initiatives are and where vaccines find themselves in the very center of public health across populations (Rodrigues & Plotkin, 2020).

Today, while the COVID-19 pandemic has disrupted global priorities and inserted some serious roadblocks into regular immunization services, it's also taught us a few things about maintaining health systems resilient during an emergency. Measles vaccination campaigns suffered quite a blow in many regions, prompting fears of outbreaks as increasingly more people became susceptible. However, in a sense, this interruption also indicates just how important it is that we have strong, adaptable health infrastructure which can keep routine vaccinations going despite emergencies. To rebound, reviving vaccination against measles is central to achieving health-related Sustainable Development Goals. Health systems, apparently, will need to be innovative so that vaccines remain in supply and public confidence is not eroded—bolstering on successes with measles and polio campaigns and learning how to meet new challenges head on (Figure 14.9).

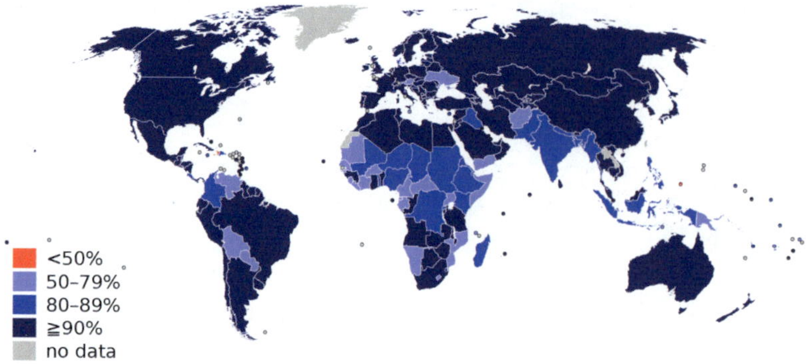

Figure 14.9. Measles vaccine.

Source: By Master Uegly - This SVG map includes elements that have been taken or adapted from this map:, CC BY-SA 3.0, https://commons.wikimedia.org/w/index.php?curid=17066839

14.3.2. Development of the Polio Vaccine

Fighting infectious diseases revolutionized medicine in the 20th century, with vaccines playing a starring role in a major way. The polio vaccine completely changed the game—it kept the virus at bay and made things much less scary. Polio was a vicious microbe back then—it could paralyze and even kill, and many families, particularly families with children, lived in perpetual fear. During the 1940s and '50s, scientists started prodding the virus with questions about how it operated and what stimulated our defense mechanisms. Some notable figures, such as Jonas Salk and Albert Sabin, contributed to the cause. Salk's vaccine, which came out in 1955, utilized a killed virus to induce immunity without infecting people with the disease—a development that eased several health fears even now (Geoghegan et al., 2020). Just after Salk's method made headlines, Sabin's oral vaccine joined the scene in the early 1960s with its own advantages. In contrast to the injected form, Sabin's OPV contained a milder live virus that triggered robust intestinal defenses—imperative for preventing the virus from spreading within. This brilliant modification powered mass immunization campaigns, especially in less-resourced settings where convenience and affordability were very important. The outcome was a sharp reduction in polio cases globally; however, as is too often the case, obstacles such as vaccine refusal and delivery challenges still arose. In many instances, the mere fact of having the vaccine did not necessarily mean that everyone enrolled, considering the combination of cultural, information, and socioeconomic factors involved (Sato, 2018). In retrospect, the history of the polio vaccine illustrates that scientific integrity and public confidence can never be a separate thing. Although these shots were extremely effective, concerns over their safety periodically erupted—prefiguring parallel fears associated with other vaccines, such as for measles. Much of the time, rumors about toxic ingredients or side effects spread, even where there was copious evidence testifying to their value (Geoghegan et al., 2020). International campaigns, such as Brazil's National Immunization Program, remind us how well-planned efforts are necessary, even in the face of challenges such as hesitancy and declines in vaccine coverage (Sato, 2018). Overall, the history of the polio vaccine is a combination of breakthroughs in laboratory work and practical problems that continue to influence the way we think about immunization programs today (Figure 14.10).

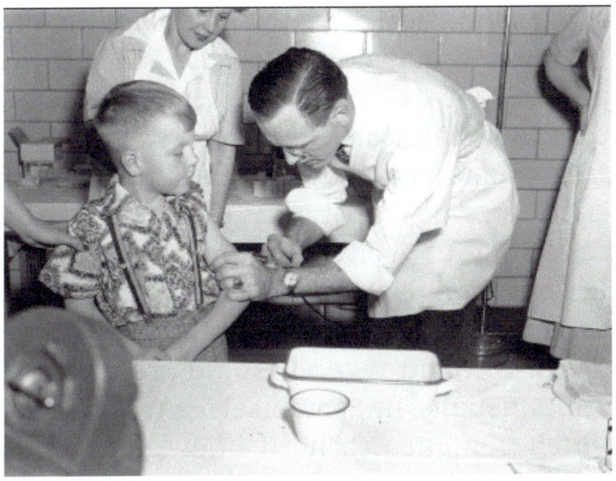

Figure 14.10. Development of the polio vaccine.

Source: https://external-content.duckduckgo.com/iu/?u=https%3A%2F%2Fimg.washingtonpost.com%2Frw%2F2010-2019%2FWashingtonPost%2F2015%2F03%2F30%2FEducation%2FImages%2FAP540426029142774903O.jpg%3Fuuid%3DWecVkNcfEeS_C_ZIuVpkiA&f=1&nofb=1&ipt=8ecb3e760b33cb9c6b0796baf6dfdc4c114c992cfcaf84036b9da245465d4c0b.

14.3.3. Current Vaccination Strategies and Recommendations

Vaccine strategies rely heavily on combining solid science with an understanding of local culture. Campaigns against measles and polio over the years have employed mass immunization campaigns aimed at reaching herd immunity levels, although the strategy is not always consistent. Children today typically receive their MMR vaccination early on, and multiple rounds of either inactivated or oral polio vaccines - a regimen adopted by medical associations such as the WHO and CDC to address weak points. But it is not always smooth; hesitancy, misinformation, and even some gummed-up logistical problems continue to emerge (Viswanath et al., 2021). More often than not, a combination of straightforward local communication and an effort to increase trust in science is responsible for maintaining progress at a steady pace. Vaccine hesitancy, intertwined with socio-political and cultural factors, tends to introduce surprise obstacles into the equation. Rumors, conspiracy theories, and outright disinformation spread on social media and sometimes even from influential individuals, eroding public trust in vaccines. For example, regions like Pakistan have experienced significant reversals in polio work because of these false narratives (Khan et al., 2020). More and more, specialists are looking to community education and mobilization—working with local influencers, providing clear information from credible health sources, and employing different forms of media—to assist in combating these myths. All of these, though cumbersome at times, are regarded as indispensable to rebuilding trust and getting everybody to value the immunization benefits. There's also the social reality aspect with the consideration of income, education level, and access to good information being a major influence on whether individuals adhere to the schedules of measles and polio vaccines recommended. Research typically indicates that marginalized groups - racial and ethnic minorities, or those struggling with poverty - have lower vaccination rates, owing in part to restricted access to healthcare and a persistent lack of trust in scientific institutions (Viswanath et al., 2021). Therefore, plans today aren't merely about dispensing vaccines; they emphasize equitable distribution and targeted interventions that overcome these structural barriers. Public health policies increasingly require a combination of medical, social, and even discursive communicative approaches to construct vaccine confidence and guarantee that all sectors of the population are protected.

14.4. Global Impact

Measles and polio impact not just health at an individual level—they transform economic, social, and even political balances across the globe. Measles and polio don't merely affect individual health—they change economic, social, and even political balances globally. In most instances, previous efforts at eradication have demonstrated that when countries roll up their sleeves as one, great things happen. Vaccine campaigns prevent deaths and relieve pressure on overcrowded hospitals, releasing money for other necessities. Children who avoid such diseases are more likely to remain in school and work harder at home, an added benefit that spreads through communities. The last push against such diseases brings up tricky challenges, which require adaptive research and monitoring on the ground to smooth over bumps in vaccine delivery and gain local confidence (Breman et al., 2011). Overall, combining various tactics is at the center of securing the world's health in the long term. There still recur outbreaks in different corners of the globe, proving that disease control is a challenge in a world where people are always on the move. Refugees, asylum seekers, and other immigrants usually find themselves tripping over obstacles when attempting to receive vaccinations, which complicates herd immunity for host nations. Various national immunization campaigns are spread wide and far between; there are some areas that provide comprehensive, extensive coverage even for migrant children, while others maintain a minimal strategy with emphasis on measles and polio only. This disparity underscores the urgent need for more harmonized vaccination schemes and improved data exchange across borders, such that gaps are avoided that could lead to renewed outbreaks (Declich et al., 2017).

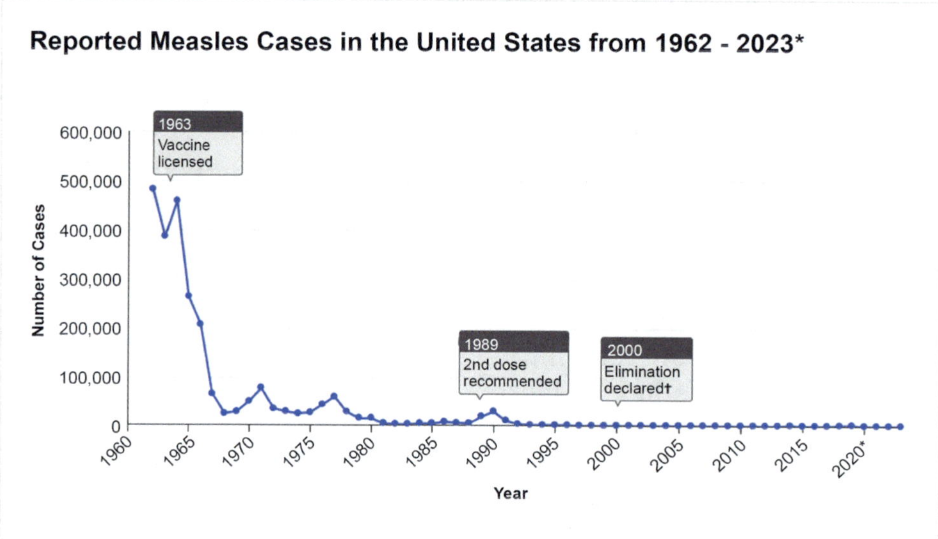

Figure 14.11. Global impact of measles and polio incidence.

Source: Centers for Disease Control and Prevention. (2025). *Map of Measles Cases in 2024 & 2025. Measles Cases and Outbreaks.*

In general, enhanced collaboration between migrant-hosting nations is necessary to maintaining these diseases at bay. Eradicating measles and polio on a world scale is dependent upon merging vaccination efforts with continuous efforts in getting vaccines more effective and within reach. Advances in science have improved vaccines to streamline them and adapt schedules, increasing their effectiveness and accommodating diverse local requirements. Simultaneously, cultural and social issues count—a community's confidence may rest on a real appreciation of local customs and beliefs. Evidence from disciplines such as anthropology and behavioral studies indicates that if local practices aren't dismissed, individuals are more likely to roll up their sleeves for a chance, bringing us nearer to complete disease eradication. Prior history with measles and polio makes a sort of map for efforts in the future, demonstrating that adaptive, adaptive research can cope with changing health threats and social demands (Breman et al., 2011). Overall, remaining vigilant and receptive to innovation is most important to contain infectious diseases (Figure 14.11).

14.4.1. Measles Incidence Rates Worldwide

In the global mix of infectious diseases, measles clearly stands out as a tricky challenge. Effective vaccines exist, yet measles cases jump up and down in different regions—often because vaccine reach, local health systems, and even political hiccups don't always line up. Sometimes the disease makes an unexpected comeback when immunization plans slip, people get uneasy about shots, or conflicts and even pandemics throw everything off-kilter. This unpredictable bounce serves as a reminder that consistent vaccine push and close monitoring of outbreaks are rather non-negotiable. And as measles is so easily transmissible, maintaining herd immunity at the correct level across the board becomes even more important to keep outbreaks at bay. Not every region or community experiences measles the same. In low- and middle-income areas, however, the disease strikes harder—mainly because vaccination rates aren't as high and healthcare systems aren't as solid. Indigenous and marginalized communities tend to carry the bulk of the burden; past neglect and lack of culturally attuned healthcare create both underreporting and less effective immunization programs (Sally et al., 2019). More often than not, these cyclical, systemic challenges render achieving universal vaccine coverage seem like an elusive dream, as measles persists in sneaking around in weak pockets. Addressing this is not simply about accelerating vaccine distributions—it is also about designing policies that get cultural contexts right and drive real health equity on the global stage. Meanwhile, measles control has been further complicated by emerging global health threats that divert resources and attention away from routine immunization. The COVID-19 pandemic impacted vaccination timetables in many countries and slowed efforts to eradicate measles, fueling fears of possible case increases (Nikolaos et al., 2021). terms, as public health officials focus on new pathogens, longstanding vaccine programs often take a backseat, as decades of advancement can be undone. It's important, therefore, to integrate measles vaccination efforts into a master plan for fighting several diseases at once. In the majority of instances, good global collaboration and adequate distribution of resources are the determinants in reducing measles transmission and getting closer to eliminating it along with other preventable diseases such as polio.

14.4.2. Polio Incidence Rates Worldwide

Vaccination campaigns have transformed our battle against infectious diseases. One of the greatest victories of the last century is the way polio cases have plummeted through mass immunization campaigns. Nevertheless, in certain regions, usually due to political instability, logistically complicated terrain, or a healthy dose of vaccine skepticism, polio persists, rendering eradication more of an uphill battle than initially anticipated. Keeping tabs on polio cases worldwide not only shows us where we've done well but also exposes the weak spots that need extra push. It's a constant balancing act between rolling out vaccines and keeping public trust intact, which has been crucial for decades (Adam et al., 2020). Even though cases of polio have plunged globally, there's an uneven spread in who gets protected. In areas with troubled health systems and economic stress, the statistics paint a different picture—reflecting wider discrepancies in access to treatment. Preventing diseases like polio isn't merely a matter of vaccine availability; it's about reaching communities, providing straightforward education, and breaking through fear and misinformation. In general, investing in immunization campaigns and health education is not negotiable if we are going to keep polio at bay. Further, when additional complicating factors such as pandemics emerge, the complex aspect of rolling out vaccines threatens to steal the limelight from polio and send its numbers back up. A balanced response that addresses root health disparities while pushing forward vaccine technology is still absolutely crucial to maintaining low infection rates (Rodrigues & Plotkin, 2020). The almost elimination of polio is an in-your-face lesson in the need for constant vaccination campaigns and international coordination. Mass vaccination drives, careful monitoring for outbreaks, and rapid intervention are all components of the arduous task of keeping totals minimal. Generally, reaching very high vaccination coverage is a must, considering that polio can easily spread among those people who have not been vaccinated. Routine checks for adverse events, even with some small hiccups in reporting, and honest interactions about vaccine safety help keep public faith strong, which is a key ingredient to any successful campaign (Adam et al., 2020). In most countries, how polio immunization is managed serves as a model for combatting other diseases such as measles that share the same challenges. Overall, the rise and fall of keeping polio in check says much about how infectious diseases are kept under control and world health is secured (Figure 14.12).

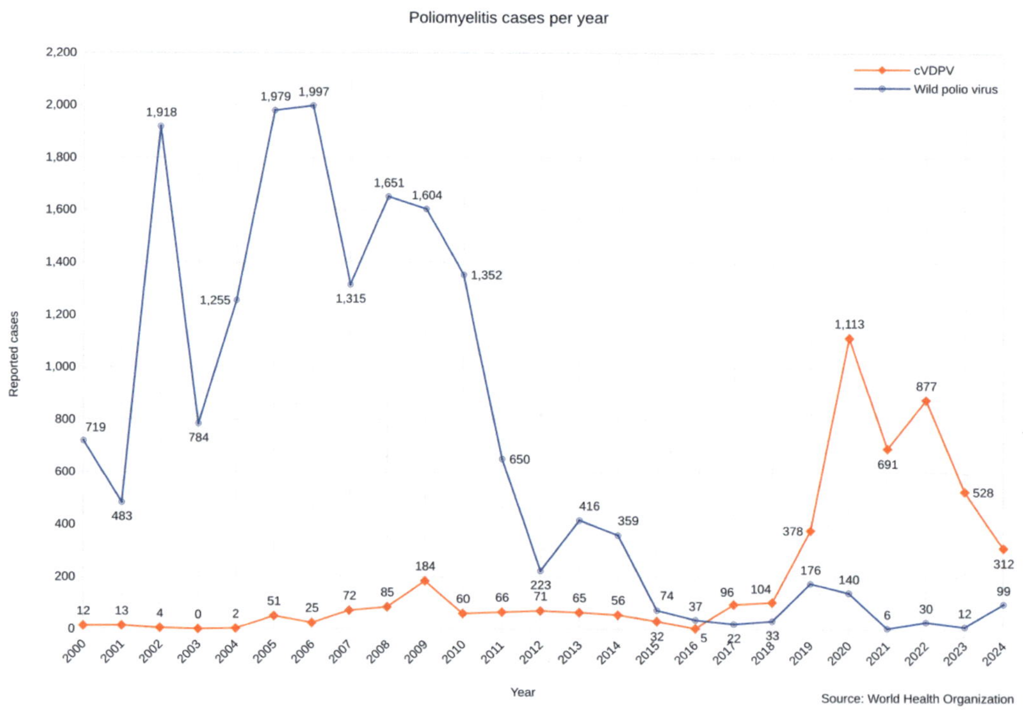

Figure 14.12. Polio incidence rates worldwide.

Source: By Bischnu - Own work based on the data on WHO's website, reproduction of the PNG version., CC BY-SA 4.0, https://commons.wikimedia.org/w/index.php?curid=161077472

14.4.3. Socioeconomic Factors Influencing Disease Spread

Public health emergencies get confused with day-to-day finance issues, shaping the way diseases such as polio and measles spread. In poorer parts of town, finding good care can be a struggle—limited budgets leave vaccines in short supply and outreach inadequate. Dirty, cramped housing and poor sanitation tend to accelerate infection rates, making outbreaks more likely; education deficits sometimes introduce conflicting messages on the value of vaccines. For instance, during COVID-19, several missed shots because of fearfulness about catching the virus in clinics and strict social limits that prove how large health emergencies can exacerbate old inequities (Matilde et al., 2021). All these economic and social barriers not only disturb routine immunizations but also keep cycles of vulnerability rolling, pointing towards interventions that dig into the more basic social triggers of disease spread. Trust among people and how communities can come together really count when vaccines fail to hit all the marks under hard economic conditions. People in economically strapped neighborhoods also end up distrusting health professionals, a sentiment that can be a booster of vaccine resistance. This is further clouded by the use of social media to present so much misinformation, particularly in individuals who might lack a good understanding of healthcare. While healthcare professionals are generally vaccination proponents, at times, they find it really challenging to dispel these established, deeply rooted myths in underserved communities (Matilde et al., 2021). When messages become unclear, communications break down, herd immunity weakens, and diseases establish a foothold. Even people who want to be vaccinated might get damaged by logistical or fiscal barriers, so it is understandable how poverty and access issues can combine to affect disease persistence beyond just personal choice or education. The way measles and polio sort of emerge and evolve becomes much more complicated when struggles with money combine with how viruses naturally change. In areas where poor vaccination coverage leaves certain groups susceptible, those gaps create entry points for ongoing transmission—and sometimes even shifts in the virus. That steady presence of disease feels a bit like it did with SARS-CoV-2, in which waning immunity and variable uptake of vaccines played a big role in what the whole disease picture ended up looking like. Limited monitoring and limited resources in poor communities can hinder outbreak identification, making rapid countermeasures difficult. Overall, these social and economic gradients not only propel immediate spread but also disrupt long-term control strategies, so our plans must integrate biological insights with the complex nature of human existence to effectively stamp out these avoidable infections.

14.5. Treatment and Management

For viruses like measles and polio, early detection and prompt supportive care can make a big difference. Generally speaking, since there aren't many specific antiviral drugs available, doctors usually focus on treating symptoms to keep complications at bay and help patients recover. In most cases of measles, which can trigger serious breathing and brain-related problems, especially among those who haven't been vaccinated, basic measures like keeping patients well hydrated, controlling fevers, and even adding vitamin A into the mix have proven useful. By way of contrast, polio is often treated by alleviating the short-term pain and working to reverse longer-term conditions such as paralysis through therapy and rehab; this combined treatment and follow-up significantly reduces the spread of secondary disease. In short, combining individual clinical treatment with a wide view of public health, no matter how occasionally erratic, is the key to reducing these diseases to a minimum and improving life in general. Central to long-term control of both measles and polio is the necessity for robust vaccination initiatives that are aimed at preventing disease earlier on instead of seeking a cure later on. Despite improvements in drugs, the truth is that, in the absence of specific antivirals, containing outbreaks hinges primarily on maintaining high levels of immunization among communities. That being said, vaccine hesitancy—often stirred up by misinformation and a general distrust in health systems—adds a tricky layer to these efforts. It becomes really important, therefore, to keep an eye on and address the circulating rumors and conspiracy theories, especially on social media where false stories can spread like wildfire (Islam et al., 2021). Health authorities are now tapping into digital platforms more than ever to share accurate facts and counter these narratives; public health campaigns that emphasize vaccine safety and build trust are absolutely crucial for maintaining herd immunity and moving toward global eradication of these diseases. Recent research breakthroughs and changes in public health policy have pushed therapy options for measles and polio slowly in new directions, especially in patients with compromised immune systems or in settings where healthcare resources are scarce. Generally speaking, treatment guidelines these days stress the need for personalized care that takes a person's overall health and risks into account—much like the customized plans used for other infections (Walewska et al., 2022).

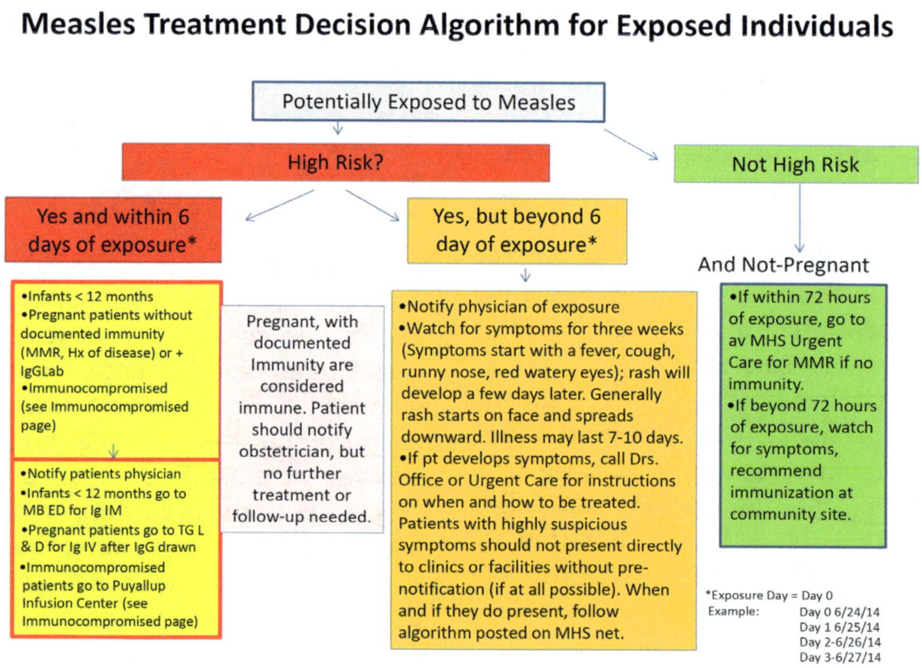

Figure 14.13. Treatment and management of measles and polio.

Source: SlideServe. (n.d.). *Measles Treatment Decision Algorithm.*

For instance, individuals with compromised immune systems might need extra preventive steps alongside standard supportive care to avoid severe disease. It's also worth noting that managing these diseases isn't only about addressing the individual; it also involves surveillance, contact tracing, and community education to catch outbreaks early. By weaving together robust vaccination efforts with appropriate supportive treatments and ongoing monitoring, current protocols aim to meet both the urgent needs of patients and the broader public health objectives in a rather flexible, yet effective, manner (Figure 14.13).

14.5.1. Treatment Options for Measles

Vaccination should be the primary defense against measles, but once a person is ill, making them well again is equally significant. In most instances, people don't receive enough vaccination or have poor immunity, so symptom management is vital. Physicians generally try to address issues such as fever, cough, and inflamed, itchy eyes to avoid complications. Kids, especially those lacking proper nutrition, can really benefit from Vitamin A, which helps lessen the severity and lowers the risk of death. Sometimes, since the virus can really weaken the body's natural defenses, antibiotics are needed to handle any extra bacterial infections that crop up. Unlike treatments for some cancers where immunotherapy has changed the game, dealing with measles still relies on treating symptoms and encouraging early care to avoid further issues (Abbass, 2023). Beyond just soothing the symptoms, our approach to treating measles picks up hints from big vaccine drives and disease-eradication efforts. Vaccines against diseases such as polio and measles have proved that firing from the outset towards immunization is essential, but where the shield of vaccine is absent, treatment must counterattack the infection outright. Today, no effective antivirals for measles exist, yet there is some interest in redirecting the body's immune system in the same manner that the COVID-19 pandemic spurred vaccine development. Overall, the global battle against novel viruses implies that improved boosting of antibody and cell immunity may open up new avenues to treat measles. All those virology and immunology learnings naturally lead us to a combination of preventive as well as treatment strategies to reduce how frequently measles attacks and how severe it becomes (Narayanan et al., 2021). Even with a strong vaccination infrastructure, measles outbreaks continue to occur, so it's critical to have rapid treatment protocols in place. In infected communities, keeping individuals hydrated, well-nourished, and managing any additional infections can prevent serious complications such as pneumonia, brain swelling, or even death. Vitamin A remains in its place as an important component of treatment, demonstrating how important proper nutrition is to recovery. It also assists when public health messages informally remind people to be aware of the early warning signs and get help in a timely manner. Just as in the fight against polio, vaccination campaigns combined with on-the-ground case management had an effect, the combination of preventive efforts and palliative treatment, even though it isn't necessarily a full-fledged cure, is instrumental in curbing the effects of measles. All of these related measures are necessary if we are to continue the momentum for the eventual eradication of measles (Abbass, 2023; Narayanan et al., 2021).

14.5.2. Treatment Options for Polio

Polio care mostly leans on supportive measures instead of a cure, simply because the virus wrecks motor neurons in a pretty destructive way. When people hit an acute case, they usually end up in the hospital just so doctors can keep an eye on their breathing; after all, the virus sometimes knocks out the muscles you need to breathe properly. In really severe cases, a breathing machine might be thrown into the mix to stop respiratory failure. Physical therapy shows up as a big help during recovery, working to keep muscles active and sidestep the deformities that paralytic polio can cause. Pain management analgesics is also key for easing the discomfort from muscle spasms and stiff joints. Even though there's no direct antiviral treatment for polio, these supportive steps, in most cases, make a tangible difference in quality of life and help ward off long-term complications. Vaccination stands as the real frontline against polio; unlike many other viruses with limited treatment options, immunization is our best bet. The introduction of the inactivated polio vaccine (IPV) and the oral polio vaccine (OPV) has reduced cases worldwide sharply—demonstrating just how critical vaccines are in the fight against the disease. Today, addressing vaccine hesitancy is all the more critical, particularly since misinformation is likely to cloud the issue for public health initiatives. Certain lessons from previous vaccine campaigns—even those grappling with COVID-19 vaccine myths—teach us that transparent communication and actual community outreach are important a lot (Islam et al., 2021). Continuing these vaccination campaigns is crucial to avoiding a resurgence and, hopefully, wiping out polio forever. Considering other contagious menaces such as COVID-19, research today continues to drive more specific treatments and vaccines—a path that could eventually define the way we deal with ailments such as polio. Although developments for emerging viruses (e.g., SARS-CoV-2) have accelerated immensely, polio's battle primarily relies on early vaccine breakthroughs and set public health measures (Nikolaos et al., 2021). There remains a sizeable gap since no antiviral drug is available for polio, a gap that progress in the fields of molecular virology and immunology may one day close. Ongoing investment in vaccine technology combined with improved public health infrastructure continues to be key to keeping ahead of polio outbreaks, particularly where healthcare resources can occasionally be a bit wobbly (Figure 14.14).

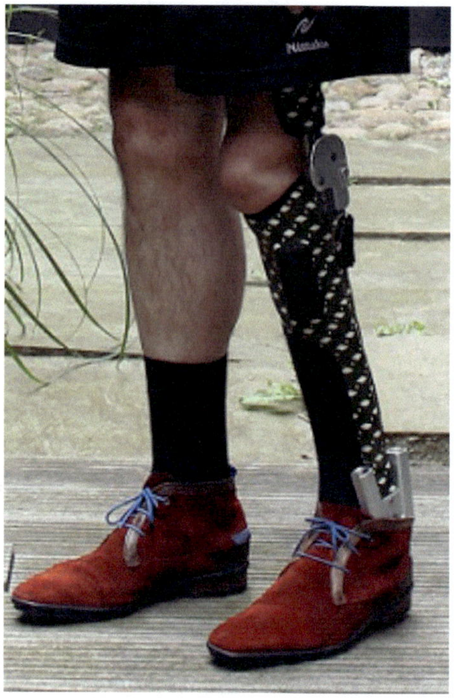

Figure 14.14. Treatment options for polio.

Source: By Orthokin - Own work, CC BY-SA 4.0, https://commons.wikimedia.org/w/index.php?curid=106968607

14.5.3. Role of Healthcare Systems in Managing Outbreaks

Prompt vaccine introductions are essential in halting outbreaks, and health systems truly need to be on the ball. As an example, for diseases such as measles and polio, mass immunization campaigns are frequently cobbled together by these systems in a rather piecemeal manner. Refugees and migrants , populations that often fall behind on routine vaccination , are left in the lurch unless there is a particular strategy. In most instances, some nations have established policies that focus on recently arrived migrants, recognizing that immunization gaps in mobile populations can be dangerous. But with national policies flying every which way and little data on what gets the job done versus what derails these efforts, it often appears better coordination is a good idea. Establishing immunization registries that are functional between borders and encouraging looser, more border-crossing collaboration can better monitor vaccines and avoid repeated shots unnecessarily, which gets that critical prevention network built up (Declich et al., 2017). Beyond just handing out shots, healthcare systems usually need to come up with smart surveillance methods to spot outbreaks quickly and respond accordingly. Generally speaking, a robust surveillance system not only guides timely vaccination efforts but also aids in picking up on cases where folks don't show typical symptoms—something we've seen with polio. New diagnostic technologies and a better understanding of the composition of viruses have, in the majority of instances, served to explain the origins and transmission of infections. Concurrently, studies of social and behavioral determinants turn out to be quite significant when addressing cultural resistance and encouraging individuals to get vaccinated. As measles and polio incidence fall to near zero in impacted regions, being vigilant while adapting vaccine strategies continues to be tough, but strictly required to ward off any resurgence (Breman et al., 2011). Healthcare systems, on their part, have to continue to innovate and remain adaptable in response to outbreak control. Lessons of previous attempts remind us to keep refining vaccine compositions, challenging the way doses are administered, and tailoring immunization schedules to accommodate the changing dynamics of disease patterns. This flexibility, even if not always without a hitch, keeps different settings and age groups effective – whether it's children, adolescents, or adults. And in addition, studies conducted in the course of vaccination campaigns have repeatedly served to highlight the particular needs and field-work challenges in specific groups of people, thus opening the door to more effective action. CombinationIncorporating intelligence from laboratory experiments, field surveys, and even common-sense community input goes a good way towards strengthening resistance against measles and polio. Ultimately, this kind of all-around engagement not only keeps progress steady toward elimination goals but also primes health infrastructures to face up to new public health threats (Breman et al., 2011) (Figure 14.15).

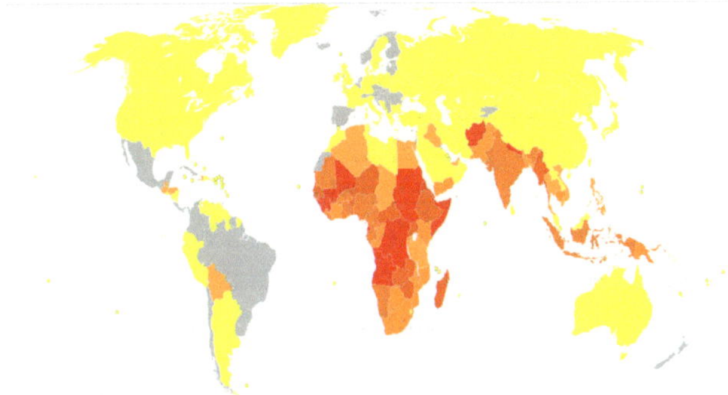

Figure 14.15. Measles outbreaks.

Source: By Chris55 - Data from World Health Organization Estimated Deaths 2012 Vector map from BlankMap-World6, compact.svg by Canuckguy et al., CC BY-SA 4.0, https://commons.wikimedia.org/w/index.php?curid=50320821

14.6. Public Health Initiatives

Vaccination and community engagement have played a central role in the battle to defeat diseases such as polio and measles. Vaccines have reduced cases by far by producing what most refer to as herd immunity—a condition where sufficient individuals are resistant that those that aren't (or cannot be vaccinated) receive some protection as an added bonus. Thanks to regular immunization campaigns, many countries have recorded sharp declines in how often these diseases come, which means fewer people fall ill or die. However, it is an ongoing task to keep vaccines from leaving the equation; communities need to remain engaged, and vaccination rates need to be maintained to avoid flare-ups. More often than not, basic surveillance and simple educational pushes that help clear up misunderstandings about vaccines are the tools that build community trust; these tactics work to counter challenges like vaccine hesitancy and gaps in access that still menace global efforts to stamp out diseases like measles and polio (Khudhair, 2020). Policies from the government also help shape how well public health programs work against infections. In most regions, mandates now necessitate vaccination for public or school activity participation, emphasizing that immunization is everyone's responsibility. Examples of global collaboration exist too—local and international governments collaborate to enhance how vaccines are transported around, so even people in remote areas are protected. New health technologies let authorities track cases in real-time; such data makes it easier to adjust strategies quickly when problems emerge. For instance, Arctic countries have shown that diverse and locally adapted policies, tuned into geographic and cultural characterestics, can really strengthen health systems. These combinationed methods give us important lessons for future immunization efforts against measles and polio (Peterson et al., 2023). Keeping the push for immunization alive definitely isn't without its hurdles. Changes in the viruses and strains that sometimes resist current vaccines mean that ongoing monitoring and new shots are needed to keep populations shielded. Social and political issues, like conflicts and a general air of mistrust—can also put pay to vaccine uptake, nudging herd immunity further out of reach. Generally, solutions for these issues require sound education, policies that incorporate all voices, and outreach that recognizes the distinct cultures. The decline in measles incidents as well as polio incidence almost to zero reminds everyone that 'steady and fact-based health steps are necessary worldwide.' Most often, this is a case not of individual protection but of protecting the community through sustained prevention and control efforts (Khudhair, 2020; Peterson et al., 2023) (Figure 14.16).

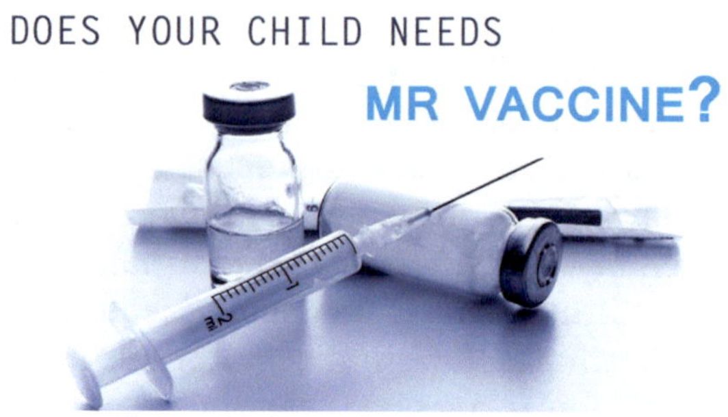

Figure 14.16. Global vaccination campaigns for measles.

Source: RXDX Healthcare. (2021). *MR Vaccine—Do You Need.*

14.6.1. Global Vaccination Campaigns for Measles

People have known for a long time that rolling out vaccines to everyone is key, especially with diseases like measles and polio. Global vaccination success isn't just about following a script; it often comes down to countries working together, smart use of resources, and getting communities on board. Measles is so contagious that vaccination rates must reach more than 95% to cut off outbreaks and provide a sort of "shelter" to the vulnerable. In reality, programs like the Measles & Rubella Initiative have worked aggressively to increase vaccine supply in low- and middle-income countries—sometimes by holding mass vaccination campaigns, occasionally by combining immunization with routine health services. On top of this, systems that quickly spot new cases are crucial, even if that means constantly alteraltering public health systems. And let's not forget, building public trust through honest education and countering misinformation (a struggle we've seen with COVID-19 too (Islam et al., 2021)) plays an equally essential role. Various areas have quite different problems with measles vaccines—mostly because of unequal healthcare infrastructure, local attitudes, and even political ebbs and flows. In a lot of poor places, things like maintaining vaccines at low temperatures, ensuring storage facilities function well, and even addressing a lack of healthcare workers complicate the entire process into a mess, much the same as the obstacles encountered with polio eradication. Occasionally, resistance in the form of vaccine hesitancy due to rumors, distrust, or misinformation spreads, and that leads to community acceptance declining, threatening those high coverage targets. COVID-19 introductions in Africa teach us that straightforward, honest communication and genuine dialogue at the community level go a great way in dispelling these fears (Islam et al., 2021). For some, engaging reliable local leaders and health workers, developing messages that resonate with local cultures, and integrating vaccination campaigns with other health initiatives have been effective, underlining the importance of adaptable and culturally sensitive solutions. Despite all these detours, global measles vaccination programs have taken significant leaps by picking up lessons from polio campaigns as well as other immunization initiatives. The push for fair vaccine distribution remains atop the list—since unequal access lets the virus lurk in pockets and slow down global elimination. Bolstering local vaccine production, expanding health facilities, and retaining well-trained immunization staff also help tackle supply and delivery woes. Also, keeping current on new data and having the ability to act fast when outbreaks seem to show up catches any gaps in coverage earlier. All of these working together create a better arrangement for handling measles shots, enhancing overall public health security, and demonstrating just how interconnected the gains and problems of measles and polio campaigns are.

14.6.2. Global Vaccination Campaigns for Polio

Eradicating polio is one of those gigantic public health puzzles that brought together international collaboration and new advances. Scientific studies propelled enhanced vaccine recipes, more intelligent delivery strategies, and novel immunization schedules – all of which improved the efficacy of vaccination campaigns. At a certain point, methods for following the virus also changed; instruments improved at detecting cases with no apparent symptoms and tracking the spread of the virus all the way down to its molecular path. That transformation assisted local health crews in pinpointing hotspots and containing outbreaks more. The work even descended into anthropology and sociology to handle cultural or religious barriers that could make people apprehensive about vaccines. Even as the number of cases declined, vaccination efforts continued, demonstrating how difficult it was to overcome the virus and why research had to continue to evolve and overcome new challenges (Breman et al., 2011). Another large part of the equation was astute financial management. A significant one of the secrets to worldwide polio vaccination achievement was shrewd financing—agencies such as the Global Alliance for Vaccines and Immunization (GAVI) combined innovative approaches when it came to organizing resources. In most instances, the coming of the International Finance Facility for Immunization (IFFIm) was a huge infusion of money immediately, allowing big clusters to be immunized sooner, reducing transmission and suppressing outbreaks much better than if the money poured in slowly. This consistent, near-predictable funding gave vaccine manufacturers and governments enough confidence to look ahead and maintain programs going along without too many bumps. It just goes to illustrate that a well-coordinated money plan can be as important as scientific advancement in advancing global vaccination initiatives (Yeh et al., 2025). CombinationIncorporating high-quality research with creative funding methods truly gets at the multi-layered battle against polio – and it positions itself within the larger battle against infectious diseases. Vaccines remain front and center, but in getting them into arms means more than possessing the shot; it requires thoughtful planning, a firm understanding of local cultures, and economic acumen to overcome both logistical and acceptance hurdles. The lessons from polio – like using molecular surveillance and engaging communities in ways that respect their unique views – offer useful pointers for handling other preventable diseases, measles for instance. Even with all the progress made, knocking out the last traces of the virus demands even stronger, flexible strategies because stubborn transmission doesn't yield easily to old methods. Therefore, consistent commitment on the part of science, money, and society is still the linchpin if world immunization goals are to become enduring public health successes (Breman et al., 2011; Yeh et al., 2025) (Figure 14.17).

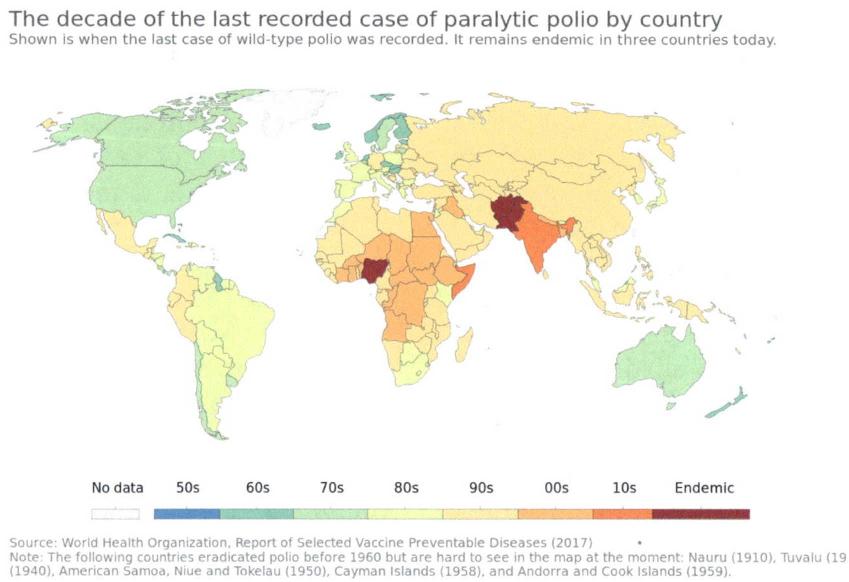

Figure 14.17. Global vaccination campaigns for polio.

Source: By Our World In Data - https://ourworldindata.org/grapher/the-decade-of-the-last-recorded-case-of-paralytic-polio-by-country, CC BY 3.0, https://commons.wikimedia.org/w/index.php?curid=86935099

14.6.3. Role of Organizations like WHO And CDC

International bodies play an enormous role when it comes to fighting infectious diseases. They appear in a chaotic, synchronized fashion to combat diseases such as measles and polio. More often than not, you'll discover that organizations such as the World Health Organization (WHO) and the Centers for Disease Control and Prevention (CDC) establish targets for vaccination, monitor epidemics, and scramble resources to increase immunization globally. They are not only conducting vaccination campaigns, they also support research initiatives, provide policy guidelines, and assist in capacity development where resources are absent. For instance, the WHO's Global Vaccine Action Plan demands that everyone gain access to vaccines, emphasizing that public health security is a shared endeavor. This type of strategy enables countries with healthcare infrastructure of any kind to leverage best practices and technical expertise. Without such a directing force, attempts at eliminating measles and polio would likely be disjointed and less successful. Confronting vaccine resistance is a significant challenge for organizations like the WHO and CDC. In the majority of situations, disinformation and misinformation are partially responsible for declining vaccination rates, particularly in some groups. They use models such as the Behavioral and Social Drivers (BeSD) to develop communication plans that are not only evidence-based but also culturally sensitive in terms of characterestics. In the US, where vaccine fake news has taken a noticeable toll on immunization schedules, the CDC has taken action to restore routine vaccination to track—navigating educational programs that are sensitive to social and behavioral factors (Chen et al., 2024). For the most part, these initiatives demonstrate that combating disease is not all about science; it's winning back public confidence and realizing that occasionally science and society must move as one. Further, organizations like the WHO and CDC extend their efforts to rectify disparities in vaccine distribution and manufacturing between regions. Whereas there have been countries that have succeeded in local vaccine production, there are still palpable gaps between supply and demand of vital vaccines across the globe (Madhavi, 2005). By maintaining oversight of the distribution, the WHO works to increase production in those areas that fall behind while establishing logistics networks that attempt to avoid supply chain disruptions. As the CDC supports such actions through tracking outbreaks and the exchange of epidemiological information to identify trouble early, their combined efforts not only seek to fortify health systems that can respond effectively to measles and polio threats but also gradually bridge immunization gaps, setting the path toward global eradication (Figure 14.18).

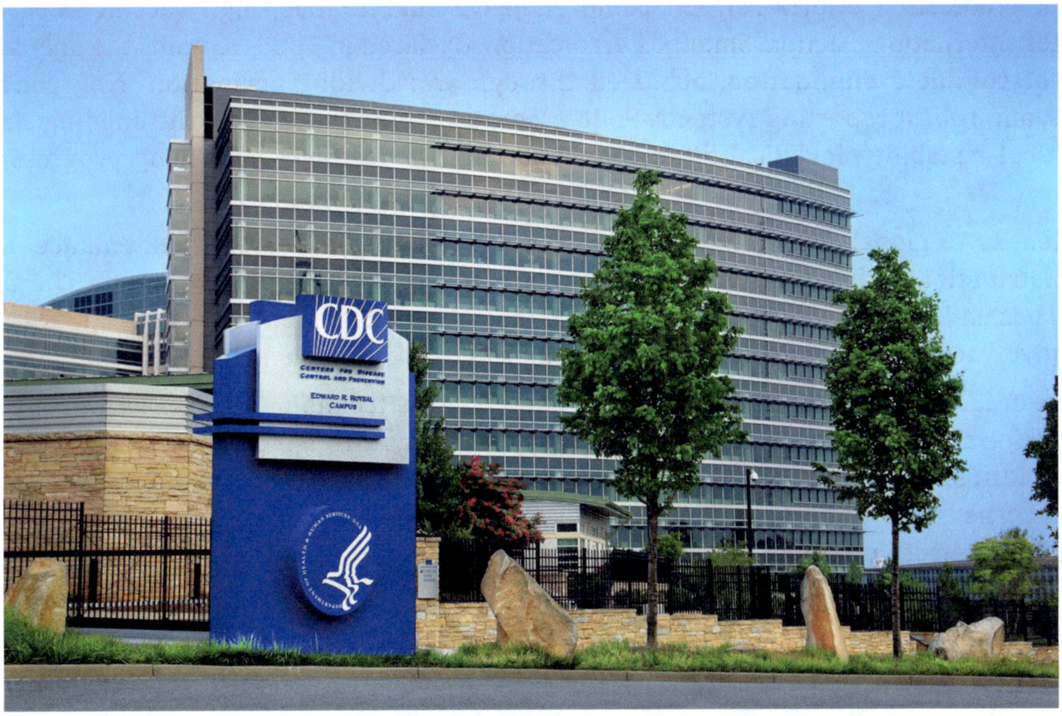

Figure 14.18. Centers for Disease Control and Prevention (CDC).

Source: By James Gathany, Centers for Disease Control and Prevention - Newsroom Image Library: Buildings & Facilities. Archived from the original on 24 June 2013., Public Domain, https://commons.wikimedia.org/w/index.php?curid=26840361

CLOSER LOOK

VACCINATION STRATEGIES AND GLOBAL ERADICATION EFFORTS

Vaccination is one of the most effective public health interventions, significantly reducing morbidity and mortality from infectious diseases. Strategic vaccination programs, combined with global cooperation, have made the eradication or control of diseases such as smallpox, polio, and measles a tangible goal.

Vaccination strategies vary depending on the disease and target population. Routine immunization provides long-term protection against endemic diseases, often beginning in infancy, as seen with the Expanded Program on Immunization (EPI) recommended by the World Health Organization (WHO). Mass vaccination campaigns are deployed during outbreaks or to achieve rapid coverage, such as the pulse polio campaigns in endemic countries. Booster doses are used to maintain immunity, while ring vaccination targets immediate contacts around detected cases, effectively controlling outbreaks of diseases like smallpox and Ebola.

Global eradication efforts rely on comprehensive surveillance, high vaccine coverage, and coordinated international action. Smallpox eradication, declared in 1980, remains the only successful example of complete elimination, achieved through worldwide vaccination, ring containment strategies, and robust reporting systems. Polio eradication efforts illustrate the ongoing challenges, with political instability, logistical difficulties, and vaccine hesitancy hindering progress in some regions.

Challenges to global vaccination and eradication include cold chain maintenance, equitable vaccine distribution, public mistrust, and the emergence of new infectious threats. The COVID-19 pandemic has underscored the importance of rapid vaccine development, international collaboration, and adaptive vaccination strategies in responding to global health emergencies.

Future eradication efforts will benefit from novel vaccine technologies, such as mRNA platforms, improved adjuvants, and thermostable formulations, as well as strengthened community engagement and health infrastructure. By combining scientific innovation with global cooperation, vaccination remains a cornerstone of disease prevention and a powerful tool for moving toward a world free of preventable infectious diseases.

Summary

People have battled measles and polio for years, with some clear wins but also a few nagging setbacks that continue to emerge worldwide. Vaccines are still the backbone of our defense, and keeping immunization programs on track will be crucial. Things took a turn for the worse with COVID-19; hence, for example, the lockdown surprised Scotland with an increase in vaccinations on time, suggesting that even public health's most agile moves can make a difference in a crisis. Meanwhile, England took a minor hit, reminding us that a major disruption can easily trip up routine services unless extra help is on hand. To summarize, it seems we need health strategies that can shift gears quickly to ensure everyone, especially the most vulnerable, stays protected (McQuaid et al., 2022). At the same time, the spread of misinformation has thrown another wrench in the works. The online world has turned into a tangled mess where wild rumors and conspiracy theories frequently hide real facts about vaccines. Studies from various places suggest that, during the pandemic, a large chunk of vaccine-related content online was off the mark, which swayed many people's views on getting immunized. This is especially troubling when it comes to diseases like measles and polio, where keeping vaccination levels high is essential to prevent outbreaks. Tackling this issue means we do not only keep sharp eyes on emerging talks but act fast to check facts and engage communities in clear, down-to-earth interactions, even if it's to repeat key points now further (Islam et al., 2021). In other words, eradicating measles and polio isn't the simple solution of just one move—it requires a combination of good vaccination programs and savvy strategies to combat misinformation and delivery glitches. Last month's issues with keeping immunizations on schedule demonstrate how having timely information and flexible policies is awfully valuable, as is understanding how social and cultural forces influence vaccine uptake. Looking into the future, there need to be efforts that are broad, sweeping, and capable of coping with unforeseen shifts. A consistent commitment at both the international and national levels is what shall ultimately enable us to hold on to our hard-won gains and push these diseases to oblivion (Islam et al., 2021; McQuaid et al., 2022).

World-wide vaccination campaigns have literally transformed the playing field as far as combatting measles and polio in recent decades. Since around 1980, children have begun getting routine shots—consider the measles vaccine (MCV1) and even the third polio shot (Pol3)—and the statistics have increased by more than double, which in most instances has resulted in a significant decline in disease cases. Much of this achievement comes from expanded immunization activities and improved supply of vaccines, supported by numerous international health initiatives. Even so, with these advances, progress has recently slowed a bit, with some areas experiencing declines, indicating that maintaining vaccines in constant supply is indeed an ongoing difficulty. , these trends call for public health interventions to shift focus toward equity, ease of access, and smarter, data-driven alterchanges to reach populations who are usually missed (Natalie et al., 2021). Understanding differences in vaccinations is important when we look at why measles and polio continue to affect vulnerable groups. Indigenous groups – for example, Aboriginal and Torres Strait Islander peoples – tend to experience a combination of historical, cultural, and systemic factors that result in them having lower immunization coverage, thus raising overall risk. Culturally sensitive health services emerge as vital in increasing immunization among such populations, as they facilitate trust building and allow for self-identification to be incorporated in data collection as well as the delivery of services. terms, closing these gaps isn't just a question of equity—it's critically important to generating the type of herd immunity necessary to finally stamp out measles and polio globally (Sally et al., 2019). Further there's the tale of children who've never even had a single dose of the diphtheria-tetanus-pertussis (DTP) vaccine. A near 75% reduction in these "zero-dose" children from 1980 to 2019 is a significant public health achievement, but the overall flattening of vaccine coverage implies that perhaps a change in strategy is in order. Few nations have reached the Global Vaccine Action Plan goals, and there are still many communities that remain vulnerable to measles and polio outbreaks. Such gaps can generally be bridged with better monitoring, stronger immunization systems, or focused outreach. Moreover, being able to keep a closer watch while taking flexible policy measures could help us catch, address, and, if possible, overcome problems like supply disruptions, stock shortages, or even some political or social obstacles. Overall, a steady commitment to equitable and complete immunization is crucial if we wish to safeguard all our children and ultimately eradicate these diseases (Natalie et al., 2021).

References

1. Abbass, M. (2023). Colorectal cancer genetics: An evolutionary tale of us. *Clinics in Colon and Rectal Surgery, 37*, 125, 126. https://www.semanticscholar.org/paper/b1d0e79d6ed931178011e1f7b8b8a6ba865bfa6d (accessed on 7 May 2025).
2. Abe, A., Adams, P., Ahmed, S., Ajariyakhajorn, R., Albrecht, M., Allen, D., Apetrei, C., et al. (2008). Macaque models of human infectious disease. *ILAR Journal, 49*(2), 220–255. https://doi.org/10.1093/ilar.49.2.220.
3. Madhavi Y (2005) Vaccine Policy in India. PLoS Med 2(5): e127. https://doi.org/10.1371/journal.pmed.0020127Biguioh, R. M., Mayaka, B., Georges, M., Miglietta, A., Pezzotti, P., et al. (2015). Vaccine coverage and determinants of incomplete vaccination in children aged 12-23 months in Dschang, West Region, Cameroon: A cross-sectional survey during a polio outbreak. *BMC Public Health, 15*, 630. https://core.ac.uk/download/54520749.pdf (accessed on 7 May 2025).
4. Bloch, E. M., Shoham, S., Casadevall, A., Sachais, B. S., Shaz, B. H., Winters, J. L., van Buskirk, C., et al. (2020). Deployment of convalescent plasma for the prevention and treatment of COVID-19. *Journal of Clinical Investigation, 130*, 2757–2765. https://doi.org/10.1172/jci138745.
5. Breman, J. G., de Quadros, C. A., Dowdle, W. R., Foege, W. H., et al. (2011). The role of research in viral disease eradication and elimination programs: Lessons for malaria eradication. *PLOS Medicine, 8*(1), e1000405. https://core.ac.uk/download/12211911.pdf (accessed on 7 May 2025).
6. Chen, C. (2024). Effects of misinformation and disinformation on vaccine hesitancy and routine vaccine uptake. *Master's Projects and Capstones*, 1773. https://core.ac.uk/download/619706192.pdf (accessed on 7 May 2025).
7. Cohen, A. F., van Gerven, J., García Burgos, J., de Boer, A., Foucher, R. A. M., Flore, H., Teitelbaum, Z., et al. (2020). COVID-19 vaccines: The importance of transparency and fact-based education. *British Journal of Clinical Pharmacology, 86*, 2107–2110. https://doi.org/10.1111/bcp.14581.
8. Coughlin, M. M., Beck, A. S., Bankamp, B., & Rota, P. A. (2017). Perspective on global measles epidemiology and control and the role of novel vaccination strategies. *Viruses, 9*(11). https://doi.org/10.3390/v9010011.
9. Declich, S., Del Manso, M., Dente, M. G., Giambi, F., et al. (2017). Immunization strategies targeting newly arrived migrants in non-EU countries of the Mediterranean basin and Black Sea. *International Journal of Environmental Research and Public Health, 14*, 459. https://core.ac.uk/download/98348059.pdf (accessed on 7 May 2025).
10. Dhalaria, P., Kumar, P., Kapur, S., Singh, A., Verma, A., Agarwal, D., Tripathi, B., et al. (2025). Path to full immunization coverage, role of each vaccine and their importance in the immunization programmed: A cross-sectional analytical study of India. *BMJ Public Health, 3, e001290.* https://www.semanticscholar.org/paper/7289b9c319cabd131429764c638a1f7927aab59d (accessed on 7 May 2025).
11. Dhochak, N., Singhal, T., Kabra, S. K., & Lodha, R. (2020). Pathophysiology of COVID-19: Why children fare better than adults? *The Indian Journal of Pediatrics, 87*, 537–546. https://doi.org/10.1007/s12098-020-03322-y.

12. Galles, N. C., Liu, P. Y., Updike, R. L., Fullman, N., Nguyen, J., Rolfe, S., Sbarra, A. N., et al. (2021). Measuring routine childhood vaccination coverage in 204 countries and territories, 1980–2019: A systematic analysis for the Global Burden of Disease Study 2020, Release 1. *The Lancet, 398*, 503–521. https://doi.org/10.1016/s0140-6736(21)00984-3.

13. Geoghegan, S., O'Callaghan, K., & Offit, P. A. (2020). Vaccine safety: Myths and misinformation. *Frontiers in Microbiology, 11*. https://doi.org/10.3389/fmicb.2020.00372.

14. Hinman, A., Tischer, A., Bruce, A. R., Jegede, A. S., Rimoin, A. W., Rubin, B. A., Daneshvar, C., et al. (2011). The role of research in viral disease eradication and elimination programs: Lessons for malaria eradication. *PLOS Medicine, 8*(1), e1000405. https://doi.org/10.1371/journal.pmed.1000405.

15. Ioannides, S. J., Beard, F., Larter, N., Clark, K., Wang, H., Hendry, A., Hull, B., et al. (2019). Vaccine preventable diseases and vaccination coverage in Aboriginal and Torres Strait Islander people, Australia, 2011–2015. *Communicable Diseases Intelligence, 43*. https://doi.org/10.33321/cdi.2019.43.36.

16. Islam, M. S., Kamal, A. M., Kabir, A., Southern, D. L., Khan, S. H., Hasan, S. M. M., Sarkar, T., et al. (2021). COVID-19 vaccine rumors and conspiracy theories: The need for cognitive inoculation against misinformation to improve vaccine adherence. *PLoS ONE, 16*, e0251605. https://doi.org/10.1371/journal.pone.0251605.

17. Jeyanathan, M., Afkhami, S., Smaill, F., Miller, M. S., Lichty, B. D., & Xing, Z. (2020). Immunological considerations for COVID-19 vaccine strategies. *Nature Reviews Immunology, 20*, 615–632. https://doi.org/10.1038/s41577-020-00434-6.

18. Khan, Y. H., Mallhi, T. H., Alotaibi, N. H., Alzarea, A. I., Alanazi, A. S., Tanveer, N., & Hashmi, F. K. (2020). Threat of COVID-19 vaccine hesitancy in Pakistan: The need for measures to neutralize misleading narratives. *American Journal of Tropical Medicine and Hygiene, 103*, 603, 604. https://doi.org/10.4269/ajtmh.20-0654.

19. Khetrapal, S., & Bhatia, R. (2020). Impact of COVID-19 pandemic on health system & sustainable development goal 3. *The Indian Journal of Medical Research, 151*, 395–399. https://doi.org/10.4103/ijmr.ijmr_1920_20.

20. Khudhair, A. (2020). Herd immunity or community immunity. *Scholarly Journal of Medical Case Reports, 8*(4), 508–509. https://www.semanticscholar.org/paper/f45c8427a96aa372f73c30a1bb0564603d1955e0 (accessed on 7 May 2025).

21. Kyriakidis, N. C., López-Cortés, A., Vásconez, E., Barreto, A., & Ortiz-Prado, E. (2021). SARS-CoV-2 vaccine strategies: A comprehensive review of phase 3 candidates. *npj Vaccines, 6*. https://doi.org/10.1038/s41541-021-00292-w.

22. Lassi, Z. S., Naseem, R., Salam, R. A., Siddiqui, F., & Das, J. K. (2021). The impact of the COVID-19 pandemic on immunization campaigns and programs: A systematic review. *International Journal of Environmental Research and Public Health, 18*, 988. https://doi.org/10.3390/ijerph18030988.

23. Machado, M. A. V., Roberts, B., Wong, B. L. H., van Kessel, R., & Mossialos, E. (2021). The relationship between the COVID-19 pandemic and vaccine hesitancy: A scoping review of literature until August 2021. *Frontiers in Public Health, 9*. https://doi.org/10.3389/fpubh.2021.747787.

24. Malande, O. O., Munube, D., Afaayo, R. N., Kisakye, A., Bodo, B., Bakainaga, A., Ayebare, E., et al. (2019). Barriers to effective uptake and provision of immunization in a rural district in Uganda. *PLoS ONE, 14*, e0212270. https://doi.org/10.1371/journal.pone.0212270.

25. McQuaid, F., Mulholland, R., Sangpang, Y., Agrawal, U., Bedford, H., Cameron, J. C., Gibbons, C., et al. (2022). Uptake of infant and preschool immunizations in Scotland and England during the COVID-19 pandemic: An observational study of routinely collected data. *PLoS Medicine, 19*, e1003916. https://doi.org/10.1371/journal.pmed.1003916.

26. Mohan, A., Temitope, R. A., Çavdaroğlu, S., Hasan, M. M., Costa, A. C. S., Ahmad, S., & Essar, M. Y. (2021). Measles returns to the Democratic Republic of Congo: A new predicament amid the COVID-19 crisis. *Journal of Medical Virology, 93*, 5691–5693. https://doi.org/10.1002/jmv.27137.

27. Nachega, J. B., Sam-Agudu, N. A., Masekela, R., van der Zalm, M. M., Nsanzimana, S., Condo, J., Ntoumi, F., et al. (2021). Addressing challenges to rolling out COVID-19 vaccines in African countries. *The Lancet Global Health, 9*, e746–e748. https://doi.org/10.1016/s2214-109x(21)00097-8.

28. Narayanan, D., Kayarohanam, S., Fuloria, S., Fuloria, N. K., Janakiraman, A., Djearamane, S., Wu, Y. S., et al. (2021). COVID-19 vaccine candidates under clinical evaluation – A review. *International Journal of Pharmaceutical Research, 17*(2). https://www.semanticscholar.org/paper/9e1b3e0941fee2d0ed733db05a1d50352af6c5b2 (accessed on 7 May 2025).

29. Peterson, M., Akearok, G. H., Cueva, K., Lavoie, J., Larsen, C. V., Jóhannsdóttir, L., Cook, D., et al. (2023). Public health restrictions, directives, and measures in Arctic countries in the first year of the COVID-19 pandemic. *International Journal of Circumpolar Health, 82*. https://www.semanticscholar.org/paper/da1216b21e66ad958323b0ed0b13515006ab0a74 (accessed on 7 May 2025).

30. Plotkin, S. A., & Levy, O. (2021). Considering mandatory vaccination of children for COVID-19. *Pediatrics, 147*. https://doi.org/10.1542/peds.2021-050531.

31. Rahmi, N., Fajri, A., Anggitamaya, A., Ekasasmita, W., Kusnaeni, K., Husain, H., & Nisardi, M. R. (2025). Mathematical analysis of polio prevention through vaccination and sanitation: Incorporating incomplete vaccination and virus carrier vectors. *ITM Web of Conferences*. https://www.semanticscholar.org/paper/8c987f3b37420332ae2107bf2c027d619378c2c8 (accessed on 7 May 2025).

32. Sallam, M., Salim, N. A., Al-Tammemi, A. B., Barakat, M., Fayyad, D., Hallit, S., Harapan, H., et al. (2023). ChatGPT output regarding compulsory vaccination and COVID-19 vaccine conspiracy: A descriptive study at the outset of a paradigm shift in online search for information. *Cureus, 15(2), e35029*. https://doi.org/10.7759/cureus.35029.

33. Sato, A. P. S. (2018). What is the importance of vaccine hesitancy in the drop of vaccination coverage in Brazil? *Revista de Saúde Pública, 52*, 96. https://doi.org/10.11606/s1518-8787.2018052001199.

34. Smatti, M., Yassine, H. M., Mbarek, H., & Boomsma, D. (2025). Understanding heritable variation among hosts in infectious diseases through the lens of twin studies. *Genes, 16*, 177. https://www.semanticscholar.org/paper/59e1d31f9dd65b41671a06a79c200db0e34e4656 (accessed on 7 May 2025).

35. Soares dos Santos, P. G., & Cury, E. R. J. (2024). Analyses of measles in Brazil in a 20-year time series: Vaccination coverage and the number of cases in children under five years old. *Concilium*. https://www.semanticscholar.org/paper/8d9507397c62651bb60380f2099f44b67fb38845 (accessed on 7 May 2025).

36. Stein, R. E. (2023). Epidemics and echo chambers: What the pandemic teaches us about beliefs, behaviors, and community. *The Journal of Plain Anabaptist Communities, 3*(2), 90–104. https://core.ac.uk/download/567892828.pdf (accessed on 7 May 2025).

37. Telenti, A., Arvin, A. M., Corey, L., Corti, D., Diamond, M., García-Sastre, A., Garry, R. F., et al. (2021). After the pandemic: Perspectives on the future trajectory of COVID-19. *Nature, 596*, 495–504. https://doi.org/10.1038/s41586-021-03792-w.

38. Trovato, M., Sartorius, R., D'Apice, L., Manco, R., & De Berardinis, P. (2020). Viral emerging diseases: Challenges in developing vaccination strategies. *Frontiers in Immunology, 11*. https://doi.org/10.3389/fimmu.2020.02130.

39. Uwishema, O., Lubanga, A. F., Torbati, T., & Onyeaka, H. (2021). Measles crisis in Africa amidst the COVID-19 pandemic: Delayed measles vaccine administration may cause a measles outbreak in Africa. *Journal of Medical Virology, 93*, 5697–5699. https://doi.org/10.1002/jmv.27150.

40. Viswanath, K., Bekalu, M. A., Dhawan, D., Pinnamaneni, R., Lang, J., & McLoud, R. (2021). Individual and social determinants of COVID-19 vaccine uptake. *BMC Public Health, 21*. https://doi.org/10.1186/s12889-021-10862-1.

41. Walewska, R., Parry-Jones, N., Eyre, T. A., Follows, G., Martínez-Calle, N., McCarthy, H. O., Parry, H., et al. (2022). Guideline for the treatment of chronic lymphocytic leukemia. *British Journal of Hematology, 197*, 544–557. https://doi.org/10.1111/bjh.18075.

42. Barder, Owen Matthew and Yeh, Ethan, The Costs and Benefits of Front-Loading and Predictability of Immunization (February 2006). Center for Global Development Working Paper No. 80, Available at SSRN: https://ssrn.com/abstract=984043 or http://dx.doi.org/10.2139/ssrn.984043 (accessed on 7 May 2025).

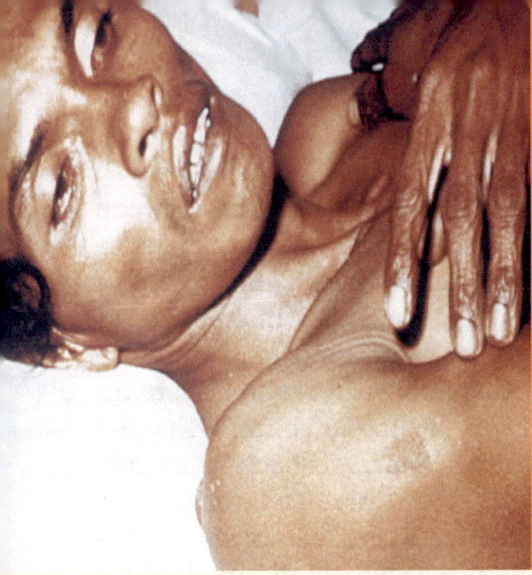

Chapter 15

CHOLERA AND TYPHOID

Contents

Introduction

Across much of the globe, infectious disease remains a significant challenge to public health, particularly in areas where clean water and adequate sanitation are scarce. Typhoid and cholera, for instance, all too frequently reach their most severe effects in poorer areas, producing high rates of disease and death. These conditions infiltrate communities by exploiting poor environmental controls and economic disparities. Humans can observe how these bacteria are transmitted—and how they function within the body—and truly that emphasizes the importance of knowing their microbial uniqueness as well as their movement through society. Because of this, health care systems everywhere are struggling with outbreaks, which in the majority of situations motivates constant research and encourages practical action like improved sanitation, vaccinations, and more open public information. Taking a closer look, the two diseases originate from gram-negative bacteria. Cholera is caused by *Vibrio cholerae* whereas typhoid fever is associated with *Salmonella enterica* serovar Typhi. Both commonly find their way into humans via contaminated water and food—a common route that binds them to common problems such as agricultural practices, handling food, and hygiene of water. In an interesting twist, *Salmonella enterica*, particularly the Typhi subspecies, appears to be quite comfortable in humans, occasionally leading to full-fledged systemic infections (Jajere, 2019). To make matters worse, these microorganisms have the ability to survive in their environment and tend to evade our defenses, owing in part to characteristics such as capsules, flagella, or secretion systems. Knowledge of these bacterial features is rather important if we are to reduce infection risks and manage outbreaks better. Antibiotic resistance further complicates the scenario, especially in low- and middle-income regions where extreme farming methods and incorrect antibiotic administration are the norm (Christy et al., 2018). In these regions, bacteria engage with residual antibiotic by-products present in animal tissue and the environment, allowing them to develop strains that can easily bypass conventional treatments. Resistance not only reduces our therapeutic choices but also frequently results in longer disease episodes and more serious complications. This fact, by and large, emphasizes the need for good-planned antibiotic stewardship, enhanced surveillance, and sound international collaboration. In the end, overcoming these challenges is about merging public health policies with actions from agriculture, clinical practice, and environmental management to reduce the burden of cholera and typhoid globally (Figure 15.1).

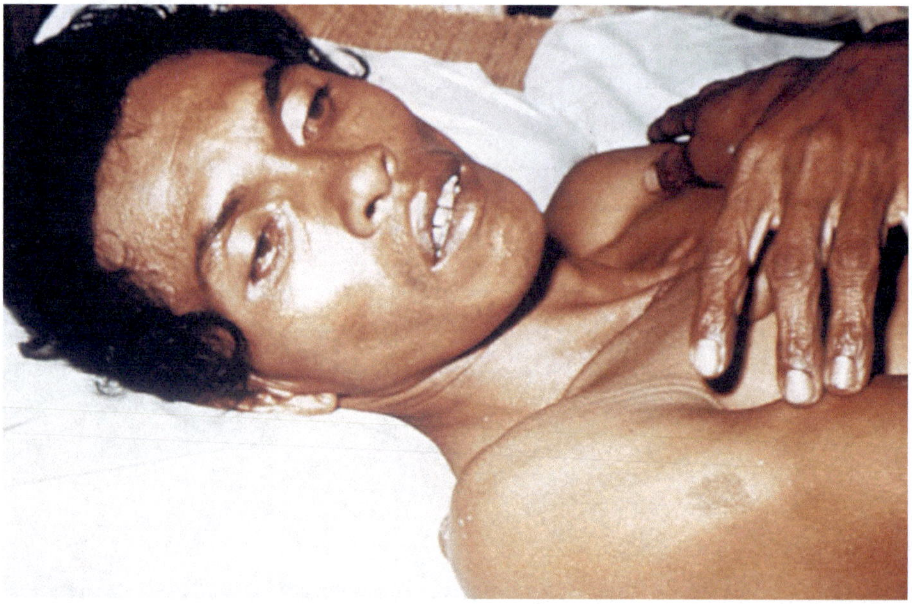

Figure 15.1. Cholera, typhoid, fever, and dysentery.

Source: By CDC - This media comes from the Centers for Disease Control and Prevention's Public Health Image Library (PHIL), with identification number #1939. Public Domain, https://commons.wikimedia.org/w/index.php?curid=4270622***Definition of Cholera***

Cholera takes effect when a person eats or drinks something that's contaminated with the *Vibrio cholerae* pathogen. At first, it may begin as a slight stomachache, only to suddenly become a potentially deadly episode of dehydration due to rapid fluid loss. More often than not, this occurs in regions where it's difficult to get hold of clean water and sanitation practices fall short—

situations aggravated by lax waste disposal. In most developing countries, for example, large landfills and open dumps release pollutants into groundwater, forming pockets in which bacteria such as *Vibrio cholerae* could proliferate. This type of pollution increases the likelihood of outbreaks among already vulnerable people, illustrating how closely environmental health is linked to disease transmission. Overall, if we consider cholera's spread, it is apparent that human activity by tampering with water quality has a significant role to play, and hence improved waste management is so important (Siddiqua et al., 2022). *Vibrio cholerae*—the same bacteria that causes cholera—lodges in the small intestine before discharging a severe toxin that interferes with regular absorption and secretion, resulting in copious watery diarrhea. Its dehydration effect can worsen very rapidly, at times, catastrophically, taking lives in hours if not immediately treated. Cholera remains an enormous challenge where there is a lack of proper sanitation. Although cholera and typhoid (the second caused by *Salmonella enterica* serovar Typhi) have the same water avenues, they unfold differently; typhoid tends to spread through a systemic infection while cholera attacks the gastrointestinal tract with explosive force. For the most part, typhoid vaccine development, particularly with those newer conjugate preparations (Jin et al., 2017), is showing progress, but the battle against cholera truly hinges on timely rehydration therapy and measures to improve water quality and sanitation. It is not merely about symptoms with cholera—it's also about the mix of epidemiologic and environmental considerations in operation. The disease is often a symptom of the wider problems that affect developing nations when their infrastructure can no longer support health demands. For instance, overflowing dumpsites and uncontrolled landfills become unwitting conduits for contamination, allowing cholera to spread more readily (Siddiqua et al., 2022). Unlike typhoid, where new vaccine strategies are being developed (Jin et al., 2017), keeping cholera at bay involves more than therapeutic medication; it requires daily modifications such as safe water, improved sanitation, and enhanced hygiene behavior. In short, cholera is a multifaceted disease that entails microbial, clinical, and socio-environmental factors, far too interrelated with the difficulties of poverty and underdevelopment.

Definition of Typhoid

Infectious diseases tend to guide the way communities respond to epidemics—typhoid fever, say, is a classic example. Brought on by *Salmonella enterica* serotype Typhi, this bacterial disease doesn't act like your run-of-the-mill airborne virus; rather, it spreads primarily through the fecal-oral route, typically slipping in on infected food or water. The microbe crawls into the intestinal lining, triggering a full-body response marked by long-lasting fever, abdominal discomfort, and a general sense of being under the weather. Its spread is tightly linked to how well a community manages sanitation and hygiene—something that, in resource-poor settings, leaves many facing ongoing challenges. For all but the most severe cases, having a clear understanding of typhoid's bacterial origins and transmission route is still central, particularly when set against other waterborne diseases such as cholera (Bell & Lewis, 2025). Typhoid usually takes one to two weeks to reveal its symptoms, and it is this delay that can really confuse preliminary diagnosis and the struggle to keep it at bay. Individuals commonly experience refractory high fevers, ongoing headaches, and generalized weakness, sometimes developing a distinctive rash referred to as rose spots in the process. If antibiotics are not given promptly, there is a risk of complications such as bleeding or perforation of the intestine, acutely doubling the risks of grave disease or death. Further there's the issue of chronic carriers, some individuals end up having *Salmonella typhi* without any visible symptoms but yet keep shedding it into their environment. This asymptomatic transmission makes it difficult to snap the cycle of transmission in communities, highlighting the importance of ongoing surveillance and enhanced cleanliness practices. All these combined make typhoid distinct from other gut infections recognized to be responsible for diarrheal disease (Arnold et al., 2019). Vigilant observations and seroepidemiologic surveys do shed light on how typhoid succeeds in surviving, particularly in low-resource settings.

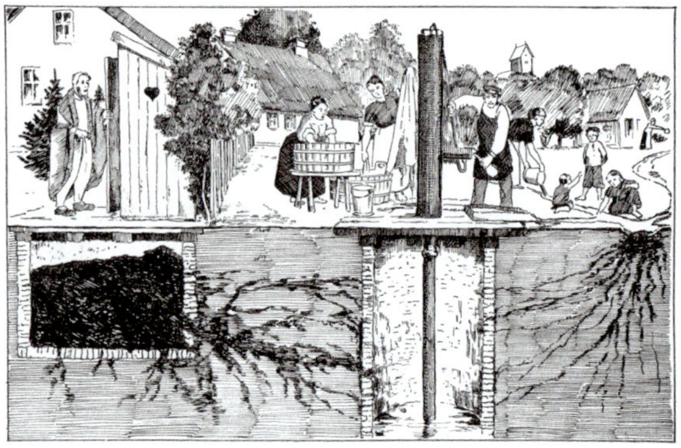

Figure 15.2. Typhoid fever.

Source: By Anonymous - Vore Sygdome; Bind II, side 116, Public Domain, https://commons.wikimedia.org/w/index.php?curid=1954765

As with other enteric microbes monitored across the globe, early introduction to typhoid tends to mirror local conditions and the quality of the public health infrastructure in the area. Long-term antibody studies tend to imply that recurrent exposures or reinfections are usual, which itself requires sustained public health initiatives, from immunization campaigns to improved water sanitation and day-to-day hygiene practices. Comparative studies even suggest that although typhoid does share some features of transmission with pathogens such as cholera, every pathogen has its idiosyncracies that require control strategies tailored especially to suit it. All these observations collectively show how rapidly transmission risks can snowball and why continuous typhoid presence is so elusive a problem for international health (Arnold et al., 2019) (Figure 15.2).

Importance of Studying These Diseases

Understanding how infections work is of monumental significance to public health, when we understand their dynamics, it is possible to create interventions that save lives and mitigate outbreaks. Ills like cholera and typhoid, which target areas where the sanitation level is not great, are excellent examples; studying them close up teaches us something about how diseases like these are transmitted, what danger is involved, and what will work best, whether that is improved vaccines or more efficient cleanup procedures. From the perspective of trends in outbreaks, it is revealed that even how we structure studies and run the numbers receives an improvement, pushing contemporary epidemiology outside its historical boundaries (Lewnard & Reingold, 2019). These enhancements, in the majority of instances, not only intensify our scientific understanding but also improve the capability to respond, ultimately reducing disease and death in the most vulnerable populations. Beyond short-term health benefits, learning about diseases such as cholera and typhoid is also essential to addressing more difficult socioeconomic issues. Throughout history, these diseases imposed a tight burden on healthcare systems in developing parts of the world—they reduced productivity and had the potential to ensnare communities in poverty through large medical expenses and lost work days. Mathematical and computational models enter the picture here, providing powerful tools to simulate the mode of spread of such infections and test various strategies of control. In countries such as Africa, where typhoid and related disease heavily hinder economic development, such models have been found to assist in designing interventions that combine many types of control to achieve the maximum overall impact (Adewumi et al., 2016). So, while this study fuels our medical information, it also contributes significantly towards supporting socioeconomic development and sustainable growth. Additionally, exploring cholera and typhoid advances the take-up of new technologies and varied data into systems utilized for tracking and responding to public health issues. New advancements in molecular diagnostics and digital epidemiology have transformed our ability to detect pathogens and follow outbreaks—often resulting in earlier interventions and a better understanding of how these incidents impact the environment. Work in these fields has even fueled innovation in techniques such as causal inference, vaccine development, and research into human microbiota. all of which contribute to improved treatment and preventive measures (Lewnard & Reingold, 2019). With ongoing shifts in threats from infectious diseases, this work equips both policymakers and health professionals with the flexible tools they require to act judiciously. Effectively, plunging into the research of cholera and typhoid ends up building strong framework structures that are capable of addressing not just renowned diseases but also upcoming challenges across the globe.

15.1. Historical Background

Infectious diseases such as typhoid and cholera have not remained constant over the years. In the 1800s, cholera outbreaks in certain regions of Asia and Europe struck communities severely, leading to the necessity of determining what was responsible for the disease and how it was transmitted. John Snow's work in London's 1854 epidemic ,where he plotted cases and attributed them to unclean water sources—set forth some initial concepts now referred to as epidemiology, and it prompted officials to reconsider sanitation. Meanwhile, typhoid fever was slowly rising as a cause for concern, particularly in crowded urban areas without proper sewage and clean water infrastructure. That century-long battle to contain these diseases illustrates how much our environment and simple public arrangements count; it even laid the foundation for contemporary solutions such as water purification, vaccination, and antibiotics. In general, these occurrences demonstrate that scientific advances and public health measures have always been twirling together, if not always in step. *Salmonella enterica* – the bacterium responsible for typhoid fever and other close cousins – has its own twist with a history as intricate as it is multifarious serovars. There are more than 2,600 identified types, some of which cling to a single host and some of which roam through several species; such diversity seriously complicates control efforts. It's fascinating, , how Salmonella evades the body's immune system with tools such as flagella, capsules, and so-called type 3 secretion systems on pathogenicity islands. It's these kinds of tricks that enable it to evolve and persist, which ultimately made typhoid fever a chronic issue in regions with poor sanitation. Despite improved hygiene overall, many of these strains of Salmonella continue to exist in food animals, and in recent times even multidrug-resistant types are cropping up (Jajere, 2019). All this serves to illustrate that combining microbiological understanding with public health measures remains crucial. The tracking of diseases such as cholera and typhoid has contributed immensely to putting together their history and making future plans. In the United States, for instance, creating national notifiable disease systems was a significant step toward monitoring outbreaks and responding more systematically. Aggregated information in annual reports provides us with a chaotic but useful glimpse at trends, patterns of outbreaks, and how control measures work over time. Consider the 2015 Summary of Notifiable Infectious Diseases—it brings together decades' worth of experience that have informed policies regarding vaccines, sanitation initiatives, and the use of antibiotics. Furthermore, these integrated systems, with all their peculiarities and small imbalances, demonstrate how indispensable historical information is in attempting to predict and control future cholera, typhoid, and other foodborne health problems (Deborah et al., 2017) (Figure 15.3).

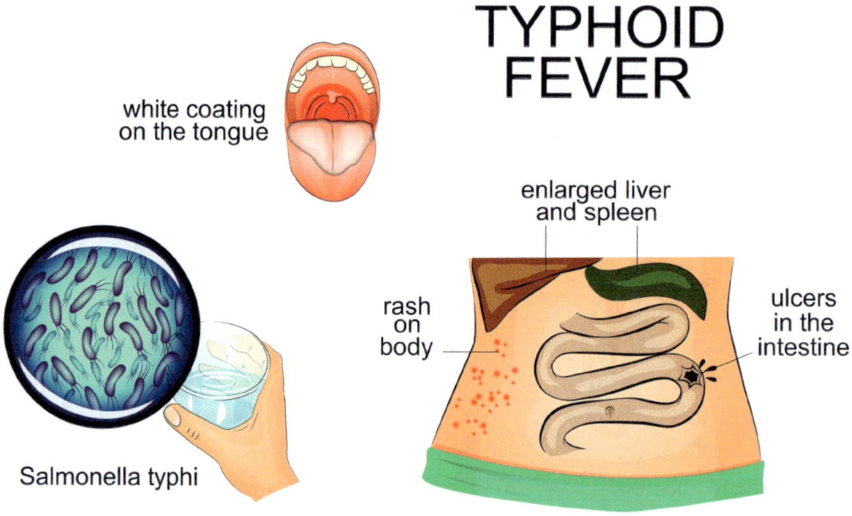

Figure 15.3. Infectious diseases like typhoid.

Source: GIDEON. (n.d.). *Typhoid Fever Illustration.*

15.1.1. Origin of Cholera

Cholera's initial history begins in India's dirty, populous Ganges Delta, where contaminated water and maintenance were day-to-day pests. City expansion and a rapid escalation in international trade shuffled things together that aided its dispersal. Close-set human habitation and inconsistent sanitation were conduits down which *Vibrio cholerae* had little difficulty moving, as expanding colonial shipping lines and military expeditions pressed it further beyond its origins. This germ, strangely enough, does well in all types of wet hideouts—even if the weather turns unexpected—so it stuck around big time. In a way, the overlap of human activity and environmental mishaps spun the perfect yarn for cholera, as with other waterborne pests, and emphasized the need for sweeping public health remedies (Bintsis, 2017). Digging deeper, cholera's origins extend beyond mere bacteria; they suggest larger changes in the way societies and governments operated during colonial periods. Colonial powers tended to be more concerned with wringing profit from areas than with getting the fundamentals of sanitation right, leaving locals exposed to rampant disease. Most scholars now contend that those early administrative decisions still resonate through our contemporary health systems. Nevertheless, some commentators point out that incomplete portions of colonial health records can distort our vision of how significant a role the disease played (Acemo Dğlu et al., 2012). This complex past illustrates the way in which old-fashioned public arrangements created lasting vulnerabilities in our battle against infections. At its very core, cholera speaks of an uncomfortable dance between nature and man. *Vibrio cholerae*, the microbe at the center of it all, prefers to make itself at home in water that is contaminated with human feces—a scenario made worse by hygiene habits. Without rigorous food safety and clean water regulations, the bacteria can truly make themselves at home in these contaminated areas. Today, professionals have moved away from just checking off risks to adopting a sophisticated, risk-based approach towards food and water safety (Bintsis, 2017). Overall, cholera's origins remind us that merging improved environmental stewardship, education, and improved infrastructure is the secret to pre-empting outbreaks in developing as well as more advanced corners of the world.

15.1.2. Origin of Typhoid

Urban sprawl with no modern solutions for water and waste provided the ideal breeding ground for typhoid fever. In much of the world, particularly densely populated developing areas—water supplies became contaminated with human waste. *Salmonella typhi*, the bacterium that causes typhoid, was able to persist in areas where clean water was virtually impossible to obtain. Consider densely populated cities with outmoded septic tanks or dodgy piped water; typhoid here spread just like its water-related relatives, cholera. Without the adequate updates and maintenance of our water, sanitation, and hygiene (WASH) infrastructure, the microbe just keeps returning (Howard et al., 2020). Retrospectively, it is clear that typhoid's origins are very much connected with hasty industrial transformation and increasing populations. For the most part, as cities expanded in the 19th and early 20th centuries, gradual improvement at clearing up the urban chaos permitted typhoid to persist—frequently in individuals who didn't even know they had it. In contrast with cholera's spectacular epidemics, typhoid smoldered along, rendering it more difficult to detect and contain. That low-grade burning compelled societies not only to reconsider sewage control but also to seek means of detecting stealthy carriers and creating vaccines. It was a delicate situation, particularly in places where healthcare and sanitation were already in tatters (Howard et al., 2020). The challenge becomes even more complicated when antibiotic resistance is involved. A few years ago, ordinary antibiotics would easily take care of typhoid, but with the current development, drug-resistant strains have cropped up. In the majority of instances, these microbes have evolved with an assortment of strategies, such as efflux pumps or enzymatic drug breakdown—rendering treatment much less certain. This resistance, in a sense, heightens typhoid's impact on public health while challenging us to combine improved hygiene and water measures with new, innovative treatments. Overall, typhoid's battle is not only about damaged pipes and sanitation but also part of a constant, never-ending fight where bacteria resist the drugs intended to halt them (Figure 15.4).

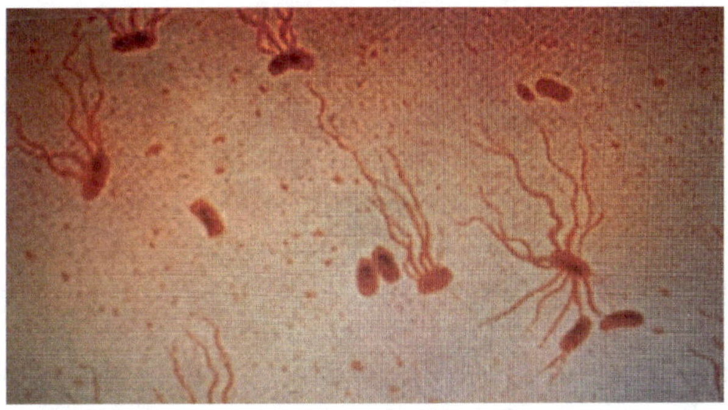

Figure 15.4. Origin of typhoid.

Source: By Microbewriter - Own work, CC BY-SA 4.0, https://commons.wikimedia.org/w/index.php?curid=106822321

15.1.3. Major Outbreaks and Their Impact

Large outbreaks disrupt communities in ways that extend far beyond simply getting people ill. In most places, diseases such as cholera and typhoid turn daily life upside down, filling hospitals and diverting resources from other pressing needs. Cholera, for instance, tends to strike large cities where water and sewage infrastructure is not strong, this subpar arrangement causes cycles of contamination and repeated reinfection. Health care services, which are already thin, barely manage to keep up with urgent care, let alone with the preventive work that is essential to shield individuals from disease in the long term. And there is also the social aspect: fear and stigma around infectious diseases drive people further apart, excluding them from basic services and further deepening social fissures. If you look at it, the spillover effects of these epidemics combination environmental concerns, social dynamics, and system failures that all need attention simultaneously. Environmental and infrastructure issues contribute significantly to how frequently and intensely cholera and typhoid hit, particularly in places where adequate sanitation and medical facilities are not available. Consider urban centers such as Lusaka in Zambia—poor drainage and waste disposal provide the ideal environment for *Vibrio cholerae* to multiply in unsanitary water. In most instances, combat against cholera here involves improving water quality and sanitation, as well as spreading the message with public health education. Typhoid fever also has much the same struggle in areas where clean water and proper hygienic practices simply do not exist. These persistent problems remind us that sustainable development, emphasizing infrastructure improvements at the grassroots level and public education on hygiene, is essential. Zambia's own initiative to eradicate cholera by 2025 demonstrates what a national effort can achieve, however, its success depends on maintaining political will and funding even after deadlines are missed (Siamalube & Ehinmitan, 2024). More generally, the sustained outbreaks throughout Sub-Saharan Africa truly underscore the importance of improved disease surveillance and more robust healthcare systems. Poor surveillance allows issues to become apparent too late, allowing outbreaks to get out of hand and even spread across borders. Economic disparities, poor health literacy, and some cultural practices can also make it difficult for communities to adopt intervention strategies. Overall, managing these emergencies requires a combination of strategies—enhancing laboratory networks, establishing local reporting mechanisms, and coordinating together within governments, international organizations, and local organizations. And boosting local vaccine and medicine manufacturing can reduce our bulk dependence on foreign supplies in emergencies. Efforts to increase public awareness and additional investment in training health workers also strengthen a more robust response, even if the process isn't always so neatly smooth. In short, only an all-encompassing, sometimes complex—, eventually human, approach will reduce sickness, save lives, curb economic impacts of these outbreaks, and safeguard public health in the long term (Hassan et al., 2024).

15.2. Causes and Transmission

In most locations, environmental conditions and disease epidemics appear to become intertwined in one way or another - consider how water problems lay the groundwork for such diseases as cholera and typhoid. These two, for the most part transmitted by water, habitually erupt in areas with poor sanitation and safe drinking water scarce. Polluted water, for example, becomes something of a reservoir for such pathogens as *Vibrio cholerae* and *Salmonella typhi*, which are propagated along the fecal-oral route. Societies that have access to polluted water caused by sewage or runoff waste are faced with much more hazards, and such conditions as overcrowding, sanitation, and inadequate infrastructure only exacerbate the situation. In the majority of instances, particularly in developing regions where water is scarce, the combination of environmental and social factors compels outbreaks to critical levels, i.e., physical infrastructure and personal practices must be addressed to stem waterborne disease (Heaviside et al., 2018). Examining further how these diseases truly occur, it's evident that contaminated food and water are the leading actors. Cholera, on the other hand, is transmitted when individuals consume food or water that's been contaminated with its bacteria, which breed very fast in water-saturated environments. Typhoid fever works more or less the same way, typically spreading through food or beverage that's contaminated with traces of fecal matter from an infected person. Fecal-oral transmission is the primary channel here, with lax handwashing and food handling contributing to the risk. In some cases of asymptomatic carriers of typhoid, individuals who have a minimal or no indication of ailing, can even unintentionally sustain the cycle. In most cases, this incident highlights the importance of clean water, proper waste disposal, and food safety awareness to interrupt the cycle of infection (Heaviside et al., 2018). Taking a step back, past events and human activities have also played an integral role in altering the way these diseases spread. Urban expansion, climate-induced migration, and even conflict may disrupt water supply and sanitation, usually triggering epidemics when populations are compelled into suboptimal living conditions. Consider, for instance, during wars or forced displacements; these situations tend to collapse access to safe water as well as sound waste disposal, thus enhancing the possibility of epidemics. As our knowledge of pathogens has increased over time, public health responses have evolved, with military and scientific developments at times even contributing to efforts to contain diseases. In particular, the formation of biological warfare strategies in the 20th century serves to remind us that knowing how pathogens are distributed is important—both to avoid unintentional spread and to combat any deliberate abuse. In most cases, tackling these issues calls for several environmental management, stronger public health systems, and global efforts to keep these dangerous outbreaks at bay (Figure 15.5).

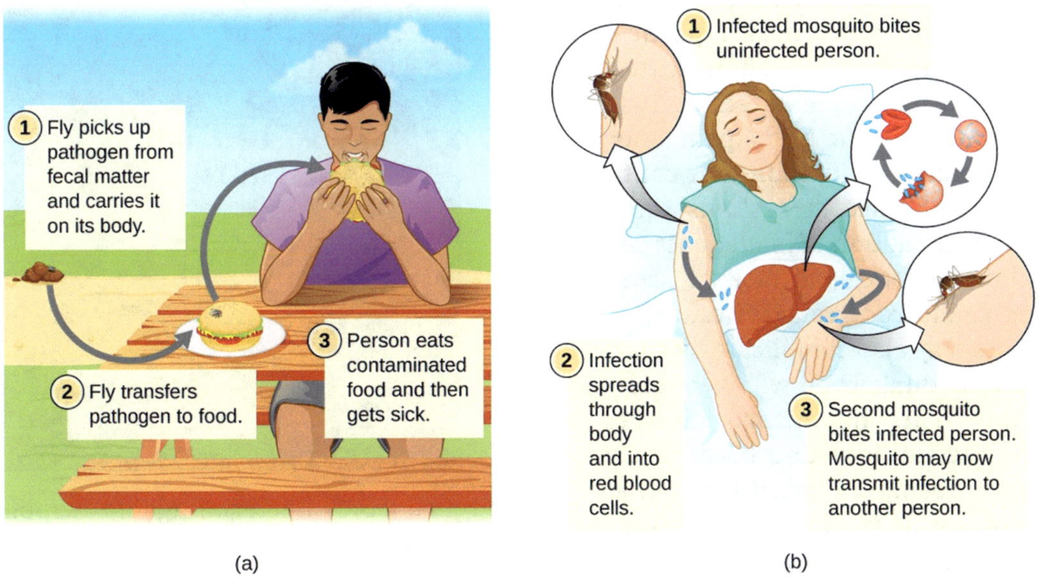

Figure 15.5. Typhoid fever causes.

Source: Philschatz. (n.d.). *Vector Transmission of Typhoid.*

15.2.1. Bacterial Agents Responsible

History indicates an complex interaction between human beings and bacteria—a kind of constant struggle influenced by constantly shifting environments and changing social behavior. Cholera and typhoid, for instance, continue to be serious threats since contaminated water serves as a public meeting ground for such pests. Consider *Vibrio cholerae*: it typically hangs around in watery places, particularly where sanitation is not what it could be, and once it gets into the small intestine, it secretes a toxin that induces massive, life-threatening diarrhea if left to its own devices. In the meantime, *Salmonella enterica* serovar Typhi gets into the lining of the gut further propagates itself around the body. The capacity of such bacteria to thrive in populations is closely linked with poor water quality and poor sanitation infrastructures. In general, knowing how such small enemies act and disseminate is central to developing improved prevention strategies within resource-constrained environments (Davison et al., 2005). Typhoid and cholera give a candid glimpse at how much waterborne bacteria can control global health, particularly in the developing world. When water for drinking or food is contaminated, both *Vibrio cholerae* and *Salmonella typhi* gain entry to produce outbreaks—a situation that continues to challenge public health systems today. In most cases, a combination of inadequate sewage disposal, poor hygiene, and lack of access to clean water is the root cause, situations that climate change may also complicate by changing the supply and quality of water, sometimes unpredictably. This haphazard mixture of environmental conditions and bacterial action guarantees that being on guard through early-detection monitoring is simply imperative. And of course, strengthening water management and sanitation methods is still a necessary step to alleviating the weight of these diseases (Heaviside et al., 2018). Examining closer how these bacteria act explains why they produce various symptoms and spread in different manners. *Vibrio cholerae*, a gram-negative, fast-moving germ, carries a potent toxin that induces massive quantities of watery diarrhea that results fairly rapidly in dehydration and electrolyte disturbances. *Salmonella typhi*, on the other hand, is more insidious, frequently infecting immune cells such as macrophages in an attempt to evade the host's defenses, resulting in a systemic febrile disease and even potentially life-threatening complications like intestinal perforation. It doesn't make matters better that some individuals can harbor these bacteria without showing any noticeable symptoms, silently driving additional transmissions. Overall, combining our knowledge of these pathogens with good public health measures, such as targeted vaccination campaigns, enhanced sanitation practices, and judicious use of antibiotics—is essential to mitigating the effects of these long-standing threats (Davison et al., 2005; Heaviside et al., 2018) (Figure 15.6).

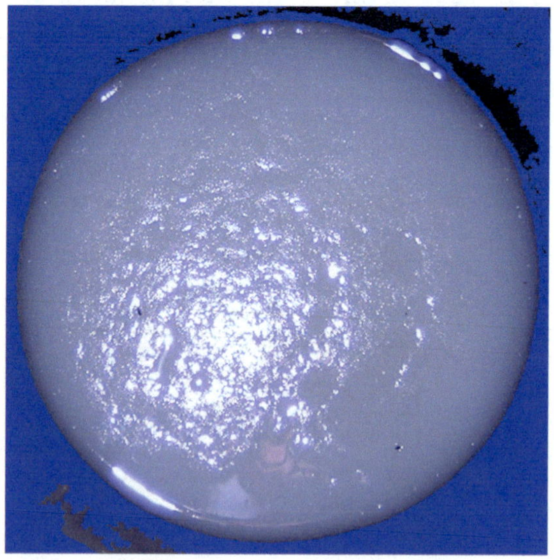

Figure 15.6. Bacterial agents responsible for cholera.

Source: By F1jmm - Own work, CC BY-SA 3.0, https://commons.wikimedia.org/w/index.php?curid=12377582

15.2.2. Modes of Transmission

Infections can spread in quite unanticipated manners—cholera and typhoid, for instance, do not have a neat, predictable scheme. Much of the time, it starts with unsanitary conditions: contaminated water finds itself playing the role of a reservoir for nasty bacteria (*Vibrio cholerae* and *Salmonella typhi*, to be exact) that infiltrate communities when humans consume it. Flies, attracted to complex and unclean spots, unwittingly pick up these pathogens and later deposit them onto food or utensils. This indirect method of transmission shows that, in crowded areas where cleanliness isn't a top priority, even seemingly minor factors can have a huge impact. It all points to the need for better water quality and stronger control over vector populations (Aditama et al., 2023). Living next to animals has the potential to trigger its own share of issues. When human housing and animal quarters are pushed tightly together—sometimes with fewer than four meters between them, the potential for germ transmission leaps alarmingly. Inadequate treatment of animal waste tends to create paths of least resistance for pathogens, impacting individuals as well as animals in regions where home and animal enclosures overlap. Poor waste management does not only end at creating short-term issues; it also contaminates soil and water, increasing the risk of infection even further. Essentially, a complex combination of environmental and economic challenges compels us to reconsider how we approach land use, sanitation, and public health (Adamu, 2019). Adding another level of complexity, both biological and environmental processes interact with each other in ways that circumvent direct human contact. For example, flies can transmit bacteria mechanically, picking them up from rot without themselves becoming infected—and depositing them on surfaces or food, causing infection when eaten. The method of transmission does this means that cleaning water alone does not suffice. Simple and low-cost interventions, such as natural repellents or bioinsecticides, like the turmeric extract that has been found to repel houseflies, provide promising solutions in resource-constrained environments. In general, these diverse mechanisms emphasize just how complicated the spread of cholera and typhoid can become, so it is important to tackle both environmental hygiene and vector control within any meaningful prevention programs (Aditama et al., 2023).

15.2.3. Environmental Factors Contributing to Spread

Cholera and typhoid tend to combine with environmental conditions in ways that are difficult to define. Water quality is important here, filthy water doesn't just happen; it winds up serving as a kind of germy hangout for bacteria like *Vibrio cholerae* and *Salmonella Typhi.* Where sanitation is inadequate and sewage disposal is poor, human excrement becomes oozing into water sources, propelling a vicious cycle that appears to drive more pollution. In most places with poor infrastructure—where open defecation and improper waste disposal prevail—water becomes a hazardous commodity very fast. At other times, natural disasters such as floods agitate the cocktail further, mixing sewage into drinking water and causing outbreaks. In many instances, upgrading such water sanitation systems is a key part of the process of ending the cycle. Food safety is also an important factor in the spread of typhoid. As *Salmonella enterica* tends to travel via food that has come from animals, even minor slip-ups in food hygiene can lead to issues that rapidly snowball, particularly when agricultural practices intensify to keep pace with our heightened demand for animal protein. As there is more antibiotic use in this type of farming, things tend to get : not just does it enhance the risk of contamination, but it also appears to facilitate the development of multiple-drug resistant strains of bacteria. The entire process from farm to fork is an important mechanism for the distribution of unwanted bacteria. Loose food safety monitoring and unsound use of antibiotics simply add to these threats (Christy et al., 2018; Jajere, 2019). terms, tighter controls on food production and the regulation of antibiotics are required to alleviate this pressure. Antibiotic resistance, driven by the environment, has proven to be another difficult challenge in the battle against both typhoid and cholera. In most developing world areas, overuse of antibiotics in medical care and agriculture—and the poor sanitation that goes along with it—seem to speed the distribution of these pesky microbes. As a case in point, animal manure can seep resistant bacteria into water and soil, and before you can say Jack Robinson, those microbes have spawned in the community and even in hospitals. This renders infections more difficult to cure, prolongs the duration that individuals endure, and can even increase the risk of mortality. Furthermore, imperfect surveillance provides an opportunity for these resistance-developing strains to proliferate in the shadows. In the majority of instances, global cooperation in addition to enhanced regulations coupled with an effort towards more responsible antibiotic use can prevent resistant cholera and typhoid-causing pathogens (Christy et al., 2018) (Figure 15.7).

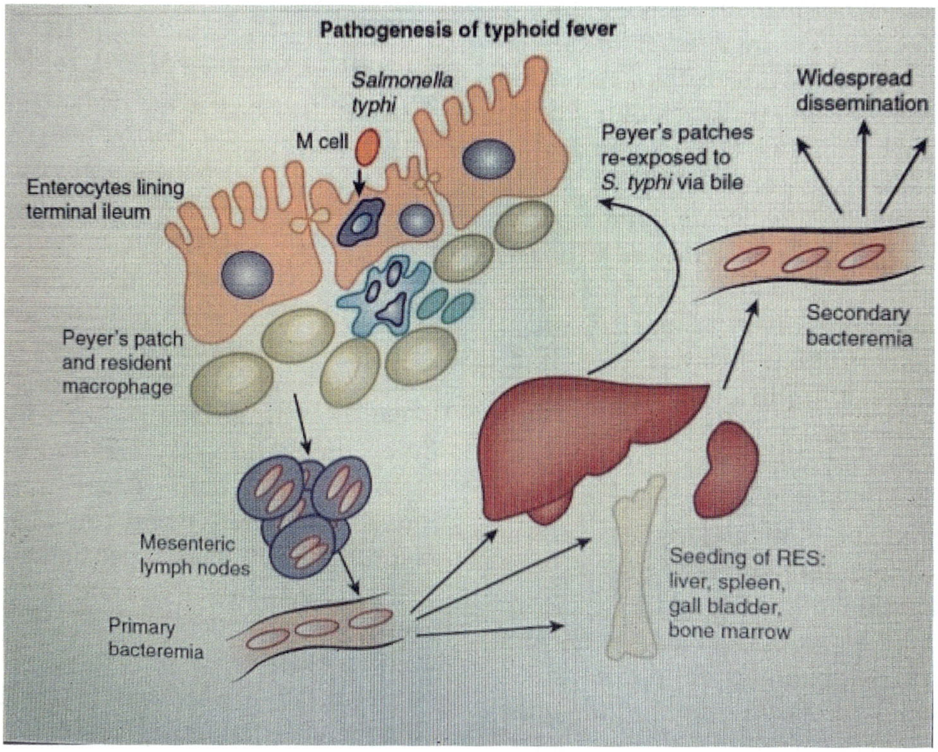

Figure 15.7. *Salmonella typhi* (typhoid fever).

Source: By Microbewriter - Own work, CC BY-SA 4.0, https://commons.wikimedia.org/w/index.php?curid=106690875

15.3. Symptoms and Diagnosis

Cholera usually strikes suddenly with a surge of watery diarrhea that people sometimes refer to as "rice-water" because it is pale and somewhat milky. In most situations the body is losing fluids so rapidly that you experience a dry mouth, sunken eyes, and skin that will not spring back, along with a morose fatigue. Vomiting and muscle spasms tend to follow along, each an indicator that the body is losing water and salt quickly. In severe cases, you may even observe hypovolemic shock and metabolic acidosis – very perilous states if not treated on time.

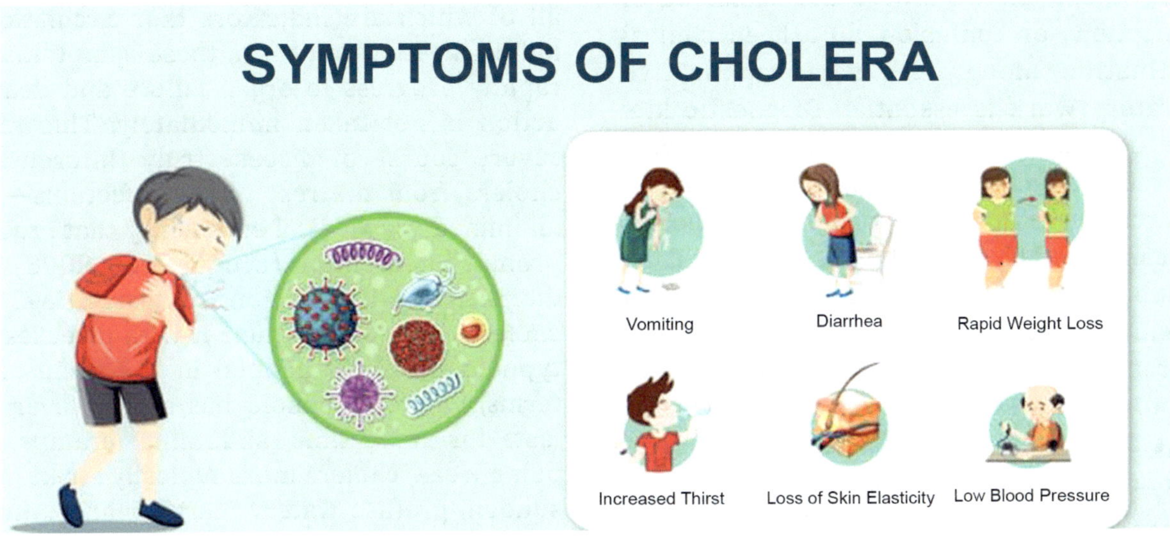

Figure 15.8. Symptoms and diagnosis of cholera.

Source: https://external-content.duckduckgo.com/iu/?u=https%3A%2F%2Fmedia.geeksforgeeks.org%2Fwp-content%2Fuploads%2F20240430124227%2FSymptoms-of-cholera-768.png&f=1&nofb=1&ipt=1690722a602712010c5fb4829c8fd5403d84ce1bcf535310774abfe63fe1f672.

GPs will usually suspect cholera in the majority of endemic circumstances or outbreak situations by simply combining the acute presentation and any recognized contact; subsequently, lab investigations such as stool culture for *Vibrio cholerae* or rapid antigen tests are used. Rapid identification is fundamental to initiate rehydration therapy, although regional limitations in lab facilities in poorer regions can essentially hamper the process (Christy et al., 2018). Typhoid fever, on the other hand, catches up with you a little more subtly. It usually begins with a persistent, high fever, a headache, and a general sense of gloom – perhaps with some abdominal pain. As the fever persists, gastrointestinal problems such as constipation or diarrhea may appear. A physical examination may indicate a heart rate slower than normal, an enlarged spleen or liver, and those characteristic "rose spots" that may show up on the trunk, although these symptoms are not always readily apparent in the early stages. Since the initial symptomatology is so nonspecific, particularly in regions where there are so many causes of fevers, physicians can have difficulty making typhoid out immediately. Lab diagnostics primarily target the isolation of *Salmonella enterica* serotype Typhi from blood, stool, or even bone marrow, and the best early warning remains blood cultures. Although tests such as the Widal are sometimes employed, they tend not to be that accurate in sensitivity and specificity. Getting the diagnosis correct as early as possible is crucial in initiating the appropriate antibiotic treatment and preventing serious complications (Christy et al., 2018). Both infections have their own set of problems when it comes to diagnosis, and their cross-over symptoms are only going to confuse the matter further. In such regions where these infections are prevalent, there's always the likelihood of co-infections or confusion, so a keen clinical examination along with some supportive laboratory work is essential. Diagnostic kits have become better for detecting *Vibrio cholerae* and *Salmonella typhi* – particularly in resource-constrained environments – although you cannot always assume that they will be available across the board. Clinicians will occasionally rely on a combination of local outbreak patterns, characteristic patterns of symptoms, and even some simple lab tests to sort out the difference. It's also necessary to continue with active surveillance and enhance laboratory facilities so outbreaks can be detected early. Overall, it is crucial to combine these diagnostic developments with robust public health measures to reduce the number of individuals who become seriously ill or die, especially among the most vulnerable groups (Christy et al., 2018) (Figure 15.8).

15.3.1. Common Symptoms of Cholera

Cholera can strike unexpectedly, giving almost no time to warn. It begins when watery stools, which are usually referred to as "rice-water" due to their white, milky appearance, suddenly appear. Individuals can also vomit, which only exacerbates the fluid loss and disrupts essential minerals in the process. Before you blink, a quick loss of fluids results in dehydration: sunken eyes, a parched mouth, and skin that simply fails to snap back like it's supposed to. Picking up on these early signs is vital, particularly where outbreaks are higher (Lockley et al., 2013). If not treated with proper rehydration, things become rapidly more serious, quickly. In most situations, the individual will begin to cramp up as the mineral balance of things such as potassium and sodium becomes crazy. The overwhelming fluid loss can even trigger shock; you may be able to detect a rapid but weak pulse, low blood pressure, and cold, moist extremities, all of which are indicators that circulation is failing. In its worst form, these symptoms can rapidly progress to organ failure and death if action is not taken immediately. This rapid, severe course of disease truly differentiates cholera from the rest of the infections—it is an immediate medical emergency that requires prompt intervention (Brown et al., 2008). Yes, diarrhea and dehydration are the red flags with cholera, but don't confuse it with diseases like typhoid that may happen in the same areas. terms, whereas typhoid has a high fever that lasts for some time, abdominal cramps, and being weak, cholera more typically strikes with sudden, profuse watery diarrhea and minimal fever. Knowing this difference is crucial because it helps shape the right treatment plans and public health responses during outbreaks. In most cases, the sharper, quicker onset of cholera means that spotting the signs early and acting fast can dramatically cut down the risks for communities exposed to contaminated water and food (Brown et al., 2008; Lockley et al., 2013).

15.3.2. Common Symptoms of Typhoid

Typhoid fever presents in a multitude of forms, and the symptoms sneak up on you slowly – this gradual onset can sneak up on you big time even though getting treated early is really crucial. A lot of people are struck with a relentless high temperature that, strangely, tends to spike in the evenings; accompanied by this is a severe feeling of fatigue and overall malaise. Many patients report persistent stomach pain, which suggests that the gut is compromised, and sometimes a headache or a loss of appetite strikes suddenly, culminating in weight loss and dehydration if not addressed. You may also observe vomiting and diarrhea appearing along with it, confusing the matter further and increasing the likelihood of other problems. In general, all these symptoms point towards a body-wide infection , so doctors need to be very cautious to distinguish it from other fever diseases in regions where such diseases are prevalent (Nurhayati, 2024). It is not uncommon for symptoms of typhoid to overlap into the grounds of other tropical diseases, so the diagnosis becomes somewhat of a mystery in fever-infested regions. For instance, although typhoid sufferers usually complain more of that nagging stomach pain and headache, dengue fever brings on rashes and muscle soreness instead. Laboratory exams can provide telling hints also – in general, typhoid typically accompanies an appreciable increase in white blood cells (leukocytosis), while dengue is more often followed by a decrease in these cells (leukopenia). In addition, if you look at the platelet levels, they tend to be higher in typhoid than in dengue, which has the reputation for having low platelets. These are small differences, yes, yet important ones for doctors attempting to identify the specific cause of a fever in areas where several diseases are rampant at the same time (Nurhayati, 2024). When it comes to infants and young children, typhoid can play somewhat differently or even strike harder at times – a reminder that symptoms are not one-size-fits-all in every age group. Convulsions can occasionally appear in small children, although they are not the most frequent symptom, suggesting potential neurological complications in this particularly vulnerable age group. Furthermore, how fever and abdominal issues persist in infants makes it imperative for physicians to intervene early to prevent severe complications such as perforation of the intestine or even septicemia. With the symptoms recurring constantly and the burden of drug-resistant strains as well, there is a definite need for constant monitoring and regular updating of treatment regimens. Particularly in areas of high incidence such as West Bengal, early diagnosis with better therapies is essentially the prime objective to slow the dissemination and enhance results for patients (Mamatkulova et al., 2024) (Figure 15.9).

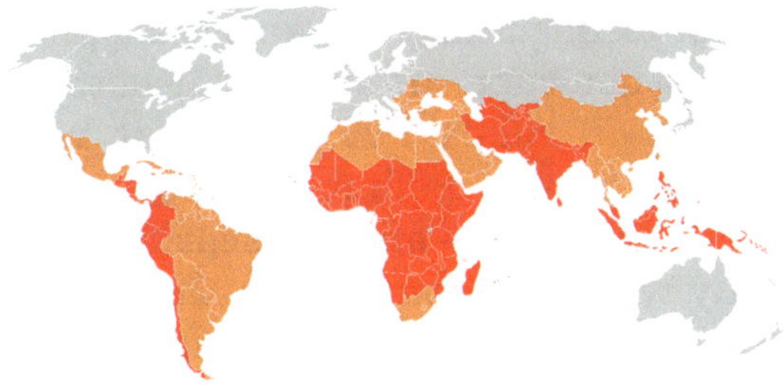

Figure 15.9. Typhoid

Source: By Percherie - CHU Rouens - Fièvre Typhoïde, CC BY-SA 3.0, https://commons.wikimedia.org/w/index.php?curid=1222560

15.3.3. Diagnostic Methods for Both Diseases

Having proper diagnoses is critically important in managing infectious epidemics; it dictates treatment options and how containment protocols get implemented. Consider cholera, for instance , the symptoms you observe in a patient may cause an initial suspicion, but laboratory testing holds the true answer. In most instances, labs extract *Vibrio cholerae* from stool samples through culture techniques , a technique that, even though it requires specialist systems, is still the gold standard for precision. RDTs have also been introduced for quicker detection in times of outbreaks, even though sometimes their sensitivity and specificity get a little into disarray. On the other hand, the diagnosis of typhoid is more challenging because *Salmonella Typhi* disseminates across the body and its symptoms become intermixed with other febrile diseases. The outdated Widal test, much depended on to detect antibodies, is plagued by problems such as cross-reactivity, resulting in unclear interpretations. In general, early blood cultures are regarded as more specific for typhoid, even though their sensitivity falls when antibiotics are in place or sampling is delayed. In summary, refining specimen acquisition and laboratory procedures is the key to improving diagnostic accuracy for both diseases. New diagnostic technology has truly transformed our strategy for distinguishing cholera from typhoid, accelerating detection and supporting outbreak surveillance in subtle but significant ways. Molecular methods – PCR, for example, which amplifies DNA targets – improve sensitivity and specificity when detecting *Vibrio cholerae* and *Salmonella typhi.* Although these techniques are not yet widespread throughout most endemic areas (largely due to expense and the requirement for solid infrastructure), they represent a hopeful path to quicker diagnosis. Research has also explored numerous smear methods as well as sample handling, again emphasizing the importance of selecting techniques during routine day-to-day laboratory processes (Karag Mülle et al., 2025). While these technologies are only gradually making their way into everyday use, they still indicate a critical necessity for standardization and training in resource-poor environments, where the effects of cholera and typhoid are particularly burdensome. Imaging and other high-tech diagnostics are beginning to contribute when assessing typhoid complications, although cholera is still sticking largely to the microbiological confirmation path. It's not typical to directly diagnose these infections using imaging, but equipment such as ultrasound or MRI may occasionally reveal typhoid's more sullied impact – for example, identifying intestinal perforations or hepatosplenic abscesses – that can influence the way a patient is treated. Current studies comparing diagnostic strategies in other infectious diseases tend to highlight the advantage of combining various methods to enhance detection precision as well as patient prognosis (Mutovkina et al., 2024). Despite a reliance on lab confirmations, combining clinical data with test findings – and adding imaging where appropriate – creates a more complete, albeit sometimes incomplete, portrait. In regions in which symptoms tend to overlap and co-infections introduce additional complexity to clinical assessment, such a hybrid approach becomes increasingly vital, underscoring the continued necessity for diagnostic tests that are available, sensitive, and really on target.

15.4. Treatment Options

Cholera treatment is simply a matter of getting liquid into the system as quickly as possible, when the body loses too much, it needs an instant solution. Oral rehydration salts accomplish this by replenishing lost electrolytes and water, a solution that in many instances becomes the cure-all. In extremely severe cases, however, physicians resort to IV fluids to increase blood volume in a matter of minutes. Antibiotics are sometimes added to reduce the duration a patient is unwell, although one must be cautious due to the increasing problem of antibiotic resistance. Insertion of nutritional care and even zinc tablets can be used to spur recovery along. It is not just individual patient care either; community interventions such as vaccination and improved hygiene measures ultimately have a big impact on cholera control. In most regions, combining treatment with prevention has been experimented with some success—integrated methods appear to function best as a whole (Greenland et al., 2013). For typhoid, the emphasis obviously falls on employing efficient antibiotics against *Salmonella typhi.* Previously, medications such as chloramphenicol were used, but with increasing resistance, substitutions including fluoroquinolones and third-generation cephalosporins are now far more prevalent. Overall, the selection of antibiotic is largely a function of local resistance patterns, a balancing act, really. Along with antibiotic treatment, supportive care in the form of hydration and adequate nutrition is necessary to allow the body to deal with typhoid's systemic impact. Occasionally, if something goes wrong—with complications such as an intestinal perforation—a surgical approach may even be required. Despite all these, antibiotic resistance still casts its shadow, demanding caution and close monitoring. Vaccination and sanitation are the other components in combating typhoid, serving to strengthen the overall disease control strategy (Korman et al., 2001).

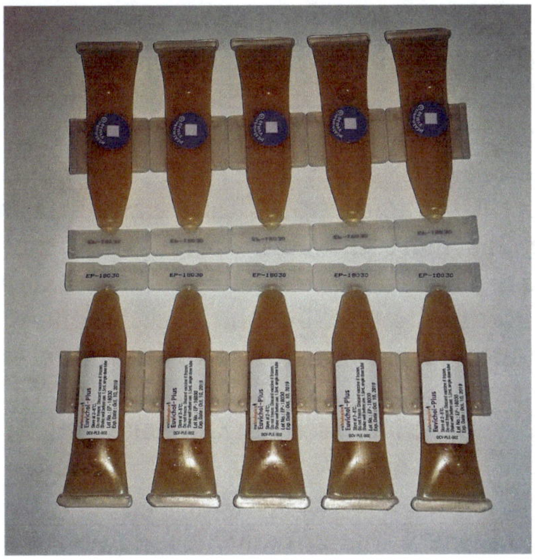

Figure 15.10. Cholera treatment antibiotics.

Source: By Mr. Ibrahem - Own work, CC BY-SA 4.0, https://commons.wikimedia.org/w/index.php?curid=78316175

Although drugs feature prominently in the treatment of the two diseases, combating these diseases in full requires going beyond the drugs. Vaccination campaigns have proved to hold a genuine promise, especially as a vital complement where medical treatments may fall short. Basic hygiene education, frequently implemented in conjunction with vaccinations, encourages individuals toward practices that interrupt the cycle of transmission. Of course, the actual effect of these measures in the real world can differ greatly—much will depend on the local environment and the resilience of the health systems in place, as some pilot schemes in Nepal have shown (Greenland et al., 2013). A glance at the past also shows that social attitudes and cultural considerations have frequently influenced public health responses, affecting quarantine policies and resource allocation in subtle ways (Korman et al., 2001). Overall, integrating medical, social, and policy-based measures appears to be the most hopeful path ahead (Figure 15.10).

15.4.1. Rehydration Therapy for Cholera

Cholera hits global health quite hard, so prompt response to its sudden, deadly dehydration is a requirement. Cholera deprives the body of fluids—, through incessant, copious diarrhea, and knowing just how that occurs is crucial before treatment can start. Rehydration therapy, which is all about replenishing lost fluids and salts, is the foundation of treatment and has reduced death rates sharply. This easy technique transformed cholera into something that could be handled even in regions with limited medical supplies. Based on the intensity, physicians could employ oral rehydration salts (ORS) or even intravenous fluids to restore balance to the body and defend against shock. It all speaks to the necessity for accessible health facilities and trained personnel, aligning with overall public health initiatives against infectious diseases (Rodrigo, 2025). In fact, implementing rehydration treatment is not as easy as it seems, particularly where pharmacy procedures are unstandardized. Research in certain areas shows that drugs are frequently distributed without prescriptions, and dispensers hardly possess complete knowledge of proper antibiotic usage. Such disarray not only complicates cholera management but also makes it difficult to work with other infections. In general, when antibiotics become used indiscriminately, they can stimulate resistance without addressing the urgent need for fluid replacement. Preventing local pharmacies and drug shops from deviating from treatment protocols—, prioritizing rehydration over unwarranted antibiotics—requires extensive training and stronger policy enforcement (Manyilizu et al., 2013). These types of programs are essential components of a complete cholera control program. Conversely, rehydration therapy is even more effective when combined with broader public health efforts to reduce fresh infections. Improved sanitation, clean water, vaccination campaigns, and education of the population all complement each other, each contributing its own part in reducing disease prevalence. This combination of medical care and disseminating practical knowledge of health has contributed to reducing worldwide mortality rates, demonstrating the way that an inexpensive, simple solution such as oral rehydration can save millions of lives. Eventually, topping up lost fluids is still very important but really comes into its own when supported by an adequate healthcare system and continued work on solving the environmental and societal issues that keep cholera infections recurring (Rodrigo, 2025).

15.4.2. Antibiotics for Typhoid

Bacterial infection treatment has improved leaps and bounds since the advent of antibiotics—they've reduced sickness and death from diseases like typhoid fever. Typhoid, caused by *Salmonella enterica* serotype Typhi, requires a rapid, sure antibiotic cure to prevent ugly complications. Previously, medications like chloramphenicol turned the tide on typhoid, cutting mortality rates way down. But with these drugs being used more, resistance started to emerge, and physicians were left struggling to find something else. Fluoroquinolones and third-generation cephalosporins are more likely to make the prescription list these days, although their success is highly dependent on your location. Although new vaccine advancements do bring some hope, antibiotics remain essential when cases strike hard. For the most part, smarter use of these drugs coupled with increased vaccine efforts is essentially the key to keeping the overall disease burden low (Rodrigues & Plotkin, 2020). The increased antibiotic resistance is turning out to be a gigantic stumbling block, particularly in low-resource settings where sanitation and decent healthcare can be fairly limited. Resistance is not solely the result of errors in medical application—uncontrolled use in agriculture, such as intensive farming to satisfy increasing protein demands, has a significant contribution as well. Such usage leaves antibiotic residues in animal products that find their way into the environment and propagate resistant bacteria everywhere. The result is a complex public health problem: drug-resistant typhoid strains that make treatment regimens more difficult, prolong disease, and increase healthcare expenses. This is a truly threatening situation that jeopardizes the hard-earned progress of combating infections, and the need is for increased stewardship initiatives, stricter regulation, and cooperation at the international level to monitor and regulate antibiotic usage (Christy et al., 2018). Without these, the effectiveness of our current antibiotics against typhoid could soon erode. Struggling against typhoid with antibiotics must be viewed as part of a comprehensive public health approach that incorporates improved surveillance, cleaner facilities, and increased vaccination. Disparities in access to vaccines and antibiotics underscore some sobering global health shortcomings, reminding us that international commitment to equitable healthcare is essential. Lessons from other vaccine campaigns indicate that combining immunization with savy, judicious use of antibiotics can truly make a difference. Through the fortification of our health infrastructures, funding research into new therapies, and heightening public knowledge about resistance problems, we can lay the ground for improved long-term control of typhoid. Ultimately, judicious use of antibiotics—and sometimes in a manner nearly married to preventive interventions—is a vital step in the battle against typhoid, both in harder-struck areas and elsewhere (Christy et al., 2018; Rodrigues & Plotkin, 2020) (Figure 15.11).

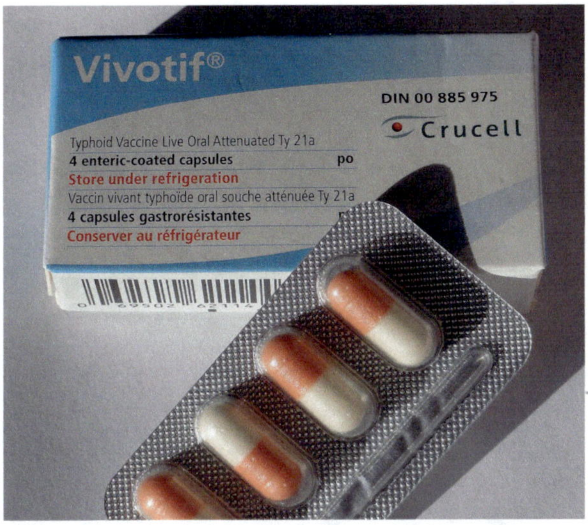

Figure 15.11. Typhoid fever treatment.

Source: By K - Own work, CC BY-SA 3.0, https://commons.wikimedia.org/w/index.php?curid=33939984

15.4.3. Importance of Early Intervention

Typhoid and cholera infections can really get going if their symptoms aren't recognized and addressed quickly enough. When treatment is administered just at the first sign of a problem, it's likely to throw the disease's natural progression into a tizzy, reducing disease and mortality associated with these waterborne pathogens. Typically, immediate treatment has cholera patients avoid that unpleasant severe dehydration, and typhoid's overall impact on the body gets diminished, which can reduce sickness time and accelerate recovery. Early diagnoses also ultimately make isolation and supportive care more effective, and that slows the spread within communities. In many cases, having snappy screening methods in regions where these infections are common bumps up the chances of catching them before they get out of hand—especially in places with limited resources, where every extra moment can lead to a worse outlook. Generally speaking, quick action is not only a must for saving lives but also a key public health move to keep outbreaks under control. Apart from benefiting people, early action also balances wider health system benefits and even certain economic benefits. Vaccinations, for instance, are extremely important in keeping typhoid and cholera at bay, although in practice unequal access can slow down global health progress. When immunizations are released quickly during outbreaks or in high-risk areas, new cases decrease while the healthcare system's burden eases up. Early shots in most cases reduce the necessity for intensive antibiotic use and, as a result, combat the growing threat of antimicrobial resistance (AMR)—a problem that tends to increase when treatment is delayed or deviates from the course. This problem is especially thorny in developing areas with poor sanitation and pervasive, at times irrational, use of antibiotics making matters even more complicated (Christy et al., 2018; Rodrigues & Plotkin, 2020). And so, it appears that prompt intervention—be it through immunization or early treatment—has multi-tiered benefits that reach across health, society, and the economy. Further there's the reality that rapid treatment and vaccination must be supported by a healthcare system that can catch problems quickly and act on them promptly. Supporting our methods of monitoring for outbreaks translates to cholera and typhoid humps being caught early, allowing teams to respond with targeted interventions and rapidly dispatch aid where required. Some grassroots educational initiatives that remind individuals of symptoms and simple hygiene can, quite understandably, get people to seek help earlier than later—no matter if there's a delay in noticing something's amiss. And, of course, worldwide cooperation comes into play here as well, particularly ensuring that poorer areas receive the aid necessary to implement such quick-response systems. Improving our diagnostic equipment as well as collaborating globally on more judicious use of antibiotics and more intelligent vaccine distribution truly addresses the numerous aspects of these diseases. , early treatment proves to be a multi-faceted approach, incorporating clinical care with social and environmental interventions—to mitigate the overall burden of cholera and typhoid globally.

15.5. Prevention Strategies

It's not just a matter of administering treatments that control cholera and typhoid—teaching people and repairing basic infrastructure counts too. These outbreaks tend to strike areas where water and sewage are inadequate, and that typically results in the food and water being contaminated. Educating people on safe food preparation, proper hand-hygiene, and the importance of clean water really reduces the rate at which these microbes spread. It's also crucial to ensure communities are provided with filtered water and improved toilets; these interventions interrupt the fecal-oral cycle that drives the infections. Vaccines, such as those for tourists traveling to high-risk areas, provide an immediate additional layer of protection while slowing down global spread. In short, where sanitation repairs, hygiene education, and immunization campaigns converge, they become the necessary building blocks for combating these diseases globally (Amicizia et al., 2019). Revisiting past and recent public health victories, it's apparent that concerted prevention efforts pay off against diseases such as typhoid and cholera. Consider China, for example, through government programs, such as mass vaccination and public health measures, over the last 70 years have cut disease rates. In most instances, long-running campaigns that encourage vaccines, improve sanitation, and improve access to care created precipitous declines in both typhoid and cholera figures; they even went so far as to explain the risk of transmission and push communities to maintain good hygiene.

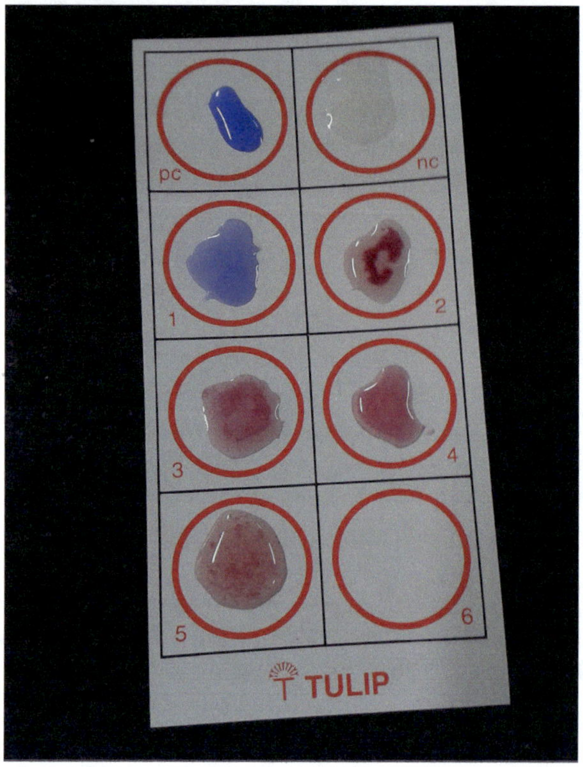

Figure 15.12. Prevention strategies for typhoid.

Source: By Sujith - Own work, CC BY-SA 3.0, https://commons.wikimedia.org/w/index.php?curid=26517466

This combination of policies not only maintained epidemics at bay but also enhanced overall health and life expectancy, demonstrating that firm government commitment and public participation are essential to successful disease prevention (Yang, 2019). Vaccination remains an important factor in the war against cholera and typhoid, particularly now when antibiotic-resistant bacteria increasingly complicate treatment. Vaccinations against *Salmonella typhi* and *Vibrio cholerae* tend to decrease not only how frequently folks become ill, but also how bad the infections are, a major benefit where health care isn't always top-notch. Although vaccines don't obviate the necessity for improved sanitation and individual cleanliness, they do provide an instantaneous, if incomplete, protective barrier, especially for higher-risk individuals and foreign travelers. Where immunization is paired with routine monitoring and rapid information exchange in most instances, this helps improve early detection and outbreak control. To summarize, this holistic strategy reduces disease and death, remains in line with international health goals, and reduces the overall disease burden that is imposed by these waterborne diseases (Amicizia et al., 2019) (Figure 15.12).

15.5.1. Vaccination Options

Preventing disease remains at the core of our collective battle against typhoid and cholera, particularly in areas where these pests are an ever-present menace and among travelers. As drug resistance grows and infections spread to new regions, it becomes rather essential to know what vaccines exist. For typhoid, vaccines are the big line of defense—as drugs take some of their old oomph away. Essentially, there are two big ones: one you swallow, using an attenuated form of the microbe, and one you receive as an injection based on a polysaccharide base. Both of these augment immunity, although the decision often has something to do with an individual's age, local patterns of disease, or just what happens to be lying around. It goes without saying that vaccine efforts work best when they're paired with improved water and sanitation , something that can easily be overlooked. Interestingly, many travelers don't get fully vaccinated, which hints at gaps in health education and policy (Atouguia & Masuet, 2021). All of this underlines the need for immunization strategies that really speak to both locals and those journeying from one place to another. Travel medicine draws a more complex picture when it comes to the rollout of vaccines, balancing protection against considerations such as cost, side effects, and sheer practicality. Most travelers begin with routine shots against hepatitis A and B because they are endemic risks, so they're usually top on the list. But once visitors are moving away from large cities, additional precautions are required – like typhoid and cholera vaccines, along with some good words about hygiene and proper eating habits. Mostly, this multi-layered approach combinations in some extra immunizations and prevention pointers that take into account the numerous hazards a traveler may encounter. Pre-travel consultations, for instance, commonly incorporate these additional steps, particularly as an unexpected onset of disease can seriously disrupt a trip and general health (Steffen et al., 2017). So whereas vaccines in isolation aren't the entire picture, they provide a pragmatic way to reduce health risks when traveling. Current research reminds us that vaccines are optimally viewed as one part of a larger public health puzzle in the battle against cholera and typhoid. In most endemic areas, typhoid vaccine programs are, more often than not, struggling with issues such as acceptance, supply chain disruptions, and the problematic challenge of integrating with other health initiatives. With drug-resistant bacteria gradually making their presence felt—due in part to the fact that more travel spreads them around—the need for effective vaccination cannot be overemphasized. Governments, global agencies, and communities are finally uniting to frame policies that enhance vaccine coverage. Over and above this, continuous research is producing new vaccines that have the potential to offer longer or even dual protection against more than one disease. Although vaccines alone aren't sufficient to eradicate these diseases outright, they are an important weapon in preventing sickness and death, particularly when combined with improved sanitation, cleaner water supplies, and increased education efforts (Atouguia & Masuet, 2021) (Figure 15.13).

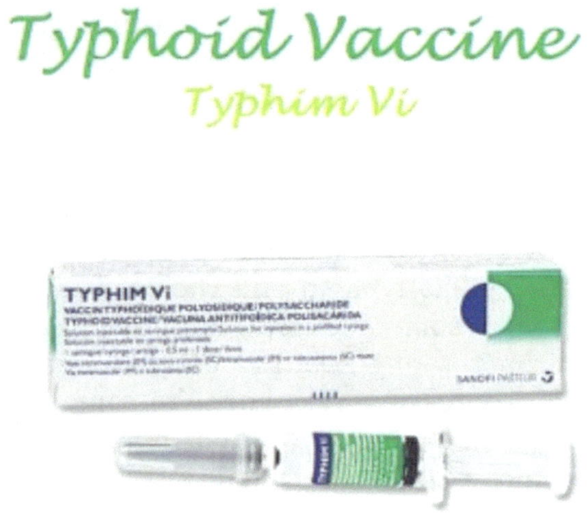

Figure 15.13. Vaccination options for cholera and typhoid.

Source: EMEDZ. (2019). *Typhoid Vaccine (Typhim).*

15.5.2. Sanitation and Hygiene Practices

The economic and demographic compositions of communities have a large influence on how individuals manage sanitation and hygiene, particularly when it comes to preventing cholera and typhoid. Less-educated and younger people tend not to be aware of the fundamentals of these diseases or the WASH practices that can assist in maintaining them at bay. For instance, one can visibly see a higher level of ignorance of the symptoms, modes of transmission, and preventive guidelines among individuals aged 18 years or less and those with minimal formal education. Poverty also has its share; families making just enough to sustain themselves tend to miss out on proper sanitation facilities and clean water supplies. In the majority of instances, enhancing public health translates to the fact that educational interventions must target such younger and disadvantaged populations in a bid for them to acquire simple practices such as water purification and latrine utilization, which are vital in disrupting the disease transmission cycle (Harry et al., 2025). Incorporating far-reaching WASH programs into public health initiatives truly raises the stakes in preventing cholera and typhoid. Consider, for example, enhancing availability of clean drinking water by installing community boreholes and public standpipes; this addresses one of the key areas where contamination sets in. Concurrently, increasing the number of latrines covered keeps open defecation to a bare minimum—another contributing factor to environmental contamination. Campaigns that encourage frequent soap hand washing and proper food handling also nip disease transmission in the bud by reducing direct transmission. Overall, these confused but sensible measures have served well in areas where local people contribute to ensuring the methods suit their lifestyle. In the majority of situations, investing in sanitation infrastructure as well as prodding behavior change constitutes the foundation of a robust defense against outbreaks in the long run (Izah et al., 2024). Slums in urban areas and refugee camps, with their overpopulation and limited resources, make sanitation and hygiene difficult to deal with. Nevertheless, if the efforts are focused and cooperative, there is a hopeful opportunity to transcend these challenges. It is not merely a matter of erecting buildings; constant pressure on education and good daily practice promotion can induce long-term changes. Local voices—either religious or community leaders—can always find a way to change habits, sometimes even balance the equation by reinforcing hygiene standards. When these efforts follow what the community will cherish anyway, acceptance and proper maintenance automatically increase. Overall, mixing infrastructure construction, continuous education, engagement of the community, and even some economic assistance is crucial in ensuring diseases such as cholera and typhoid are contained, especially among the most vulnerable (Harry et al., 2025; Izah et al., 2024) (Figure 15.14).

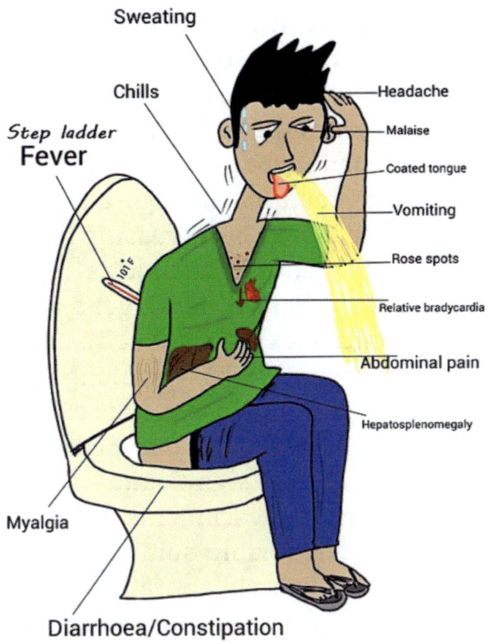

Figure 15.14. Sanitation and hygiene practices.

Source: https://commons.wikimedia.org/wiki/File:Typhoid_patient.JPG

15.5.3. Public Health Initiatives

Upgrading the quality of water and increasing sanitation are now the default play for combating cholera and typhoid. In Nigeria, for instance, water becomes through industrial spills, agricultural runoff, and rather lazy waste management. The goal isn't simply to eradicate bacteria – these solutions typically reduce long-term disease by reducing our everyday contact with bad stuff. Local initiatives at pollution prevention and primary hygiene always come into play, complementing behavior modification that persists in the long run. When good governance is accompanied by these local drives, vulnerable populations experience fewer outbreaks associated with tainted water (Vosa et al., 2025). How intestinal infections spread over time and geographically really illustrates how we require public health interventions that address local heterogeneities. Consider Zhejiang Province in China: clustering of enteric fever and other diarrheal conditions is an open invitation for tailored responses. Officials there are even resorting to spatio-temporal modeling – which sounds perhaps a bit exotic – to identify high-risk areas and reallocate resources where they are most needed. All of these variables, such as population density, urban configuration, and even local temperature, go into the shaping of these responses. In the majority of scenarios, evidence-informed strategies enable officials to implement context-relevant campaigns—be it vaccination campaigns, sanitation improvements, or health education—that collectively reduce the burden of cholera and typhoid (Zhu et al., 2023). Sustaining these public health achievements requires a combination of tough regulation, technological advancement, and a healthy measure of community education. Regulatory actions must be enforced stringently to eliminate pollution that compromises water safety, while new wastewater treatment technology (which, in all honesty, is a game changer) assists in keeping microbial threats under control. Concurrently, educating people on proper hygiene, safe food handling, and the importance of clean water is just as vital. When governments, NGOs, and local communities unite, even when things are a little rough around the edges sometimes—it provides a strong foundation for intelligent monitoring and rapid responses to the emerging threats. Overall, this multi-layered response has the potential to decrease rates of cholera and typhoid globally and makes clean water and good sanitation a genuine cornerstone of public health (Zhu et al., 2023; Vosa et al., 2025).

15.6. Global Impact

Cholera and typhoid cause more harm than personal health—they disrupt entire societies and economies, primarily in areas where clean water is not available and sanitation is poor. We recognize vaccines reduce sickness and death, and they play a central role in making health more equal; however, despite new vaccines and improved programmes, many vulnerable individuals remain excluded. For the most part, such a gap requires intensified global action to roll out immunization in regions where these diseases hold on so stubbornly (Rodrigues & Plotkin, 2020). It's usually said in vaccine fairness debate that addressing these matters instills trust in local healthcare systems and stabilizes society, and it can facilitate long-term growth. Meanwhile, there is another issue simmering on the horizon—antibiotic resistance. The inappropriate use of antibiotics, both in hospitals and farms, has accelerated this problem, particularly in areas of the globe where regulations are sort of loose. Large-scale livestock production, fueled by the demand for greater animal protein, also contributes to the problem by spreading antibiotic-resistant bacteria through our food and surroundings. Resistant bacteria complicate treatment, lengthening diseases, increasing healthcare expenditures, and, unfortunately, resulting in more fatalities. In general, antibiotic resistance pays no attention to borders, so nations must unite in better surveillance, intelligent antibiotic usage, and strong stewardship programs to control these supermicrobes (Christy et al., 2018). To summarize, combating cholera and typhoid is about working on several fronts—making vaccines, sanitation, and our management of antibiotics better. Epidemics in a single location can rapidly become wider public health issues, which is a reminder that quick detection and immediate action truly do count. Poverty, education, and available local infrastructure also significantly impact the spread of these diseases and how they affect communities. That's why governments, international agencies, and community groups have to collaborate to provide sustainable solutions that both treat the symptoms and address the causes of these diseases. Through collaboration across the world and more equitable sharing of resources, we can control these diseases more effectively and reduce their effect on health, economies, and societies overall (Christy et al., 2018; Rodrigues & Plotkin, 2020) (Figure 15.15).

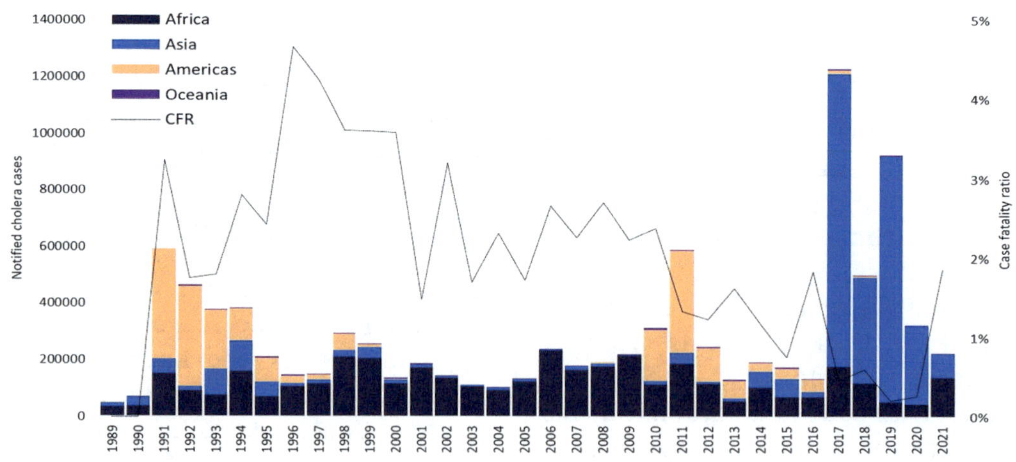

Figure 15.15. Global Impact of cholera and typhoid.

Source: World Health Organization. (n.d.). *Cholera Global Epidemic Curve.*

15.6.1. The effect of cholera on developing countries

Cholera in less-developed countries isn't only a health matter—it bleeds into daily life and the economy in ways not easily overlooked. Simple issues such as inefficient water supplies and rundown sanitation provide entry for outbreaks, particularly in densely populated neighborhoods. Local hospitals and clinics, that are not equipped to handle unforeseen patient inflows, become clogged, so other critical health services are neglected. This disparity, in the majority of instances, results in greater disease and even greater mortality, eventually decelerating productivity and hindering economic progress.

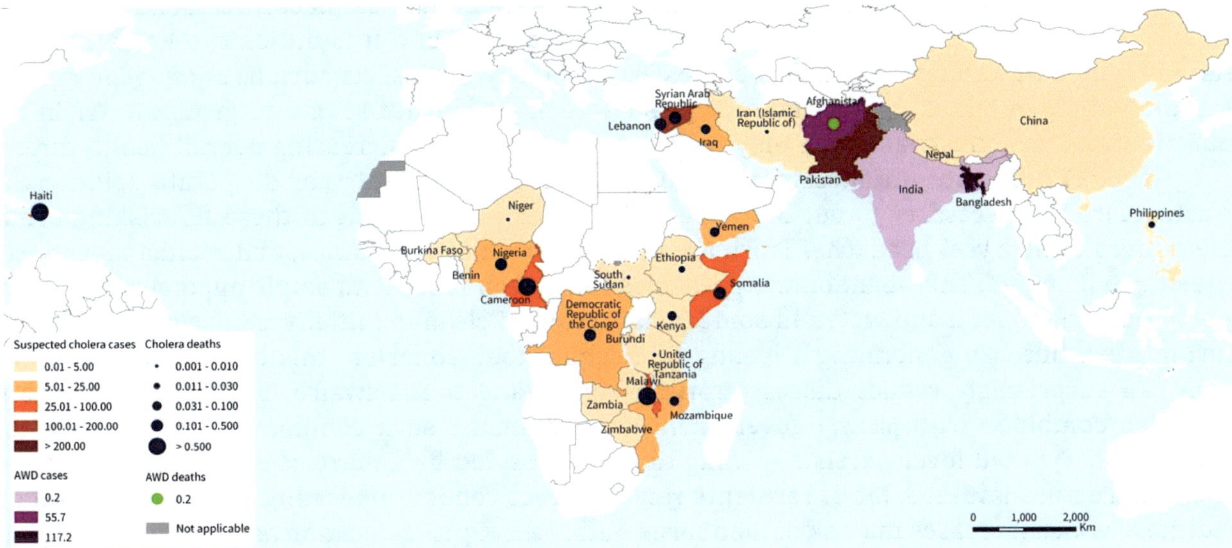

Figure 15.16. The effect of cholera on developing countries.

Source: World Health Organization. (n.d.). *Cholera Global Map.*

A combination of interventions, including access to clean water, sanitation facilities, and strengthened healthcare infrastructure (Metsopkeng et al., 2023), is needed to address these issues. Natural and traditional medicine sometimes dances onto the scene as a promising substitute when conventional drugs are unavailable. For instance, there's increasing curiosity about plant extracts—Moringa varieties, that is—that appear to deliver a knockout punch on *Vibrio cholerae*, cholera's germ. Experiments report that *Moringa oleifera* and *Moringa stenopetala* act differently; at times they kill off the bacteria completely and at times only decelerate it, depending on what part of the plant is used and how it's prepared. Interestingly, roots and seeds tend to need the least amount of medicine to work effectively, which suggests their usage as a complementary therapy in cholera management. In essence, combining these traditional remedies with orthodox methods may present a budget-friendly and locally available remedy where resources are limited (Metsopkeng et al., 2023). Cholera's persistence in these areas indicates an urgent necessity for reliable water management and sanitation policies that will endure. Resources such as GIS mapping of the groundwater recharge areas have the potential to identify locations with potential access to safe drinking water and pressure more targeted interventions against outbreaks. But only a small number of individuals in those impacted communities have access to safe water and adequate sanitation, a gap that unmistakenly underlies broader systemic problems. That shortage drives health emergencies and provokes enormous economic losses—not just from ballooning healthcare expenses but also from lower work productivity. Overall, the alignment of infrastructure improvements with public health education and intelligent policy reforms seems necessary to reduce cholera's far-reaching effects (Adesogan et al., 2022) (Figure 15.16).

15.6.2. Typhoid's Prevalence in Urban Areas

Hasty urban expansion in most low- and middle-income nations has produced sprawling settlements with rudimentary services lacking in them. In such densely populated places, residents frequently lack safe water, decent sanitation, or effective waste management. It is difficult to keep the place clean in cramped dwellings, and this provides an easy entry for insects such as *Salmonella typhi*—the same pathogen that causes typhoid. Typically, weak pit latrines seep into groundwater in the area, and rampant industrialization only makes the water dirtier, increasing overall health threats (Amegah, 2021). Despite the messiness of the picture, it's apparent that desperate solutions in infrastructure are necessary to cut the cycle. Solid waste management in these flourishing urban areas proves to be a real headache. Trash accumulates in unofficial dumps, and municipal services frequently fall behind. This abandonment provides rodents and flies with ample opportunity to carry typhoid bacteria to food and water. In some instances, local cleanup initiatives have stumbled upon clearing trash but also generating a feeling of neighborhood cohesion; this type of neighborhood action can surprisingly reduce disease transmission (Rangeti & Dzwairo, 2021). Lack of public knowledge combined with patchy government support makes such community initiatives all the more crucial. Typhoid fever persists to cling to city slums, fed by a maze of environmental, social, and infrastructure issues. A lot of residents rely on street vendors operating in less-than-sanitary conditions, which increases the risk of foodborne outbreaks. Open defecation and limited availability of clean water complicate matters further, trapping the population in a chain of contamination that's difficult to break. Harsh living conditions and deep-seated poverty result in families being unable to meet even minimum water treatment or hygiene standards. In general, addressing typhoid in these densely populated environments requires a combination of improved infrastructure, public education, and bottom-up mobilization to incrementally enhance overall health outcomes (Amegah, 2021; Rangeti & Dzwairo, 2021).

15.6.3. Economic Implications of Outbreaks

Disease outbreaks such as cholera and typhoid don't only cost hospitals a lot of money—they disrupt entire communities. When the bad times arrive, many people take days off work due to disease or even long-term disabilities, which also reduces overall productivity and slows economic development. Emergency patients flood the hospital, siphoning precious resources away from other essential treatments, quickly overwhelming the hospital. Governments are then compelled to allocate money into stopgap measures—vaccination campaigns and sanitation improvements that could otherwise have initiated long-term development. This type of financial pressure is most acutely experienced in low- and middle-income regions, where unstable infrastructure and delayed disease detection merely perpetuate the poverty and repeated epidemics cycle (Lewnard & Reingold, 2019). Occasionally, waterborne disease crises stir economic stability even more, particularly in areas with political turmoil. For example, in some areas of the Middle East, war and disrupted water systems conspire to increase the frequency and severity of outbreaks. When clean water is difficult to obtain for agriculture, industry, or even just day-to-day consumption, local economies suffer. Individuals tend to become apprehensive about purchasing from local markets if there is a whiff of contamination, and this erosion of consumer trust further depresses economic activity. Additionally, as humanitarian aid and foreign assistance costs rise, communities may become trapped in a dependence that undermines their long-term recovery and growth plans (Alsubih et al., 2023). In all but a few instances, that combination of political upheaval and increasing outbreaks truly hypercharges economic risks. Globally, the persistent challenges of cholera and typhoid outbreaks remind us of the importance of smarter public health investments and more subtle disease surveillance. More often than not, when epidemiological action gets ahead of things early, they nip in the bud the huge economic costs of widespread sickness. New diagnostic technology combined with analytics has been a goldmine, accelerating response and reducing the eventual social cost of epidemics. Regions with strong health security continue to hum their economic engines even during difficult times, whereas places with patchy surveillance and low care capacity lag behind. By interweaving more robust preventive strategies and refining epidemiologic models, we safeguard not only public health but also build economies' resilience against the intermittent shocks of infectious disease epidemics (Lewnard & Reingold, 2019).

CLOSER LOOK

WATERBORNE TRANSMISSION AND ENVIRONMENTAL RISK FACTORS

Waterborne diseases are caused by pathogenic microorganisms transmitted through contaminated water, affecting millions worldwide. Common pathogens include bacteria (Vibrio cholerae, Salmonella typhi), viruses (hepatitis A, rotavirus), and protozoa (Giardia, Cryptosporidium). Understanding the mechanisms of waterborne transmission and associated environmental risk factors is critical for prevention and public health interventions.

Transmission occurs primarily via ingestion of contaminated water, but it can also happen through recreational exposure or use of unsafe water for food preparation and hygiene. Poor sanitation, inadequate sewage treatment, and the presence of fecal matter in drinking water sources significantly increase the risk of outbreaks. Flooding, heavy rainfall, and natural disasters can exacerbate contamination, leading to large-scale epidemics, as seen in cholera outbreaks in flood-affected regions.

Environmental factors play a central role in the persistence and spread of waterborne pathogens. Warm temperatures can promote bacterial growth, while stagnant or slow-moving water provides ideal conditions for protozoa and virus survival. Urbanization and population growth often strain water supply systems, leading to overcrowding and insufficient water treatment. Rural areas may face additional challenges, such as reliance on open wells, rivers, or ponds that are susceptible to contamination.

Human behaviors, including poor hand hygiene, inadequate food handling, and unsafe water storage, compound environmental risks. Climate change further intensifies these challenges by altering rainfall patterns, increasing the frequency of extreme weather events, and affecting water quality and availability.

Preventive strategies focus on ensuring safe drinking water, proper sanitation, hygiene promotion, and community awareness. Point-of-use water treatment, chlorination, and improved sewage management can significantly reduce disease incidence. Monitoring water quality and implementing early warning systems are essential for outbreak prevention.

Waterborne diseases are closely linked to environmental and behavioral factors. Addressing these risks through infrastructure development, public health education, and climate-resilient water management is vital for safeguarding communities and reducing the global burden of waterborne infections.

Summary

Cholera and typhoid don't simply disappear with a rapid clinical solution—there's a whole mess of problems behind them. Inadequate sanitation, inconsistent access to clean water, and a fragile public health infrastructure all contribute, and in countries like Nigeria, unequal resource distribution combined with political issues makes it even more difficult. The diseases persist because they mark larger, underlying issues. In the majority of instances, enhancing daily hygiene, having more individuals vaccinated, and providing our healthcare systems with a genuine shot in the arm are actions that can prove to be beneficial. Even better, addressing issues such as poverty and education—topics that may not be directly related— benefits us in the long term. Various industries must collaborate and the government needs to step up its monitoring for any meaningful change (Abubakar et al., 2022). On top of all that, increasing antibiotic resistance is making treatment a headache. terms, overuse and misuse of antibiotics—either out in farms or in less-restricted clinics—has created recalcitrant strains that do not respond to our standard medications. Not only does this cloud up treatment regimens but also makes disease persist longer and unfortunately increases the chances of death. With the way our health is interconnected with animal and environmental health, a One Health strategy becomes virtually unavoidable. Reinforcing regulations, monitoring antibiotic use more closely, and even collaborating globally are all important steps to maintain current treatments effective and smother possible resistance problems (Christy et al., 2018). Without sorting this out, our efforts against these diseases could unravel. Taking a step back, controlling cholera and typhoid involves not just addressing immediate health requirements but also reconsidering the social and environmental contexts that allow the diseases to spread. Investing in health infrastructure—ensuring everyone has access to clean water, proper sanitation, and good public health education—is the actual backbone here. Meanwhile, improved management and additional funding for our health system enable us to act on outbreaks more quickly. It's about the understanding that infections, resistance to drugs, and problems such as poverty and poor education all get intertwined, so the one-dimensional solution won't suffice. In the end, the coordinated, long-term strategy supported by the high political will and participation of the community is what will reduce both cases' quantity and the cruel toll of cholera and typhoid globally (Abubakar et al., 2022; Christy et al., 2018).

Combating cholera and typhoid involves seeing beyond the diseases themselves. You must think about how societal and infrastructural problems contribute to these health issues. Nigeria, for instance—is poverty paired with an unequal distribution of resources, and so many are left vulnerable despite some areas being wealthy. Lots of individuals find themselves in situations that allow the pathogens to fall through the cracks; lack of access to clean water, inadequate sanitation, and poor health systems all combine to render prevention and early treatment a difficult decision. A combination strategy, starting from overarching policies and in the local setting, should invest in water, hygiene, sanitation, and healthcare to respond to the actual hardships of the vulnerable populations (Abubakar et al., 2022). Climate and weather variations, in most instances, simply add fuel to the fire. Warming temperatures, unpredictable rainfall, and an increase in extreme weather events weaken drinking water supplies and sanitation facilities, allowing outbreaks to occur. In developing regions, where water management may be quite tenuous, such changes further pollute supplies and, at times, drive individuals to migrate unexpectedly. Increasing such as surveillance and rapid-track responses is sort of critical if outbreaks are to be detected in time. Overall, ensuring that there is plenty of safe water and proper sanitation, supported by effective monitoring, becomes an important step as the climate becomes increasingly unpredictable (Nichols et al., 2018). All considered, cholera and typhoid persist because social disparities, substandard infrastructure, and environmental changes are interwoven. In general, a balanced plan that increases health financing, distributes resources more equitably, and bolsters healthcare provision is essential, particularly in areas struggling with political and demographic pressures. At times, tying adjustments in health services to shifts in social and environmental policies opens the door to a more comprehensive, collaborative war against these diseases. By pushing digital health systems a little harder and engaging communities slightly more, answers can be faster and more representative. Emphasizing improved water quality and sanitation together with simpler access to treatment could be our very best strategy to reduce the burden of cholera and typhoid over time (Abubakar et al., 2022; Nichols et al., 2018).

References

1. Abubakar, I., Dalglish, S. L., Angell, B., Sanuade, O. A., Abímbọ́lá, Ṣ., Adamu, A. L., Adetifa, I., et al. (2022). The Lancet Nigeria Commission: Investing in health and the future of the nation. *The Lancet, 399*, 1155–1200. https://doi.org/10.1016/s0140-6736(21)02488-0.
2. Acemoğlu, D., Johnson, S., & Robinson, J. A. (2012). The colonial origins of comparative development: An empirical investigation: Reply. *American Economic Review, 102*, 3077–3110. https://doi.org/10.1257/aer.102.6.3077.
3. Adams, D. A., Thomas, K., Jajosky, R. A., Foster, L., Baroi, G., Sharp, P., Onweh, D. H., et al. (2017). Summary of notifiable infectious diseases and conditions–United States, 2015. *MMWR Morbidity and Mortality Weekly Report, 64*, 1–143. https://doi.org/10.15585/mmwr.mm6453a1.
4. Adamu, U. (2019). Non-implementation of Planning Laws and Its Resultant Consequences as a Basis for Zoonotic Diseases Transmission among Urban Livestock Keepers in Potiskum Town, Yobe State, Nigeria. *The International Journal of Humanities & Social Studies, 7*(8). https://doi.org/10.24940/theijhss/2019/v7/i8/HS1908-038
5. Adesogan, S. O. (2022). Harnessing our available resources for sustainable development in rural areas of developing countries. *Engineering and Applied Science Letters, 5*(1), 18–26. https://www.semanticscholar.org/paper/c4d003361e2ec9ffb0236554739be46139a6e557 (accessed on 7 May 2025).
6. Adewumi, A., Adewumi, A., Fatumo, S. A., Fatumo, et al. (2016). Computational and mathematical modelling: Applicability to infectious disease control in Africa. *Asian Journal of Scientific Research, 9*(3), 88–105. https://core.ac.uk/download/603238311.pdf (accessed on 7 May 2025).
7. Aditama, W., Zulfikar, Z., Khairunnisa, K., & Arianto, B. (2023). Efektivitas ekstrak kunyit (*Curcuma longa*) sebagai bioinsektisida alami untuk menghalau lalat rumah (*Musca domestica*). *Journal SAGO Gizi dan Kesehatan.* https://www.semanticscholar.org/paper/8b2e81ad758d4701dea5e9355bf1b275ffb509a3 (accessed on 7 May 2025).
8. Alsubih, M., El Morabet, R., Hrynzovskyi, A., Khan, et al. (2023). Epidemiology study of diarrhoea, cholera, typhoid, hepatitis A, and hepatitis E in the Middle East and North Africa region. https://core.ac.uk/download/587227742.pdf (accessed on 7 May 2025).
9. Amegah, A. K. (2021). Slum decay in Sub-Saharan Africa. *Environmental Epidemiology, 5*, e158. https://doi.org/10.1097/ee9.0000000000000158.
10. Amicizia, D., Micale, R. T., Pennati, B. M., Zangrillo, F., Iovine, M., Lecini, E., Marchini, F., et al. (2019). Burden of typhoid fever and cholera: Similarities and differences. Prevention strategies for European travelers to endemic/epidemic areas. *Journal of Preventive Medicine and Hygiene, 60*, E271–E285. https://www.semanticscholar.org/paper/58aa87636ce8dd07eb4c4f23408aa2fac0c4eedd (accessed on 7 May 2025).
11. Arnold, B. F., Cooley, G. M., Costantini, V., Goodhew, et al. (2019). Entomopathogen antibody dynamics and force of infection among children in low-resource settings. *eLife, 8*, e45594. https://doi.org/10.7554/eLife.45594.
12. Atouguia, J., & Masuet Aumatell, C. (2021). Typhoid fever infection–Antibiotic resistance and vaccination strategies: A narrative review. *Travel Medicine and Infectious Disease, 40*, 101946. https://doi.org/10.1016/j.tmaid.2021.101946.

13. Bell, C., & Lewis, M. (2025). The economic implications of epidemics old and new. https://core.ac.uk/download/pdf/7089767.pdf (accessed on 7 May 2025).
14. Bintsis, T. (2017). Foodborne pathogens. *AIMS Microbiology, 3*, 529–563. https://doi.org/10.3934/microbiol.2017.3.529.
15. Brown, G. V., Leder, K., Matchett, E., O'Brien, D. F., et al. (2008). Disease in returned travelers and immigrants/refugees: The 6-year experience of two Australian infectious diseases units. *Journal of Travel Medicine, 13*(3), 145–152. https://doi.org/10.1111/j.1708-8305.2006.00106.x.
16. Buj, V., Kedenge, S., Kim, J., Ngongo, S., et al. (2014). Community health workers and stand-alone or integrated case management of malaria: A systematic literature review. *The American Journal of Tropical Medicine and Hygiene, 91*(3), 461–470. https://doi.org/10.4269/ajtmh.14-0086.
17. Davison, N. (2005). The role of scientific discovery in the establishment of the first biological weapons programmers. https://core.ac.uk/download/135022.pdf.
18. Greenland, K., Gautam, O., & Velleman, Y. (2013). An opportunity not to be missed: Vaccination as an entry point for hygiene promotion and diarrheal disease reduction in Nepal. https://core.ac.uk/download/75783161.pdf (accessed on 7 May 2025).
19. Hassan, H. K., Adigun, O. A., Manirambona, E., Olaleke, N., Abioye, M. S., Lucero-Prisno, D. E. III, et al. (2024). Mitigating the escalating threat of infectious disease outbreaks in tropical Africa: A perspective examination of challenges and strategies for future preparedness. *Beni-Suef University Journal of Basic and Applied Sciences.* https://www.semanticscholar.org/paper/eded8d62cc86a1d52bb632bde78ffb5b03eae6ec (accessed on 7 May 2025).
20. Heaviside, C., Lake, I., & Nichols, G. (2018). Climate change and water-related infectious diseases. *Atmosphere, 9*(11), 385. https://doi.org/10.3390/atmos9110385.
21. Howard, G., Bartram, J., Brocklehurst, C., Colford, J. M., Costa, F., Cunliffe, D., Dreibelbis, R., et al. (2020). COVID-19: Urgent actions, critical reflections, and future relevance of 'WaSH': Lessons for the current and future pandemics. *Journal of Water and Health, 18*, 613–630. https://doi.org/10.2166/wh.2020.162.
22. Izah, S. C., Etim, N. G., Alaka, O. O., Nwachukwu, B. C., & Joshua, G. (2024). Public health interventions for cholera control and prevention: Water, sanitation, and hygiene (WASH) perspective. *Greener Journal of Epidemiology and Public Health, 12*(1), 1–15. https://www.semanticscholar.org/paper/0ea36a36be619f27b0e81f7da8af0b943872438e (accessed on 7 May 2025).
23. Jajere, S. M. (2019). A review of *Salmonella enterica* with particular focus on the pathogenicity and virulence factors, host specificity, and antimicrobial resistance including multidrug resistance. *Veterinary World, 12*, 504–521. https://doi.org/10.14202/vetworld.2019.504-521.
24. Jin, C., Gibani, M. M., Moore, M., Juel, H. B., Jones, E., Meiring, J., Harris, V., et al. (2017). Efficacy and immunogenicity of a Vi-tetanus toxoid conjugate vaccine in the prevention of typhoid fever using a controlled human infection model of *Salmonella Typhi*: A randomized controlled, phase 2b trial. *The Lancet, 390*, 2472–2480. https://doi.org/10.1016/s0140-6736(17)32149-9.
25. Karagülle, M., Arslan, F. Z., Ozcan, B., & Gedik, A. (2025). A comparison of different transfer techniques in evaluating specimen adequacy in FNAB: An unexplored topic. *Diagnostic*

Cytopathology, 53(5), 251–255. https://www.semanticscholar.org/paper/70a17b0d89bec842bcbd8a79bfd3cfe1d81e7a31 (accessed on 7 May 2025).

26. Korman, G. (2001). When heredity met the bacterium: Quarantines in New York and Danzig, 1898–1921. https://core.ac.uk/download/5132727.pdf (accessed on 7 May 2025).

27. Lewnard, J. A., & Reingold, A. L. (2019). Emerging challenges and opportunities in infectious disease epidemiology. *American Journal of Epidemiology, 188*(5), 873–882. https://doi.org/10.1093/aje/kwy264.

28. Lockley, T. J. (2013). Black mortality in antebellum Savannah. *Social History of Medicine, 26*(4), 633–652. https://core.ac.uk/download/19444204.pdf (accessed on 7 May 2025).

29. Mamatkulova, N., Jayaraman, R., Periasamy Bharathi, S., Jothimani, K., Abdul, G. S., Balakumar, G., & Peter, I. D. A. (2024). Typhoid fever: A comparison among various age group people. A detailed case report and review. *ТЕНДЕНЦИИ РАЗВИТИЯ НАУКИ И ОБРАЗОВАНИЯ.* https://www.semanticscholar.org/paper/7d14266118cd933cf6c8e21707ae7cf4d3ab72ab (accessed on 7 May 2025).

30. Manyilizu, V. S., & Minzi, O. M. (2013). Application of basic pharmacology and dispensing practice of antibiotics in accredited drug-dispensing outlets in Tanzania. https://core.ac.uk/download/pdf/18410778.pdf (accessed on 7 May 2025).

31. Manyi-Loh, C. E., Mamphweli, S., Meyer, E. L., & Okoh, A. I. (2018). Antibiotic use in agriculture and its consequential resistance in environmental sources: Potential public health implications. *Molecules, 23*, 795. https://doi.org/10.3390/molecules23040795.

32. Metsopkeng, C. S., Bricheux, G., Donnadieu, F., Nana, P., Ripoche, I., Tchinda, N., Agbor, G., et al. (2023). Bactericidal and bacteriostatic effects of four different parts of two plants' Moringa extracts against *Vibrio cholerae* and *Salmonella typhi*, and some phytochemical properties. *Journal of Advances in Microbiology, 23*(9). https://www.semanticscholar.org/paper/416d6986ac3707c7d2acdfe30929b0c6de323dff (accessed on 7 May 2025).

33. Mutovkina, N. I., Cheremisin, V. M., Kamyshanskaya, I., Mishchenko, A. V., Zakharova, A. V., Grishko, P., Trofimov, S., et al. (2024). The efficiency of MRI in the diagnostic of esophageal cancer in comparison with CT and endoscopic ultrasound. *Journal of Oncology: Diagnostic Radiology and Radiotherapy.* https://www.semanticscholar.org/paper/b8205ab666ff827f99848b2e20c8965ac9bb37b6 (accessed on 7 May 2025).

34. Nichols, G., Lake, I., & Heaviside, C. (2018). Climate change and water-related infectious diseases. *Atmosphere, 9*, 385. https://doi.org/10.3390/atmos9100385.

35. Ntumba, H. C. K., Taty, N., Mako, S., & Batumbo, D. (2025). Assessment of knowledge, attitudes, and practices regarding cholera among people living in a cholera-endemic health zone in the Democratic Republic of the Congo. *BMJ Open, 15,* e091360. https://www.semanticscholar.org/paper/afb15e4e867b82d5ce270cc0087781f32c0ace0d (accessed on 7 May 2025).

36. Nurhayati. (2024). Comparison of clinical symptoms and laboratory findings in typhoid fever and dengue fever patients. *International Journal for Research in Applied Science and Engineering Technology, 12.* https://www.semanticscholar.org/paper/7fd7b7deab22c367cc135f1e848b8f717481ff08 (accessed on 7 May 2025).

37. Rangeti, I., & Dzwairo, B. (2021). Guide for organizing a community clean-up campaign. In *IntechOpen eBooks*. https://doi.org/10.5772/intechopen.94515.

38. Ranjbar, R., & Farahani, A. (2019). *Shigella*: Antibiotic-resistance mechanisms and new horizons for treatment. *Infection and Drug Resistance, 12*, 3137–3167. https://doi.org/10.2147/idr.s219755.

39. Rodrigues, C. M. C., & Plotkin, S. A. (2020). Impact of vaccines: Health, economic, and social perspectives. *Frontiers in Microbiology, 11*. https://doi.org/10.3389/fmicb.2020.01526.

40. Siamalube, B., & Ehinmitan, E. (2024). Cholera-free Zambia 2025: A distant dream or an achievable reality? *Public Health Open Access, 8*(2), 1–6. https://www.semanticscholar.org/paper/72738b9502dcf4562cc40060c6610b3951274da5 (accessed on 7 May 2025)

41. Siddiqua, A., Hahladakis, J. N., Al-Attiya, W. A. K. A. (2022). An overview of the environmental pollution and health effects associated with waste landfilling and open dumping. *Environmental Science and Pollution Research, 29*, 58514–58536. https://doi.org/10.1007/s11356-022-21578-z.

42. Soares, R. R. (2025). On the determinants of mortality reductions in the developing world. https://core.ac.uk/download/pdf/6820092.pdf (accessed on 7 May 2025).

43. Steffen, R. (2017). Travel medicine—Prevention based on epidemiological data. *Transactions of the Royal Society of Tropical Medicine and Hygiene, 85*(3), 156–162. https://core.ac.uk/download/85211134.pdf (accessed on 7 May 2025).

44. Stucchi, R. S. B., Lopes, M. H., Kumar, D., & Manuel, O. (2018). Vaccine recommendations for solid-organ transplant recipients and donors. *Transplantation, 102*, S72–S80. https://doi.org/10.1097/tp.0000000000002012.

45. Vosa, O., Salibi, G., & Tzenios, N. (2025). Water pollution and its impact on human health in Nigeria. *Special Journal of the Medical Academy and Other Life Sciences, 3*(2). https://www.semanticscholar.org/paper/61540819475fe25731ae5ad2da37e9a50b6582b2 (accessed on 7 May 2025).

46. Yang, W. (2019). Dramatic achievements in infectious disease prevention and treatment in China during the past 70 years. *Zhonghua liu xing bing xue za zhi = Zhonghua liuxingbingxue zazhi, 40*(12), 1493–1498. https://www.semanticscholar.org/paper/9390b50a73aef9d183a4183780749442b780013c (accessed on 7 May 2025).

47. Zhu, Z., Feng, Y., Gu, L., Guan, X., Liu, N., Zhu, X., Gu, H., et al. (2023). Spatio-temporal pattern and associated factors of intestinal infectious diseases in Zhejiang Province, China, 2008–2021: A Bayesian modeling study. *BMC Public Health, 23*. https://www.semanticscholar.org/paper/aa352773ee6a417e6979eeaa00688e25f52a239e (accessed on 7 May 2025).

INDEX

B

C

J

K

L

M

N

O

P

T

U

V